USMLE™ Step 3 Qbook

Third Edition

OTHER BOOKS BY KAPLAN MEDICAL

USMLE™ Step 1 Qbook, Third Edition

USMLE™ Step 2 CK Qbook, Third Edition

USMLE™ Step 2 Clinical Skills, Third Edition

USMLE™ Step 3 Qbook

Third Edition

KAPLAN

PUBLISHING

New York • Chicago

Editorial Director: Jennifer Farthing
Editor: Cynthia C. Yazbek
Production Artist: Maria Warren
Cover Designer: Carly Schnur

Published by Kaplan Publishing, a division of Kaplan, Inc.
888 Seventh Ave.
New York, NY 10106

Printed in the United States of America

September 2006

10 9 8 7 6 5 4 3 2

ISBN-13: 978-1-4195-5152-9
ISBN-10: 1-4195-5152-3

Test-Taking and Study Strategies Guide

Author

Steven R. Daugherty, Ph.D.
Director of Education and Testing
Kaplan Medical
Rush Medical College
Chicago, IL

Contributor

Judy A. Schwenker, M.S.
Director of Study Skills
Kaplan Medical

USMLE Step 3 Qbook

Editor-in-Chief

Elissa Levy, M.D.
New York, NY

Editors

Michael S. Manley, M.D.
Director, Medical Curriculum
Kaplan Medical
Department of Neurosciences
University of California–San Diego

Leslie D. Manley, Ph.D.
Director, Medical Curriculum
Kaplan Medical
Departments of Neurosciences and Pharmacology
University of California–San Diego

Contributors

David J. Anschel, M.D.
Prasad S. Adusumilli, M.D.
Timothy S. Bollom, M.D.
Dragana Bugarski-Kirola, M.D.
Judith U. Cope, M.D., M.P.H.
Maryellen Flaherty-Hewitt, M.D.
Shashank Mishra, M.D.
Charles Park, M.D.,
Adam C. Urato, M.D.
Vesna Petronic-Rosic, M.D.
Eric Rudin, M.D.
Neil D. Sherman, M.D.
Marie Sicari, M.D.
Sam Siddighi, M.D.

Senior Vice President, Kaplan Medical

Rochelle Rothstein, M.D.

Executive Director of Curriculum

Richard Friedland, D.P.M.

Medical Curriculum Manager

Sonia Reichert, M.D.

Managing Editor

Kathlyn McGreevy

Production Manager

Michael Wolff

Production Editor

William Ng

AVAILABLE ONLINE

Free Additional Practice

kaptest.com/booksonline

As owner of this guide, you are entitled to get more practice online. Log on to kaptest.com/booksonline to access additional practice questions.

Access to this selection of online USMLE™ Step 3 practice material is free of charge to purchasers of this book. When you log on, you'll be asked to input the book's ISBN number (see the bar code on the back cover). And you'll be asked for a specific password derived from the text in this book, so have your book handy when you log on.

For any Test Changes or Late-Breaking Developments

kaptest.com/publishing

The material in this book is up-to-date at the time of publication. However, the USMLE™ may have instituted changes in the test after this book was published. Be sure to carefully read the materials you receive when you register for the test. If there are any important late-breaking developments—or any changes or corrections to the Kaplan test preparation materials in this book—we will post that information online at kaptest.com/publishing.

Feedback and Comments

kaplansurveys.com/books

We'd love to hear your comments and suggestions about this book. We invite you to fill out our online survey form at kaplansurveys.com/books. Your feedback is extremely helpful as we continue to develop high-quality resources to meet your needs.

Contents

Preparing for and doing well on the USMLE Step 3 are essential requirements on the road to becoming a practicing physician. The skills needed for preparation and execution on multiple-choice tests have little to do with the day-to-day practice of medicine but are necessary hurdles that you must surmount to advance in your medical career. Take heart—this task is not insurmountable; there have been many ahead of you. It only requires some knowledge of techniques, a little planning, a dash of impertinence, and above all, patience. This guidebook is intended to help you with this process.

- The first chapter was developed to help you gain a better understanding of the exam, including the clinical case simulations (CCS). It describes the overall purpose of the exam, as well as its structure and design, and offers crucial insights to help you do your best on test day.
- The *Test-Taking and Study Strategies Guide* section offers practical suggestions to help you make the most of your preparation time and to avoid common pitfalls in the exam itself. (We've also included advice on how to approach the USMLE's new FRED™ software interface.) This section summarizes the key study and test strategies that have helped thousands of students achieve their maximum score. As you read it, think about the way that you study and the way you take exams. Consider your options and make the choices that work best for you.
- The *Qbook Practice Tests* contain a total of 850 Step 3–style questions divided into test blocks of 50 questions each. These blocks are designed to give you a sense of how the actual exam is constructed. Each test is followed by comprehensive explanations of both the correct and incorrect answer choices. We recommend that you wait until you compete your review of a subject area before taking an exam, that you take each exam in the allotted one-hour time frame, and that you do not look at the answers until you have completed a test. Following each test, review why each answer is correct and why each distractor is wrong. This will provide you with the information needed to answer other similar questions on the same topic. There are two exams each in Psychiatry, Surgery, and Neurology; three in Obstetrics/Gynecology; and four each in Internal Medicine and Pediatrics. A list of standard lab values can be found on pp. 601–602 for easy reference.

Good luck on your Step 3 exam!

Kaplan Medical

| SECTION ONE |

Test-Taking and Study Strategies Guide

Chapter One: Inside the USMLE Step 3 Exam

ABOUT THE USMLE

The United States Medical Licensing Examination (USMLE) consists of three steps designed to assess a physician's ability to apply a broad spectrum of knowledge, concepts, and principles and to evaluate the physician's basic patient-centered skills.

Step 1 (multiple-choice exam)—This exam is designed to test how well the examinee understands and applies concepts integral to the basic and clinical sciences.

Step 2 (two separate exams)—The Step 2 Clinical Knowledge (CK) is a multiple-choice exam designed to determine whether the examinee possesses the medical knowledge and understanding of clinical science considered essential for the provision of patient care under supervision. The Step 2 Clinical Skills (CS) is a separate, "hands-on" exam that tests the examinee's clinical and communication skills through his/her ability to gather information from patients, perform a physical examination, communicate the findings to the patient, and write a patient note.

Step 3 (multiple-choice exam)—This exam assesses the examinee's ability to apply medical knowledge and the understanding of biomedical and clinical science essential for the unsupervised practice of medicine, with emphasis on patient management in ambulatory settings.

The results of the USMLE are reported to medical licensing authorities in the United States and its territories ("state boards") for use in granting the initial license to practice medicine. The examination serves to provide a common basis for evaluation of all candidates for licensure. The USMLE is sponsored by the Federation of State Medical Boards (FSMB) and the National Board of Medical Examiners (NBME).

ABOUT THE USMLE STEP 3 EXAM

The USMLE Step 3 is the last in a series of the three USMLE examinations that all physicians desiring a license to practice medicine in the United States are required to pass. After successfully completing the three steps of the USMLE, a physician is eligible to practice medicine in an independent, unsupervised setting (some period of U.S. postgraduate training is also required).

Note

The test focuses on the management approach to a particular situation and refrains from quizzing the test-taker about the pathophysiology, molecular mechanisms, or long-term management issues of disease processes.

This test is not a more advanced and detailed version of the Step 2 CS and CK exams. Understanding this concept is key to this challenging exam. Step 3 tests whether a physician can not only assimilate data and diagnose clinical conditions, but also has acquired the ability to make individual clinical decisions about patient management.

How can the Step 3 test all first-year interns if they are working in such varied subspecialty settings? The same concepts that medicine house-officers learn about managing a diabetic with heart failure can be equally applied to the postsurgical patient with heart failure.

How Step 3 Is Different

Unlike the Step 2 exams, Step 3 evaluates the physician's ability to perform certain tasks that are related to the clinical management of patients. In a typical case scenario, the test-taker must go beyond making the diagnosis (which is often implicit in the question itself) and make clinical *management decisions* to help the patient. The interpretation of laboratory data, imaging results, points of the history, and even the physical examination is pertinent only insofar as it assists in the correct clinical management of the patient.

Note

There are three clinical encounter frames found in the Step 3 exam:

- Initial care
- Continuing care
- Urgent care

Clinical Encounter Frames

Multiple choice and case simulation questions are presented in clinical encounter frames. There are three clinical encounter frames used in the test: initial care, continuing care, and urgent care. The encounter frame determines the amount of knowledge you have about the patient's history, as well as clinical and laboratory test results. Most important, it will determine how you proceed with management of the patient.

For example, if the question describes a long-standing patient of yours with a history of repeated hospitalizations for asthma who presents with shortness of breath, you would approach her symptoms differently than if she were presenting for the first time to a clinic complaining of periodic dyspnea or if she presented to the emergency department while having an acute asthma attack. The majority of test items (60 to 70 percent) describe patients in a continuing care framework.

Note

There are four clinical settings seen on the Step 3 exam:

- Satellite health center
- Office
- Inpatient facility
- Emergency department

Clinical Settings

In addition to the clinical encounter frame, it is important to know the clinical setting, where you are seeing the patient. On the Step 3 exam, there are four clinical settings: satellite health center, office, inpatient facility, and emergency department. As with the encounter frame, knowing the clinical setting will also contribute to your management decisions. For example, consider the following case scenario:

> A 49-year-old man presents to you complaining of 30 minutes of crushing substernal chest pain. He reports that the pain radiates to his left arm and is associated with severe nausea. He has a history significant for diabetes mellitus, and he has a strong family history of coronary artery disease. On arrival, vital signs are normal, and a loud S4 is heard on cardiac auscultation. What is the next step in management of this patient?

Obviously, this patient needs urgent care. But what is most appropriate? Should an EKG be obtained? Should cardiac enzymes be sent for evaluation? Should the patient be given heparin or sent immediately to the cardiac catheterization laboratory for revascularization? All of these are potentially correct options, but without specifying the clinical setting, you have no idea how limited you may be in diagnostic and therapeutic options. So if the goal is to see that all physicians should know to check vital signs and order an EKG, the question will specify a setting where revascularization is not an option (e.g., an office setting).

The USMLE Step 3 Content Description and Sample Test Materials Guide (found at www.usmle.org) gives complete descriptions of what diagnostic and therapeutic options are available in each setting. The descriptions will also be provided on test day. However, when in doubt, rely on your own logical reasoning skills. It is unlikely that you would be expected to perform an invasive procedure in an office setting, and it is unlikely that a patient presenting to the emergency department would need only a quick check of his vital signs before being released.

Physician Tasks

For any given clinical encounter frame in a clinical setting, there is a finite number of skills or abilities on which a test-taker may be challenged. The six physician tasks that are tested on the Step 3 exam are representative of what all physicians at the intern level should know.

Task 1: Obtaining a history and performing a physical examination

Tests: Your ability to pick out key facets of the history or physical exam and relate them to the presenting problem or condition

Task 2: Using laboratory and diagnostic studies

Tests: Your ability to select the appropriate test in a clinical situation, interpret the results of such tests, and/or anticipate likely test results given clinical data

Task 3: Formulating the most likely diagnosis

Tests: Your ability to determine the diagnosis and use it to manage the patient

Task 4: Evaluating the severity of the patient's problems

Tests: Your ability to assess a patient and make critical evaluations and prognosis decisions

Task 5: Managing the patient

Tests: Your ability to manage a patient in the following four areas:

- Health maintenance, i.e., implementing preventative measures by identifying risk factors
- Clinical intervention, i.e., knowing appropriate postsurgical/postprocedural management and followup
- Clinical therapeutics, i.e., properly utilizing pharmacotherapeutic options
- Legal/ethical and health care system issues, including patient autonomy, physician-patient relationships, and managed care protocols

Task 6: Applying scientific concepts

Tests: Your ability to identify processes responsible for an underlying condition and to interpret results of clinical or epidemiologic experiments

PROBLEMS/DISEASES ON THE TEST

The Step 3 problem/disease list can be accessed at the USMLE website at usmle.org. The list is organized at the system level according to the *International Classification of Diseases*, 9th Revision, *Clinical Modification* (ICD-9-CM). It is subdivided according to presentation categories and includes disorders, health problems, and issues relating to health maintenance. Although this list may not include everything on the test, it identifies many of the clinical problems you should be prepared to encounter in one or more of the frames cited.

STEP 3 EXAMINATION STRUCTURE

The USMLE Step 3 is a two-day computerized examination. The first day-and-a-half tests your knowledge by using a total of 480 traditional multiple-choice questions in a format similar to that of the computerized Steps 1 and 2 CK exams. Note that it has 20 questions fewer than that offered in previous years.

Note

For more information about the new FRED software, which will replace the USMLE software for the Step 3 exam in the fall of 2004, refer to pages 23–24.

Save the Perfectionism

No matter how well prepared you are for the USMLE Step 3 exam, you will get many questions wrong. This is not an exam where you can expect to know every answer. Remember, 65 to 70 percent gives you a passing score.

The first day of testing includes 336 multiple-choice items divided into blocks of 48 items. A total of 60 minutes is allowed for completing each block of questions, for a maximum of seven hours of testing. A minimum of 45 minutes of break time and an optional 15-minute tutorial complete the eight-hour day. Extra break time can be gained by completing question blocks or the tutorial before the allocated time.

The second day includes 144 items divided into four blocks of 35–50. You will have 45 to 60 minutes to complete each of these blocks. The second day also includes four hours for the nine clinical case simulations (CCS), preceded by a 15-minute tutorial. As for the first day, a minimum of 45 minutes of break time is allocated for the day.

Step 3 at a Glance

Examination Length: Two days

Question Types and Numbers: 480 traditional multiple-choice questions; 9 clinical case simulations

Breakdown by Day:

Day 1: 336 multiple-choice items divided into eight 60-minute blocks of 48 items each. Minimum of 45 minutes of break time and an optional 15-minute tutorial.

Day 2: 144 multiple-choice items divided into four 45–60-minute blocks of 35–50. Four hours for the nine 20-minute clinical case simulations (CCS), preceded by a 15-minute tutorial. 45 minutes of break time.

Tip: Extra break time can be gained by completing question blocks or the tutorial before the allocated time.

Clinical Case Simulations

The cases for this component of the exam are designed to simulate the physician-patient encounter, from presentation through initial management, diagnostic testing, and treatment. The challenge of the CCS is twofold:

1. You need to manage the case itself. The management steps are case-dependent and based on acceptable standards of care. It is assumed that you will have reviewed the management of the most common presenting complaints during your year of internship and/or during the course of your Step 3 review.
2. These questions require you to manage a presented patient by initiating actions, such as ordering tests or transferring the patient to another setting. For most of the case, the computer will *not* cue you on what to do—*you* must decide independently what you need to do and the sequence in which it should be done.

Each case can be divided into three parts: the case introduction, vital signs, and initial history (first 1 to 2 minutes); the management of the case (10 to 12 minutes maximum, often less); and the conclusion of the case (last 5 minutes).

Case Introduction Screen

During the first part of the case, you are not allowed to do anything other than read the first three screens. The first screen is called the case introduction and provides a one- or two-sentence description of the patient's chief complaint. It will also indicate the patient's location at presentation, as well as the time of day. At this point, the patient's complaint usually will be too nonspecific to begin establishing a differential diagnosis in your mind. After reading this screen, simply click the **OK** button.

Vital Signs Screen

The second screen is called the initial vital signs screen and gives you the presenting vital signs. Recognize that these vital signs may be the most important indicator of whether this is an acute-emergent or a chronic-stable situation. You should scan them quickly for abnormalities before hitting the **OK** button.

Initial History Screen

The initial history screen will give you a comprehensive description of the history of present illness, past medical history, family history, social history, and review of systems. It is likely that you'll have to scroll through this section. You should read it carefully, as it will present key diagnostic information. This history is sufficiently detailed so that by the time you finish reading the paragraph of "History of Present Illness," you will usually be able to establish a short differential diagnostic list. The remainder of this screen, including the past medical history, family history, social history, and review of systems, may help you further narrow your differential. As you review this screen, you should jot down what you think are the most important facts or clues. At the end of the initial history, click the **OK** button; this will mark the end of the prompted section of the case.

Case Management

At this point, you enter the second stage of the case. There are four buttons at the top of the interface that define this stage. These four options, which allow you to manage the case, remain operational until there are five minutes of case-time left, at which point they are no longer accessible and you are automatically brought to the final stage.

Clicking on the **History/Physical** button allows you to order a followup history, as well as either a comprehensive or directed physical exam.

The **Write Orders/Review Chart** button brings up a number of other chart options, including an order sheet, progress notes, vital signs, lab reports, imaging studies, other tests, and a treatment record.

Other than the order sheet on which you can type in orders, the remaining buttons show you what you've already done or show you data that you have already seen.

The **clock button** allows you to manipulate the **case time clock**. This is a completely separate function from the real-time clock that is found in the bottom right-hand part of the screen throughout the case. In real test time, you have up to a maximum of 20 to 25 minutes to manage the case from beginning to end. But to get results or schedule a time to reevaluate the patient, you'll need to move the case time clock ahead. This button accesses four options:

1. Move the clock to a selected time so that you can get specific results back.
2. Move the clock automatically to when the first result comes back. This is a convenient shortcut that you'll probably use often. Remember, though, that the first test results might not come back for a while, and the patient may need to be tended to in the interim.
3. Indicate a specific time to reevaluate the patient.
4. Ask the patient to call you if he or she is having any problems. (Use this option least often, as it represents a very passive management style.)

Note

Although the CCS will take about 25 percent of your scheduled exam time, it currently accounts for only about 20 percent of your score.

Note

The order sheet is where you would "order" counseling and advise the patient regarding smoking cessation, dietary habits, sexual practices, etc.

Other Multiple-Choice Questions

The first day-and-a-half of more standard multiple-choice questions is a stronger contributor to your overall result than the CCS. Don't get so caught up worrying about the CCS that you forget about the rest of the exam!

The format of the multiple-choice questions is like that you've seen before on the Step 1 and Step 2 CK exams, but the case management perspective you need to take is entirely different. We'll go into more detail on how to handle these in the strategy chapters that follow.

SCORE REPORTING

The USMLE program recommends a minimum passing score for each exam. Currently, the passing score as set by the USMLE program is 184 for Step 3. This corresponds to answering 60 to 70 percent of the items correctly.

Your score report includes the mean and standard deviation for recent administrations of the exam.

There will also be a two-digit score on your score report. This two-digit score is derived from the three-digit score and is used in score reporting to meet requirements of some medical licensing authorities that the passing score be reported as 75. The graphical profiles that appear on the back of your individual Step 3 score report are provided as an assessment tool for your benefit and will not be reported or verified to any third party. The profiles summarize relative areas of strength and weakness to aid in self assessment. Percentiles are not provided in connection with USMLE scores.

Eligibility

Medical school graduates who have passed Steps 1, Step 2 CK, and Step 2 CS are eligible to take the USMLE Step 3 exam.

REGISTRATION FOR STEP 3

For registration and more information, contact:

FSMB
Department of Examination Services
P.O. Box 619850
Dallas, TX 75261-9850
Website: http://www.fsmb.org
Telephone: (817) 868-4041
Fax: (817) 868-4098
Email: usmle@fsmb.org

or your state **medical licensing authority** (see the USMLE website at usmle.org.).

The Steps to Take Step 3

Obtain application materials from FSMB/Medical licensing authority.

Complete your application materials.

Receive a Scheduling Permit verifying your eligibility and authorizing you to schedule the examination.

Follow the instructions on your Scheduling Permit to schedule your test date at a Prometric test center. Center locations are available at www.prometric.com.

On the scheduled dates to take the examination, bring your Scheduling Permit and identification as described on your Scheduling Permit to the Prometric test center.

EXAMINEES WITH DISABILITIES

Reasonable accommodations will be made for USMLE examinees with disabilities who are covered under the Americans with Disabilities Act (ADA). If you wish to apply for test accommodations, you must send your official request and documentation at the same time that you apply for the exam. See the USMLE website for more information.

THE TWO DAYS OF THE EXAM

1. Plan to arrive 30 minutes early at the Prometrics Center so that you are not rushed and have time to get organized.
2. Don't forget your identification! You will need it to sign in at the exam site.
3. Once you sign in, you will be given a locker to store your personal items and assigned to a computer station.
4. Remember that you will have 11 hours to complete 480 items in the first day and a half. These questions will be presented in one-hour blocks of 48 questions the first day, and 45–60 minute blocks of 35–50 questions the second day. The CCS fills the second half of the second day.
5. On each exam day, you will have a minimum of 45 minutes of break time to be used for lunch, bathroom needs, or just to rest.
6. Have a schedule for your test and break time. Remember that if you complete a block early, you can use that time as additional break time.
7. Be aware that if you leave the exam room *during* a block, it will be marked as an irregularity in your testing session. Therefore, stop and consider after each block whether you want a bathroom break.
8. If you don't know the answer, guess!
9. Between the first and second days of the exam, if you can, forget about the day you just had and relax. Work hard to stop yourself from opening up your textbooks and reviewing material and looking up the answers to the questions you recall from the exam. This is not usually a positive experience. Students are more likely to remember questions that they got wrong. Recalling and reviewing questions at this point is likely to dent your confidence and not help you to feel positive about your exam performance.
10. After the exam, *relax*! You definitely deserve it.

FOR MORE INFORMATION

- See the USMLE *Bulletin of Information* and the USMLE website at USMLE.org. Changes can occur after the *Bulletin* is released, so monitor the USMLE website for the most current information about the test.
- Refer to the FMSB website.
- Run the sample Step 3 test materials and tutorials provided at the USMLE website.

Chapter Two: **Study Strategies**

MAKING GOOD CHOICES IS THE KEY TO SUCCESSFUL EXAM PREPARATION

Effective preparation for the USMLE Step 3 is about making choices. At each stage of the preparation process you need to choose the strategies that will most likely lead you to success and stick with them.

Everyone has a different way of studying. Some people prefer a quiet room and total focus on the work at hand; others can study with noise and confusion around them. However, there are some well-recognized ways to study any material effectively that will enable you to learn and retain the most information in the shortest time. The best way to retain information is to be *active* in your own learning process.

Active use of material that you learn increases retention and facilitates recall. Repetition makes memories. Each instance of recall produces a new memory trace, linking it to another moment of life and increasing the chance for recall in the future. Memory is dynamic. Recall actually changes neuronal structures. To be truly useful, a piece of information needs to be triangulated, connected to a number of other concepts or, better yet, experiences. Meaning, not mere information, is your goal.

The key to the Step 3 exam is knowing what to do or say in presented situations. Content knowledge is essential, but the focus of the test is on whether or not you can take the correct action based on what you know. Being able to say what should be done next in presented situations is the hallmark of this exam.

Rereading textbooks from cover to cover and underlining—yet again, in a different color—every line on every page is not an efficient way to learn. You need to focus on the material most likely to appear on the examination. Studying that material through active application is the best way to enhance your understanding and retention of the information. Remember, your goal is to reach beyond "knowing" to "knowing what to do."

The following study techniques will help you develop better ways to prepare for the exam, but remember, learning for retention and use requires active involvement.

CHOOSING WHAT TO STUDY (AND WHAT TO IGNORE)

How can you possibly know what is likely to be on your examination? There are a number of approaches.

1. First, talk to clinical faculty. They often have seen past exams or have reviewed an item analysis and can tell you the topics most likely to appear on the examination. Often, they have talked to other students in previous years and have accumulated some insight as to what issues are more likely to be tested.

2. Talk to students and colleagues who took the examination in past years. Do they remember some topics being particularly "hard hit"? Students who took the exam in the past cannot tell you what will be on the exam that you will take, but they can direct you to the high-yield content areas that you must make sure to master.

   However, be cautious. Candidates typically overestimate how much of their weakest area was on the exam. They are most likely to recall tested content that they got wrong.

   Also, beware of the trap of "studying for the last exam"—exam content differs from year to year. This year's exams will be very different from last year's. And within any given year, your exam will be different from that of others. This is especially true now that the exam is computerized.

3. Use the NBME booklet for study guidance and take advantage of the CD-ROM practice disk sent with your Step 3 application confirmation. These questions can also be downloaded from the USMLE's website (www.usmle.org). These practice questions will indicate the content structure of the exam, but each exam may have sections not covered. Be sure to check these sources.

   Every year new topics are added to the content outline and some older ones are eliminated. The good news is that this USMLE book contains a general outline of everything that can be tested on the exam. The bad news is that as you peruse the outline, you will soon realize that there is more content indicated than any one person can possibly master in detail.

4. Remember that this is a primary care exam. The examiners want you to deal with each presented problem, but to do so within the context of a long-term perspective. If you are preparing for one of the procedure-based medical specialties such as radiology or surgery, your instincts as to what is the best answer may be different from what the examiners are looking for. Spend some time getting used to how primary care physicians think.

5. In general, topics begin to appear on the exam two to three years after they reach prominence in the scientific/lay community. Any interesting medical topic that appeared in the literature at least two years ago is a candidate for inclusion on the exam.

Study Tip

The exam changes from year to year, and exams will be different from test taker to test taker.

Study Tip

More content is covered on Step 3 than can possibly be mastered by one human being. Choose your study areas wisely.

The Primary Care Perspective

The exam is geared to the long-term perspective of primary care. Learn to answer questions from the primary-care point of view.

DECIDING HOW TO STUDY

Mastering the material you must learn for this exam is a three-stage process. These stages parallel the functional organization of memory.

1. **You must learn basic terms and definitions**. This provides the core vocabulary to understand the content being tested. This stage is a matter of simple recognition and memorization. Terms and definitions are learned by the use of associational memory. This is the level where mnemonics can be useful.

2. **You must learn central concepts for each of the test's subject areas**. This stage is a matter of being able to explain the meaning of concepts, how they are used, and how they connect with other concepts. Understanding the cross-linkages within subjects and across subjects will serve you well over the course of the exam. Your basic mental task here is that of reconstructive memory, learning to recall concepts in terms of how things fit together. At this stage, the practice of recalling one concept facilitates the recall of other related ideas. Patterns begin to emerge. This is the level at which diagrams, tables, and pictures can be most helpful. For this stage of preparation, some students find it useful to go back and review some of the basic USMLE Step 2 material. Don't shy away from doing this. If you discover gaps in your basic knowledge base, go back and reacquaint yourself with the material.

3. **You must be able to apply the concepts in presented clinical settings and recognize what concepts are most important in mini-case presentations.** This is the hardest stage of preparation, the one that is most central to the exam, but the one that most students neglect. Remember that the exam will test not only whether you understand general concepts, but also how well you can make use of them in specific situations. Achieving your best possible score depends on knowing not only what concepts mean, but also how they should be applied in a given medical situation. The task at this level is that of reasoning, understanding the implications of presented information and being able to choose the appropriate action from the available options. At this level, study/discussion groups and doing practice questions can be most helpful.

Your method of study and your study schedule should be arranged to allow you to master each of these stages in turn. Having the time to master the necessary material at all three of these levels requires some forethought and planning.

Study Tip: Work Your Plan

Set up a study schedule and stick to it.

As you make your decisions about how you will study, the following suggestions may be helpful:

1. Be organized. Set up an organized study schedule and adhere to it. The two biggest dangers when preparing for the exam are as follows:
   a. Spending too much time on one area or ignoring one subject altogether, and
   b. Allowing study time to be eroded by other obligations.

   If you are going to do your best, you must lay out a plan of action and then defend the time you need to execute the plan. Decide how much time you will study each day and put your time in like it is a job. Schedule regular breaks and keep them. Stick to your schedule. Plan your work and work the plan.
2. Identify your weak areas by taking the diagnostic exam or by using information from your own experience. Begin your study plan with your weak areas and plan to cover those at least twice before the exam.

   It is easy to discover your weak areas. In addition to the results of your diagnostic exam, watch your own reaction to each subject. Whatever subjects or subject areas you like the least are probably the ones in which you are the weakest. Those subjects that you like the most are the ones in which you are likely the strongest. Do not entirely neglect your strong areas, but allocate less time to them. This can be difficult. Research suggests that, left on their own, most students study what they know best and give less time to subjects that make them uncomfortable. This is basic reward and punishment—spending time on what makes us feel good and avoiding what makes us feel bad. Doing well on the exam means reversing this process. Spend the most time on the subjects that make you the most uncomfortable.
3. Keep your sessions short; no more than an hour to an hour-and-a-half with a 10- to 15-minute break. Your concentration declines significantly after an hour or so. Sitting longer will provide only minimal return. In addition, the break time allows the short-term memory to be consolidated into long-term memory, which, of course, is the goal. The key is not how long you spend studying, but being efficient, getting the most out of the time.
4. Do not reread textbooks from cover to cover. Use review books that consolidate the information for you.
5. Limit the number of information sources from which you study. Select *one* main review book for each subject. Trying to master several sources is confusing and time-consuming. If you have several books, use one as your primary study material and the others as backup to clarify points as needed. Especially as your exam gets closer, resist the temptation to buy each new review book you see your friends using. Too many study sources creates overload, and overload stifles comprehension. Choose your study materials and stick with them.

HIGHLY EFFECTIVE STUDY METHODS

Each person has his or her own preferred way of studying. You will have to decide what will work best for you. High-yield study methods all have one feature in common. The more active you are with the material, the more content you will ultimately retain. Remember, your goal in studying is not just to put in the most time but to be efficient, to get the most out of your time. Many of the best students make use of the following active learning techniques:

1. One of the best study techniques is to **pose questions** to yourself as you review material. Perhaps you'll want to jot them down on index cards to share with others and to practice later. By asking yourself questions you are framing the material, challenging yourself to focus on key areas, and, in the long run, developing many of the questions you will see on the examination. Your goal is not to learn knowledge for general use, but to be able to answer exam questions. Your study strategy should reflect this.

   The ultimate goal here is to move you from thinking like a student answering questions to thinking like a faculty member who is writing questions. By this process, you "get into" the heads of the question writers and begin to understand what makes a good question and the issues likely to be at the core of presented questions.

2. **Use graphs and charts** to enhance your comprehension of the material. A picture is worth a thousand words. Practice reading graphs, charts, and tables because this is important for the USMLE. Try abstracting the salient facts quickly from a graph or chart. This may be expedited by using a plain sheet of paper to cover unneeded information, lines, etc., and to focus your attention on selected information.

3. A multiple-choice exam requires you to choose among options. Design your study to prepare you for this task. Do not learn everything you can about a particular test, disease, or procedure. Rather, focus on the key differentiating features. What would cause you to select this test instead of another? The exam will not reward you for knowing all details, only for knowing those that differentiate. Organize your study by grouping things into classes (i.e., type of drug), and then focus on the essential element that allows you to choose within the class.

4. Practice **paraphrasing** material to highlight important information. Paraphrasing means processing the material you have read; telling yourself what is important and unimportant as you read through it, and summarizing the key content in your own words. Pretend that you are the teacher who is in charge of presenting the content. What would you choose to emphasize? What would you leave out if you were short on time? How would you explain the concept to someone new to the field? Remember, if you can say it in your own words, then you really know it. Second, the art of paraphrasing will allow you to answer questions with extensive information in the stem, such as case histories, much more efficiently. Many students say the most difficult part of the USMLE is getting through the large volume of reading required for each question. When you are paraphrasing, do not treat every piece of information with the same emphasis, but decide what is important and what is not. Developing this skill will also be helpful as you progress through your medical career.

5. Creating **summary notes** is a good way to facilitate this paraphrasing process. Summary notes are your personal representation of key points in a way that makes sense to you. Summary notes should run parallel to your primary study material and should serve to annotate, illustrate, and amplify the key points of that material. The physical action of simply writing the notes tends to reinforce learning and aid long-term retention. Once completed, summary notes provide a ready guide for those times when you re-review the material.

6. **Study with friends or colleagues in groups of four or five.** The best groups comprise people with a range of expertise. Try to form a group where each person's weakness is complemented by the strength of someone else in the group.

Study Tip

Think like the question writer and ask yourself questions as you study.

Study Tip

Use graphs and charts as you study to prepare for the USMLE Step 3.

Study Tip

If you can say it in your own words, you really know it.

The goal of these study groups is not to show your colleagues how much you know. Rather, it's to find the holes in your knowledge while you still have time to correct those gaps. Don't be afraid to tackle the tough topics. With the aid of your study group, things will make sense much sooner than they will on your own. Challenge each other. Pose hypothetical situations and seek agreement as to the best answers.

7. **Plan your study time for a distributed practice review.** For most efficient studying, avoid cramming and plan to re-review key material on a regular basis. Repeated exposure to material over time leads to more thorough retention than one massive concentrated exposure.
8. **As you re-review, remember that active learning is best.** This means avoiding simply reading the same page of notes over and over. Instead, use key words as mental triggers and tell yourself as much as you can about the issue you are studying. For example, don't simply reread the treatment protocol for asthma. Rather, tell yourself about asthma care as if you were explaining it to someone else, and then check yourself against your notes.

Using Practice Questions

Doing practice questions is essential in your preparation for taking a multiple-choice exam. Your goal here is to test yourself, but also to learn good question-answering habits. As you do questions, examine whether you got them right, but more importantly, look at *why* you got the question right or wrong. Did you not know the content? Then that's your cue that more study is needed. Did you misread the question? Then evaluate how you misread it and learn how the question-writer wants you to read it.

When you do your practice questions, do them under a time limit similar to the actual exam. In general, your rule should be one minute per question. You will have more time per question during the actual exam, but training yourself for the shorter time frame will reduce the pressure you feel from the clock during the real Step 3 exam. Get used to the time constraint. It is one of the unchangeable realities of the USMLE.

When doing practice questions, avoid these common mistakes:

- Do not just do questions without preparatory studying. Review material first until you feel you know it, and then use questions to test yourself. Learning the answers to hundreds of questions that you may not see on the exam will not help you prepare. If you study by doing questions before you are ready, you will erode your self-confidence and fail to develop key linkages within the material. At the start of your exam preparation, most of your time should be spent studying, with only a little time devoted to doing and reviewing practice questions. As your study time progresses, and you feel more comfortable with the material, you should start spending more time on questions. Right before you take your exam, most of your preparation time should be spent on questions.
- You do not do questions to learn content, but to practice the skills of answering questions. Questions should drive you back to study more. If you get a question wrong, after you look at the annotated answers, open your study material to the section the question was about and review the key information. Consider questions a sample of your knowledge. If you missed a question, then there is likely other information in that topic area that you need to review.
- Do not get into the habit of lingering over a question or thinking about it for an extended period of time. You do not have this luxury on the real exam. Remember that you have just over one minute per question. You should spend about 75 percent of that time reading and analyzing the question stem, and the other 25 percent selecting an answer. Be honest when you do not know an answer; move on, and look it up when you are finished.

- Do not do questions individually. Do them in clusters under time pressure, with 5 to 10 as a minimum. This will get you used to moving from question to question. Do not look up answers after each question. Instead, check yourself after you have done the full set of questions.
- When you start working on questions, do not panic if you do not get the correct answers. Learn from your mistakes. Questions are a part of the study process; they help you see what else you need to learn. You will get better at questions as your studying continues.

Try this exercise:

1. Cover up the options to the question and read the question stem. Pause at each period and paraphrase what you have read.
2. Think about what would make a good answer
3. Now cover the question and reveal the options. Select from the options without looking back at the question stem. With practice, you will get faster, and this strategy will become a habit.

This strategy forces you to get the information out of the question as you read it and does not allow you to waste time by going back and rereading. Remember, you only have time to read each question once. Learn to make that time reading as efficient as possible.

A PROVEN ROUTINE FOR HANDLING EACH QUESTION

Increasingly, the exam is not just about regurgitating facts but about applying those facts in a clinical context. To handle these types of questions your response pattern must not simply be "read, answer," but "read, *think*, answer." You must train yourself to take this crucial moment of thought on each question. Give yourself time to reflect and call to mind the key facts that will help you answer the question. Many questions require you to make multiple determinations to arrive at a correct answer. You must take a reflective moment on each question to allow yourself the time for this cognitive processing. Read the question, call to mind what you know, and then proceed to select an answer. Approach each question with the assumption that you know the answer, and then muster your knowledge to attack it.

The mental task of selecting an answer on a multiple-choice exam is different from the task you face when you make decisions in clinical medicine. In the day-to-day practice of medicine, when selecting a laboratory test, arriving at a diagnosis, or finding the best treatment option, you want to carefully consider all of the options and be sure about your choice. A patient's health, and perhaps life, is in your hands. Before making a choice, most people report that they want to feel as close to 100 percent certainty as they can. For the USMLE exams, you do not have the time to wait for this level of certainty. You must train yourself to make your choice within the time allotted.This often means choosing an answer even when you are not completely sure. If you wait for that absolute feeling of inner certainty, you will take too long. Don't wait until you are sure. Make your choice as soon as you have identified a clear best guess. Then move on to the next question. Remember, there is always another question coming.

THE WEEK BEFORE THE EXAM

During the last few days before the exam, you should be tapering off your studying and getting into mental and physical shape.

1. This is not the time for cramming in new material, but time to organize and integrate what you already know. Work on making what you know more accessible.

2. Review key words, phrases, and concepts. Look over your summary notes one more time. This is the time to drill yourself on essential information. The key is to practice recall, not simply read over the material again. What you need to know is probably already in your head. Your task now is to train yourself to access it when you need it. Doing practice questions is a good way to reinforce your recall skills. Only remember, practice questions are often harder than the questions on the real exam. Do not panic if you do not get them right. Use them to clarify your understanding of key details.

3. Have an honest conversation with yourself and decide what you will not know. No one can know everything that is asked on this exam. Be honest with yourself about what you do and do not know. Knowing that you do not know something gives you more of a sense of control on the exam and makes you less likely to panic when you encounter the material and/or to waste time on questions you are not likely to get correct. When you come to a question that you know that you do not know, simply mark your favorite letter and move on!

4. Get yourself onto the right time schedule. Wake up every day at the same time you will need to on the day of the exam. This will get your circadian rhythm coordinated with the exam schedule. Do not nap between 8:00 AM and 5:00 PM. Otherwise, you will accustom your body to shutting down during critical exam hours. If you get up at the right time each day, you will also find it easier to fall asleep at night. By getting into the proper sleep–wake cycle, you will find it easier to get to sleep the night of the exam as well.

5. You should be getting a sufficient amount of sleep. For most people that means at least six to seven hours a night. Sleep is an essential time for your brain to consolidate what you have learned. You need sleep; it makes you a more efficient learner when you are awake.

6. Take some time each day to relax. Have a good meal. Take a walk in the fresh air. Find time for exercise. The change of pace will refresh you, and the physical activity will help you relax and sleep at night.

7. Consider the impact of your personal relationships. Family responsibilities and obligations can be very distracting. The week before the exam you should avoid family confrontations and any stressful relationships. Your focus should be on the exam and nothing else. The other parts of your life can wait.

8. If you haven't done so already, visit the Prometrics Center where you will be taking the exam. It will be indicated on your exam entry ticket. This will ensure you know how to get there and how much time you should allow for the commute. You can see where you should park, and see what the computer setup is like.

9. If you have not yet done so, review the tutorial on the official USMLE CD-ROM. Become familiar with the interface, the location of key information on the screen, and how to navigate between screens. If you walk into the exam familiar with the exam, you will not have to use any of your valuable break time to do this on test day.

Test-Taking Tip

When you come to a question that you do not know, simply mark your favorite letter and move on!

THE DAY BEFORE THE EXAM

1. **Take the day off from all studying.** This is your day to relax and gather your strength before the main event. Get out of bed at the same time you will have to get up the next day, and then treat this day as a vacation day to reward yourself for all your hard work. If you must study, limit yourself to reviewing your own notes and flashcards.

2. **Have some fun.** Go for a walk. Listen to your favorite music. Go see a good comedy or an action movie that will allow cathartic release. Go shopping. Spend time with a significant other. Do whatever you like. You have worked hard and deserve it.
3. **Make sure that you have checked out the basics for the exam:**
   - Have you worked through the USMLE CD-ROM tutorial?
   - Do you know where the exam is being given and how to get there?
   - Do you have alternative transportation if, for example, your car does not start?
   - Do you trust your alarm clock to wake you up in time? If not, make arrangements with friends as a backup. You want to be sure to wake up rested, refreshed, and on time.
   - Lay out what you'll need for your exam before you go to sleep. This includes your photo identification, scheduling permit, and confirmation number, as well as any personal items like eyeglasses. While you're at it, don't forget to pack a lunch!
4. **Call your friends and classmates and make some plans to celebrate after the exam is over.** You'll need to blow off some steam anyhow, and talking with colleagues will remind you that you are not in this by yourself.
5. **Be sure to do some physical activity**. Just taking a walk for an hour will help relax you.
6. **Get a good night's sleep**. To help you sleep, consider a hot bath or warm milk. Avoid taking sleeping medication as it may leave you groggy in the morning.

THE TWO DAYS OF THE EXAM

These are not the most important days of your career, but just another hurdle on your way to becoming a licensed physician. Keep it in perspective. Treat the exam like what it is: a routine mechanical exercise. You are not a doctor for this day, but an assembly-line worker. Rather than making cars or toasters, you are answering questions. Deal with each question as you come to it, make your choice, and then move on.

No matter how well prepared you are for the USMLE Step 3 exam, you will get many questions wrong. This is not an exam where you can expect to know every answer. Remember, seventy percent gives you a better than passing score.

Doing well on this exam means spending your time on those questions you are most likely to get correct, and not wasting time on questions you are likely to get wrong. Two minutes spent on a question that you get wrong is two minutes wasted. Approach every question assuming that you will be able to answer it correctly. If you discover that you cannot arrive at a clear answer, admit it, make a choice, and move on to the next question. The core idea is a simple one. You know you will get some questions wrong. Therefore, choose which ones they will be and spend your time on those questions for which your probability of a correct answer is higher.

Test-Taking Tip

Although it's important, the CSS counts for only 20 percent of your score, so don't forget about the multiple-choice sections.

We find that most students focus on the clinical case simulations (CCS) portion of the Step 3 exam, which you will face on the afternoon of the second day. Although the CCS is important for your overall score, it is not the most important part of the exam. Although the CCS will take about 25 percent of your scheduled exam time, it currently accounts for only about 20 percent of your score. Proportionately, the first day-and-a-half of more standard muliple-choice questions is a stronger contributor to your overall result. Don't get so caught up worrying about the CCS that you forget about the rest of the exam!

Suggestions for handling the CCS portion of the exam are found in the first chapter of this study guide and on the Kaplan CD-ROM. The following chapter offers advice on how to handle the non-CCS portion of the exam.

Chapter Three: **Test-Taking Strategies**

THE TESTING CENTER

Try to arrive 30 minutes early at the Prometrics Center so that you are not rushed and have time to get organized. Don't forget your identification! You will need it to sign in at the exam site. Once you sign in, you will be given a locker to store your personal items and assigned to a computer station.

Remember that you will have 11 hours to complete 480 items in the first day and a half. These questions will be presented in one-hour blocks of 48 questions the first day and half-hour blocks of 36 questions the second day. The CCS fills the second half of the second day. On each exam day, you will have a minimum of 45 minutes of break time to be used for lunch, bathroom needs, or just to rest.

Day 1

Question Block	Break Time at End of Block
Block 1	No break
Block 2	5-minute break
Block 3	5-minute break
Block 4	30-minute lunch break
Block 5	No break
Block 6	10-minute break
Block 7	Done!

Day 2

Question Block	Break Time at End of Block
Block 1	No break
Block 2	No break
Block 3	5-minute break
Block 4	No break
Block 5	No break
Block 6	30-minute lunch break
CCS Cases 1–3	5-minute break
CCS Cases 4–6	5-minute break
CCS Cases 7–9	Done!

This is just one possible schedule for your break time. If you'd like a different schedule, that's fine. The important thing is to have a schedule! Remember that if you complete a block early, you can use that time as additional break time. You should also be aware that if you leave the exam room *during* a block, it will be marked as an irregularity in your testing session. Therefore, stop and consider after each block whether you want a bathroom break.

MULTIPLE-CHOICE QUESTION STRATEGIES

Some students have their own personal strategies for dealing with multiple-choice exams. If you have a method that you are comfortable with, stick with it. However, many people find the following set of recommendations helpful. Our experience shows that your best strategy is to follow this advice:

- **Start with the beginning of the question block and work your way to the back of it.** This means start with the first question and do each question, in order, until you come to the last question. The idea here is to get into a rhythm that will carry you through the exam. This rhythm will help create what one psychologist calls a "flow" experience. The flow experience is a state of optimal concentration and maximal performance.
- **Do not skip any questions.** If you don't know it when you come to it, you are not likely to know it later. Skipping around wastes time and can end up confusing you as to where you are in the exam. Deal with each question as you come to it. Answer it as best you can, and move on to the next question.
- **Limit your use of the question-marking feature to a few questions in each question block.** Of course, you should answer each question as you come to it, but you may want to double-check yourself on a few questions. The marking feature lets you return to review and reconsider questions where you would like more time. However, marking more than a couple of questions makes it hard to keep track of how many you want to revisit. Keep track of the questions you do mark by writing the question number and any option you have been considering on your whiteboard. You simply may not have time to go back and look at questions you have marked, especially if you mark a lot of them. Use the marking feature to keep yourself from getting bogged down, not to hold yourself back.

Test-Taking Strategy

Used correctly, question marking will let you double-check questions where you have a high probability of getting the answer correct. Misused, marking causes you to not give a question your full attention the first time around.

- **Remember that you can only return to questions within the current question block.** Once the time has expired on any given question block, you can no longer access any of the questions within it.
- **Be cautious about changing answers.** In general, your odds of changing a correct answer to a wrong one are so much higher than the reverse that it is simply not worth the risk. If you change an answer, you are most likely making it wrong! Your first impulse is usually the correct one. Stay with it unless some clear insight occurs to you. If you are not sure, leave your first answer.
- **If you finish a question block with time left over, go back and check only those answers that you have previously marked.** Checking almost always leads to changing and tends to reduce your score. If you have a spare moment, make sure that you have entered an answer for every question in the block and then relax. Sit, take a break, and mentally prepare yourself for the next block of questions. Focus on the questions to come, not the ones that are past.
- **Segment your time so that you know how much you have left, and so that you do not find yourself rushed at the end.** As each block begins, you know how much time you have and how many questions you must answer in that time. Spend a moment getting a sense of how much time you have per question. If the block contains 50 questions, you have just over one minute per question (72 seconds). If the block contains 25 questions, you have 144 seconds per questions. Fewer questions does not mean that you will have more time, however. You have fewer questions because the examiners calculate that the ones they gave you will take longer to do.
- **Whatever the number of questions in the block, some questions will take more time and some less.** Work on your pacing from the beginning of the question block. Check your watch every ten questions to make sure you are on the correct pace to finish. If you pace yourself throughout the block, you should not be squeezed for time at the end.

Test-Taking Tip

If you find yourself thinking, "Maybe I'm taking too long on this question," you are. As soon as you think this, stop, mark your best guess, and move on to the next question.

- **Keep moving.** Do not spend a lot of time on individual questions. Research has shown that students spend the most time on questions that they get wrong. If you find yourself spending a lot of time on a question, this is your indication that you do not know the answer.
- **During the breaks between question blocks, try to relax and not think back over the exam.** The desire to recall questions is strong but not helpful. Those questions are in the past. Focus on relaxing and making the most of your break. Remember, you will

always tend to remember those questions you got wrong. Thinking back over these questions will just convince you that you do not know anything. This puts you in a bad frame of mind and leads to negative thoughts that only make the remainder of the exam more difficult. Be glad one set of questions is behind you. Forget about them, and think about something more pleasant.

THE KAPLAN METHOD: THREE TRIES FOR AN ANSWER

You have three chances after you read the question to get it right. If you cannot get a clear answer using these three attempts, you do not know the answer. Mark your favorite letter and move on to the next question. The key to this strategy is that you always know what you are going to do next. This helps you feel in control and reduces anxiety.

Step 1: Read the Question

This may seem trivial, but studies have shown that most students look at the answers first. Questions cause anxiety and answers provide the solution, so many people go right for the solution. However, you cannot pick the correct answer until you know what you are being asked.

Superior students generally spend about three-fourths of their time reading the question and just one-fourth choosing from the given options. Poorer students tend to reverse this time allocation, spending less time on the question and more on the options. Time reading the question is time well spent. More time on the question means more time spent thinking.

- Read the question and pick out key words. Key words are diagnostic information, abnormal values, indications of gender or race, and any qualifying terms.
- Read carefully enough so that you only have to read the question once. Going back over the question takes time. Read for comprehension the first time.

Paraphrasing is the key to effective reading. Because the exam is administered on computer, you can no longer underline key facts, circle abnormal findings, or make notes in the margins. To compensate, superior test-takers continuously summarize the key information briefly while reading the question. This allows you to look to the options with a sharp focus on the key elements and lessens the need to go back to reread it while examining the choices. Look at the following question to see how this is done.

A 75-year-old smoker and alcohol abuser is hospitalized for evaluation of a squamous cell carcinoma of the larynx. On his second hospital day, he complains of sweating, tremors, and vague gastrointestinal distress. On physical examination, he is anxious and has a temperature of 101 F, heart rate of 104/min, BP of 150/100 mm Hg, and a respiratory rate of 22 breaths/minute. Later that day, he has three generalized tonic-clonic seizures. The most likely cause of his seizures is

(A) alcohol withdrawal
(B) brain metastasis
(C) febrile seizure
(D) hypocalcemia
(E) subdural hematoma

Answer: A

The mental paraphrasing for this question might be as follows:

An old man with laryngeal cancer who smokes and drinks too much has sweats, tremor, anxiety, and some GI problems—he has three seizures a few days after admission. What's causing the seizures?

Paraphrasing is the mental equivalent of underlining. It helps you select what's important and keep those key facts in mind while you are evaluating possible answers. Like most test-taking skills, it also takes practice. If you practice paraphrasing material when you study, you will find that you have developed the basics to answer questions. Paraphrase each time you work with questions to gain skill and confidence.

Step 2: The Prediction Pass

After reading the question, stop. Before looking at the options, try to come up with an answer. We call this the prediction pass because you are trying to think like the question-writer and predict the correct answer. By the USMLE's own rules, questions are written so that any expert in the field can come up with the correct answer without having any options present.

With the correct answer in mind, you are less likely to be led astray by distractors. Remember, they are supposed to distract you and convince you to pick the wrong answer. If you see the answer you thought of, scan the other answers to be sure that it is the best. Then pick it and move on to the next question.

Step 3: The Selection Pass

After reading the question, look down through all of the distractors, in order (A, B, C, D, E, F, G, etc.). If you see a correct answer, pick it. This is the selection pass. If the answer seems obvious and direct, good. Do not trick yourself into thinking the question must be tricky or more difficult.

Most answers will be clearly correct. If you find yourself making up a long story why one option is better than another, stop yourself. You are probably wrong. *The correct answer should be clearly correct.* If two answers seem to be almost the same, then neither one is correct. Once you have identified what looks like the best answer, choose it and move on to the next question.

Step 4: The Final Pass

If, after reading through the options, you are still not sure of the answer, you have one final try: the final pass. At this stage, rather than trying for a correct answer, you are eliminating those you know to be incorrect. Using this strategy, you can usually eliminate all but two of the options.

When you have narrowed your choices down to only two options, you have now arrived at the most crucial moment of the exam. The correct action at this point is to pick one of the two answers and move on to the next question. If you are really unsure of the correct answer, which one you pick does not matter. With two options to choose from, you have a 50 percent chance of getting the question correct, rather than the 20 percent chance you started with.

Make a choice. Many people waste time at this point by not choosing. Some people, when they have eliminated all but two answers, go back and reread the question in hopes of finding some information that will help them choose between the two options. Time spent talking with students and watching their thought processes during the exam suggests that this is the wrong strategy. When students reread a question at this point, they tend to add to it or pick out single features that help them feel better about choosing one of the answers. However, it does not help them pick the right answer. By adding assumptions to the question, students may feel more confident but they are really mentally rewriting the question to be one that they feel more comfortable answering. The answer they pick is then the right answer to the question that they envision, but not necessarily for the actual question presented.

Questions with a large number of options should be handled the same way as all "single best"–type questions. The only difference is that you do not get a final pass as it would eat up too much time. That means these questions usually take less time to handle if done correctly.

Remember

Not answering a question counts as a wrong answer.

If after these three passes: prediction pass, selection pass, and the final pass, you still are not sure of the answer, your best option is to guess. At this point, mark any letter and move on to the next question. *Not answering counts the same as a wrong answer.*

Remember, the key to doing well on this exam is to train yourself to make choices. If you do not know an answer, admit it, make your best guess, and move on to the next question.

UNDERSTANDING FRED™: HOW TO USE THE NEW USMLE™ SOFTWARE

The new NBME software, known as FRED™, will replace the USMLE software for the Step 3 exam in the fall of 2004. FRED will replace the Step 2 CK software when the Step 3 transition is complete, and it will not be used for Step 1 until sometime in 2005.

Note

You *do not* have to use the new FRED features. If you discover that they are distracting you, then the right solution is simple: Ignore the new features and place your concentration where it belongs—on the exam question.

The FRED software provides four significant changes from the usual test delivery software: *1*) a new window that shows answers within a block, *2*) the ability to highlight and/or strike out, *3*) the ability to annotate a question, and *4*) categorization within the display of normal laboratory values to make them easier to access.

Show Answers Window

In the NBME software, students could review their answer choices within a given block by clicking on the ITEM REVIEW button at the bottom of the screen. In the new FRED software, the ITEM REVIEW button is gone. In its place is a window down the left-hand side of the screen that lists the question number and any answer given to each question in the block. This enables students to track where they are in the block and provides an easy way to make sure they have answered every question in the block.

Highlight/Strike Out Options

One of the most consistent complaints from students when the USMLE moved from the paper-and-pencil mode to a computer-based presentation was the loss of the ability to underline key words within the question stem and to cross out answer choices that were decided to be incorrect. The FRED software gives both of these abilities back to students. The key to these new functions is a button at the top of the screen that allows student to select HIGHLIGHT, STRIKEOUT, or neither.

Note

Highlighting can be very useful when creating a symptom list in a long clinical case item or for making sure that some significant feature of the presented information is remembered at the end of the question.

Highlighting feature

When HIGHLIGHT is turned on, you can use your mouse to highlight in yellow a section of text. This yellow highlighting will remain even after you move your mouse onto something else.

Used appropriately, highlighting can also keep you engaged and make sure you are actually taking content out of the question rather than just reading without retention. Highlighting can help to draw you into the details and avoid the mental mistake of skimming over the question without focusing on the presented details.

Note

Don't use the strikeout feature on every question, but only on the questions where you are trying to improve your odds by eliminating options.

Note

The annotation window is probably more trouble than it's worth. It takes time to write a note. Your best approach is always to deal with each question as you come to it and then move on. Look forward, not backward.

Note

If you do not know your normal lab values, spend five minutes a day on these until they are part of your reflexive knowledge base. You need to know these for the exam, but also for medical practice. Committing these lab values to memory will facilitate your performance in both arenas.

Strikeout feature

When STRIKEOUT is turned on, text in options that you click on with your mouse will be faded from black to a grayish color. This moves them to the background (while not completely removing it from view) and provides a clear visual indication that you have ruled out that option as a choice. If you can read the options and select the best answer directly, you will not need to use the strikeout feature. If one answer looks best, pick it and move on.

Annotation Window

FRED provides a window in which you can write question-specific comments. You can use this annotation feature to create a symptom list or to remind yourself of something if you desire to revisit the question.

Categorized Lab Values

As with the NBME software, FRED gives you the ability to look up the reference ranges for standard laboratory values, which may be presented as a part of your question stem. Previously, these lab values were presented as a long list that blocked out much of the screen. FRED groups the lab values into categories such as blood, cerebrospinal, hematologic, and sweat and urine. When you click on each category, you will be shown the lab values and reference ranges only for that category. This reduces the size of the list you have to scan and makes a particular value easier to find.

Although the categorization of the lab value reference ranges is an improvement to the previous presentation, looking up lab values still takes time. Every time you click on the LAB VALUES button, you are pulling yourself away from your focus on the question. Our advice, therefore, is what it always has been: *Learn your normal lab values so you do not have to look them up*. You should know these already before you walk into the exam. If you forget a reference range, the LAB VALUES button is there to help you. But consider this button a safety net. It is there to bail you out if you need it, but do not plan to use it.

Other Minor Changes

In addition to these major changes, FRED repositions important buttons and information on your screen. The exam clock has been moved from the upper right to the upper left corner of the screen. All navigation buttons have now been consolidated at the top center of the screen. This includes the buttons for moving forward to the next question, back to the previous question, lab values, as well as the new highlight/strikeout and annotation features.

Putting all the buttons in the same place and at the top of the screen makes the FRED interface a bit more intuitive and easier to use. And because the exam questions are at the top of the screen, moving all key buttons to the top of the screen allows the student to focus on one portion of the screen rather than having to look for the necessary buttons at the periphery. This narrowing of focus tends to help with concentration.

Chapter Four: **Physical and Mental Preparation**

PHYSICAL PREPARATION

The USMLE Step 3 is a big event. Like an athlete preparing for a big race, you want to approach it fully prepared—both physically and mentally. It's a long two days. The following information consists of test-taking training tips to help you prepare for your test-taking marathon.

All-day examinations are physically stressful. What can you do to help decrease this stress? Get in training. At least one month before the exam, begin the plan described below.

- **Get enough rest.** Although you may be tempted to study late into the night and right up to the moment before the examination, this strategy can backfire and hurt you. The brain needs rest. By shutting off factual input, you foster the assimilation of information into long-term memory and allow time for making connections that help the integration, retention, and recall of information. In the week before the exam, you should be getting at least six and one half hours of sleep a night.
- **Eat right.** While preparing for the exam, have good solid meals. Protein, carbohydrates, and some fats are all important. However, do not overeat or eat very late, because this will impair your sleep. Breakfast on the big day should be no more than cereal with fruit, a bagel, toast, or another complex carbohydrate source. Avoid heavy breakfasts to avoid the subsequent "crash" that many people experience at a crucial time in the first or second question block!

  Likewise, keep sugar or simple carbohydrate equivalents, such as candy, to a minimum at this time. Hard candy, not chocolate, can be useful as a pick-me-up during the examination. If you normally drink coffee in the morning, drink coffee the morning of the exam. You don't want to trigger a caffeine-withdrawal headache. Eat light lunches, salads, simple sandwiches, and nonalcoholic drinks to avoid after-lunch sleepiness. Schedule and eat meals as a part of your study time. These meals serve as breaks that give you a chance to recharge and be more efficient in your studies.
- **Get some exercise**. The exam requires you to be in good physical condition because you will be sitting for long periods of time and want to avoid muscle fatigue resulting in neck, back, or leg aches. As part of your preparation, start an exercise program and stick with it, no matter how difficult. Your regimen should include stretching and aerobic exercise, such as brisk walking or bike riding. The night before the exam, exercise, on a more moderate scale, should continue. Besides the physical benefit, exercise can also help to decrease your anxiety.

MENTAL AND EMOTIONAL PREPARATION

People differ tremendously in their reaction to test situations. Some appear to sail through—confident and calm—while others experience mental and physiologic symptoms of test anxiety such as insomnia, nausea, muscle twitching, or increasing inability to concentrate. If you have serious concerns about test anxiety, don't wait until the day before to seek help. Deal with the problem so anxiety doesn't increase as exam day approaches and your options for dealing with it decrease to zero. This is a situational problem, and effective treatment is available.

Here are some suggestions for how to deal with test anxiety and some exercises that may help you to cope.

1. **Avoid negative thoughts and feelings.** Negative self-talk such as, "There is no way I can pass this exam," can be distracting and produce more anxiety about the test. Focusing on avoiding failure is a recipe for failure. Focus instead on achieving success.
2. **Make anxiety your friend.** A degree of anxiety on the day of the examination is not only natural but also beneficial. How often have you heard of people responding well beyond their daily abilities when pushed to the limits psychologically? However, there is no need for you to push yourself to the limits, but to simply be a little tense and anticipatory on exam day. Incapacitating anxiety will destroy your ability to pass. We have heard many individuals say, "I knew everything, I even taught my peers, but I didn't pass. I don't understand it." Anxiety may do this to you!
3. **Seek help if necessary.** If you find that your studying is being overwhelmed by your anxiety, the most useful thing you can do may be to seek counseling. Talking to someone about your anxiety is not a waste of time if your study time is unproductive due to that anxiety. Get help to be more productive.
4. **Be aware of obsessive thoughts.** If you find yourself focusing on your inability to answer questions, the volume of material, or doubts about your ability to pass the exam, try giving yourself something else to think about. Keeping your mind focused on a small task at hand, such as the information you are currently studying, will help you avoid letting obsessive thoughts distract you.
5. **Make a study schedule.** Purchase a calendar and write out which subjects you will study and a time frame for each. Leave room for breaks and free time. This helps you gain control over your life and your studying. Following a schedule gives you structure, which makes you more efficient and reduces stress.
6. **Improve your attention control.** Awareness is like a searchlight. Whatever you direct your attention to is pretty clear, but other things and events tend to fade into the periphery. Try directing your attention separately to sights, sounds, the feelings in your hands, feet, etc. Your awareness can shift very quickly from one focus to another; however, you can only be fully aware of whatever is in your realm of focus at that moment. Use this fact to redirect your wandering thoughts and feelings by focusing your attention. In time this will allow you to quickly de-emphasize extraneous thoughts by redirecting them to simple bodily functions. Keep in mind how attention works:
   - You can attend to only one thing at a time.
   - Attention is voluntary and immediate, focus on *now*. The future has no role to play.
   - You can monitor your own attention.
   - Attention can be redirected.
   - Focusing on other things that are more relevant can redirect irrelevant attention.
   - You cannot pay attention continuously to one thing without breaks.
7. **Use visualization.** Spend a few moments thinking back to a crisis situation that you handled beautifully. Perhaps it was a medical emergency or a family quarrel where you intervened and helped solve the issue. It can be any type of crisis in which you took charge successfully. Recall how strong and in control you felt, how effectively you controlled a bad scene, even what the setting was like. Reflect on the event to recall it in as much detail as you can. Each day while you are studying, spend 5 to 10 minutes revisiting this past event until you are able to bring it back in your mind with great clarity and detail. Now, when

you feel an anxious feeling welling up, take a mental time-out and revisit this scene. When you do, all the emotions of that day will also return and replace those anxious feelings.

8. **Use an affirmation card.** Take 30 minutes or so to write a series of statements on an index card. The statements should describe what you believe are your greatest personal strengths, character traits, and talents. You might state that you are a deeply empathetic person or that you are very good at solving problems. It doesn't matter what you write down, as long as you believe each statement is true and that you are proud of that skill, personality aspect, or talent. Once you have created the card, keep it with you as you study and practice with test questions. When anxious feelings begin to intrude, take out the card and read through it slowly, realizing the truth of what you have written. With practice, this process will help focus you and lessen negative thoughts.
9. **Take a mental "time out".** If anxious or angry thoughts interfere while you are practicing with questions, try this exercise. Close your eyes; take some slow, deep breaths; and flex, then relax first the muscles in your neck, then your shoulders, then your lower limbs. Use a 1-2-3 count for each inhaled and exhaled breath to keep your breathing deep and even. The whole process will only take a few minutes and will help you reduce the physical symptoms of anxiety and allow you to return to the test with a calm, focused state of mind.
10. **Learn and practice deep breathing techniques.** It can be difficult to focus your attention when you are anxious; however, deep breathing can help. With enough practice during stressful events, this technique will become second nature during the exam.
11. **Use "time out" during the exam.** If necessary, to break the anxiety loop during the exam, back away from the mouse and keyboard and take a few deep breaths. Thirty seconds of rest will seem like thirty minutes in the middle of the exam. Try timing yourself and see how long it feels. By taking very little time away, you get a lot of mental rest. When the exam becomes too much, the best strategy is often not to push yourself to concentrate harder, but to back off and rest for a few moments. You will find that when you return to the exam, your anxiety will be reduced and the questions will make more sense.

THE USMLE STEP 3 EXAMINATION: DOS AND DON'TS

DOS

DO recognize that you have three chances to get every question right: recall, selection, and final passes. If you can't get a good answer after these three tries, guess and move on.

DO take advantage of the CD-ROM computer-based testing practice disk that will be sent with your Step 3 application confirmation. You also will have the option of practicing at a Kaplan Center near your home.

DO be organized. Set up an organized study schedule and adhere to it. Plan your work and work the plan.

DO be sure to make up questions while you study (use index cards) and form a study group to review important content.

DO understand that Step 3 is a primary care exam. Think about the full range of the patient's needs, not just the presenting problem.

DO know that not all of the questions on the exam will count. Anywhere from 30 to 35 questions on the exam are included so they can be pretested and evaluated for use in later exams. In addition, as many as 10 to 15 other questions may be eliminated from the scored pool after the exam results are reviewed.

DO make sure your selected answer matches *all* the information presented in the question. All answers are somewhat likely; you want to pick the one *most* likely.

DO be prepared for questions that make you think. Answers that are not immediately obvious often come to you if you just stop and reflect for a few seconds.

DO remember when you have the question down to two choices, you need to pick one and move on. Lingering over the question tends to result in making the wrong choice.

DO practice questions only after mastering the underlying material. Always do questions in clusters and within a time limit.

DO taper off your preparation before the exam to give yourself a chance to rest up mentally and physically.

DO make sure to take care of yourself. Suffering doesn't help anyone.

DON'TS

DON'T just practice questions without preparatory studying. Review material first until you feel you know it, and then use questions to test yourself.

DON'T do practice questions individually. Do them in clusters of a minimum of 5 to 10 to get yourself used to moving from question to question, and don't look up answers after each question.

DON'T get into the habit of lingering over a question or thinking about it for an extended period of time. You do not have this luxury on the real exam.

DON'T just memorize material. Learn and understand how to apply the content in presented scenarios. Very little of the exam will test rote memory for basic facts. If this is your preparation, you will not pass.

DON'T reread your textbooks from cover to cover. You need to focus on the material most likely to be on the examination. Talk to others who have taken the exam to see how they prepared, and talk to faculty. Download the Step 3 Content Description and Sample Test Mateials document from the USMLE website.

DON'T assume commercial review books and practice exams are current. A good rule of thumb is that whatever appears in most of the review books is probably important, and whatever appears in just one book is most likely peripheral.

DON'T be afraid to face your weak or least-liked areas. Take pretests and/or diagnostic exams to help you narrow down strengths and weaknesses. Begin your study plan with your weak areas and plan to cover those at least twice before the exam. Do not entirely neglect your strong areas, but leave them to a time closer to the examination.

DON'T expect traditional exam tricks, shortcuts, or buzzwords to point you to the correct answer. The USMLE has put great effort into eliminating these cues from the exam.

DON'T get caught by distractors. They may be partially right answers, but not the best answer. Common misconceptions, incomplete knowledge, and faulty reasoning will cause you to select a distractor.

DON'T substitute reading the last line of the question for reading the whole question. This can cause you to miss important information or point you to distractors intended to confuse the issue.

DON'T linger over questions that you do not know. Move on and use the time to answer the questions that you do know. Keep moving, keep moving, keep moving.

DON'T change an answer. Your odds of changing a correct answer to a wrong one are so much higher than the reverse that it is simply not worth the risk.

A FINAL COMMENT

This is not a test of your intelligence or even of how good a doctor you will be. This is a test of your capacity to apply concepts and understand what is appropriate in a stepwise management of patients within the constraints of a computerized exam. Planning, preparation, practice, perseverance, and patience will lead you to your best score. Good luck, and remember, we're here to help.

| SECTION TWO |

Qbook Practice Tests

Internal Medicine: **Test One**

1. A 42-year-old woman with poorly controlled insulin-dependent diabetes mellitus comes to the office complaining of a 5-day history of increasing left ear pain and fullness. She denies subjective fevers or any otorrhea of the affected ear, but does describe a decrease in hearing on the left. She denies any recent swimming. Although she has used a glucometer in the past, she has not checked her glucose at home in several weeks. Her temperature is 37.7 C (99.9 F). Physical examination reveals tenderness of the left auricle, particularly with manipulation of the tragus. There is no fluctuance, but significant erythema extending approximately 4 cm onto her left face. Examination of the left external auditory canal reveals significant edema and squamous debris. A portion of the tympanic membrane remains visible and appears intact and mobile. The remainder of the examination is within normal limits. Blood glucose level is 312 mg/dL. The most appropriate next step in management is to

   (A) administer oral corticosteroids to reduce swelling of the external auditory canal

   (B) admit her to the hospital for treatment with intravenous antibiotics, control of serum glucose, and initiate topical treatment with antibiotic drops to the left ear

   (C) initiate oral antibiotic therapy with amoxicillin

   (D) initiate oral antibiotic therapy with ciprofloxacin

   (E) perform a left myringotomy and initiate topical treatment with antibiotic drops to the left ear

2. You are seeing an active 39-year-old woman in the office. She has always been athletically inclined and has been involved in multiple sports during her high school and college years. She still exercises regularly to keep in shape. From many years of pounding the pavement, she has had an early development of degenerative joint disease. She has reported various aches and pain that is usually resolved with acetaminophen and rest from her activities. However, the past 6 months have been particularly hard on her. She comes in to your office for evaluation of hand stiffness and increasing fatigue that does not seem to be responding to her usual treatments. On further questioning, she reports increasing early morning stiffness that gets better during the day. It seems to affect both her hands equally and she swears that her fingers are swelling as well. She has had a 5-lb weight loss over the last 2 months that she attributes to a loss of appetite. Physical examination confirms swelling and point tenderness mostly over her proximal interphalangeal joints bilaterally. No nodules are present. X-rays are performed and show erosions of several joints. Laboratory studies show an elevated erythrocyte sedimentation rate, C-reactive protein, and rheumatoid factor. The most appropriate pharmacotherapy at this time is

   (A) celecoxib

   (B) ibuprofen

   (C) infliximab

   (D) low-dose prednisone

   (E) methotrexate

3. A 35-year-old woman comes to the office for the first time. She has recently switched jobs and her new employer's insurance has you as her primary care provider. She is here to get acquainted and hands you copies of her most recent medical records. She reports no active medical issues except for patellofemoral syndrome that she occasionally takes acetaminophen for. Past medical history reveals that she contracted hepatitis C from a blood transfusion during pregnancy 12 years ago. She has already been immunized for hepatitis A and B. On review of medications, she takes acetaminophen 500 mg rarely, vitamin A 4000 I.U. each day, which she heard is good for her vision, and a daily multivitamin fortified with iron. In terms of her ob-gyn history, she had 2 children, is up to date with Pap smear, and has regular menses without heavy flow. There is no report of any major surgeries except for the cesarean section of her second child. She tells you her last medical doctor told her that she should never drink again and that she should keep up with her exercises, as she is 15 pounds overweight. Concerned about her liver disease, she asks you if there are any changes that she should make in her daily routine. Based on her history, you should tell her that she should

(A) be fine if she drank 1 to 2 drinks of alcohol from time to time

(B) discontinue acetaminophen and start ibuprofen 800 mg PO tid for the patellofemoral syndrome

(C) discontinue the multivitamin fortified with iron

• (D) discontinue the vitamin A

(E) take herbal remedies as they are natural and safer

4. A 52-year-old married man comes to the clinic because of a 1-year history of impotence. He admits that he used to smoke and drink occasionally but he has recently "cut down on both." He denies any particular stressors in his life. His marriage is stable and his sex life was always great before this. This is causing some concern, even though his wife has been very supportive and understanding. Physical examination and routine laboratory studies reveal no abnormalities. He is unable to give some answers when you ask him about spontaneous erections. In order to establish what is wrong with the patient and proceed with further treatment you should

(A) advise him that no further investigation is needed

• (B) order nocturnal penile tumescence testing

(C) order a standard EEG

(D) perform an abdominal CT

(E) refer him to a psychiatrist

5. A 40-year-old woman comes to the office for evaluation of muscle weakness and rash. She complains of proximal muscle weakness to the point that sometimes she has to use her arms to climb herself up to a prone position. She has also noticed the development of dysphagia, mild visual changes, vague midepigastric abdominal pain, and several "interesting rashes." She has poikilodermata macules in a "V" shaped area on her upper anterior torso. On her periorbital area, there is a violaceous eruption with moderate edema. There is also a violaceous erythematous papule overlying the dorsal interphalangeal and metacarpophalangeal areas. She has periungual telangiectasias. Her overall hands appear fissured, scaly, hyperkeratotic, and hyperpigmented akin to the appearance of a mechanic's hand. The cutaneous manifestation in this patient that is pathognomonic for this patient's condition is

(A) Gottron papules; violaceous erythematous papules overlying the dorsal interphalangeal areas

(B) heliotrope rash; violaceous eruption with periorbital edema

(C) "mechanic's hand"

(D) periungual telangiectasias

• (E) shawl or V-sign; poikilodermata macules in "shawl" distribution over shoulder, arms, and upper back

6. A 42-year-old type 2 diabetic woman comes to the emergency department worried that she has an infection of her left foot. She remembers accidentally stubbing her left great toe against the corner of a wall 24 hours ago. She has been following up regularly with her primary care physician and is compliant with her medications. Her temperature is 37.0 C (98.6 F), blood pressure is 130/80 mm Hg, pulse is 70/min, and respirations are 16/min. Her left foot is swollen, erythematous, and warm to the touch. A stat complete blood count reveals no leukocytosis and no left shift, while an erythrocyte sedimentation rate is normal as well. X-rays of the foot show no evidence of fractures, cortical disruption, or periarticular inflammation. Acting on a hunch, you take a Semmes-Weinstein 10-gauge monofilament wire and probe her skin. She is found to be neuropathic. You then place the patient supine with the involved lower extremity elevated for 10 minutes and watch as the swelling and redness disappear. The most likely condition in her foot is

    (A) cellulitis
    (B) Charcot foot
    (C) gout
    (D) malingering
    (E) osteomyelitis

7. A 65-year-old man is admitted to the hospital with a 1-week history of a productive cough and 3 days of fever and chills. He has hypertension that is well controlled by lisinopril and a 40 pack-year history of tobacco abuse. His temperature is 39.0 C (102.2 F), blood pressure is 110/70 mm Hg, pulse is 90/min, respirations are 20/min, and oxygenation is 93% on room air. Physical examination shows decreased breath sounds at the left lung base with dullness to percussion. A chest x-ray shows a left lower lobe infiltrate with a small pleural effusion. You diagnose him with community-acquired pneumonia and begin therapy with appropriate antibiotics. He is clinically improved on hospital day 1, but on hospital day 2, the patient has recurrent fever with increasing respiratory distress and oxygen requirement. Repeat chest x-ray shows increase in the pleural effusion. A lateral chest x-ray shows 15 mm of layering fluid and you decide to perform a thoracentesis. During the procedure you remove 100 mL of thick, turbid, yellow-white fluid. The fluid is sent for analysis. While you wait for the results, you should advise the patient that:

    (A) The appearance of the fluid is consistent with a lung abscess and he will need surgery to drain the abscess.
    (B) The effusion is likely secondary to a malignancy that may not have been initially apparent on the chest x-ray secondary to the effusion, so he may need a chest CT.
    (C) The fluid may reaccumulate, so a follow-up chest x-ray will need to be done in 2 to 3 days to reevaluate the situation.
    (D) You have removed all of the fluid that was causing his increased respiratory difficulty and he should improve rapidly.
    (E) You will arrange for a chest tube to be placed to allow for further drainage of the fluid.

8. A 64-year-old man is brought to the emergency department because of shortness of breath. His medical history is significant for coronary artery disease, hypertension, and diabetes. His current medications include metoprolol, digoxin, and NPH insulin. He has no allergies to medications. His temperature is 37.0 C (98.6 F), blood pressure is 110/68 mm Hg, pulse is 78/min, and respirations are 28/min. On examination, he is anxious appearing. He has jugular venous distension. His cardiac rhythm is regular and a soft ejection murmur can be heard over the cardiac base. There are audible rales half way up both lung fields. He has 2+ pitting edema of the lower extremities bilaterally. A chest radiograph shows perihilar air space disease. The most appropriate pharmacologic intervention at this time is administration of intravenous

(A) etomidate
(B) labetalol
(C) midazolam
(D) morphine
(E) propranolol

9. A 23-year-old woman comes to the clinic because of palpitations for the past 18 hours. She has no medical history. Her only medication is an oral contraceptive pill. She describes a rash to sulfa-containing agents and denies tobacco, alcohol, or drug use. On examination, she is anxious appearing. Her temperature is 37.0 C (98.6 F), blood pressure is 102/67 mm Hg, pulse is 109/min, and respirations are 24/min. Her cardiac rhythm is irregular. No murmurs can be heard. Her lungs are clear to auscultation bilaterally. An electrocardiogram shows atrial fibrillation. The most appropriate next step in management is to order a

(A) cardiac stress test
(B) serum thyroid-stimulating hormone level
(C) transesophageal echocardiogram
(D) urine hCG level
(E) ventilation-perfusion scan

10. A 27-year-old man comes to the emergency department complaining of substernal chest pressure radiating to his jaw and left arm, associated with shortness of breath and diaphoresis, without relief for the past 30 minutes. He has a past history of asthma for which he uses a beta-agonist inhaler infrequently and denies any history of hypertension. He denies any family history of coronary artery disease. He admits to occasional cocaine and marijuana use and reports using both "recently." His blood pressure is 170/95 mm Hg, pulse is 110/min, and respirations are 20/min. A chest x-ray is normal. Initial laboratory studies show a leukocyte count of 8000/mm^3, a hematocrit of 42%, and a platelet count of 280,000/mm^3. Serum electrolytes are within normal limits. Cardiac enzymes are sent and are currently pending. An electrocardiogram shows an ST-segment elevation of 2 mm in leads V_2 to V_4. The most appropriate next step is to administer

(A) aspirin and beta-blockers
(B) aspirin, benzodiazepines, and nitrates
(C) aspirin and calcium-channel blockers
(D) benzodiazepines alone
(E) beta-blockers alone
(F) beta-blockers plus heparin

11. An 87-year-old woman with dementia is admitted to the hospital from her nursing home with a cough and difficulty breathing. On admission, her temperature is 39.1 C (102.4 F), blood pressure is 95/60 mm Hg, pulse is 110/min, respirations are 24/min, and her oxygen saturation is 93% on room air. She has dry mucous membranes, deep furrows in her tongue, and jugular venous pulsations are not visible at 30 degrees. She also has crackles at her right lung base. Laboratory studies show

Leukocytes	18,000/mm^3 with a left shift
Hemoglobin	13.5 g/dL
Platelets	356,000/mm^3
Urea nitrogen	25 mg/dL
Creatinine	0.6 mg/dL

A chest x-ray is consistent with pneumonia and she is started on levofloxacin. Over the next few days, her mean arterial pressure remains in the 70s and her creatinine rises to 4.5 mg/dL. Urine sodium is 50 mEq/L. The urine is spun and examined. The most likely finding is

(A) eosinophils
(B) "muddy brown" granular epithelial cell casts
(C) red cell casts
(D) red cells, numerous, without casts
(E) white cell casts

12. A 46-year-old woman with type 1 diabetes mellitus, hypertension, hyperlipidemia, and depression comes to the emergency department because of progressive weakness of her arms and legs over the past 7 days. She says, "I am unable to get up out of my chair or off the toilet seat and I have also been unable to walk." She denies any past neurological history, and her diabetes has been under control. She recalls that her primary physician had recently increased the dosage of one of her medications, but she is unable to remember which one. She takes furosemide, ranitidine, nefazodone, simvastatin, and alprazolam. Her temperature is 37.0 C (98.6 F), blood pressure is 150/80 mm Hg, pulse is 72/min, and respirations are 16/min. The neurological examination confirms proximal weakness of her upper and lower limbs although her reflexes are brisk and normal. Some muscular tenderness is also noted. A chest x-ray and electrocardiogram are normal. Laboratory studies show

Sodium	139 mEq/L
Potassium	4.4 mEq/L
Chloride	99 mEq/L
Bicarbonate	30 mEq/L
Blood urea nitrogen	13 mg/dL
Creatinine	0.4 mg/dL
Serum glucose	233 mg/dL
Leukocyte count	5700/mm^3
Hemoglobin	10.9 g/dL
Hematocrit	32.6%
Platelets	228,000/mm^3
HbA1c	5.4
Total bilirubin	0.4 mg/dL
Direct bilirubin	0.1 mg/dL
ALT	389 U/L
AST	638 U/L
Alkaline phosphatase	638 U/L
Albumin	3.4 g/dL
CPK	20,209 U/L
CK-MB	1
Troponin	<0.15

You administer a normal saline infusion intravenously and you follow the abnormal laboratory studies. In addition you should discontinue the patient's

(A) alprazolam
(B) furosemide
(C) nefazodone
(D) ranitidine
(E) simvastatin

13. A 48-year-old man is admitted to the coronary care unit because of an acute inferior myocardial infarction. Two hours after admission you notice that his blood pressure is 85/55 mm Hg and pulse is 45/min with sinus rhythm. The most appropriate initial therapy is to

(A) administer atropine sulfate 0.6 mg
(B) administer dobutamine, 0.35 mg/min
(C) administer isoproterenol, 5.0 µg/min
(D) administer normal saline 300 mL over 15 min
(E) immediately insert a temporary pacemaker

14. A 35-year-old chronic alcoholic comes to the emergency department after vomiting bright red material and having a syncopal episode. His blood pressure is 95/60 mm Hg and pulse is 110/min. You insert a large bore nasogastric tube and notice that there is red-tinged fluid draining. Physical examination shows multiple vascular spider angiomata and a distended abdomen with shifting dullness. The results of his laboratory studies are not yet available. The most appropriate next step in management is to

(A) administer propranolol 10 mg PO
(B) give the patient normal saline 500 mL over 15 min
(C) have an interventional radiologist place a transjugular intrahepatic portosystemic shunt (TIPS)
(D) perform endoscopy immediately
(E) prepare the patient for the operating room for shunt surgery

15. A 22-year-old healthy woman comes to the office for her annual physical examination. She reveals that she has had amenorrhea for the past 11 months. She recently lost 6.5 kg (13.4 lb) intentionally by diet and exercise. She has never been pregnant, and though sexually active, is not attempting to become pregnant. Her medical history is unremarkable, and she is taking no medications. She is 167 cm (66 in) tall and weighs 53.5 kg (117 lb). Her blood pressure is 123/75 mm Hg and pulse is 64/min. The rest of the examination is normal. Laboratory studies show

Serum total thyroxine	8.4 µg/dL (normal 5-12 µg/dL)
Serum thyroid-stimulating hormone	1.7 µU/mL (normal 0.5-5.0 µU/mL)
Serum prolactin	35 ng/mL (normal less than 20 ng/mL)
Serum luteinizing hormone	1.4 mU/mL (normal 5-22 mU/mL, follicular or luteal phase)
Serum follicle-stimulating hormone	1.2 mU/mL (normal 5-15 mU/mL)
Serum beta human chorionic gonadotropin	Negative

The most appropriate next step in the management is to

(A) begin low-dose dopamine agonist therapy
(B) initiate oral contraceptive pills for estrogen replacement and contraception
(C) order MRI or CT scan of the head
(D) reassure her that amenorrhea is associated with weight loss and will resolve spontaneously
(E) start radiation therapy to the brain

16. A 91-year-old woman is being discharged home from the hospital after being admitted for an acute myocardial infarction. The hospital course has been uncomplicated and the patient is nearly back to baseline status on discharge day. Her past medical history is significant for osteoporosis and a fractured hip 2 years ago. The patient also fell most recently 2 months ago, but sustained no injuries. The patient will be returning to her home, where she has lived alone for the past 40 years. She has one son who lives several hours away. In addition to medication counseling with the pharmacist, this patient needs

(A) determination of do not resuscitate status
(B) evaluation of the home by a nurse for possible hazards and new needs
(C) a live-in companion
(D) nursing home placement
(E) wheelchair delivery

17. A 62-year-old woman comes to the office for a followup visit for hypothyroidism. She has no complaints at this time. She has been a patient of yours for years and was diagnosed with hypothyroidism 2 years ago during a workup for depressive symptoms. She takes thyroxine and a daily multivitamin. Her blood pressure is 140/90 mm Hg and pulse is 72/min. She weighs 280 lb and is 5 ft 5 in tall. Physical examination is normal. Her thyroid-stimulating hormone level is 0.360 mU/L. The most appropriate next step in management is to

(A) decrease the dose of L-thyroxine
(B) discontinue her L-thyroxine therapy
(C) increase the dose of L-thyroxine
(D) make no changes in her current therapy
(E) obtain a free thyroxine index (FTI) to determine her thyroid status more accurately

18. A 20-year-old man comes to the student health clinic with complaints of feeling "blah" and having a sore throat for the past 7 days. He states that he has also had low-grade fevers and body aches. His temperature is 38.1 C (100.6 F). Physical examination shows an erythematous pharynx with exudates, enlarged cervical lymph nodes, and a palpable spleen tip. The presence of atypical lymphocytes on laboratory studies would suggest

(A) herpes gingivostomatitis
(B) an infection with the Epstein-Barr virus
(C) an infection with group A streptococcus
(D) an infection with the varicella zoster virus
(E) mucocutaneous candidiasis

19. A 52-year-old woman comes to the emergency department complaining of shortness of breath. She has a medical history significant for a "heart murmur" and hypertension. She is on no medications and describes "throat swelling" with penicillin. Her temperature is 37.0 C (98.6 F), blood pressure is 123/89 mm Hg, pulse is 103/min, and respirations are 28/min. On examination, she has jugular venous distension. There is a loud ejection murmur at the cardiac apex and rales bilaterally in both lung fields. Her chest radiograph shows perihilar air-space disease. An electrocardiogram shows sinus rhythm and left ventricular hypertrophy. The most appropriate next diagnostic step is to order a

(A) cardiac stress test
(B) CT scan of the chest
(C) transesophageal echocardiogram
(D) transthoracic echocardiogram
(E) ventilation-perfusion scan

20. A 39-year-old woman comes to your office because of a "skin problem." She is in good physical health and her only complaint is that she started getting acne about 6 months ago. She cannot understand why this is happening to her now because she never had any problems with her skin, not even in her teenage years. On inquiring what makes her acne worse she answers "just about everything" and then lists heat, cold, spicy foods, alcohol, exercise; even the makeup she has been using for many years has started bothering her. She admits to trying some over-the-counter acne medication from the drug store, but that didn't cause any improvement. There is a diffuse pink flush that extends over her central face and few erythematous papules on the chin. You take a closer look and notice multiple tiny telangiectases on the sides of her nose and the cheeks. The most appropriate topical treatment to prescribe at this time is

(A) augmented betamethasone cream
(B) azelaic acid cream
(C) metronidazole cream
(D) terbinafine cream
(E) tretinoin cream

21. A 45-year-old man comes to see you at the office for psoriasis of the hands that appeared about 6 months ago. The diagnosis was at that time confirmed with a skin biopsy by your colleague who is now on vacation. You check the patient's chart and note that he has no other significant medical problems. Last time he saw your colleague, 3 months ago, he was advised to use calcipotriol cream in combination with betamethasone cream. Unfortunately, this has not really controlled the skin lesions well and the patient is upset. He is a waiter in a fine restaurant and this skin condition may cost him his job. On examination, there are multiple well-demarcated, red, scaly plaques on the dorsal hands. The fingernails have diffuse coarse pitting, and the perionychium is red and scaly. You think his fingers are a little swollen because his wedding ring is cutting deep into his fourth finger. You ask him if he has had any joint pain recently and the patient recalls having morning stiffness of the hands that improved with some exercise maybe a couple of times weekly over the past 6 months. He used to be able to remove his wedding ring prior to that. The most appropriate next step in management is to

(A) start the patient on local PUVA therapy
(B) start the patient on oral methotrexate
(C) switch to topical anthralin
(D) switch to topical calcipotriol ointment alternating with betamethasone ointment
(E) tell him to move to the shore and get lots of sunlight

22. A 35-year-old man with a known history of hepatitis C cirrhosis is admitted to the hospital because of abdominal pain and altered mental status. The pain is diffuse and began sometime during the previous day. He also reports having some loose stool. Other history is difficult to obtain due to his altered mental status. His temperature is 38.1 C (100.6 F), blood pressure is 98/60 mm Hg, pulse is 60/min, and respirations are 20/min. His examination shows spider angiomata, palmar erythema, and gynecomastia. He has an enlarged spleen and a very distended abdomen with a fluid wave and his abdomen is diffusely tender without rebound or guarding. He appears somnolent and is oriented to name and place only. Laboratory studies show

Sodium	138 mEq/L
Potassium	4.7 mEq/L
Chloride	103 mEq/L
Bicarbonate	22 mEq/L
Urea nitrogen	4 mg/dL
Creatinine	0.9 mg/dL
Leukocytes	15,000/mm^3
Hematocrit	32%
Platelets	90,000/mm^3
Prothrombin time	20 sec

The most appropriate study at this time is

(A) an abdominal CT scan with oral and intravenous contrast
(B) paracentesis, with inoculation of blood culture bottles
(C) stool for culture, *C. difficile* toxin, and fecal leukocytes
(D) supine and upright abdominal films
(E) ultrasound of the abdomen

23. A 55-year-old man with diabetes comes to the office for followup after an emergency department visit for chest pain. He reports that he developed left-sided chest pressure with feelings of indigestion over the preceding 2 weeks that lasted 10 to 20 minutes in duration. There was no radiation to the left arm or neck. He initially attributed the feeling to indigestion and took over-the-counter antacids to some relief. On further questioning, he also admits to escalation of symptoms for 2 days prior to the emergency department visit, shortness of breath on exertion, and diaphoresis with onset of chest pressure. He hands you the emergency department documents that indicate he was observed in the cardiac observation unit for a full 24 hours before discharge. Serial electrocardiograms showed a transient 1.5-mm ST elevation in the anterior leads but no Q waves. However, CK-MB and troponin levels were negative. Discharge diagnosis was unstable angina and he was advised to start aspirin once a day and to follow-up with his primary medical doctor for further management. To risk stratify the patient further, you note that he has never smoked, his blood pressure is 150/80 mm Hg with a pulse of 72/min, and he has no prior history of myocardial ischemia. You review several recent laboratory studies that indicate a fasting glucose of 140 mg/dL, HbA_1c 7.2, and a total cholesterol of 285 mg/dL with HDL 32 mg/dL and LDL 221 mg/dL. The most appropriate next step in the management of his unstable angina is to

(A) continue current care with aspirin at 325 mg once daily and follow up closely
(B) discontinue aspirin and start clopidogrel
(C) schedule him for coronary angiography
(D) start therapy with lovastatin
(E) start therapy with nifedipine

24. A 34-year-old African American woman with recurrent urinary tract infections comes to the emergency department complaining of right flank pain, which has been recurrent during the past year and has worsened during the past few hours. She complains of mild nausea yet no vomiting. She says that a doctor once told her that she has "stones." No one in her family has a history of stones. Vital signs are: temperature 37.2 C (99.0 F), blood pressure 140/88 mm Hg, pulse 98/min, and respirations 28/min. She has mild right costovertebral angle tenderness and mild right lower quadrant tenderness on deep palpation. Her leukocyte count is 12,500/mm^3. Laboratory studies are otherwise normal including serum calcium and uric acid. Urinalysis with microscopy shows moderate RBCs, moderate WBCs, and few bacteria yet no crystals. An x-ray of the kidney, ureters, and bladder shows a 2 × 2 cm staghorn calculus overlying the right renal shadow. A diagnosis of struvite nephrolithiasis is made. The organism that is most commonly cultured from these stones is

(A) *Escherichia coli*
(B) *Klebsiella pneumoniae*
(C) *Proteus mirabilis*
(D) *Pseudomonas aeruginosa*
(E) *Staphylococcus aureus*

25. To test the efficacy of a new shot for preventing a specific strain of the Asian flu, 100 volunteer subjects were all given shots at the start of flu season. These 100 subjects were then followed forward over the next 4 months, along with a matched group of 100 volunteers who were not given shots. A total of 68 cases of the flu were recorded across both groups, with the distribution by group displayed in the table below.

	Shot	No shot	Totals
Flu	23	45	68
No flu	77	55	132
Totals	100	100	200

The study included the statement chi-square = 10.77, df = 1, $p \leq 0.05$. A 36-year-old man brings a copy of this study to your office and asks what the chance of avoiding the flu would be if he were to be given the flu shot. The best response is:

(A) "At your age, we don't even need to talk about flu shots."
(B) "I can't really evaluate the results of the study until I know where you got it."
(C) "If you want the shots, let's give it a try."
(D) "Ninety-five percent of the patients who had the shot benefited from the treatment."
(E) "The flu shots are effective at eliminating 95% of the usual flu symptoms."
(F) "The study suggests that taking the flu shot will cut your risk of getting the flu in half."
(G) "The study was conducted on volunteer subjects and the results might not be the same for you."
(H) "You don't really need the shot because you have less than a 50% chance of getting the flu."

26. A 39-year-old woman has right-sided neck pain that radiates down her left arm. The pain is only partially relieved with NSAIDs, which you prescribed at her previous visit. A CT scan of the neck is obtained and confirms your suspicion of cervical stenosis. In addition, you notice a 0.6-cm nodule on the left lobe of the thyroid that is not palpable on physical examination. She has no significant medical history and has never undergone neck irradiation. She has no family history of thyroid cancer. Her thyroid-stimulating hormone level is within normal limits. The most appropriate next step in management is to

(A) determine T_3 and free T_4 levels
(B) repeat the CT scan in 3 to 6 months
(C) repeat the physical examination in 6 months
(D) send her for a thyroid uptake scan
(E) send her for an ultrasound guided biopsy

27. A 67-year-old postmenopausal woman with coronary artery disease, stable angina, congestive heart failure with an ejection fraction of 30%, and hyperlipidemia comes to the office for her regularly scheduled 3-month examination. Her blood pressure is 130/70 mm Hg, pulse is 93/min, and respirations are 18/min. Physical examination is normal. Her LDL cholesterol is 129 mg/dL and her HDL cholesterol is 45 mg/dL. The pharmacotherapy that should be prescribed at this time that has been shown to decrease mortality is

(A) atorvastatin
(B) digoxin
(C) diltiazem
(D) estrogen
(E) isorbide mononitrate

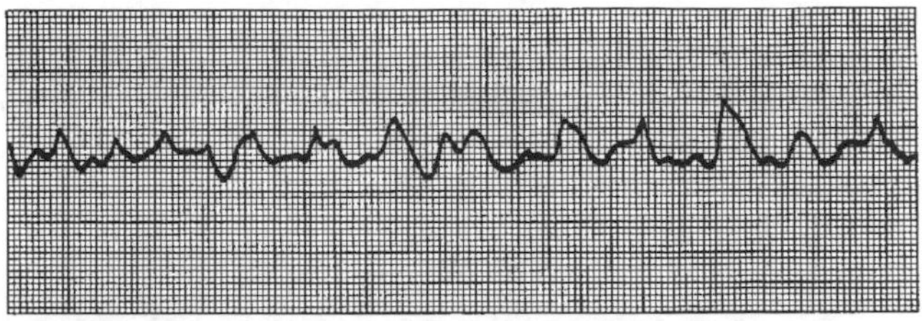

28. A 52-year-old man comes to the emergency department complaining of crushing substernal chest pain and shortness of breath. As you are interviewing the patient, he suddenly becomes unresponsive. The electrocardiographic findings are shown. You do not feel a pulse. You quickly stabilize his airway and begin chest compressions. A nurse begins ventilating the patient with an ambu-bag and face mask. The most appropriate next step in management is to

(A) amiodarone load
(B) defibrillate at 200 J
(C) intubate immediately
(D) push adenosine
(E) push epinephrine

29. A 47-year-old man with hypertension comes to the office complaining of increased urination, headaches, joint pain, and occasional blurry vision. On further history you learn that he has also noticed that his gloves and shoes no longer seem to fit properly. His blood pressure is 140/70 mm Hg, pulse is 83/min, and respirations are 18/min. Physical examination reveals a moderately obese male with coarse facial features, a protruding jaw, and multiple skin tags. His hands and feet appear larger than normal. The most appropriate initial diagnostic study to establish a diagnosis is

(A) fasting glucose
(B) insulin-like growth factor level
(C) an MRI of the brain
(D) random growth hormone level
(E) a 24-hour urine cortisol

30. A 62-year-old man with diabetes, hypertension, and hyperlipidemia comes to the emergency department because of chest discomfort and shortness of breath. He describes the discomfort as 8 out of 10 on a pain scale and says that it is really more of a substernal "chest pressure." His takes aspirin, metoprolol, NPH insulin, and furosemide. He appears anxious. His temperature is 37 C (98.6 F), blood pressure is 110/87 mm Hg, pulse is 64/min, and respirations are 22/min. His cardiac rhythm is regular and his lungs are clear to auscultation bilaterally. At this time you should order

(A) a chest radiograph
(B) a CT scan of the chest
(C) an electrocardiogram
(D) a transesophageal echocardiogram
(E) a transthoracic echocardiogram

31. A 55-year-old Caucasian woman with no previous medical problems comes to the clinic because of an enlarging pigmented nodule on her right calf. Since the lesion is suspicious, an excisional biopsy is performed and the diagnosis comes back as a nodular malignant melanoma, 5 mm in thickness. The patient admits to "baking in the sun" as a teenager at the New Jersey shore and states that her father also had a melanoma in his 50s. She works as a postal delivery person and wears shorts on a daily basis, chronically exposing her legs to the sun "300 days of the year" for the last 30 years. The factor that is the most important in predicting this patient's prognosis is

(A) a family history of malignant melanoma
(B) a history of blistering sunburns
(C) a history of chronic daily sun exposure
(D) the depth of the lesion as measured on histologic examination
(E) the type or classification of melanoma, i.e., nodular versus superficial spreading type

32. A 54-year-old woman with coronary disease with prior myocardial infarction, hypertension, diabetes, and hyperlipidemia comes to the emergency department because of chest pain and shortness of breath. She is a current smoker and has a 40 pack-year history of tobacco use. Her current medications include metoprolol, aspirin, NPH insulin, lovastatin, and furosemide. Her temperature is 37.2 C (99.0 F), blood pressure is 108/55 mm Hg, pulse is 59/min, and respirations are 23/min. Her cardiac rhythm is regular with a prominent S_4 and rales are audible at both lung bases. She has no jugular venous distension. An electrocardiogram shows sinus rhythm with ST-segment depression laterally. She has already received aspirin. The next most appropriate pharmacologic intervention is to administer

(A) diltiazem, intravenously
(B) heparin, intravenously
(C) metoprolol, intravenously
(D) phenylephrine, intravenously

33. A 58-year-old woman with metastatic lung cancer and hypertension is admitted to hospital because of chest pain and shortness of breath. She is recently status post-left-lower lobectomy and radiation therapy. Her post-operative course has been complicated by recurrent pericardial effusions, requiring repeated drainage. Her current medications include verapamil and furosemide. An electrocardiogram taken in the emergency department shows a sinus tachycardia. A transthoracic echocardiogram shows no effusion, a thickened pericardium, and physiology consistent with constrictive pericarditis. Her temperature is 37.2 C (99.0 F), blood pressure is 98/67 mm Hg, pulse is 102/min, and respirations are 26/min. Based on the available information, on physical examination you would expect to find

(A) an increase in jugular venous pressure with inspiration
(B) inspiratory stridor
(C) jugular venous flattening
(D) muffled cardiac sounds
(E) tracheal deviation to the right

Items 34-36

A 47-year-old woman was admitted to the hospital for severe abdominal pain. She has a long history of vague abdominal complaints and has been hospitalized three times in the previous 12 months for similar complaints. She has a past medical history that is also significant for hypertension and diet-controlled diabetes mellitus. Three days ago she experienced the onset of severe abdominal pain, mid-epigastric, radiating to her back. She vomited once and then slept, albeit with much discomfort overnight. The following morning she had tremendous abdominal pain after eating her breakfast, and once again vomited brown-black fluid. She called 911 and was brought to the hospital emergency department by ambulance. She reports that she has had similar symptoms in the past but other hospitals have failed to find any etiology for her pain. On examination, she is an obese woman who appears to be in mild distress. Her vital signs are unremarkable except for a temperature of 37.3 C (99.1 F). Her abdomen is diffusely tender to palpation with guarding.

34. The most appropriate diagnostic study at this time is

(A) an abdominal CT scan
(B) an HIDA scan
(C) liver function tests with amylase and lipase levels
(D) no study is indicated based on her previous abdominal history
(E) a right upper quadrant ultrasound

35. Liver function tests show

Alkaline phosphatase	450 IU/L
Direct bilirubin	3.4 mg/dL
Serum glucose	180 mg/dL
Amylase	267 mg/dL
Serum calcium	8.8 mg/dL
Lipase	101 mg/dL
SGOT	45 IU/L
SGPT	33 IU/L

A right upper quadrant ultrasound shows a distended common bile duct and an abdominal CT scan reveals stranding and inflammatory changes in the pancreatic head. The most appropriate management at this time is

(A) continuous infusion of intravenous opioids
(B) daily abdominal CT scans to evaluate for pancreatic necrosis
(C) intravenous antibiotics
(D) intravenous fluids and *nil per os* status
(E) surgical debridement

36. That evening, the patient is noted to have a temperature of 39.7 C (103.4 F). Her blood pressure and pulse are within normal range. Her physical examination is unchanged. The most appropriate next step in management is to

(A) draw blood cultures and await results
(B) draw blood cultures and initiate ampicillin, gentamicin, and metronidazole therapy
(C) draw blood, urine, and sputum cultures and await results
(D) obtain an urgent abdominal CT scan
(E) start ampicillin, gentamicin, and metronidazole therapy

37. A 61-year-old man with coronary disease and a history of two prior myocardial infarctions, hypertension, and diabetes is brought to the emergency department because of chest pain and shortness of breath. His takes aspirin, simvastatin, metoprolol, and NPH insulin. His temperature is 37.0 C (98.6 F), blood pressure is 90/60 mm Hg, pulse is 87/min, and respirations are 26/min. His cardiac rhythm is regular and his lungs are clear to auscultation bilaterally. His jugular venous pulse is elevated, and his extremities are cold and clammy. An electrocardiogram shows sinus rhythm with ST-segment elevation in leads II, III, and aVF. Based on the available information, the next most appropriate diagnostic step is to order

(A) a cardiac stress test
(B) a chest radiograph
(C) an electrocardiogram with right-sided leads
(D) a green dye cardiac output measurement
(E) a ventilation-perfusion scan

38. A 68-year-old man with long-standing hypertension, depression, and gout comes to the office with complaints of decreased appetite and right upper quadrant pain. He was recently diagnosed with hyperlipidemia, which you elected to treat pharmacologically. His current medications include aspirin, atenolol, furosemide, sertraline, and lovastatin. His temperature is 37.0 C (98.6 F), blood pressure is 118/78 mm Hg, pulse is 58/min, and respirations are 16/min. On examination, his cardiac rhythm is regular with occasional premature beats. He has moderate right upper quadrant tenderness to palpation without rebound or guarding. Rectal examination shows guaiac-negative stool. Routine laboratory studies show that his ALT and AST are now 120 mg/dL and 100 mg/dL from their previous values of 23 mg/dL and 20 mg/dL, respectively. The most appropriate management at this time is to

(A) add hydrochlorothiazide to his medical regimen
(B) administer intravenous lidocaine
(C) discontinue his aspirin
(D) discontinue his lovastatin
(E) increase his atenolol dosage

39. A 43-year-old man is brought to the emergency department following a motor vehicle accident. He was an unrestrained passenger in a head-on collision. He has no known medical history or allergies to medications. He has a chest contusion without rib fractures. His blood pressure is 90/50 mm Hg, pulse is 112/min, and respirations are 26/min. An electrocardiogram shows sinus rhythm with pulsus alternans and a right bundle branch block. A transthoracic echocardiogram shows a pericardial effusion with tamponade physiology. On physical examination you expect to find

(A) an Austin-Flint murmur
(B) a mill wheel murmur
(C) a pericardial rub
(D) pulsus paradoxus
(E) tracheal deviation

40. A 25-year-old woman comes into the office because of an exacerbation of her psoriasis over the past week. She has a long history of psoriasis that has been well controlled with topical steroid and calcipotriene ointment. Approximately 2 weeks ago she had sore throat, fever, cough, and headache, which she treated with bed rest, acetaminophen, and large doses of vitamin C. Since then, those symptoms have subsided slowly but she noted an abrupt increase in the number of red, itchy lesions on her chest and back resembling her previous psoriatic lesions. She denies any changes in topical or oral medications and says that she has not consumed alcohol and has had no changes in her psychosocial situation. On examination, there are numerous well-demarcated, erythematous, thick-scaled, drop-shaped papules involving mostly her trunk and proximal extremities. There are fewer similar lesions on her lower extremities. Oral mucosa is within normal limits. She otherwise appears well with no hepatosplenomegaly. She most likely has

(A) contact dermatitis due to new bed sheets
(B) guttate psoriasis due to streptococcal antigen
(C) a hypersensitivity reaction due to a large dose of vitamin C
(D) a multiple fixed drug eruption from acetaminophen
(E) pityriasis rosea due to streptococcal antigen

41. A 34-year-old man comes to the office complaining of 13 months of chronic diarrhea and a 15-pound weight loss over the last 6 months. He has no significant past medical history and denies alcohol and drug use, recent travel, or sick contacts. His temperature is 37.0 C (98.6 F). Physical examination is normal and fecal occult blood test is negative. Laboratory studies are positive for IgA antiendomysial antibodies. You send him for a small bowel biopsy that shows villous blunting along with lymphocytic and plasma cell infiltration. The most appropriate next step in management is to

(A) prescribe antibiotic therapy
(B) prescribe pancreatic enzyme replacement
(C) prescribe prednisone therapy
(D) recommend folic acid replacement
(E) recommend a gluten-free diet

42. A 35-year-old quadriplegic decides that he has had enough and wants to end his life with dignity. His plea is that there is no future for him and that there is no hope of a cure. He refuses to take food and resents the idea that the hospital is trying to force-feed him. He files a suit against the hospital. The most likely outcome would be that the courts would

(A) comply
(B) deny the patient's wishes
(C) dismiss the case as the patient failed to discuss the matter with his family before filing a suit
(D) order the hospital not to force-feed the patient
(E) refer the matter to a subcommittee

43. A 37-year-old woman comes to the office for a pre-employment physical examination. She has no medical history and takes no medications. She drinks one to two drinks each week, does not smoke cigarettes, and denies ever using illicit drugs. She also denies ever taking herbal medications or supplements and has never had a blood transfusion. Her physical examination is normal. The employment form that you need to fill out asks for a set of laboratory studies that show

Hemoglobin	13 g/dL
Leukocyte count	5700/mm^3
Platelets	270,000/mm^3
Hematocrit	31%
Sodium	145 mEq/L
Potassium	4.5 mEq/L
Chloride	100 mEq/L
Bicarbonate	24 mEq/L
Glucose	106 mg/dL
Creatinine	1.0 mg/dL
BUN	17 mg/dL
Total protein	6.9 g/dL
Albumin	4.1 g/dL
Total bilirubin	0.9 mg/dL
Direct bilirubin	0.4 mg/dL
Alkaline phosphatase	73 U/L
AST	30 U/L
ALT	71 U/L
INR	1.1

The most appropriate next step in evaluation of her transaminase level elevation is to

(A) order an abdominal ultrasound
(B) order serum antinuclear antibodies
(C) refer her for a liver biopsy
(D) repeat the transaminase levels in 1 to 2 months

44. Two days after a right total hip replacement a 74-year-old woman develops acute-onset shortness of breath and right-sided pleuritic chest pain. She denies any sputum production or cough. Her temperature is 37.0 C (98.6 F), blood pressure is 140/70 mm Hg, pulse is 133/min, respirations are 28/min, and oxygen saturation is 92% on 6 L by nasal canula. Electrocardiogram reveals sinus tachycardia rate of 133 without S-T changes. A chest x-ray is most likely to show

(A) Hampton hump
(B) lobar consolidation
(C) normal findings
(D) a unilateral elevated hemidiaphragm
(E) Westermark sign

45. A 20-year-old college student comes to the clinic for a routine physical examination. She has no complaints at this time. She has spent most of her summers in Florida and admits to multiple sunburns each year. She tells you that her mother has recently been diagnosed with melanoma on the lower leg. On examination, she has reddish brown hair, a light complexion, hazel-green eyes, and numerous small, light brown, flat macules on her face, shoulders, and V of the neck. Similar lesions are also seen on bilateral dorsum hands and a few on her arms. Her posterior trunk, abdomen, and lower extremities are within normal limits. At this time it is most important to

(A) give her a clean bill of health and recommend that she come back in 1 year for follow-up
(B) give her sunscreen and tell her to stay out of the sun to avoid increasing the number of freckles
(C) offer her catalogs selling UV protective clothing
(D) offer her chemical peels to remove her freckles
(E) provide pamphlets and education about melanoma

46. A 58-year-old woman with mental retardation, cerebral palsy, and a seizure disorder is admitted to the hospital because of difficulty breathing, high fevers, and diaphoresis. She is unable to verbalize coherently but her caregiver tells you that her mental status right now is at baseline. Her temperature is 39.0 C (102.2 F), blood pressure is 148/70 mm Hg, pulse is 90/min, and respirations are 20/min. She has significant drooling from the mouth and coarse inspiratory crepitations diffusely throughout the lung fields. A chest x-ray shows a right lower lobe infiltrate. Laboratory studies show

Leukocyte count	15,000/mm^3 with a neutrophil bandemia of 8.0%
Hemoglobin	12.4 g/dL
Hematocrit	36.8%
Platelets	318,000/mm^3

You admit her for pneumonia and begin treatment with ceftriaxone and azithromycin.

To improve antibiotic coverage for this patient's pneumonia the most appropriate antibiotic to add is

(A) cefpodoxime
(B) ciprofloxacin
(C) clindamycin
(D) nafcillin
(E) vancomycin

47. A 48-year-old Caucasian woman comes to the clinic because of nocturnal coughing that has been preventing her from sleeping. She produces a moderate amount of sputum, but denies any fever or weight loss. She does not smoke cigarettes, has no pets, and denies any previous respiratory problems. She bought an air humidifier to use in the room to help her cough but with no benefit. Her temperature 37.0 C (98.6 F), blood pressure is 140/80 mm Hg, pulse is 72/min, and respirations are 16/min. Her breath sounds are coarse and you think you can hear a mild expiratory wheeze in the left lung field. Otherwise she has good air entry. Her sinuses are not tender to palpation. You decide to do a spirometry test using an albuterol nebulizer in your office, and the results are shown in the figure and table below.

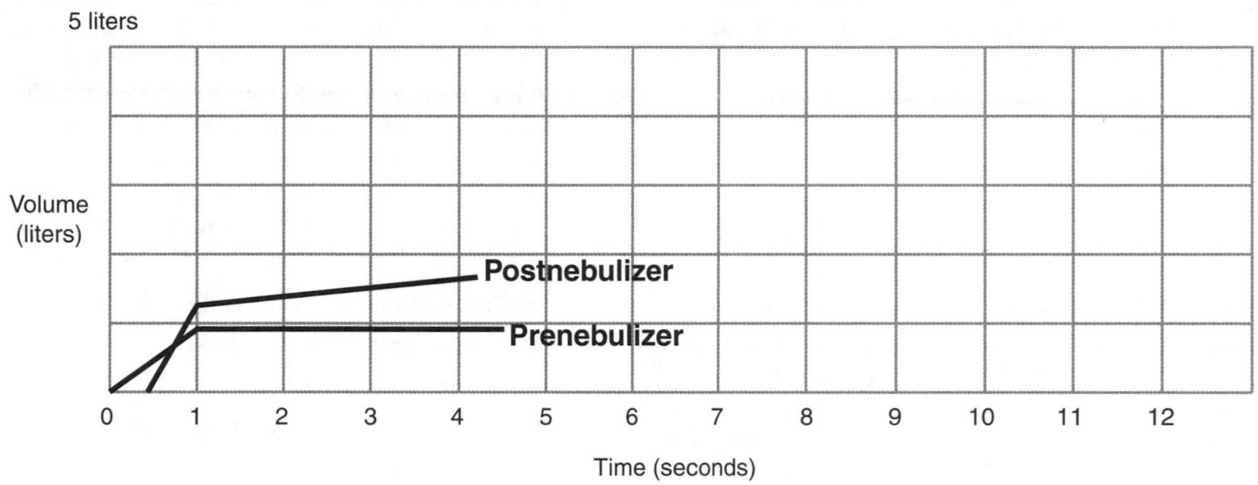

Measurements	Prenebulizer	Adult Predicted Normals	Postnebulizer	% Change from Pre- to Postnebulizer
FVC/L	0.85	2.45	1.24	145
FEV_1/L	0.94	1.97	1.44	153
% FEV_1	98.2	79.5	68.4	86

The most appropriate next step in management is to

(A) prescribe an antitussive agent and ask to see her in 1 week

(B) prescribe an albuterol metered-dose inhaler and ask to see her in 1 week

(C) prescribe a 14-day course of clarithromycin and ask to see her on completion of the course

(D) prescribe both an albuterol metered-dose inhaler and a 14-day course of oral clarithromycin and ask to see her in 1 week

(E) prescribe an albuterol metered-dose inhaler and observe the patient using it in your office and prescribe a spacer if necessary if the patient is not using it effectively

48. A 78-year-old Portuguese woman is admitted to the hospital because of an acute confusion state. Her daughter tells you that the patient has increased agitation, disorientation, and has had a loss of appetite over the past 2 days. She denies any chest or abdominal pain, vomiting, or fevers. She had a total knee replacement 3 years ago. Her temperature is 37.8 C (100.0 F), blood pressure 140/60 mm Hg, pulse is 72/min, and respirations are 16/min. Physical examination is normal. A head CT scan, electrocardiogram, and chest x-ray are normal. Laboratory studies show

Leukocyte count	13,300/mm^3
Hemoglobin	12.3 g/dL
Hematocrit	36.0%
Platelets	222,000/mm^3

Urinalysis shows proteinuria and some cast cells, and is positive for leukocyte esterase and nitrites. She is admitted for a urinary tract infection and started on intravenous ciprofloxacin. Overnight you are called to see the patient because her blood pressure is 70/40 mm Hg. She is drowsy but arousable and physical examination is unchanged. Her temperature is 37.2 C (99.0 F). An electrocardiogram is also unchanged from the previous one. The most appropriate next step in evaluation is to order

(A) a CT scan of abdomen
(B) an MRI of the brain and abdomen
(C) a portable abdominal x-ray
(D) a portable chest x-ray
(E) a retrograde micturating cystourethrogram

49. A 68-year-old Asian woman comes to the emergency department because of 24 hours of shortness of breath. She has a past medical history of depression and hypothyroidism for which she takes fluoxetine and L-thyroxine. She smokes a pack of cigarettes per day. A chest x-ray shows left upper lobe bronchofibrotic changes and mild kyphosis. She is admitted to the hospital and started on oxygen, intravenous ceftriaxone and azithromycin, albuterol and ipratropium nebulizers, and intravenous methylprednisolone. She continues to take her L-thyroxine. She makes an excellent recovery with this management. On the day of discharge you advise her to continue with the L-thyroxine, antibiotics, albuterol and ipratropium nebulizers, and low-dose oral steroids. She is agreeable to smoking cessation. In view of her new medications and her medical history the most important nutritional advice you can give at this time is to

(A) avoid drinking tea and coffee
(B) eat plenty of fish
(C) keep well hydrated
(D) take calcium carbonate with added vitamin D daily
(E) take ferrous sulfate

50. A 32-year-old woman comes to the emergency department complaining of diffuse body aches and generalized abdominal pain. She also reports that her urine is darker than usual. She admits to a long history of polysubstance abuse and has been using crack cocaine for the last 2 days. The remainder of her past medical history is unremarkable except for a bilateral tubal ligation 6 years ago. Her temperature is 36.8 C (98.2 F), blood pressure is 110/70 mm Hg, and pulse is 110/min. Physical examination shows a soft, nonrigid abdomen, no costovertebral angle tenderness, and a normal pelvic examination. Urea nitrogen is 60 mg/dL, creatinine is 2.5 mg/dL, and creatine kinase is 7500 U/L. A urine dipstick is 4+ for blood and there is a normal sediment. The most appropriate next step in management is to

(A) administer copious intravenous hydration in addition to sodium bicarbonate
(B) administer copious intravenous hydration only
(C) order a CT scan of the abdomen
(D) send a urine culture and prescribe antibiotics
(E) send her for abdominal x-ray films

Internal Medicine Test One: Answers and Explanations

ANSWER KEY

1. B
2. E
3. C
4. B
5. A
6. B
7. E
8. D
9. B
10. B
11. B
12. E
13. A
14. B
15. C
16. B
17. A
18. B
19. D
20. C
21. B
22. B
23. D
24. C
25. F
26. C
27. A
28. B
29. B
30. C
31. D
32. B
33. A
34. C
35. D
36. B
37. C
38. D
39. D
40. B
41. E
42. B
43. D
44. C
45. E
46. C
47. E
48. A
49. D
50. A

1. **The correct answer is B.** The patient presents with the classic signs and symptoms of otitis externa. In this case, there is evidence for progression to a left facial cellulitis. Although otitis externa is often treated on an outpatient basis with antibiotic drops to the external auditory canal, one should be concerned about possible complications in diabetic patients or other immunocompromised patients, including facial cellulitis or abscess or progression to malignant otitis externa with subsequent osteomyelitis of the temporal bone. Poor control of serum glucose (in this case >300 mg/dL) is a predictor of progression of the infection. Therefore, the most appropriate course of action is to treat the patient with IV antibiotics with good coverage for pseudomonas (the most common pathogen), initiate immediate control of serum glucose with an appropriate insulin regimen, and begin topical treatment.

   Treatment with corticosteroids would likely exacerbate the patient's serum glucose and inhibit the patient's normal immune response to the infection and is therefore incorrect (**choice A**).

   Treatment with oral antibiotics alone amoxicillin (**choice C**) or ciprofloxacin (**choice D**) is unlikely to resolve an otitis externa in this patient, although ciprofloxacin is a better anti-pseudomonal agent than amoxicillin.

   A myringotomy (**choice E**), or incision of the tympanic membrane, is commonly performed for the treatment of acute otitis media, but has little role in the treatment of otitis externa. Physical examination revealed an intact and "mobile" tympanic membrane, indicting that the presence of middle ear fluid (characteristic of an otitis media) was unlikely.

2. **The correct answer is E.** Medications for RA can be broadly categorized into four classes: nonsteroidal antiinflammatories (NSAIDs), corticosteroids, disease-modifying antirheumatic drugs (DMARDs), and analgesics. When erosions are present, a DMARD is required. Methotrexate is an effective and inexpensive DMARD for the treatment of RA and as such would be an excellent choice for our patient. Methotrexate is a folic acid antagonist that can achieve response rates of 50 to 60%. A major concern is hepatic toxicity that can be limited by dose adjustment, periodic liver function testing, and addition of pyridoxine.

   Celecoxib is a cyclooxygenase 2 (COX-2) inhibitor (**choice A**). It is found to be no more efficacious than conventional NSAIDs like ibuprofen (**choice B**) in RA treatment. The only advantage is an overall lower gastrointestinal toxicity than ibuprofen as there is no COX-1 inhibition. It should be noted that only celecoxib is approved in RA and osteoarthritis, whereas rofecoxib is only approved for osteoarthritis and acute pain. When erosions are present, however, a DMARD is required and the above medicines are insufficient.

   Infliximab (**choice C**) is a tumor necrosing factor alpha inhibitor (TNF-α). It is postulated that the TNF-α plays a key role in joint inflammation and host defense. Infliximab itself is a chimeric (human/mouse) anti-TNF-α monoclonal antibody. In studies, it has shown significant benefits as a DMARD alongside methotrexate. Since its release, the use of infliximab has been linked to the occurrence of tuberculosis. It is now recommended to test for tuberculosis and treat if necessary prior to initiating this drug. One of the major drawbacks of this medicine is the high cost and other well-proven cheaper alternatives would be a better bet.

   Low-dose prednisone (**choice D**) is excellent to gain rapid control of disease activity, reduce symptoms when DMARD treatment is inadequate, or when there are multiple drug failures. In addition to systemic use, local injections intraarticularly can be done for isolated joint swelling. However, this is not used initially as there is potential for long-term side effects.

3. **The correct answer is C.** In a recent review article, chronic liver disease was reported to be the 10th leading cause of death in the United States. Hepatitis C is the most frequent etiology of chronic liver disease. As there is no cure for this condition except for liver transplantation, preventive measures are extremely important in retarding the progress of liver disease. Discontinuing the multivitamin fortified with iron is the correct choice. Patients with chronic liver disease have a propensity for secondary hemosiderosis. It is reported that up to one third of patients have high serum iron levels. The etiology of this process is unknown although there are many postulated reasons from liver cell injury, acute-phase reaction, ineffective body use of iron stores, and increased uptake in the gastrointestinal system. Interestingly, some recent studies link failure of interferon therapy to high iron concentrations. It should be stated that there are no conclusive studies indicating that dietary iron supplementation is harmful, but it is generally recommended to avoid unless iron deficiency is present.

   Abstinence from alcohol is the cornerstone of preventive strategies for patients with chronic liver disease (**choice A**). Alcohol is synergistic with hepatitis C in promoting the continued damage of hepatic cells. Abstinence may have some effect in letting the liver regenerate and heal itself to some degree. It should be strongly encouraged for patients to seek program assistance if drinking is still continued. Alcohol cessation seems to be one of the most important factors in retarding the process to live cirrhosis. You should not tell the patient that she can drink any alcohol. Abstinence must be encouraged.

All medications should be evaluated for their potential hepatotoxicities. It should be remembered that many drugs are metabolized or detoxified through different enzymatic pathways in the liver. A common drug class with known hepatotoxicity is the nonsteroidal antiinflammatory drugs (NSAIDs). NSAIDs can cause idiosyncratic liver toxicity and even failure (**choice B**). Several case studies have linked ibuprofen use with more than 20-fold increases in liver function values. Acetaminophen is also hepatotoxic when ingesting more than 2 grams per day. Unlike NSAIDs, acetaminophen toxicity is dose-dependent and more predictable and is a safer choice.

Vitamin A is also a known hepatotoxin in high doses (**choice D**). Case reports have shown liver failure when patients have taken more than 100,000 IU per day. Failure has also been reported with dosages of 25,000 IU per day but this is much less common. Most multivitamins contain only 4000 IU of vitamin A, which is well within the safe range for daily consumption. Patients with chronic liver disease should be advised to keep vitamin A levels well below 25,000 IU per day.

There is a long list of herbal remedies that can be hepatotoxic (**choice E**). A short list includes echinacea, mistletoe, niacin, senna fruit extracts, valerian root, "Bush" herbal teas, and comfrey. Every herbal supplement and over-the-counter remedy should be scrutinized for potential hepatotoxicities as well. Interestingly, there is some evidence that milk thistle may have a protective effect on hepatic cell membranes with no reported adverse consequences as of yet.

4. **The correct answer is B.** In order to diagnose and treat chronic impotence the presence or absence of nocturnal penile tumescence needs to be established. The best way to do it is using all-night sleep recording.

   No further investigation (**choice A**) is inappropriate since there are obviously unanswered questions.

   Ordering a standard EEG (**choice C**) is not going to address the problem of presence or absence of erections.

   Performing an abdominal CT (**choice D**) in a patient who has no medical complaints and whose workup and physical are unremarkable is not justified before doing a polysomnogram. It can be done afterward if there is a suspicion of a process in the lower abdomen.

   Referral to a psychiatrist (**choice E**) may be done after everything else is ruled out.

5. **The correct answer is A.** Dermatomyositis (DM) is an idiopathic autoimmune disorder that is characterized by an inflammatory myopathy and various cutaneous manifestations. Overall incidence is rare with a prevalence of 1 to 10 cases per million. Average age of onset is in the 40s with predilection for women. Mortality used to be near 50% but with more modern medicines, mortality has been decreased to less than 10%. Early recognition is important and the cutaneous manifestations are important in the overall diagnosis of DM. Gottron papules are the pathognomonic manifestation of DM. The eruption described above can also be located on the elbow or knee joints. Gottron sign is a symmetric, nonscaling, violaceous, erythematous macule or papule, often atrophic appearing in the same distribution of Gottron papules.

   Heliotropes are considered a characteristic manifestation of DM (**choice B**). Heliotropes are located in the upper palpebra of the eyes. Along with Gottron papules/sign, a heliotrope is part of the classification criteria for DM according to rheumatology guidelines.

   Mechanic's hand (**choice C**) is also characteristic of DM but not a pathognomonic manifestation of DM.

   Periungual telangiectasias (**choice D**) are also considered a characteristic manifestation but are not included in the classification criteria for DM. It is only suggestive of DM.

   The shawl or V-sign is characteristic and suggestive of DM but not part of the classification criteria for DM (**choice E**).

   In summary, the classification criteria for DM is to have a skin lesion of Gottron sign or papule or heliotropes, along with 4 of 8 additional criteria including: *1*) proximal muscle weakness; *2*) elevated serum creatine kinase or aldolase level; *3*) muscle pain on grasping or spontaneous pain; *4*) myogenic changes on EMG; *5*) positive anti-Jo-1 antibody test; *6*) nondestructive arthritis or arthralgias; *7*) systemic inflammatory signs (temperature, elevated C-reactive protein, or sedimentation rate); and *8*) pathologic findings compatible with inflammatory myositis. (Tanimoto K, et al. J Rheumatol 1995;22:4)

6. **The correct answer is B.** Charcot foot is a pedal neuropathic joint disease that can mimic cellulitis or gout. In the clinical stage or acute inflammatory stage there is erythema, edema, and increased temperature to the affected foot. This is followed by the fragmentation stage or the acute Charcot stage where there are periarticular fractures particularly of the tarsometatarsal joint, joint dislocation, instability of the joint, and the formation of a deformed foot. The coalescence stage or the subacute stage finds reabsorption of bone debris. In the final reparative stage or chronic stage, there is fusion of bone fragments and the deformed foot is stable. By the description above, the patient is in the clinical or acute inflammatory stage. The most appropriate therapy for her would be limiting her weight bearing, possibly in a total contact cast or a prefabricated pneumatic walking brace, along with very close observation and follow-up. This condition is associated with diabetic neuropathy, tabes dorsalis, spinal cord injury, pernicious anemia, and peripheral nerve injury.

   Cellulitis is suggested by the erythema, swelling, and warmth of the involved extremity (**choice A**). However, the disappearance of the infectious signs with lower extremity elevation is not consistent with an infectious process.

   Gout is suggested also by the erythema, swelling, and warmth (**choice C**). One of the most common sites of inflammation is the great toe (podagra). Once again, the disappearance of the infectious signs on feet elevation is not suggestive of this process.

   Malingering (**choice D**) is when a patient presents under false pretenses for the purposes of some kind of gain. There is nothing in her history suggestive of this disorder.

   Osteomyelitis (**choice E**) is always important to rule out in any diabetic with soft tissue infection. Any ulcer should be probed to see if it reaches the bone. An extremely elevated sedimentation rate can be suggestive of an infectious process of the bones but overall has low sensitivity. Plain film x-ray is an important modality in the evaluation of osteomyelitis. Sometimes, a plain film x-ray can lag behind clinical presentation and if a clinician has high clinical suspicion for osteomyelitis despite a negative plain film x-ray, considerations should be given to an MRI or an indium-111 leukocyte scan.

7. **The correct answer is E.** Effusions are common complications of pneumonia. They usually resolve with appropriate antibiotic coverage of the underlying infection; however, they may become complicated, as in this case. The increasing size of the effusion with clinical deterioration suggests a complicated effusion and further evaluation with thoracentesis is warranted. The finding of pus in the pleural space requires definitive drainage of the fluid. Since the fluid is not dependent on the lateral chest x-ray, loculations are not likely and a chest tube is likely to be of benefit. If loculations were suspected, surgical drainage may be necessary.

   The appearance of fluid that layers easily on chest x-ray is not consistent with a lung abscess (**choice A**). Lung abscess presents with air fluid levels in the lung parenchyma.

   Although the patient is a smoker and sometimes effusions can hide other pulmonary pathology, malignant effusions are more likely to be serous and may be hemorrhagic. The effusion is likely secondary to a malignancy that may not have been initially apparent on the chest x-ray secondary to the effusion, so the need for a chest CT (**choice B**) is unlikely, given that the clinical picture is highly suggestive of pneumonia.

   The fluid will likely reaccumulate, but the quality of the fluid seen during the thoracentesis should lead you to seek additional treatment and not simply repeat a chest x-ray. Therefore, the fluid may reaccumulate, so performing a follow-up chest x-ray in 2 to 3 days (**choice C**) is incorrect.

   Although the patient will likely have clinical improvement shortly after the procedure, this is likely to be secondary to decreased volume in the pleural space. This diagnostic thoracentesis (**choice D**) may therefore have a therapeutic effect but should not be considered definitive therapy for this problem and is incorrect.

8. **The correct answer is D.** Morphine will have two beneficial effects in this patient with congestive heart failure: it will help reduce anxiety, and also dilate the venous bed, decreasing myocardial preload, and thereby alleviating the congestive failure.

   Etomidate (**choice A**), a steroidal agent used in the induction of general anesthesia in patients with a compromised cardiovascular system, has no role in the medical management of congestive failure.

   Labetalol (**choice B**), a mixed alpha and beta antagonist, should also not be used in the setting of acute congestive failure given the risk of exacerbating the disease.

Midazolam (**choice C**), a benzodiazepine, is a reasonable choice for anxiolysis. However, given that anxiety is not the main pathology in this case, it is inappropriate as a first-line agent.

Propranolol (**choice E**), a nonselective beta antagonist, should not be administered in the setting of acute congestive failure given the potential to worsen symptoms. Further, the patient is already on a beta antagonist with reasonable heart rate and blood pressure control.

9. **The correct answer is B.** The standard workup for new-onset atrial fibrillation is a serum thyroid-stimulating hormone (TSH) level in an effort to screen for hyperthyroidism. A serum TSH level is the most sensitive screen for hyperthyroidism.

Given that the patient is young and without risk factors for coronary disease, it is unlikely that a stress test (**choice A**) will provide any useful information. Further, while a myocardial infarction remains in the differential for causes of new-onset atrial fibrillation, it is only very rarely implicated.

A transesophageal echocardiogram (**choice C**) can be used to detect the presence of a left atrial thrombus prior to cardioversion in a patient with atrial fibrillation for over 48 hours. This patient has had her dysrhythmia for less than this period, and medically does not need cardioversion. If cardiac abnormalities need to be assessed (as is done during the workup of new-onset atrial fibrillation), a surface echocardiogram is more appropriate.

Pregnancy, as assessed by a urine hCG level (**choice D**), is not a risk factor for the development of atrial fibrillation.

A ventilation-perfusion scan (**choice E**) is used in the diagnosis of a pulmonary embolus (PE). While a PE can cause atrial fibrillation, there is no reason to suspect one in this instance.

10. **The correct answer is B.** Cocaine is associated with a number of cardiovascular complications including stroke, myocarditis, and arrhythmias. However, the most common is probably an acute ischemic coronary syndrome. Cocaine may induce this effect by *1*) vasospasm, *2*) increased oxygen demand, and *3*) increased thrombotic tendency, e.g., platelet aggregation and thromboxane production. This patient's presentation is entirely consistent with this syndrome, especially in the absence of other risk factors for "typical" CAD. Although more recent (i.e., within the past few hours) use is more strongly associated with ischemia, last use may have even been days prior. First-line therapy is aspirin to counteract the platelet-activating effects noted above; nitrates for vasodilation; and benzodiazepines to reduce blood pressure, heart rate, and anxiety. If myocardial infarction is present, the patient should receive thrombolytics or undergo percutaneous coronary intervention (e.g., angioplasty).

Beta-blockers (**choices A, E, and F**) are contraindicated and result in unopposed alpha-adrenergic stimulation supported by human and animal data; this includes combined alpha and beta blockade seen with beta-blockers (e.g., labetalol).

Aspirin and calcium-channel blockers (**choice C**) are a reasonable alternative if the other medications are contraindicated; pure alpha- blockers may also be useful.

Benzodiazepines alone (**choice D**) are inappropriate because this patient is most likely having an acute ischemic coronary syndrome and requires antiplatelet therapy with aspirin, vasodilatation with nitrates, and benzodiazepines to reduce blood pressure, heart rate, and anxiety.

11. **The correct answer is B.** Acute tubular necrosis is the most common cause of acute renal failure in the hospital setting. Risk factors include hypotension, sepsis, surgery, and nephrotoxic agents. This patient presented with features consistent with hypotension secondary to volume depletion and sepsis and is at risk for ATN. Levofloxacin is not commonly associated with renal failure, especially if dosed appropriately for creatinine clearance. The diagnosis of ATN is supported by an elevated urine sodium (typically >40 mEq/L) and fractional excretion of sodium (typically over 2%); these are both indicators of loss of sodium through loss of tubular function. By contrast, prerenal azotemia should have intact tubules and low urine sodium and an FANA <1%. Urinalysis is also helpful; typical findings of ATN are muddy brown granular and epithelial casts resulting from necrosed tubules, although the sediment may be bland or show only hyaline or granular casts.

Eosinophils (**choice A**) would be more consistent with allergic interstitial nephritis, although not necessarily diagnostic, a much less common cause of renal failure.

Numerous red cells alone without casts (**choice D**) are consistent with hematuria, which may be from a number of causes, but is not associated with ATN.

Red cell casts (**choice C**) and dysmorphic red cells are virtually diagnostic of glomerular disease; tubular function is usually preserved in these cases and therefore the diagnosis would not be consistent with the high urine sodium.

White cell casts (**choice E**) may be associated with pyelonephritis and interstitial nephritis, but not specifically with ATN.

12. **The correct answer is E.** The patient has myopathy due to rhabdomyolysis secondary most likely to the simvastatin that had recently been increased. The other medications would not cause this. Rhabdomyolysis may also be due to strenuous exercise and alcohol myopathy as well as with simvastatin. It often presents with dramatic and painful muscle weakness. Before starting a patient on this medication you should obtain baseline LFTs. LFTs should be monitored as well as symptoms suggestive of myopathy. If the AST or ALT rises to three times the normal level or myopathy occurs, then the medication should be stopped.

    Alprazolam (**choice A**) can cause drowsiness, ataxia, and withdrawal seizures. It is not typically associated with rhabdomyolysis.

    Furosemide (**choice B**) can cause orthostatic hypotension, hypokalemia, and hypernatremia. It is not typically associated with rhabdomyolysis.

    Nefazodone (**choice C**) can cause dry mouth, blurred vision, and constipation. It is not typically associated with rhabdomyolysis.

    Ranitidine (**choice D**) can cause jaundice and arrhythmias. It is not typically associated with rhabdomyolysis.

13. **The correct answer is A.** The combination of sinus bradycardia and hypotension suggests a vagal response in the setting of an acute myocardial infarction. Administration of atropine is the treatment of choice. If the bradycardia and hypotension persist after the administration of atropine 2.0 mg in divided doses then a temporary pacemaker is indicated (**choice E**).

    Isoproterenol (**choice C**) should be avoided in patients with acute myocardial infarction since it increases myocardial oxygen consumption and thus intensifies ischemia.

    Volume replacement (**choice D**) or inotropic support with dobutamine (**choice B**) may be required if hypotension persists after correction of the bradycardia, but neither are indicated as initial therapy.

14. **The correct answer is B.** This patient is most likely bleeding from esophageal varices. He has decompensated liver disease as manifested by ascites. Other potential sources of gastrointestinal bleeding include peptic ulcer disease, portal gastropathy, and Mallory-Weiss tear. The patient is hemodynamically unstable and needs resuscitation with fluids, which should be the first step.

    Propranolol (**choice A**) is indicated for the management of esophageal varices because it lowers portal hypertension but has no role in the acute bleeding varices.

    A transjugular intrahepatic portosystemic shunt (TIPS) (**choice C**) may be considered if endoscopic therapy is unsuccessful.

    The patient will need endoscopy (**choice D**) because of the high risk of continued active bleeding or recurrent bleeding only after he is hemodynamically stable. Endoscopic therapy is as effective as surgical shunting (**choice E**) for the management of variceal hemorrhage but is easier to perform and has much lower complications rate.

15. **The correct answer is C.** This woman has hyperprolactinemia in the absence of medications, pregnancy, or hypothyroidism, and therefore needs further investigation. It is essential that an MRI or CT scan of the head be performed to rule out a large sellar mass causing "stalk" hyperprolactinemia by interrupting the inhibitory dopaminergic tone between the hypothalamus and the pituitary gland. MRI provides the highest resolution for visualizing the anatomy of the sellar area but is more expensive than CT. CT is acceptable for excluding a large sellar mass and is the imaging procedure of choice in a patient who cannot undergo MRI because of claustrophobia or the presence of metal implants. The MRI scan in this patient revealed a 2.5-cm sellar mass extending superiorly to the optic chiasm, which, on histologic examination was shown to be a dysgerminoma. Therapy for this disorder is surgery followed by radiation.

    If the patient had been given therapy with a dopamine agonist (**choice A**), such as bromocriptine or cabergoline, on the assumption that she had a microprolactinoma, she may have experienced visual loss as the dysgerminoma enlarged.

    Oral contraceptives (**choice B**) might be a reasonable second choice of therapy for a patient with a microprolactinoma, but such therapy should not be initiated before the radiologic study of the head.

    Although hypothalamic amenorrhea (**choice D**) is a possibility in this patient because of her recent weight loss, it is a diagnosis of exclusion, which cannot be made in the presence of a high serum prolactin level.

Radiotherapy (**choice E**) should be used only in patients with progressive disease who don't respond to other forms of therapy.

16. **The correct answer is B.** This patient is being discharged from the hospital after a serious illness. She is elderly, solitary, and has a history of falls. It is essential that her home be evaluated for safety issues and special needs prior to discharge. Assessment of the patient's ability to live alone at home must be made with the input from the patient, family, and medical staff.

The resuscitation status (**choice A**) is recorded in the medical chart of all patients that are admitted to the hospital. This decision is ideally made prior to admission by the patient or by the patient's durable power of attorney if she is not competent to make that decision. This is not an issue at this time. Now that the patient is being discharged, a safe home environment must be ensured.

A live-in companion (**choice C**) is but one option for the care of an elderly patient. All options should be explored to see what is best for this patient.

Nursing home placement (**choice D**) is but one option for the care of an elderly patient. All options should be explored to see what is best for this patient.

A wheelchair (**choice E**) may be necessary and this needs to be assessed before discharge. This is just one part of an overall assessment of discharge needs.

17. **The correct answer is A.** The patient's TSH is low suggesting oversuppression with L-thyroxine. When this happens, the dose should be decreased, not increased (**choice C**) and the TSH repeated in 3 months time. There is a strong relationship between circulating thyroid hormone and pituitary secretion of TSH. Therefore, measurement of serum TSH is important in the management of patients receiving L-thyroxine.

Discontinuing her L-thyroxine therapy (**choice B**) is not the best management as it should be decreased and then she should be reevaluated. Discontinuing it would revert her to a hypothyroid state.

Making no changes in her current therapy (**choice D**) is incorrect because her TSH levels are low suggesting that there is oversuppression caused by L-thyroxine, which should be decreased. Every attempt should be made to treat her hypothyroidism with as low a dose of L-thyroxine as possible because of its side effect of osteoporosis.

Obtaining a free thyroxine index (FTI) to determine her thyroid status more accurately (**choice E**) is unnecessary since it is not as sensitive as a TSH level for detecting mild states of excess thyroid hormone.

18. **The correct answer is B.** EBV mononucleosis is characterized by a 2 to 3 day prodrome of malaise and anorexia that leads to an abrupt febrile illness with pharyngitis and splenomegaly in 50 to 75% of cases. On peripheral blood smear, leukopenia may be seen but an atypical lymphocytosis (10% of total lymphocyte count) is seen.

Herpes gingivostomatitis (**choice A**) can cause sore throat but not hematological changes or splenomegaly.

Group A streptococcus (**choice C**), though characterized by exudative pharyngitis and cervical lymphadenopathy, does not have the hematological changes.

The case scenario does not mention a dermatomal distribution rash and so without this information, infection with the varicella zoster virus is unlikely (**choice D**).

Mucocutaneous candidiasis (**choice E**) is characterized by white coating on the tongue and buccal mucosa; it is also known as thrush.

19. **The correct answer is D.** On the basis of the available information, this patient has congestive failure from aortic stenosis. It is therefore appropriate to request a transthoracic echocardiogram to investigate this further.

A cardiac stress test (**choice A**) will not provide useful information in the evaluation of aortic valvular disease.

A chest CT scan (**choice B**) will not provide useful information in the evaluation of possible aortic valvular disease.

A transesophageal echocardiogram (TEE) (**choice C**) is typically not used as the first diagnostic tool in the echocardiographic evaluation of aortic stenosis. Because the aortic valve is an anterior structure, the transthoracic approach is able to provide excellent information in the evaluation of aortic stenosis.

A ventilation-perfusion scan (**choice E**) is used in the diagnosis of a pulmonary embolism, which is not consistent with this patient's clinical picture.

20. **The correct answer is C.** This patient has the typical presentation of rosacea (it is also called acne rosacea), an inflammatory disorder predominantly affecting the central face. It is seen almost exclusively in adults, only rarely affecting patients under 30 years of age. Rosacea is seen

more often in women, but those most severely affected are men. It is characterized by the presence of erythema, telangiectases, and superficial pustules, but is not associated with the presence of comedones. Rosacea only rarely involves the chest or back. There is a relationship between the tendency for pronounced facial flushing and the subsequent development of rosacea. Often, individuals with rosacea initially demonstrate a pronounced flushing reaction. This may be in response to heat, emotional stimuli, alcohol, hot drinks, or spicy foods. As the disease progresses, the flush persists longer and longer and may eventually become permanent. Papules, pustules, and telangiectases can become superimposed on the persistent flush. Rosacea may be complicated by various inflammatory disorders of the eye, including keratitis, blepharitis, iritis, and recurrent chalazion. These ocular problems are potentially sight-threatening and warrant ophthalmologic evaluation. Acne rosacea can generally be treated effectively with oral tetracycline in doses ranging from 250 to 1000 mg/d. Topical metronidazole or sodium sulfacetamide has also been shown to be effective. Topical therapy is not effective treatment for ocular disease.

Fluorinated topical glucocorticoids, such as augmented betamethasone cream **(choice A)** should be avoided since chronic use of these preparations may actually elicit rosacea.

Azelaic acid cream (**choice B**) is used for the treatment of disorders with hyperpigmentation. It competitively inhibits the enzyme tyrosinase, thus preventing melanin synthesis. It is most commonly prescribed for patients with melasma and postinflammatory hyperpigmentation. It is not used to treat rosacea.

Terbinafine cream (**choice D**) is a naftifine derivative that is used as an oral or topical medication in the treatment of fungal infections of the skin, hair, and nails. Some patients with seborrheic dermatitis may benefit from used topical antifungals, which reduce the yeast *Pityrosporum ovale* in the scalp and on the skin, but it is not used for the treatment of rosacea.

Tretinoin cream (**choice E**) is used in the treatment of acne that has a marked comedonal component. It causes moderate to severe irritation of the skin and diffuse scaling which subsides after 2 to 3 weeks of daily application. This would be extremely irritating to use in a patient who has rosacea, and there is no indication since this woman has no comedones.

21. **The correct answer is B.** This patient has psoriatic arthritis and should be started on oral methotrexate. Psoriatic arthritis is often accompanied by pitting of the nails and recalcitrant periungual skin lesions when the interphalangeal joints are affected. These patients need treatment for both the arthritis and the skin lesions, preferably with an agent that will do both and thus ensure compliance of the patient to the treatment regimen (complicated treatment protocols with multiple oral and topical medications have very low yield of compliance in patients). Methotrexate is an effective agent, especially in patients with associated psoriatic arthritis. Liver toxicity from long-term use limits its use to patients with widespread disease not responsive to less aggressive modalities. The synthetic retinoid acitretin has been shown to be effective in some patients with severe psoriasis but is a potent teratogen, thus limiting its use in women with childbearing potential. The evidence implicating psoriasis as a T cell-mediated disorder has created a new perspective relating to the treatment of psoriasis. Based on this presumed disease mechanism, immunomodulatory therapy utilizing cyclosporine has proven to be highly effective in selected patients with severe, crippling, and potentially life-threatening disease.

Local PUVA therapy would possibly improve the skin lesions in this patient, but not the psoriatic arthritis (**choice A**). Ultraviolet light is an effective therapy for patients with widespread psoriasis. The ultraviolet B (UV-B) spectrum is effective alone, or may be combined with coal tar (Goeckerman regimen) or anthralin (Ingram regimen). The combination of the ultraviolet A (UV-A) spectrum with either oral or topical psoralens (PUVA) is also extremely effective for the treatment of psoriasis, but long-term use may be associated with an increased incidence of squamous cell cancer and melanoma of the skin.

Anthralin (**choice C**) is very effective in the treatment of psoriasis, and has the longest published remission periods induced by a topical medication in this disease, but will not have an effect on the arthritis of this patient. In addition, it leaves brown-purple spots on the treated skin due to oxidation and that would not be acceptable for a man in his profession.

Most patients with localized plaque-type psoriasis can be managed with midpotency topical glucocorticoids, although their long-term use is often accompanied by loss of effectiveness (tachyphylaxis). To prevent tachyphylaxis, alternating use with a topical vitamin D analog (calcipotriol) is recommended. Dry, thick, scaly plaques should be treated with ointment vehicles, and thinner, sensitive, intertriginous areas with cream vehicles. Switching from a cream vehicle to an ointment vehicle in this patient (**choice D**) will not affect the psoriatic arthritis. In addition, many patients dislike using ointments on their hands because of the greasy, tacky film they leave behind.

Moving to the shore and getting lots of sunlight (**choice E**) may be a tempting proposal but it is inappropriate to ask of a patient who suffers from a relatively mild chronic disease to completely change his lifestyle and uproot himself and, possibly, a family when so many other treatment options for psoriasis and psoriatic arthritis exist.

22. **The correct answer is B.** Spontaneous bacterial peritonitis (SBP) is a frequent complication of cirrhosis and large ascites. This patient presented with the classic symptoms of fever, abdominal pain, and altered mental status. The latter is often overlooked, but is common. Diarrhea, ileus, and hypotension can be other manifestations and rebound tenderness can be present if cases are severe. It is important to note, however, that patients may present without any symptoms. The diagnostic procedure of choice is paracentesis, which can be done safely in most cases even with an elevated PT. Diagnosis of SBP is made by cell count with a polymorphonuclear leukocyte count of >250. Yield of cultures is increased if blood culture bottles are inoculated by the bedside.

A CT scan of the abdomen is often a very useful test for abdominal pain; in this case, for example, an abscess, hepatoma, or colitis. A CT scan would also be able to show ascites but would not be able to demonstrate infection, therefore an abdominal CT scan (**choice A**) is incorrect.

Sending stool for the above studies (**choice C**) as well as testing it for occult blood would in general probably be helpful, but as noted above diarrhea may be one of the manifestations of SBP.

Of the other imaging studies, supine and upright abdominal films (**choice D**) may be appropriate if an obstruction or perforation is expected, but otherwise would probably be unhelpful as for most diagnoses.

An abdominal ultrasound (**choice E**) would help detect biliary ductal dilation or cholecystitis, which is not as likely; as well as confirming the presence of ascites, but will not help diagnosis infection in the fluid.

23. **The correct answer is D.** Unstable angina is a presentation of atherosclerotic coronary artery disease with severe luminal narrowing involving one or more coronary arteries. Approximately 90% of cases fall into this category while the remaining are nonischemic or noncardiac pain with minority having rare vasospastic or Prinzmetal angina. Unstable angina is thought to be an episodic reduction in coronary blood flow due to superimposed platelet-fibrin thrombus on disrupted atherosclerotic plaque. Long-term goals include stabilization and prevention of progression of underlying atherosclerotic disease. With an LDL of 221, the patient should be started on a statin, as he should strive for a goal LDL <100. With an HDL <36, he should also be strongly recommended to increase his exercise level as well. Consultation with a dietician should be considered to educate or reinforce proper heart-healthy and diabetic-appropriate diet.

Just continuing his aspirin (**choice A**) is not a good idea as aggressive risk management is warranted to prevent progression of his unstable angina. Aspirin should definitely be continued as studies show it can reduce the relative risk of acute MI and death in patients with unstable angina by up to 50%.

Clopidogrel (**choice B**) works through platelet adenosine diphosphate (ADP) receptor antagonism. This option should be considered if the patient is found to have aspirin sensitivity. Results from the Clopidogrel in Unstable Angina to Prevent Recurrent Ischemic Events (CURE) trial suggests more efficacy when combining aspirin and clopidogrel but at a cost of higher risk of nonintracranial bleeding complications.

Coronary angiography (**choice C**) is generally accepted as appropriate for patients who continue to report symptoms despite aggressive management, escalation of symptoms or their severity, or hemodynamic instability. At this point, the patient should be managed conservatively by managing his risk factors to their fullest extent.

Blood pressure control is paramount in patients with unstable angina. The best choices are beta-blockers or ACE inhibitors. Nitrates are also useful in reducing the frequency of angina. Calcium-channel blockers are not frequently used, and short-acting dihydropyridines such as nifedipine (**choice E**) are contraindicated as they can increase heart rate and the risk of acute MI.

24. **The correct answer is C.** *Proteus mirabilis* is the most common organism associated with struvite (magnesium-ammonium-phosphate) stones. These stones are caused by recurrent urinary tract infection with urea-splitting organisms. Organisms such as *Proteus* possess the enzyme urease, which splits urea thus creating the alkaline urinary environment necessary for struvite stones to form.

Escherichia coli (**choice A**) is the organism most commonly associated with urinary tract infection. It is also sometimes found in association with struvite stones.

Klebsiella pneumoniae (**choice B**) is also associated with struvite stones, however less commonly than *Proteus.*

Pseudomonas aeruginosa (**choice D**) is not a common urinary pathogen and is not associated with struvite stone formation.

Staphylococcus aureus (**choice E**) is also not a common urinary pathogen and does not cause struvite stones.

25. **The correct answer is F.** Twenty-three percent of those given the flu shot got the flu, whereas 45% of those not given the shots got the flu, based on the data presented as a part of the study. This is approximately a 50% reduction in the number of cases when the two groups are compared.

Flu shots have been shown to be effective at reducing the incidence of flu in most adult groups. Age (**choice A**) is no reason to exclude this patient from the benefits of the intervention.

The study can be evaluated on the merits of the study design and data that are described. Publication in a prestigious source does not guarantee a better study. Nor does publication in a more obscure source mean that the study results are less meaningful. A doctor is expected to be able to evaluate the results for himself or herself, and not merely accept what is published in a reputable journal as some absolute truth (**choice B**).

Simply agreeing to the shots without any explanation of the study's results is nonresponsive and inappropriate (**choice C**).

This answer uses the p value, the indicator of statistical significance, as an index of clinical significance. The p value gives the chance that an error was made in rejecting the null hypothesis. It does *not* give the chance that an individual patient will benefit, nor does it give the percentage of patients who will benefit (**choice D**).

To continue the comment from choice D, the p value also does not tell the percent of symptoms that will be relieved (**choice E**).

Volunteer subjects are unlikely to bias a study examining the efficacy of a preventive shot. Although it is remotely possible that subjects that are either especially susceptible or especially impervious to the flu were the study participants, there is no evidence suggesting that this might be the case (**choice G**).

Although those without the shot do have less than a 50% chance of getting the flu (**choice H**), the risk reduction (50%) between the group who got the shot and the one who did not is sufficient to justify the use of this intervention.

26. **The correct answer is C.** Thyroid nodules that are not palpable do not need to be biopsied since they are rarely clinically significant. Rather, reexamining the thyroid gland at a later date to ensure that the size has not increased is all that is needed. If the patient had a history of neck radiation or family history of cancer, some might opt for a more aggressive approach.

Measurement of thyroid hormones (**choice A**) is not necessary. This patient has a normal TSH, which should discourage you from ordering further thyroid function tests.

This nodule is likely not clinically significant. There is no proven benefit to fine-needle biopsy of nonpalpable nodules. Followup CT scan of the neck (**choice B**) is therefore not indicated. CT scan of the neck is useful in evaluation of possible tracheal compression secondary to a goiter.

Thyroid uptake scans (**choice D**) are typically not indicated in the evaluation of a euthyroid patient. Thyroid uptake scanning is useful in the hyperthyroid patient to differentiate a hyperfunctioning nodule from the diffuse increased activity seen in Graves disease.

A thyroid ultrasound can be helpful in improving the yield of fine-needle aspirations. Biopsy of a nodule that is not palpable but is visible with ultrasound (**choice E**) is not advised since these nodules are rarely clinically meaningful.

27. **The correct answer is A.** Atorvastatin has been shown to decrease mortality in coronary artery disease. In a patient with known CAD, diabetes, or multiple risk factors for heart disease, the goal LDL cholesterol is below 100 mg/dL. New data suggest that statin medications might also have a role in coronary plaque stabilization post MI. Our patient's LDL cholesterol is too high since she has known CAD.

Digoxin (**choice B**) is a drug that is useful in CHF since it decreases morbidity and improves CHF-related symptoms. It does not decrease overall mortality in patients with CHF but it remains a useful adjunctive medication in management of symptomatic patients.

Calcium-channel blockers, such as diltiazem (**choice C**), have not been shown to decrease the risk of death in patients with coronary artery disease and are therefore not first-line agents in management. They serve as important adjunctive therapy in those patients who cannot tolerate a beta-blocker because of underlying asthma or COPD. They are also helpful in the management of patients with difficult to manage blood pressure.

Estrogen replacement (**choice D**) remains a controversial topic in medicine. HRT may be an option for patients with symptomatic menopause and CAD, but it is no longer recommended routinely as a medication to prevent cardiovascular mortality. Recent studies have shown an increased mortality initially when starting HRT only to be followed by a decreased mortality a few years into treatment. The increase in mortality may be due to prothrombotic effects of estrogen. Future data will likely clarify this issue further.

Nitrates (**choice E**) should be incorporated into the management of all patients with angina to minimize symptoms. They are an important part of the management of coronary artery disease. That being said, there is no conclusive evidence that nitrates decrease mortality in heart disease.

The interventions that have been shown to decrease mortality in CAD are the following: aspirin, beta-blockers, ACE inhibitors, statins. Other medications which lower LDL cholesterol are likely helpful as are medications that increase HDL cholesterol. Smoking cessation and blood pressure management are also vital.

28. **The correct answer is B.** This patient is having a V-fib arrest. When encountering this situation, you need to remember your ACLS protocols. The V-fib algorithm advises that CPR begin until the defibrillator is ready. As soon as you have the defibrillator, three shocks should be administered at 200 J, 300 J, then 360 J. After the three shocks are delivered, the patient should be intubated (**choice C**).

Amiodarone (**choice A**) has started to replace lidocaine as the medication to be used in conjunction with epinephrine and shocks in V-fib. After the initial three shocks are given and the patient is intubated, 1 mg of epinephrine (**choice E**) should be given. The patient should then be shocked again with 360 J. If a more stable rhythm is not achieved, amiodarone is then loaded over a prolonged period.

Adenosine (**choice D**) has no role in the management of V-fib. Adenosine is useful in the management of stable supraventricular tachycardia to help identify the underlying rhythm (a-fib versus PSVT versus junction tachycardia versus MAT).

29. **The correct answer is B.** This patient has acromegaly, which is an excess of growth hormone. This is evidenced by increased hand and foot size and coarse facial features with a protruding jaw. Other features like tooth space narrowing and macroglossia can be present. Impaired glucose tolerance is often present, as is diabetes. The test of choice to diagnose this condition is insulin-like growth factor, which is elevated to greater than five times the normal limit.

Fasting glucose (**choice A**) should be measured since acromegaly is associated with insulin resistance and diabetes but it is not the test of choice for diagnosis of this patient's primary problem.

An MRI of the brain (**choice C**) would likely reveal a pituitary mass. Around 90% of patient with acromegaly have a pituitary tumor. The diagnosis of acromegaly should be made serologically before the radiographic workup is initiated.

Random growth hormone levels (**choice D**) are not recommended since patients have a normal daily fluctuation of GNRH and growth hormone. Growth hormone levels can also fluctuate with exercise and acute illness. Therefore, normal patients can have a falsely elevated growth hormone level and an affected person can have a false normal growth hormone level.

This patient has features classically associated with acromegaly. A 24-hour cortisol (**choice E**) collection would help us in the diagnosis of Cushing syndrome. Cushing syndrome can be associated with insulin resistance and weight gain but does not share other features associated with acromegaly.

30. **The correct answer is C.** Based on the available data, this patient is likely having myocardial ischemia. It is always important to obtain an electrocardiogram in such an instance to evaluate whether the patient is having elevation of his ST segments, which would then mandate a trip to the catheterization laboratory for thrombolysis or angioplasty.

A chest radiograph (**choice A**) is unlikely to provide any useful information, especially in the setting of clear breath sounds bilaterally.

A chest CT (**choice B**) will not provide any useful information in this instance, especially given that the patient has clear breath sounds bilaterally.

A transesophageal echocardiogram (**choice D**) is not an appropriate first test in the diagnosis of myocardial ischemia.

A transthoracic echocardiogram (**choice E**) is not an appropriate first test in the diagnosis of myocardial ischemia.

31. **The correct answer is D.** The most important factor in the prognosis of any patient with melanoma is the thickness of the lesion as measured from an excisional biopsy. The thickness helps determine the appropriate treatment options as well as the long-term prognosis. For instance, in situ lesions (lesions confined to the epidermis) should have a 100% survival. Lesions less than 0.76 mm have approximately 96 to 98% survival over 5 years, whereas lesions 0.76 to 1.49 mm thick have an 86 to 90% survival rate over 5 years. Larger lesions 1.50 to 3.99 mm thick have a 66 to 70% 5-year survival rate and so on.

A family history (**choice A**), a history of blistering sunburns (**choice B**), and a history of chronic daily sun exposure (**choice C**) are all very important risk factors in developing melanoma but do not help predict the long-term prognosis of a patient with melanoma.

The different types or classifications of melanoma (**choice E**) cannot be compared in terms of prognosis. They are clinicohistologic types separating malignant melanoma into location, into racial preponderance, or into shape. These differences have nothing to do with overall prognosis.

32. **The correct answer is B.** In the presence of ongoing myocardial ischemia as presented above, it is important to anticoagulate patients in an effort to inhibit intracoronary clot formation and progressive ischemia. Aspirin provides an antiplatelet effect. Heparin is used to inhibit the clotting cascade.

Intravenous diltiazem (**choice A**), a calcium-channel antagonist, has no proven benefit in the treatment of myocardial ischemia not related to coronary vasospasm (Prinzmetal angina).

Intravenous metoprolol (**choice C**), a selective beta-1 antagonist, is not indicated since this patient has a reasonable blood pressure and excellent heart rate control.

Intravenous phenylephrine (**choice D**), an alpha-1 agonist used in the treatment of hypotension related to vasodilation, is not indicated here since the patient is not hypotensive.

33. **The correct answer is A.** One of the classic physical findings of constrictive pericarditis is an increase in jugular venous pressure with inspiration, Kussmaul sign. This is believed to be a result of increased right-sided pressure exerted by the noncompliant pericardium as the heart is moved inferiorly by the descending diaphragm during inspiration.

One would not expect to see jugular venous flattening (**choice C**) with constrictive pericarditis. Conversely, constrictive pericarditis is associated with poor right ventricular compliance, and hence, with an elevated jugular venous pressure.

Inspiratory stridor (**choice B**) is associated with an upper airway obstruction, which is not associated with constrictive pericarditis.

Muffled cardiac sounds (**choice D**) can be associated with pericarditis associated with a pericardial effusion. However, we are told that no effusion is present on echocardiography making this physical finding unlikely.

Tracheal deviation (**choice E**), which is a hallmark of conditions such as tension pneumothorax, is not associated with constrictive pericarditis.

34. **The correct answer is C.** The most appropriate diagnostic intervention at this time is to order liver function tests with amylase and lipase levels. This patient presented with the classic signs and symptoms of pancreatitis. This entity is very common on general surgical services and the presentation of the disease is actually quite varied. For this patient, her vomitus, abdominal pain, age, and recent history all suggest gallstones or gallstone pancreatitis. Therefore, a full set of liver function tests with amylase and lipase levels is indicated. One of the gravest errors that can be made in medical practice is that of "labeling." This patient has had multiple previous visits to the hospital with no diagnosis made.

An abdominal CT scan (**choice A**) may be indicated depending on the results of the screening chemistries.

HIDA scan (**choice B**) is a quick and effective method for determining whether a patient has gallstones or gallbladder disease. Again, very useful if the chemistries point toward the gallbladder as the etiology for this patient's pain.

The tendency is to ascribe her visits to some psychological issue rather than to medically evaluate her. Therefore, offering no diagnostic study (**choice D**) is incorrect.

If chemistries suggest a hepatic or cystic cause for the pain, right upper quadrant ultrasound (**choice E**) would be an excellent modality to evaluate the ducts and gallbladder.

35. **The correct answer is D.** The most appropriate management at this time is intravenous fluids and *nil per os* status. This patient has gallstone pancreatitis. Her amylase and lipase are elevated and an RUQ ultrasound

shows stones. The standard therapy for this entity is bowel rest, hydration, and pain control as needed

A continuous infusion of intravenous opioids (**choice A**) is not indicated since, although the patient will have pain, it can easily be controlled with an "on demand" or "as needed" method. Continuous opiate infusions promote bowel immotility and constipation.

A daily abdominal CT scan to evaluate for pancreatic necrosis (**choice B**) is not routinely done. At most institutions, a CT scan is obtained a few days after diagnosis to evaluate for a worsening phlegmon or necrosis

Intravenous antibiotics (**choice C**) are only indicated if there is evidence of pancreatic necrosis or the patient develops a fever after the diagnosis pancreatitis is made. There is a substantial amount of clinical literature validating this approach to treating pancreatitis.

Surgical debridement (**choice E**) is indicated in cases of very severe necrosis that is worsening or is suspected to be a focus for bacteremia and sepsis.

36. **The correct answer is B.** The most appropriate management at this time is to draw blood cultures and initiate ampicillin, gentamicin, and metronidazole therapy. Intravenous antibiotics are only indicated if there is evidence of pancreatic necrosis or if the patient develops a fever after the diagnosis of pancreatitis is made. There is a substantial amount of clinical literature validating this approach to treating pancreatitis. The appropriate sequence of events is to draw blood cultures prior to initiating therapy in order to maximize chances of detecting an organism.

Drawing blood cultures and awaiting results (**choice A**), although partially correct, fails to address the key issue of instituting some type of therapy. The same is true for drawing blood, urine, and sputum cultures (**choice C**). Sending lab tests is not the same as a therapeutic intervention and a patient with pancreatitis that spikes a temperature requires intervention.

Although obtaining an abdominal CT scan (**choice D**) is important and should be done to assess any necrosis or progression of the phlegmon, it should not come prior to initiating antibiotic therapy.

Starting ampicillin, gentamicin, and metronidazole therapy (**choice E**) without drawing blood cultures is inappropriate because it is important to determine what organisms are present.

37. **The correct answer is C.** Evidence of isolated right-sided heart failure (increased jugular venous pressure with clear lungs) in the setting of electrocardiographic evidence of inferior wall ischemia suggests right ventricular ischemia/infarction. One of the better ways to evaluate for this pathology is to obtain an electrocardiogram with right-sided leads and look for ST-segment elevation in V_4.

A cardiac stress test (**choice A**) should not be considered in a patient such as this with active ongoing myocardial ischemia.

A chest radiograph (**choice B**) will provide little diagnostic help in the setting of clear lungs in this instance.

A green dye cardiac output measurement (**choice D**) is a method of obtaining a cardiac output measurement without placing a Swan-Ganz catheter. However, given that one could predict that cardiac output is diminished based on the exam, it will be of minimal benefit in this instance. This measure is also unable to distinguish between isolated left and right ventricular failure.

A ventilation-perfusion scan (**choice E**) used in the diagnosis of pulmonary embolism is of no benefit in the diagnosis of myocardial ischemia.

38. **The correct answer is D.** HMG-CoA reductase inhibitors such as lovastatin used in the treatment of hyperlipidemia can be associated with liver dysfunction. Therefore, in the setting of unexplained elevation in AST and ALT suggesting liver toxicity, it is prudent to discontinue lovastatin while the precise etiology of the liver dysfunction is investigated further.

Since we are not told of any historical data or physical findings to suggest volume overload, adding a hydrochlorothiazide, a second diuretic, to this patient's medical regimen (**choice A**) is not warranted.

Despite the patient's occasional premature beats, lidocaine (**choice B**) is not warranted in this instance. It will also not help in the management of the patient's liver dysfunction. Further, one could argue that lidocaine should not be given to a patient with hepatic dysfunction since it is primarily metabolized in the liver.

Aspirin is not associated with liver toxicity. Therefore, discontinuing aspirin (**choice C**), as would be helpful in the setting of gastritis, will be of no benefit in this instance.

Given that the patient has a reasonable blood pressure and excellent heart rate control, an alteration in his atenolol regimen (**choice E**) is not warranted.

39. **The correct answer is D.** Pulsus paradoxus describes the phenomenon where the normal drop in systemic blood pressure with inspiration is exaggerated in the presence of a condition such as pericardial effusion, especially with tamponade physiology.

An Austin-Flint murmur (**choice A**) is a murmur best heard at the cardiac apex resulting from a regurgitant jet with aortic insufficiency. It is not associated with pericardial effusion or tamponade.

A mill wheel murmur (**choice B**), a murmur characteristic of air embolism, is not associated with pericardial effusion or tamponade.

A pericardial rub (**choice C**) is associated with pericarditis, which can be associated with a pericardial effusion. However, since this patient's effusion is acute and traumatic in nature, a pericardial rub will likely not be present.

Tracheal deviation (**choice E**) in the setting of a trauma victim is typically seen with a tension pneumothorax. However, in this instance we are told that the patient does not have any rib fractures, and are not given any other information to suggest the presence of this pathology.

40. **The correct answer is B.** Streptococcal antigen and guttate psoriasis is correct because this type of psoriasis usually occurs as an abrupt eruption following some acute infection, such as a streptococcal pharyngitis. It occurs mostly in patients under age 30. Recurrent episodes are likely. If penicillin or cephalosporin fail to eradicate it, rifampin should be tried.

Contact dermatitis due to new bed sheets (**choice A**) is unlikely because contact dermatitis usually appears as large plaques or patches of lichenified, erythematous, pruritic lesions with small amount of scales. In this case, since this patient was resting in bed, contact dermatitis would most likely involve her back or front, but not both sides equally.

Large doses of vitamin C and hypersensitivity reaction (**choice C**) is incorrect because vitamin C has not been reported to cause hypersensitivity reactions. In addition, hypersensitivity reactions tend to have systemic manifestations including fever, fatigue, lymphadenopathy, and hepatosplenomegaly.

Acetaminophen and multiple fixed drug eruptions (**choice D**) is incorrect because fixed drug eruption lesions tend to be violaceous, flat patches without scale.

Streptococcal antigen and pityriasis rosea (**choice E**) is incorrect because the etiology of pityriasis rosea has not been clarified. In addition, pityriasis rosea usually initiates with a large erythematous or dusky violaceous plaque with none or small amount of scale (herald patch). Pityriasis lesions tend not to be pruritic.

41. **The correct answer is E.** This patient has celiac sprue. This condition is more common than previously believed. It is a hypersensitivity to gluten, which is a protein found in wheat, barley, rye, and oats. The IgA antiendomysial antibody is a serological test with a specificity of 99% and sensitivity of about 85%. Small bowel biopsy would reveal blunting of villi and lymphocytic and plasma cell infiltrates. Patients typically respond to a gluten-free diet.

Tropical sprue is an infectious disease found in those patients who travel to tropical areas. Therapy includes antibiotics (**choice A**) and folic acid (**choice D**). This patient's lack of recent travel and positive antiendomysial antibody makes this diagnosis less likely.

Patients with chronic pancreatitis and cystic fibrosis can develop pancreatic insufficiency. This patient doesn't have a history of cystic fibrosis. Chronic pancreatitis is associated with pain. Since this patient's history is not consistent with either of these disorders, he would not benefit from pancreatic enzyme replacement (**choice B**).

Refractory cases of celiac sprue may respond to a course of prednisone (**choice C**). Steroids should be reserved for cases resistant to diet modification. Other inflammatory conditions causing diarrhea such as inflammatory bowel disease and eosinophilic gastroenteritis also respond to prednisone.

42. **The correct answer is B.** Notwithstanding that the patient has a right to deny treatment, quadriplegia by itself is not a terminal condition, nor is it a progressive malady. The state will therefore deny the patient's request.

The courts will not acquiesce to the plaintiff's request (**choice A**).

Discussing the matter with the family (**choice C**) is of no consequence, as the patient is an adult individual who has the mental ability to make a decision.

The courts cannot command health care personnel to deny food to the patient (**choice D**). Most physicians believe that intravenous fluids and tube feedings are interventions, and that withholding both or either has to be considered after pondering all the hazards and advantages. Families as a whole generally regard tube feeding to be part of basic care, and that it should not be withheld or discontinued, as it smacks of discrimination against the susceptible and impaired.

The courts do not resort to appointing committees (**choice E**) in these cases, as they rely on testimony from expert witnesses to fathom the patient's malady, treatment, and prognosis. Expert witnesses are physicians who have specialized knowledge and expertise that would subserve the court in resolving disputes.

43. **The correct answer is D.** Finding an asymptomatic elevation in liver enzymes, especially ALT, is very common. An isolated elevation in ALT, which is less than 3 to 5-fold greater than normal, does not require an extensive workup. Rather, repeat testing in 1 to 2 months is sufficient. Abstinence from alcohol or suspect medications should be recommended. Alternatively, if the elevation of ALT is greater than 3 to 5 times normal, if there are stigmata of chronic liver disease, or if there is bilirubin level or clotting time abnormalities, a complete work-up should be undertaken. Persistent elevations should be more completely evaluated because they may indicate undetected chronic liver disease.

An abdominal ultrasound (**choice A**) is indicated in those patients who have had a serological workup for the etiology of their liver test abnormalities and the etiology remains unclear. It is helpful in defining the architecture of the liver and identifying any space-occupying lesions that might account for the serological abnormalities. Ascites can be seen. Liver and spleen size is easily measured. Doppler flow studies can be performed with the ultrasound to evaluate the hepatic blood flow.

Serum antinuclear antibodies (**choice B**) are positive in autoimmune hepatitis (especially in type 1 disease). This is a condition characterized by extrahepatic autoimmune disease, female predominance, and positive ANA and anti-smooth muscle antibody. Classic appearance of spider nevi, hepatomegaly, cutaneous striae, acne, and hirsutism suggests the diagnosis. Patients often present jaundiced although about 20% can have normal skin color.

Liver biopsy (**choice C**) can be helpful in the evaluation of liver disease but the decision of when to biopsy is not always clear. Certainly, a patient who has persistent liver function test abnormalities and no clear diagnosis by serology or history needs to have a biopsy to make a diagnosis. Liver biopsy is also helpful in determining the amount of damage that the liver has already suffered which can be important in the decision.

44. **The correct answer is C.** This patient likely has a pulmonary embolus (PE) as evidenced by the proximity to high-risk surgery, tachypnea, tachycardia, and hypoxemia. The chest x-ray is not the test of choice to diagnose PE. A CT scan or a V/Q scan are the most appropriate tests to order. A normal chest x-ray in this setting is helpful in the diagnosis of PE in that it helps exclude other causes of acute hypoxia and pleuritic chest pain such as pneumothorax and rib fracture.

About 10% of pulmonary emboli result in infarction. Infarction, and subsequent intraparenchymal hemorrhage, may result in a lateral opacity known as a Hampton hump (**choice A**). This is not a common finding on chest x-ray after a pulmonary embolus.

A lobar consolidation (**choice B**) would classically be associated with pneumonia. This patient has shortness of breath and pleuritic chest pain, but lacks fevers and productive cough. She also reports acute onset of these symptoms, which is not consistent with pneumonia.

Signs of diminished lung volume may be present on the affected side of a patient with a pulmonary embolus. Elevation of the hemidiaphragm (**choice D**) and linear or patchy atelectasis can all be signs of volume loss.

Prominence of the central pulmonary artery with local oligemia is a rare finding with pulmonary embolus. This finding is known as Westermark sign (**choice E**).

45. **The correct answer is E.** Pamphlets and education about melanoma is correct. About 1 in 72 Americans will develop a melanoma. It occurs most often in light-complexion people. Other etiologies include light eyes, blond or red hair, occurrence of blistering sunburns in childhood, heavy freckling, and tendency to tan poorly and sunburn easily. In addition, the incidence of melanoma increases in first-degree relative.

Clean bill of health (**choice A**), sunscreen and avoidance of sun (**choice B**), UV protecting clothing (**choice C**), and chemical peels (**choice D**) are all good advice for this young female patient; however, they are not the most important recommendation in this setting of new melanoma diagnosed in the patient's mother.

46. **The correct answer is C.** This patient has pneumonia, which is covered by ceftriaxone for streptococcal pneumonia (community acquired) and azithromycin for atypical pneumonia coverage. She also has a history of mental retardation, seizure disorder, and cerebral palsy, which places her at an increased risk of aspiration pneumonia. She also probably has an aspiration pneumonia in view of the right-sided lower lobe infiltrate.

For aspiration pneumonia she would need good *anaerobic* coverage for organisms originating in the mouth and the best antibiotic choice here is clindamycin.

Cefpodoxime (**choice A**) is a third-generation cephalosporin that has no anaerobic coverage and only comes in the oral form, which would counteract any aspiration precautions you begin.

Ciprofloxacin (**choice B**) is a fluoroquinolone that has gram-negative coverage, which ceftriaxone is already covering. But it has no anaerobic coverage.

Nafcillin (**choice D**) is an antistaphylococcal penicillin and ceftriaxone already has gram-positive coverage.

Vancomycin (**choice E**) should be held off until the sputum Gram stain shows gram-positive cocci in cluster formation consistent with methicillin-resistant *Staphylococcal aureus* infection (MRSA) which currently has no coverage.

47. **The correct answer is E.** This patient has reversible airway disease, which is evident in the spirometry test as an improvement in FVC (forced vital capacity) from 22% predicted to 51% predicted after albuterol treatment. Greater than 50% improvement is suggestive of reversible airway disease. The nighttime cough is also suggestive of asthma. There is also an underlying acute bronchitis secondary to a recent viral infection. This is improving in view of the reduction in sputum production. The best management would be to prescribe albuterol and observe that she can use the metered-dose inhaler effectively, using a spacer if necessary.

An antitussive agent for the cough alone (**choice A**) may treat the coughing symptoms but not the cause of these symptoms.

Simply prescribing albuterol as a metered-dose inhaler and discharging the patient without observing her inhaler technique (**choice B**) means that the patient could have poor technique at home. This rarely results in any symptomatic improvement and lends itself to poor compliance by the patient.

Taking the patient's temperature is important. In adults with acute bronchitis, antibiotics are not indicated unless there is an active pneumonia. She is afebrile today and denies any fevers in the past, and so an antibiotic such as clarithromycin (**choices C and D**) is not indicated at this time.

48. **The correct answer is A.** The patient was hospitalized for an uncomplicated pyelonephritis most likely due to *E. coli* and was started on an intravenous course of ciprofloxacin. She then became hypotensive on the ward. A cardiogenic origin of the hypotension is unlikely because of the unchanged electrocardiograms. Prompt imaging is now required to ensure absence of an obstructive uropathy. The best choice to delineate abdominal soft tissue would be a CT scan of the abdomen as opposed to a portable abdominal x-ray (**choice C**).

An MRI (**choice B**) is contraindicated because of her total knee replacement. In any case, an MRI of the brain is likely to be normal in view of the recently normal head CT. Additionally, at this stage the abdomen can be imaged adequately by a CT scan rather than an MRI, thereby reducing the degree of irradiation exposure.

A chest x-ray (**choice D**) would not affect your management of the hypotension unless there was an underlying pneumonia. This is unlikely in view of the recently normal chest x-ray in the emergency department and the normal breath sounds throughout her hospital stay.

A retrograde micturating cystourethrogram (**choice E**) is inappropriate here because it is normally used to investigate the presence of retrograde urinary reflux during micturition.

49. **The correct answer is D.** This patient is at high risk of developing osteoporosis and at an increased risk of fractures. Her risk factors for osteoporosis include her Asian race, age greater than 55 years (most likely postmenopausal), her smoking history, the L-thyroxine medication, and now the start of possible long-term steroid therapy (since long-term steroid therapy inhibits bone cell growth and decreases concentrations of calcium and vitamin D). The best nutritional advice would be for her to begin calcium and vitamin D to offset the risk of osteoporosis.

Avoiding tea and coffee (**choice A**) is a less aggressive maneuver in reducing osteoporosis. Caffeine studies found that greater than 2 cups/day increased the risk of hip fracture, while 1 cup/day did not. Another study on tea found that older women who drank tea had a higher bone mineral density.

Fish and animal protein (**choice B**) have high acid and phosphorus loads. Bone responds to acid by releasing calcium to buffer the acid breakdown products of protein. Demineralization of bone increases the risk of osteoporosis.

Good hydration (**choice C**) is good advice regardless of the circumstances, but is not aggressive enough in osteoporosis prevention.

Since there is no indication of iron deficiency anemia, ferrous sulfate supplementation (**choice E**) is not indicated.

50. **The correct answer is A.** This patient has rhabdomyolysis secondary to crack cocaine abuse. Rhabdomyolysis is an entity that is caused by multiple and diverse factors. It is commonly seen after crack cocaine binges. This is complicated by acute renal failure secondary to the nephrotoxic effects of myoglobin. IV hydration is the mainstay of treatment with alkalinization of the urine using $NaHCO_3$ in the hope of keeping myoglobin in solution.

    In the setting of acute renal failure, IV hydration alone (**choice B**) is not sufficient and should be accompanied by alkalinization of the urine.

    The presence of blood in the urine with no RBCs is typical of myoglobinuria rather than kidney stones, which would possibly show a sediment. Therefore, a CT abdomen looking for stones is not justified (**choice C**).

    Urine culture and antibiotics (**choice D**) are only indicated in the setting of a urinary tract infection, which is not suspected in this clinical setting.

    Similarly, abdominal x-ray films (**choice E**) would not reveal any finding. They might be appropriate in the setting of kidney stones, which typically present with flank pain.

Internal Medicine: **Test Two**

1. A 33-year-old man is brought to the emergency department complaining of "sharp" and "stabbing" chest pain that radiates from his sternum to between his shoulder blades. He describes one episode of fainting following the onset of this pain. He has Marfan syndrome with a known dilation of the aortic root, and hypertension. He is on no medications and denies any allergies to medications. His blood pressure is 178/87 mm Hg in his right arm, 99/67 mm Hg in his left arm, and his pulse is 99/min. Physical examination shows a regular cardiac rhythm with a I/IV diastolic murmur at the lower left sternal border. His breath sounds are clear bilaterally. An echocardiogram shows a dissection of the thoracic aorta with the dissection flap involving the left subclavian artery. The most appropriate immediate intervention is to administer

   (A) aspirin
   (B) heparin
   (C) labetalol
   (D) phenylephrine
   (E) sodium nitroprusside

2. A 19 year-old man comes to the student health center as a walk-in patient and is assigned to a female colleague of yours but requests to be seen by a male physician because of a "very sensitive problem." He says that something appeared on "his private area" about 4 to 6 weeks ago and it may be genital warts. He has no past medical history and does not take any medications. He has recently become sexually active with a single partner and has regularly used condoms as birth control. He is very upset that this has happened just as he started his sexual activities and wonders if he could have "caught it" from his girlfriend. You inspect his genital area and note that he is not circumcised. On the entire circumference of the coronal sulcus of his penis there are multiple, asymptomatic, firm, white, dome-shaped papules. Each one is less than 1 mm in diameter. It is appropriate to advise the patient that:

   (A) He has allergic contact dermatitis from the condoms and should change to a nonallergenic brand.
   (B) He has a *Candida* infection and he should be treated with nystatin cream.
   (C) He has genital warts and he should be treated with liquid nitrogen.
   (D) He has irritant contact dermatitis secondary to retention of smegma in the coronal sulcus and he should be circumcised.
   (E) This is a normal finding and no treatment is indicated.

3. A 32-year-old African American woman comes to the clinic for a preemployment physical examination. She has no complaints. Her medical records reveal that 6 months ago she had an episode of erythema nodosum that resolved uneventfully with a week of bed rest and nonsteroidal antiinflammatory drugs. At the time, her chest x-ray revealed bilateral hilar lymphadenopathy. An electrocardiogram, ophthalmologic examination, liver function tests, serum calcium, and 24-hour urine calcium determination were all within normal limits. You repeat the chest x-ray and find that the bilateral hilar lymphadenopathy is unchanged. Routine laboratory studies are normal and she has no physical symptoms of disease. At this time the most appropriate treatment for this patient is

(A) ibuprofen 400 mg PO every 6 hours for 6 to 8 weeks
(B) intravenous prednisone 1 mg/kg/day for 10 days, followed by oral prednisone for 4 to 6 weeks
(C) methotrexate 15 mg weekly for 6 to 8 weeks
(D) no treatment is indicated at this time
(E) oral prednisone 40 mg a day for 6 to 8 weeks

4. A 38-year-old Japanese woman comes to the office complaining of a dark patch on her face that has been getting darker in recent years. She initially started getting small dark spots in that area when she was a teenager, and by her early 30s, it had covered the greater part of her left eyelids and cheek. It is no longer growing in size, but has become a few shades darker since, and a similar patch appeared on the white of her left eye about 5 years ago. The lesion is not symptomatic. Her mother told her that similar spots were occasionally encountered in her countrymen but she has not noticed them as much since she has immigrated to the United States. On inspection, you note confluent bluish gray macules extending from the left upper eyelid to the left midcheek with dark blue pigmentation of the lateral left sclera. Malignancies reported to occur in association with this lesion are

(A) melanoma of the skin and the eye
(B) melanoma of the skin, eye, and brain
(C) melanoma of the skin only
(D) melanoma and nonmelanoma skin cancers
(E) predominantly nonmelanoma skin cancers, although melanoma can also occur

5. A 63-year-old obese woman with diabetes mellitus and asthma is admitted to the intensive care unit with fever and respiratory failure. She was just discharged from the hospital 3 days earlier when she had been admitted for a severe exacerbation of asthma precipitated by an upper respiratory tract infection. Today, a chest x-ray shows pulmonary edema and signs of parenchymal consolidation. On admission, you note a large erythematous patch on her lower abdomen. Within 24 hours hemorrhagic bullae develop and progress to form large necrotic ulcerations with yellow-green purulent exudate covering the base, and undermined borders. Laboratory studies show

Erythrocyte sedimentation rate	110 mm/h
Leukocytes	4800/mm^3
Neutrophils	70%
Bands	15%
Lymphocytes	5%
Eosinophils	2%
Monocytes	7%

Blood cultures: Gram stain shows many gram-negative rods (preliminary)

Based on the clinical appearance and laboratory results the most appropriate initial treatment is

(A) intravenous antibiotics and surgical debridement
(B) intravenous antibiotics only
(C) oral antibiotics and surgical debridement
(D) oral antibiotics only
(E) surgical debridement only

6. A 23-year-old woman comes to the urgent care clinic for the evaluation of a "rapid heart beat." She describes two prior episodes of this heart rhythm. She has no prior medical history, and is on no medications. She denies any allergies to any medications. Her temperature is 37.2 C (99.0 F), blood pressure is 112/67 mm Hg, pulse is 131/min, and respirations are 25/min. Her cardiac rhythm is regular and her breath sounds are clear to auscultation bilaterally. An electrocardiogram shows a paroxysmal, supraventricular tachycardia (PSVT). The most appropriate management at this time is

(A) administration of intravenous heparin
(B) administration of a loading dose of digoxin
(C) carotid massage
(D) immediate cardioversion

7. You get a phone call in the morning from one of your patients with complaints of a fever and generalized malaise. The patient is a 26-year-old woman you saw 3 weeks ago with complaints of dysuria. A urine culture grew >100,000 CFU of *E. coli* which was sensitive to the antibiotic that you prescribed for her. The dysuria resolved, but she has had a fever with shaking chills for the past 24 hours and is wondering if she still has the infection. Her past medical history is significant for a prolonged hospitalization during childhood following a motor vehicle accident during which she fractured her femur and sustained a splenic laceration that required splenectomy. She is otherwise healthy. Her fevers have been as high as 40.0 C (104.0 F). She denies any rash, headache, ear pain, neck stiffness, cough, shortness of breath, sore throat, runny nose, abdominal pain, vaginal discharge, nausea, vomiting, diarrhea, dysuria, hematuria, or urinary frequency. She is visiting her sister who lives 3 hours away in the same state, and asks you what she should do. You advise her to

(A) come to your office that evening so you can examine her and thus guide her treatment better
(B) drink plenty of fluids and take acetaminophen as needed for fever; she likely has a viral syndrome and her symptoms should resolve in the next few days
(C) find the name of a local pharmacy and you will call in an antibiotic with broader coverage for her likely recurrent urinary tract infection
(D) seek medical attention at the nearest acute care facility so they can do another urine culture
(E) seek medical attention immediately at the nearest hospital

8. A 35-year-old homeless man comes to the emergency department because of a 3-week history of fatigue, malaise, and difficulty in breathing. He also reports a nonproductive cough with occasional vomiting and decreased appetite. The patient denies any weight loss or night sweats, but did notice being "quite warm" lately. He tells you that he was diagnosed with AIDS 2 years ago and his last CD4 cell count was done 2 months ago and was 150/mm^3. He takes no medications and admits to occasional alcohol and cocaine use. His temperature is 37.6 C (100.0 F), blood pressure is 130/70 mm Hg, pulse is 105/min, and respirations are 30/min. His pulse oximetry saturation is 92% on room air. On examination, the patient appears to be in respiratory distress with coarse breath sounds over both lung fields. A chest x-ray shows bilateral diffuse interstitial infiltrates. His arterial blood gas on room air had a pH of 7.35, a PaO_2 of 65 mm Hg and a $PaCO_2$ of 30 mm Hg. The most appropriate next step in the management is to

(A) admit him to the hospital for therapy with intravenous azithromycin
(B) admit him to the hospital for therapy with intravenous steroids if the lactate dehydrogenase is greater than 500 U/L
(C) admit him to the hospital for therapy with intravenous trimethoprim-sulfamethoxazole
(D) admit him to the hospital for therapy with intravenous trimethoprim-sulfamethoxazole and prednisone
(E) discharge him with a daily dose of oral trimethoprim-sulfamethoxazole and follow up within the next 72 hours

9. A 45-year-old African American man comes to the office because of pruritic papules on his penis for over 1 month. The patient describes himself as a "typical male who sleeps around" but states he always wears a condom and denies ever having genital warts before. He also vehemently denies giving or receiving oral sex and cannot imagine how he got the "white spots" in his mouth or on his penis for that matter. He has no other medical problems to date. Physical examination shows multiple papules on his penis, white lacy streaks on his buccal mucosa, and papules on his wrists and shins. After performing a skin biopsy, the most appropriate next diagnostic study to order is

(A) ANA
(B) a complete blood count
(C) a hepatitis panel
(D) an HIV test
(E) a viral load

10. A 28-year-old man comes to the clinic with questions about exposure to sexually transmitted diseases. One of his previous partners contacted him with information that she had tested positive for chlamydia. She is one of his three sexual partners in the past 6 months. He is wondering if he should be treated. He has no symptoms. As part of the appropriate management you should

(A) prescribe ceftriaxone intramuscularly
(B) prescribe ciprofloxacin orally
(C) prescribe metronidazole orally
(D) recommend that he get HIV testing and the hepatitis B immunization series
(E) tell him that no treatment is indicated because he is asymptomatic and he does not need to tell his other partners

Items 11-12

A 48-year-old obese woman comes to the emergency department because of painful swelling of the left ankle. She says that the pain came on suddenly and was so severe that it woke her from sleep. She cannot recall injuring it or changing anything in her bedtime routine, which includes having a glass of wine, removing her make-up, and settling down with a "trashy" book. She is generally healthy, except for an episode of cholelithiasis last year and nephrolithiasis 6 months ago. Her last menstrual period was 2 years ago and she says that she is in a monogamous sexual relationship. Her temperature is 39.5 C (103.1 F), blood pressure is 130/90 mm Hg, and pulse is 82/min. Her left ankle is warm, tender, and swollen. The skin overlying the joint is erythematous, tense, and shiny. She is unable to bear weight on her left foot.

11. The procedure/study most likely to establish the underlying cause of the joint pain is

(A) arthrocentesis and joint fluid examination under a polarizing microscope
(B) arthrocentesis and PCR of the joint fluid
(C) cervical, pharyngeal, and rectal cultures
(D) a technetium radionuclide bone scan
(E) an x-ray of the ankle

12. The finding that would best indicate that indomethacin is the appropriate treatment is

(A) diffuse increase in technetium uptake around the ankle on the bone scan
(B) a fracture of the fibula and a displaced fracture of the medial malleolus
(C) intracellular gram-negative diplococci in the cervical, pharyngeal, and rectal cultures
(D) negatively birefringent crystals under a polarizing microscope
(E) spirochetal DNA by PCR

13. A 45-year-old man was diagnosed with the human immunodeficiency virus 2 years ago upon routine screening for a life insurance plan. He has had no treatment thus far because he feels "perfectly healthy all the time." Today, however, he is complaining of a 1-day history of a painful rash on his back and down the length of his left leg. He admits to being fearful of having Kaposi sarcoma since he saw the popular movie years ago where a famous actor develops Kaposi sarcoma and thinks "it's the stigma of AIDS." He says he will do anything to make the rash disappear even if it means taking numerous pills everyday. On inspection, the rash is made up of grouped vesicles on an erythematous base, crusted papules, and eroded areas scattered over his left sacrum and left leg. He states he was recently very "stressed out" at work but denies any recent illnesses or other medical problems. At this time the most correct statement about his condition is:

(A) This patient has herpes zoster and requires oral acyclovir for 7 to 10 days.

(B) This patient has herpes zoster and requires topical acyclovir applied every 2 hours during waking hours for the next 7 to 10 days.

(C) This patient has Kaposi sarcoma and needs to be referred to a dermatologist for a biopsy and further treatment options.

(D) This patient has Kaposi sarcoma (KS) and needs to be tested for HHV-8 (human herpes virus 8), the culprit of KS, to confirm the diagnosis.

(E) This patient has Kaposi sarcoma, which shows a poor prognosis in untreated HIV-positive patients. This patient needs to be referred to an infectious disease specialist to start appropriate therapy for his HIV.

14. A 42-year-old man is brought into the emergency department after a sudden fall that occurred when he was jogging. He was reported to have lost consciousness and sustained an injury to his forehead. He is adamant that he had no prodromal symptoms and that he did not trip. He does mention occasionally feeling short of breath but has never felt lightheaded before. It was confirmed from an eyewitness that there was no seizure activity and that he had lost consciousness for less than a couple of minutes. He has a history of a "murmur" that he routinely takes antibiotics for when he visits his dentist. He is on no medications. His blood pressure is 110/58 mm Hg and he has a slowly rising pulse. The point of maximal impulse, although not displaced, has a heaving quality to it. The aortic component of the second heart sound appears to be diminished. There is an ejection click and a rasping ejection systolic murmur heard over the right second intercostal space. The cardiac valvular lesion responsible for this patient's condition is

(A) aortic stenosis

(B) mitral regurgitation

(C) mitral stenosis

(D) pulmonic stenosis

(E) ventricular septal defect

15. A 45-year-old man is admitted to the hospital with altered mental status. The patient carries a diagnosis of multiple myeloma and has been undergoing therapy at the local hospital. The patient is otherwise healthy and was diagnosed 3 months ago with his disease. His family reports that they found him in the kitchen confused and wandering around with a spoon in his hand. On examination, the patient is disheveled but in no acute distress. His blood pressure is 140/90 mm Hg, pulse is 100/min, and respirations are 18/min. He is afebrile. Physical examination is remarkable for brisk deep tendon reflexes bilaterally. The diagnosis of hypercalcemia is made. It is determined that the patient will require long-term management of this problem. However, he now requires acute therapy. The most appropriate next step in management is to

(A) administer bisphosphonate therapy, orally

(B) administer calcitonin therapy, intravenously

(C) administer corticosteroid therapy, intravenously

(D) administer saline, intravenously, and then furosemide

(E) begin hemodialysis

16. For the past year you have been treating a 55-year-old man for hypertension and have provided a program to help the patient lose weight. He has followed the weight loss program for the past few months and has managed to lose just over 10 pounds. During a follow-up visit, his weight has increased by 5 pounds after this initial success. When questioned about the weight gain, the patient reports that he is going through a "messy divorce" and has, consequently, been eating more than he should. You encourage him to continue with his weight loss program and offer to provide additional counseling to deal with the stress of the divorce. One month later, you receive a subpoena asking you to appear at the local county courthouse to testify about the patient's medical condition as a part of the divorce proceedings. The patient's health will be used to estimate life expectancy and to fix alimony payments based on projected earnings. At this point you should

(A) appear at the courthouse at the scheduled time, but only to read a prepared statement about the importance of the physician-patient relationship
(B) appear at the courthouse at the scheduled time, but refuse to answer any questions about the patient
(C) appear at the courthouse at the scheduled time, answer any general questions about the patient, but refuse to answer questions about the patient's health
(D) appear at the courthouse at the scheduled time, but refuse to answer any questions asked by the court
(E) appear at the courthouse at the scheduled time, answer any questions asked using "Yes" or "No" responses, but do not volunteer any information about the patient
(F) contact the American Medical Association's Department of Ethics to obtain guidance on the prevailing legal standards
(G) ignore the subpoena
(H) contact the patient and discuss his willingness to have you testify
(I) notify the court that you will not appear to testify

17. You are called to the emergency department to admit a 25-year-old with insulin-dependent diabetes mellitus because of diabetic ketoacidosis. His vital signs are: temperature 37.0 C (98.6 F), blood pressure 110/65 mm Hg, pulse 98/min, and oxygen saturation 97%. He appears dehydrated. The rest of his examination is normal. Laboratory studies show

Sodium	129 mEq/L
Potassium	4.5 mEq/L
Chloride	98 mEq/L
Bicarbonate	16 mEq/L
BUN	30 mg/dL
Creatinine	1.2 mg/dL
Glucose	900 mg/dL
Anion gap	20

The physician in the emergency department tells you that the patient is on insulin drip and she is going to start hypertonic (3%) saline to treat the patient's hyponatremia. Regarding the management of this patient's sodium level, you should tell the emergency room physician that

(A) demeclocycline should be administered
(B) hypertonic saline is appropriate
(C) no treatment is needed, as the patient is asymptomatic
(D) no treatment is needed, as the sodium level is normal
(E) restriction of fluid intake will correct the sodium level

18. A 28-year-old woman comes to the office for a pre-employment physical examination. She is healthy and has no medical problems. She does not smoke or drink alcohol. Physical examination and routine laboratory studies are normal. A PPD is placed and 2 days later shows a 16-mm induration. The patient was never tested with PPD before and does not recall being exposed to tuberculosis. A chest x-ray shows no abnormalities. At this time the most appropriate management is to

(A) admit the patient to the hospital and put her in respiratory isolation
(B) explain that no treatment is indicated, as she does not have tuberculosis
(C) obtain sputum specimens for AFB stain and culture
(D) start isoniazid daily for 9 months
(E) start isoniazid, rifampin, and pyrazinamide daily for 9 to 12 months

19. A 29-year-old woman comes to the emergency department complaining of right calf pain for 2 days with swelling and redness. Her temperature is 38.5 C (101.3 F), blood pressure is 150/90 mm Hg, and pulse is 97/min. The right calf is swollen and tender. Homans sign is positive. The rest of her physical examination is normal. Doppler of the lower extremity shows a deep venous thrombosis above the knee. You begin therapy with intravenous heparin and admit her to the hospital. Three days later her laboratory studies show a protein S deficiency. The most appropriate management at this time is to

(A) discharge the patient on aspirin
(B) discharge the patient on dipyridamole
(C) start warfarin, and once INR is therapeutic, discharge the patient on warfarin for 3 to 6 months
(D) start warfarin, and once INR is therapeutic, discharge the patient on warfarin for 1 year
(E) start warfarin, and once INR is therapeutic, discharge the patient on warfarin for life

20. A 47-year-old woman with no past medical history comes to the clinic because of fatigue and loss of energy for the past few months. She also complains of polydipsia and polyuria. Her physical examination is normal. A random plasma glucose level is 237 mg/dL. The most appropriate next step to confirm the diagnosis of diabetes mellitus in this patient is to

(A) order a fasting plasma glucose
(B) order a fasting plasma insulin and fasting plasma glucose
(C) order a glucose tolerance test
(D) order hemoglobin A_{1C}
(E) repeat the random plasma glucose

21. A 66-year-old heavy smoker with diabetes mellitus is admitted to the hospital for new-onset chest pain. A myocardial infarction is ruled out and he is ready for discharge the following morning. While taking a shower he notices a worsening of a groin rash he has had for a few weeks. He tells you that it usually itchy but never painful. On examination you find a macerated, red, slightly scaly rash on the inside of the thighs that is sparing the testicles. The borders of the large plaques are slightly raised but there are no vesicles or satellite lesions. At this time the most correct statement about his condition is:

(A) His age most likely caused this candidal infection since it only occurs in postpubertal male patients.
(B) His diabetes mellitus most likely caused this fungal infection or tinea cruris; it is best treated with antifungal creams with activity against *Candida* species as well as dermatophytes.
(C) His diabetes mellitus most likely caused this fungal infection or tinea cruris; it is best treated with antifungal creams with activity against dermatophytes only.
(D) His smoking habit most likely caused this bacterial infection since smokers are prone to bacterial infections; it is best treated with topical antibiotics for 5 to 7 days.
(E) His smoking habit most likely caused this fungal infection since smokers are prone to them; it is best treated with topical steroid to calm down the inflammation and pruritus.

22. A 71-year-old man with diabetes mellitus and recurrent episodes of dizziness over the past few months is brought to the emergency department after a syncopal episode. He said that he felt lightheaded and nauseated before he fainted; however, he denies any chest pain or shortness of breath. This episode is similar to his previous episodes of dizziness except that he "fainted" this time. His only medication is metformin. There is no evidence of myocardial infarction at this point. While the patient is still in the emergency department he complains of another episode of dizziness, you check a rhythm strip which shows absent QRS complexes every fourth beat. The PR interval is consistent from beat to beat. P waves are present at regular intervals. The episode resolves spontaneously. The most appropriate next step in management is to

(A) administer atropine, intravenously
(B) administer isoproterenol, intravenously
(C) insert a permanent pacemaker
(D) insert a temporary pacemaker
(E) observe as no further treatment is indicated at this time

23. A 76-year-old man with metastatic prostate carcinoma comes to the emergency department complaining of generalized weakness and fatigue for the past few weeks. His temperature is 37.0 C (98.6 F), blood pressure is 100/60 mm Hg, and pulse is 90/min. He appears pale and cachectic and has scattered petechiae on his lower extremities. Examination of the chest and abdomen is normal. Stool guaiac is strongly positive. The rest of his physical examination, including a neurologic examination, is normal.

Laboratory studies show

Leukocyte count	$3000/mm^3$
Hemoglobin	7.3 g/dL
Hematocrit	22%
Platelet count	$20,000/mm^3$
Prothrombin time	12.6 sec
INR	1.1
Partial thromboplastin time	29.5 sec
Fibrinogen	350 mg/dL

You order 2 units of blood to be transfused. The most appropriate next step in management is to

(A) do not transfuse platelets as this patient's platelet count is >20,000
(B) give cryoprecipitate
(C) give DDAVP
(D) transfuse 4 units of fresh-frozen plasma
(E) transfuse 4 units of platelets

24. A 71-year-old man with hypertension, diabetes mellitus, and osteoarthritis comes to the emergency department with left knee pain and swelling, redness and limitation of movement, fever, chills, nausea, and vomiting for the past few days. He denies any history of trauma to the knee. He takes metformin, lisinopril, and allopurinol. His temperature is 38.8 C (101.8 F), blood pressure is 180/100 mm Hg, and pulse is 94/min. The left knee is swollen, tender, and red with effusion and limitation of movement. The rest of his physical examination is normal. An x-ray of the left knee shows osteoarthritic changes. Laboratory studies show

Leukocyte count	18,000/mm^3
Hemoglobin	12 g/dL
Hematocrit	36.2%
Platelets	230,000/mm^3

The most appropriate next step in management is to

(A) check his uric acid level
(B) do knee joint arthrocentesis
(C) reassure the patient that this is most likely a flare-up of his osteoarthritis and discharge him on pain medications
(D) start intravenous antibiotics
(E) start intravenous colchicine

25. A 72-year-old African American woman comes to the office on a winter morning complaining of dry, itchy skin for several months. She denies taking any new medication and continues to use the same personal hygiene products and detergents as before. She has diet-controlled diabetes, hypertension, and chronic right-hip pain for which she takes nonsteroidal anti-inflammatory drugs and gets physical (hydro) therapy 2 to 3 times a week. Her current medications are valsartan ibuprofen and a daily multivitamin. You examine her skin and notice that her upper body is fine. The skin is smooth with good shine and appropriate turgor. On the other hand, the skin below her waist is dry, ashy, and with fine cracks that are erythematous and have a "crazy pavement" pattern on the anterior shins. In addition to regular use of a moisturizing emollient, to prevent this condition from recurring you should advise her

(A) that it will go away without treatment once the weather gets warmer
(B) to change her brand of detergent
(C) to discontinue the ibuprofen
(D) to discontinue the valsartan
(E) to discontinue the physical (hydro) therapy

26. A 35-year-old woman comes to your office complaining of foul-smelling discharge from a toe on her foot. She had multiple ingrown toenails as a teenager and finally had partial destruction of the nail matrix on the left big toe done at age 20. Six months ago she noticed tenderness of the skin surrounding the toenail but it resolved without treatment. About a month ago, the tenderness reappeared, and soon thick, yellow discharge started draining from one edge of the nail. She has no other medical problems and is not on any medication. She denies allergies to medications. On physical examination, the nail of the first left toe is thin, dystrophic, and with multiple horizontal ridges. The posteromedial perionychium is erythematous and edematous. On pressure, a drop of yellow purulent discharge emerges from beneath the proximal cuticle. You suggest radiographic and imaging studies to rule out osteomyelitis. An x-ray of the foot shows a 1-cm sclerotic erosion of the left first distal phalanx and two small pieces of sequestered bone in the adjacent soft tissue. Gadolinium-enhanced magnetic resonance imaging shows increased uptake in the area of the bone erosion with a normal distal interphalangeal joint. The most appropriate initial treatment for this patient is

(A) amputation of the distal phalanx
(B) intravenous antibiotics
(C) intravenous antibiotics and surgical debridement of the bone
(D) oral antibiotics
(E) oral antibiotics and surgical debridement of the bone

27. A 33-year-old man from the local meatpacking factory comes to the emergency department with a painful skin infection that started the prior day. He had cut his right thumb with a butcher's knife several days earlier and started having chills and a fever the prior morning. He also noticed that his right thumb had become tender, swollen, and red. He has no other medical problems and his only medication is a daily multivitamin. On examination, this is a towering 6-foot tall man of 200 pounds in mild distress. He has a temperature of 38.0 C (100.4 F) and pulse of 100/min. On his right thumb there is a 2-cm linear laceration covered by serohemorrhagic crust. Surrounding it are confluent bright red, tender plaques with a shiny, glistening surface. There is no regional lymphadenopathy. Leukocyte count is 10,000/mm^3 with a marked left shift. The most appropriate treatment for this patient is

(A) intralesional triamcinolone acetonide 5 mg/mL monthly for 3 months
(B) local surgical debridement
(C) penicillin 500 mg PO qid for 7 to 10 days
(D) terbinafine 250 mg PO qd for 3 months
(E) topical Neosporin ointment

28. A 25-year-old man with exercise-induced asthma comes to the emergency department with shortness of breath after a basketball game. His temperature is 37.0 C (98.6 F), blood pressure is 110/60 mm Hg, pulse is 96/min, respirations are 24/min, and oxygen saturation is 94% on room air. He is in mild respiratory distress. Auscultation of the chest reveals diffuse wheezing. The most appropriate next step is to provide

(A) inhaled albuterol
(B) inhaled beclomethasone
(C) inhaled cromolyn sodium
(D) intravenous aminophylline
(E) intravenous methylprednisolone

29. A 35-year-old woman comes to the emergency department with epigastric pain radiating to the back and vomiting. She has no significant medical history, takes no medications, and occasionally has a glass of wine. Her vital signs are: temperature 38.0 C (100.4 F), blood pressure is 118/74 mm Hg, and pulse is 104/min. There is an absence of bowel sounds and there is severe epigastric tenderness with voluntary guarding. An upright chest radiograph is normal. Laboratory studies show

Leukocyte count	14,000/µL
Amylase	2482 U/L
Lipase	18,756 U/L
Alkaline phosphatase	189 U/L
Aspartate aminotransferase (AST)	88 U/L

The most appropriate diagnostic study at this time is

(A) abdominal computed tomography
(B) abdominal ultrasonography
(C) endoscopic retrograde cholangiopancreatography (ERCP)
(D) oral cholecystography
(E) upright and supine abdominal radiographs

30. A 58-year-old woman comes to the office for a routine visit. She has a history significant for depression and migraine headaches. She was also recently diagnosed with hyperthyroidism. She is now complaining of a "racing heart," increased sweating, and anxiety. Her current medications include amitriptyline and acetaminophen as needed. She has no allergies to medications. She appears anxious. Her temperature is 37. 0 C (98.6 F), blood pressure is 112/67 mm Hg, pulse is 105/min, and respirations are 25/min. Her cardiac rhythm is regular, and her lungs are clear to auscultation bilaterally. The most appropriate pharmacologic intervention at this time is to

(A) start the patient on ketoconazole
(B) start the patient on nitroglycerin
(C) start the patient on nitroprusside
(D) start the patient on propylthiouracil
(E) start the patient on spironolactone

31. A 27-year-old military recruit comes to the clinic with a 3-day history of a nonproductive cough, sore throat, fever, and myalgias. His temperature is 38.5 C (101.3 F), blood pressure is 120/70 mm Hg, pulse is 85/min, and oxygen saturation is 98% on room air. Auscultation of the chest reveals crackles in the bases bilaterally. The rest of his physical examination is normal. Laboratory studies show a normal leukocyte count with positive cold agglutinins, normal lactate dehydrogenase, and normal chemistries. A chest x-ray shows diffuse interstitial infiltrates. The most appropriate next step in management is to

(A) administer erythromycin, intravenously
(B) begin therapy with oral erythromycin
(C) begin therapy with oral trimethoprim-sulfamethoxazole
(D) order a high-resolution CT scan of the chest
(E) order pulmonary function tests

32. You are seeing a 68-year-old man with alcoholism and depression in the hospital who is being treated for a right leg deep venous thrombosis. His current medications include intravenous unfractionated heparin, a multivitamin, and thiamine. He has a 60 pack-year history of tobacco use, and currently smokes a pack per day. His temperature is 37.2 C (99.0 F), blood pressure is 122/67 mm Hg, pulse is 76/min, and respirations are 19/min. His cardiac rhythm is regular, and his breath sounds are clear bilaterally. While reviewing his laboratory data, you notice that his platelet count has been gradually diminishing from an admission value of 240×10^6/µL to 100×10^6/µL today. The most appropriate next step in management is to

(A) administer cryoprecipitate
(B) change the unfractionated heparin to low molecular weight heparin
(C) immediately discontinue heparin
(D) transfuse platelets
(E) transfuse whole blood

33. A 60-year-old man with hypertension and diabetes comes to the emergency department complaining of generalized numbness and weakness. His regular medications include atenolol, metformin, and triamterene, which was recently added for better blood pressure control. His blood pressure is 110/60 mm Hg and pulse is 60/min. Auscultation of the chest reveals scattered crackles. An electrocardiogram shows flattened P wave with prolonged QRS complex. Laboratory studies show

Sodium	138 mEq/L
Potassium	6.5 mEq/L
BUN	16 mg/dL
Creatinine	1.0 mg/dL

The most appropriate next step in management is to

(A) administer calcium gluconate
(B) administer dextrose and insulin
(C) administer nebulized albuterol
(D) administer sodium polystyrene sulfonate
(E) perform emergent hemodialysis

34. A 56-year-old woman with a fever of unknown origin and spontaneous bacterial peritonitis is intubated in the intensive care unit. She has a history of a seizure disorder that began at age 22 after head trauma. She has been off phenytoin for 8 years now without any recurrences. Her blood pressure is 90/70 mm Hg on fluid boluses, and she has a pulse of 125/min. Cultures and a chest x-ray are pending. Her creatinine is 1.0 U/L, hematocrit is 44%, and leukocyte count is 23,000/mm^3. You want to initiate antibiotic therapy, and you remember that the antibiotic that should not be used due to her seizure disorder is

(A) cephalexin
(B) clindamycin
(C) imipenem
(D) levofloxacin
(E) ticarcillin/clavulanic acid

35. A 26-year-old man comes to the office complaining of shortness of breath, a cough, and arthralgia for several days. He has had no previous illnesses. He has never smoked cigarettes and has had no exposures to irritant fumes or chemicals. He works at a local pet shop and part of his responsibilities is cleaning out birdcages. His temperature is 37.2 C (99.0 F), blood pressure is 125/65 mm Hg, and pulse is 82/min. Auscultation of the chest reveals bilateral fine crackles. PaO_2 is 65 mm Hg at rest. A chest x-ray shows reticular opacities at the lung bases and a patchy infiltrate at lower right and left mid lung. The most appropriate next step in management is to

(A) measure angiotensin-converting enzyme level
(B) obtain a sputum sample for culture and sensitivity
(C) perform a lung biopsy
(D) prescribe a 3-week course of inpatient therapy with intravenous doxycycline
(E) recommend that he eliminate exposure to the birds

36. A 74-year-old woman is admitted to the hospital for a right total hip replacement. The surgery and few days hospital course is uneventful. You go to examine her on the day of discharge, and, while in her hospital room, she develops acute-onset shortness of breath and right-sided pleuritic chest pain. Her temperature is 37.0 C (98.6 F), blood pressure is 140/70 mm Hg, pulse is 133/min, respirations are 28/min, and oxygen saturation is 92% on 6 L by nasal cannula. An electrocardiogram shows sinus tachycardia at a rate of 133/min without S-T changes. A stat portable chest x-ray is clear without evidence of active disease. The most appropriate next step in management is to

(A) extend her hospital stay for oxygen therapy
(B) obtain a ventilation-perfusion scan
(C) order a spiral CT of the chest
(D) order a venogram
(E) send her for a pulmonary angiogram

37. A 37-year-old man comes to the office complaining of back pain that started 24 hours earlier while he was chopping wood in his backyard. The pain is localized to his lower back with no radiation. He denies any fever, muscle weakness, numbness, trauma, recent weight loss, or bowel or bladder incontinence. He is in good health and has never been hospitalized. He does not smoke or drink alcohol and has one female sexual partner with whom he uses condoms. His temperature is 37.0 C (98.6 F), blood pressure is 111/74 mm Hg, and pulse is 76/min. Physical examination shows some slight tenderness to palpation in the lumbosacral area but has full range of motion of his back. He has 5/5 strength in both the lower and upper extremities as well as intact sensation to pinprick and light touch. His reflexes are 2+ and symmetric and a straight leg test is negative. The remainder of the physical examination is unremarkable. The most appropriate management of this patient is to

(A) advise complete bed rest for 2 weeks
(B) obtain an orthopedic consult
(C) order a lumbosacral x-ray
(D) order an MRI of the spine
(E) recommend a gradual return to activities along with acetaminophen for pain control

38. A 64-year-old woman comes to the office for her first time. She hands you an old chart that indicates that she has type 2 diabetes, depression, and carpal tunnel syndrome and takes metformin, enteric-coated aspirin, and paroxetine. She has no known drug allergies. She does not smoke, drink alcohol, or use recreational drugs. She is happily married and works as a sales representative. Her father had diabetes and her mother had coronary artery disease. Review of systems is negative other than occasional headaches that are relieved by acetaminophen. Her blood pressure is 170/102 mm Hg. She reports that her previous doctor detected an elevated blood pressure on her last several visits, but had not yet begun medication. The remainder of her physical examination is unremarkable. At this time, the most appropriate antihypertensive agent to use for this patient is

(A) benazepril
(B) clonidine
(C) felodipine
(D) hydrochlorothiazide
(E) losartan
(F) metoprolol

39. A 34-year-old woman comes to the emergency department complaining that her throat is "very sore." Her past medical history is significant for paroxysmal supraventricular tachycardia and previous right knee arthroscopic surgery. She smokes 1 pack of cigarettes per day but does not drink alcohol. Her vital signs are: blood pressure 130/70 mm Hg, pulse 110/min, respirations 12/min, and oxygen saturation of 96% on room air. In the examination room, she is sitting upright in bed with her head turned to the ceiling slightly. She is able to answer all of your questions without too much difficulty, although she does so slowly as she pauses occasionally in obvious discomfort. Her voice is slightly muffled and occasionally some saliva runs out of the corner of her mouth. You shine a light in her mouth and see that her palate and oropharynx show moderate erythema. Her tonsils are slightly enlarged with no exudates. The most appropriate next step in management is to

(A) examine her pharynx more closely with the assistance of a tongue depressor because of concern for her airway
(B) prescribe antibiotics for her bacterial tonsillitis and reassure her that this will begin to resolve in 2 to 3 days
(C) reassure her that she likely has a viral URI that will take some time to run its course
(D) refer her to an otolaryngologist for biopsy of a possible throat lesion within the next several days.
(E) try to avoid further manipulation but alert an otolaryngologist and anesthesiologist to evaluate her under anesthesia with the potential need for intubation

40. You have been taking care of an obese 57-year-old man with hypertension, asthma, and type 2 diabetes for the past 2 years. His hypertension is well controlled with losartan and hydrochlorothiazide and he has not had any problems with his asthma ever since he started taking montelukast regularly. As for his diabetes, he has had problems controlling his blood sugar level despite a good diet regimen, daily exercise, and glyburide. This has been a problem ever since he developed diabetes 15 years ago, and of all the medications he tried, glyburide has been doing the best job. He has some microvascular disease and makes sure to wear comfortable shoes and avoid trauma to his legs. Last week, he noticed several spots on his shins that he is sure were not there before. He does not remember injuring himself over the past couple of weeks and wonders where they came from. His blood pressure is 135/90 mm Hg and pulse is 80/min. Fasting blood glucose level is 150 mg/dL. On both anterior shins there are several pink plaques with a yellowish hue 1 to 3 cm in diameter. The center of the larger plaques is somewhat atrophic, with no hairs and some telangiectases traversing it. At this time the most correct statement about his skin condition is:

(A) It is a side of effect of montelukast treatment and changing to a drug from a different category will hasten its resolution.

(B) It is an idiopathic skin condition unrelated to his other diseases and medications, and there is no successful treatment available.

(C) It is often seen in patients with hypertension and can be successfully treated with topical corticosteroids regardless of the stage of disease.

(D) It is often seen in patients with poorly controlled diabetes, and although they can be treated with topical or intralesional corticosteroids, some permanent scarring will remain.

(E) It is often seen in patients with poorly controlled diabetes, and better control of his blood glucose levels will eventuate in its resolution.

41. A 65-year-old retired man comes to the office because of corns on the palms and soles that have been increasing in number over the last 5 years and are becoming a nuisance because they cause discomfort when he walks or tries to do some work around the house. His wife and he recently moved to a smaller house to better suit their needs. This was a difficult decision because they had spent their entire marriage in their previous home, but hoped moving out of an urban environment would give them more peace and comfort. He enjoyed renovating the new house, although he would have been much happier if it were not for the corns bothering him so much. He tells you that he has been pretty healthy all of his life despite his physically demanding work, and has only 2 years ago started taking blood pressure medication and an occasional sleeping pill. His medical history also includes a basal cell carcinoma removed from his lower back 3 years ago. You examine him and find that he is a fit, well-developed man. His blood pressure is 130/85 mm Hg, pulse is 70/min, and respirations are 12/min. There are numerous 1 to 2-mm punctate keratoses on the thenar and hypothenar eminence, as well as on the soles, especially on the heel and metatarsals. On the trunk and proximal thighs you note multiple hyper- and hypopigmented macules. There is a 1×1 cm scaly, erythematous patch with a pearly, threadlike border on the right buttocks adjacent to an old linear surgical scar. The most important initial screening question in the diagnostic evaluation of this patient's skin disease is:

(A) "How long have you been married to your wife?"

(B) "What kind of cleaning solutions did you use when renovating your new home?"

(C) "What kind of work did you do before you retired?"

(D) "What medications are you taking for your blood pressure and sleeping problem?"

(E) "When was the house you moved to built?"

42. A 20-year-old man comes to the office 10 days after his return from Haiti complaining of fever, abdominal pain, and yellow eyes. He was well for his entire 3-week trip, but 2 days after his return he developed anorexia, followed by fevers as high as 39.1 C (102.4 F). Over the subsequent days, his abdomen began to hurt, with the pain mostly localized to the right upper quadrant. He vomited several times, had some loose stools, and noticed that "the white part of my eyes looks yellow." He tells you that he does not drink alcohol but uses marijuana "occasionally," had an unprotected sexual encounter with a woman in Haiti, and denies any injection drug use. His temperature is 38.1 C (100.6 F), blood pressure is 105/65 mm Hg, pulse is 110/min, and respirations are 15/min. He appears uncomfortable but is in no acute distress. Physical examination shows hepatomegaly (liver edge soft but felt 4 to 5 cm below the right costal margin), right upper quadrant abdominal tenderness, and scleral icterus. Serum antibody testing confirms the diagnosis of acute hepatitis A infection. At this time the most correct statement about this patient's condition is:

(A) Hepatitis A is largely a sexually transmitted disease, so his sexual partners should be evaluated for possible asymptomatic infection.
(B) His risk of developing chronic hepatitis from this infection is roughly 75%.
(C) Most cases of hepatitis A are transfusion-related, so that was the likely means of transmission.
(D) Since the mode of spread of hepatitis A virus is fecal-oral, he likely contracted the illness from an exposure on his recent trip.
(E) Treatment of his infection with ribavirin will decrease the length of the illness.

43. A 56-year-old woman without significant past medical history comes to the office for a periodic routine physical examination. She has no complaints at this time. She does not smoke cigarettes and has an "occasional" glass of wine with dinner. She has had normal annual screening mammograms since she turned 50. Routine laboratory studies are normal except for a calcium level of 11.1 mg/dL and an elevated PTH level. The most likely diagnosis is

(A) multiple myeloma
(B) osteoporosis
(C) parathyroid adenoma
(D) parathyroid carcinoma
(E) squamous cell carcinoma

44. A 27-year-old woman with a long history of type 1 diabetes is admitted to the hospital because of lethargy. Her significant other accompanies her and reports that she has had a history of poor glycemic control with neuropathy, retinopathy, and long-standing nausea and abdominal pain "due to diabetes." They had gone out for dinner and had two mixed drinks; she does not usually drink alcohol. Later that night, she stumbled and hit her forehead against a wall. There was no loss of consciousness. She is currently taking 30 units of NPH insulin in the morning and 15 units in the evening with a short-acting insulin sliding scale. She has not had any recent changes in her insulin regimen. On arrival to the hospital, she is afebrile, has a blood pressure of 130/80 mm Hg, pulse of 110/min, and respirations are 14/min. She complains of feeling slightly nauseous and sleepy. She is diaphoretic and has a small abrasion on her forehead. A brief neurologic examination is remarkable for lethargy, and is otherwise normal. An intravenous line was placed in the field. A finger-stick glucose level is 38 mg/dL. The most appropriate management at this time is

(A) a CT scan of the head
(B) dextrose 5%, continuous infusion
(C) dextrose 50%, followed by D5W infusion with further monitoring over several hours
(D) dextrose 50%, followed by NS infusion
(E) glucagon
(F) normal saline
(G) orange juice

45. A 67-year-old man is brought to the emergency department with chest pain and shortness of breath. His medical history is significant for a 100 pack-year history of tobacco use, adenocarcinoma of the lung with known metastases to the liver, and hypertension. His current medications include verapamil. His temperature is 37.2 C (99.0 F), blood pressure is 90/60 mm Hg, pulse is 112/min, and respirations are 25/min. Physical examination shows jugular venous pressure elevation and pulsus paradoxus. His cardiac rhythm is regular with muffled sounds and his lungs are clear to auscultation bilaterally. Based on the available information, you request an electrocardiogram and expect to see

(A) left ventricular hypertrophy
(B) a new left bundle branch block
(C) peaked T waves
(D) a prolonged QT interval
(E) pulsus alternans

46. A 30-year-old woman comes to the office because of a 3-month history of nonspecific joint pain. She has no significant past medical history. Past surgical history is significant for repair of the umbilical hernia. Postoperatively, her pain control was difficult according to her and she stayed in the hospital for 2 days. Now she describes diffuse pain throughout her hands, knees, and neck and states that she aches all over. She indicates that the pain is always present but is worse after activity. She has morning stiffness lasting approximately 1 hour. She has tried several analgesic medications and herbal medications with no improvement. Physical examination is normal except for numerous symmetric tender points. Laboratory studies and radiographs of joints and bones are unremarkable. The most likely cause of this patient's pain is

(A) fibromyalgia
(B) hypothyroidism
(C) polymyalgia rheumatica
(D) polymyositis
(E) rheumatoid arthritis

47. A 20-year-old man comes to the clinic stating that for the past 2 days there has been "something draining from my penis." He describes the fluid as thick, dark, and foul smelling. He has already discolored one pair of underwear. He denies any pain or fever but does complain of burning with urination. Although he is initially reluctant to confide in you, he finally admits to having unprotected intercourse with a new partner about 1 week ago. His temperature is 36.6 C (97.9 F). Physical examination shows that he is circumcised and there are no external lesions on his glans penis or coronal sulcus. There is a thick, brown, purulent discharge from his urethra. His testicles are within the scrotum and without masses or tenderness. Rectal examination reveals a firm, nontender, small prostate. There is no discharge with prostatic massage. After you take a culture swab of the urethra, you perform a Gram stain, which shows Gram-negative diplococci within polymorphonuclear leukocytes. The most appropriate next step in management is to

(A) administer 1 g of PO azithromycin
(B) administer 125 mg of IM ceftriaxone and 1 g of PO azithromycin
(C) administer 200 mg of PO acyclovir for 7 days
(D) administer 2.4 million units of IM penicillin G
(E) provide the patient with literature on safe sexual practices
(F) wait for culture results to return prior to treatment

48. On a Friday afternoon a 65-year-old woman comes to the office because of shortness of breath. You have cared for her primary care medical needs for the last 10 years and know that this patient has no history of respiratory problems. You recall she recently had a total hip replacement by a local orthopedic surgeon. The patient tells you that she has been well since her surgery 12 days ago. She has been resting at home without doing much activity because her daughter is staying with her. The patient noted that early this morning she awoke short of breath with moderate pain in her chest with deep inspiration. The pain subsided but she has been unable to comfortably breathe throughout the day. A review of her current medication list reveals she is on her usual antihypertensive medication (hydrochlorothiazide) and estrogen replacement therapy. On physical examination the patient is laboring to breathe and appears to be in mild distress. Respirations are shallow and 25/min. Her blood pressure is 140/76 mm Hg, pulse is 112/min, and peripheral O_2 saturation is 82%. On examination of her lungs you appreciate no crackles or rhonchi. Both lungs have symmetric breath sounds. The cardiac examination is unremarkable with the exception of the aforementioned tachycardia. The right arthroplasty incision is intact with no surrounding erythema or drainage noted. The right foot and ankle are swollen and there is tenderness with calf palpation. The most appropriate next step in management is to

(A) administer an albuterol nebulizer treatment because she likely has a component of reactive airway disease that will respond to bronchodilators
(B) administer 1 g of an intramuscular cephalosporin because this patient likely has contracted a community-acquired pneumonia
(C) administer 10 mg of oral warfarin because she is likely in a hypercoagulable state and is at risk for deep venous thrombosis
(D) alert the hospital that you will be admitting this patient and she will likely require an intensive care bed, a workup for a probable pulmonary embolus, and immediate heparinization
(E) inform the patient that she likely has postoperative atelectasis and needs to do home deep-breathing exercises to improve her pulmonary status

Items 49-50

A 28-year-old woman comes to the office because she is "finally ready for the big guns" to get rid of her acne. She has been a patient of yours since childhood, and over the years you have treated her with benzoyl peroxide gel, topical tretinoin, topical erythromycin, and oral tetracycline, minocycline, and erythromycin. She has never been satisfied with the results of these agents, and you have discussed isotretinoin with her in the past, but she always said "next time." Physical examination shows multiple large and inflamed cysts and nodules on her face, back, and chest.

49. The most appropriate next step is to

    (A) check her records for previous lipid, CPK, and glucose levels and liver function tests; if normal give her a prescription for isotretinoin
    (B) do a urine pregnancy test; if negative give her a prescription for isotretinoin
    (C) do a urine pregnancy test; if negative tell her to take another pregnancy test on the second day of her next period or 11 days after her last unprotected intercourse, and then if negative, prescribe isotretinoin
    (D) obtain lipid, CPK, and glucose levels and liver function tests, and if normal give her a prescription for isotretinoin
    (E) order pelvic ultrasonography; if there is no visible fetus, give her a prescription for isotretinoin

50. The appropriate steps are taken. You should explain to her that while she is taking isotretinoin she should

    (A) avoid all physical activity
    (B) be cautious when driving or operating any vehicle at night
    (C) make sure to use one form of birth control; it should be an effective one, such as an injectable/implantable contraceptive product
    (D) not donate blood until 3 weeks following discontinuation of the drug
    (E) take a multivitamin with vitamin A
    (F) wax her legs and underarms instead of shaving

Internal Medicine Test Two: **Answers and Explanations**

ANSWER KEY

1. C
2. E
3. D
4. B
5. B
6. C
7. E
8. D
9. C
10. D
11. A
12. D
13. A
14. A
15. D
16. H
17. D
18. D
19. E
20. A
21. B
22. C
23. E
24. B
25. E
26. C
27. C
28. A
29. B
30. D
31. B
32. C
33. A
34. C
35. E
36. B
37. E
38. A
39. E
40. D
41. C
42. D
43. C
44. C
45. E
46. A
47. B
48. D
49. C
50. B

1. **The correct answer is C.** Aortic dissections quite often present in the presence of hypertension. Uncontrolled hypertension can lead to the propagation of a dissection leading to rupture of end-organ ischemia. Therefore, controlling blood pressure in the setting of an aortic dissection is crucial. However, it is also important to ensure that cardiac contractility does not increase as a compensatory response to the blood pressure decrease, because the increase in contractility can also cause a propagation of the dissection. Therefore, an agent such as labetalol with both alpha antagonistic (vasodilation) and beta agonistic (prevents an increase in cardiac contractility) properties is used in the treatment of an aortic dissection.

   Aspirin (**choice A**), with its antiplatelet action, has no role in the acute management of an aortic dissection.

   Heparin (**choice B**) should not be administered in the setting of a dissection given the risk of aortic rupture.

   Phenylephrine (**choice D**) should not be used in the setting of an aortic dissection since an increase in blood pressure can lead to propagation of the dissection. It is important to note that the diminished left arm blood pressure is artifactual in that the left subclavian artery is involved in the dissection.

   Sodium nitroprusside (**choice E**), a potent vasodilator, should not be used alone since the compensatory increase in cardiac contractility can cause propagation of the aortic dissection.

2. **The correct answer is E.** Pearly penile papules are pearly, white, dome-shaped papules occurring circumferentially on the coronal margin and sulcus of the glans penis. Occasionally, lesions are also present on the penile shaft. Pearly penile papules are not uncommon. Patients usually present around the age of 20 to 30 years concerned these are condylomata or are referred as treatment-resistant venereal warts. These lesions should be differentiated from papillomas, hypertrophic sebaceous glands, and condyloma acuminatum. No treatment is necessary, only reassurance. If treatment is desired, laser ablation is best.

   Allergic contact dermatitis (**choice A**) from condoms is a variant of latex allergy and presents with pruritic, moist, weepy, crusted red patches on the glans and shaft of the penis. It is best treated with mild- to moderate-potency topical steroids and use of latex-free condoms.

   Candida infection (**choice B**) of the glans and prepuce (*Candida* balanoposthitis) presents with moist red plaques and cheesy-white exudate in uncircumcised men. It may be asymptomatic or cause itching and burning. Treatment is with topical nystatin or other antifungal creams.

   Genital warts (condyloma acuminatum) (**choice C**) usually present as flesh-colored to red sessile or filiform papules with a verrucous surface on the glans or shaft of the penis. They can also be present on the surrounding anogenital skin. They vary in size and shape from less than 1 to 5 mm or more and are haphazardly distributed in the affected areas. Sometimes they attain gigantic proportions (giant condyloma of Buschke and Lowenstein). Treatment modalities include liquid nitrogen, topical podophyllotoxin, topical imiquimod, topical cantharidin, and laser therapy.

   Irritant contact dermatitis secondary to retention of smegma in the coronal sulcus (**choice D**) presents with persistent itchy, burning, red, scaly patches and plaques on the glans penis. It is an uncommon finding and circumcision is recommended to prevent progression to squamous cell carcinoma.

3. **The correct answer is D.** This patient has asymptomatic pulmonary sarcoidosis with no extrapulmonary involvement and no treatment is indicated at this time. Sarcoidosis is a granulomatous disease of unknown etiology. Up to two thirds of patients who present with sarcoidosis will experience resolution or improvement in symptoms or radiographic abnormalities over the following several years, with chronic disease developing in only a minority of patients. Because of the waxing and waning nature of the illness, and the lack of controlled studies, it has been difficult to prove that glucocorticoids actually improve outcome. Initial evaluation after diagnosis should include an ECG, ophthalmologic examination, liver function tests, serum calcium, and 24-hour urine calcium determination. The asymptomatic patient with no evidence of clinical or radiological progression should be followed closely without treatment. Erythema nodosum is the most common nonspecific cutaneous finding in sarcoidosis and is associated with a good prognosis, with the sarcoidosis involuting within 6 months of onset in 80% of cases.

   Ibuprofen (**choice A**) is sometimes used in the treatment of erythema nodosum associated with otherwise asymptomatic sarcoidosis. Many cases will resolve with bed rest only.

   Intravenous prednisone (**choice B**) is not used for the treatment of sarcoidosis.

   Methotrexate (**choice D**) has been used successfully (as have chloroquine and hydroxychloroquine) in the treatment of severe mucocutaneous sarcoidosis and in patients who either do not respond to prednisone or have serious side effects.

Symptomatic patients and those with progressive objective deterioration warrant a trial of prednisone, 30 to 40 mg PO qd for 6 to 8 weeks (**choice E**). When therapy is effective, a clinical and radiological response is obtained in 2 to 4 weeks. If no response is obtained in 4 to 8 weeks, it is reasonable to discontinue treatment gradually.

4. **The correct answer is B.** This patient has nevus of Ota, an oculodermal melanocytosis. Typical lesions are coalescing and confluent bluish gray macules with accompanying scleral pigmentation on one side of the face. Areas innervated by the first (ophthalmic), second (maxillary), and occasionally third (mandibular) branch of the trigeminal nerve are affected. Approximately half of the lesions are present at birth, with the remainder becoming evident in childhood or puberty. Histologically, darkly pigmented, spindle-shaped, dendritic melanocytes are present in the upper and mid dermis. Nevus of Ota is most prevalent in Japan, where the incidence approaches 1%. Other ethnic groups and races may be affected, but less commonly. It is several times more common in women than in men. Physiologic and environmental factors may alter the pigmentation in nevus of Ota. Fatigue, emotional excitement, insomnia, and unusually cold or warm weather may increase intensity of color. Hormonal variations during menstruation and menopause may induce darkening. Spontaneous regression may occur. Apart from the skin, nevus of Ota frequently involves the eye and the central nervous system. Melanoma may arise within nevus of Ota, in the skin, choroid, brain, orbit, iris, ciliary body, and optic nerve. Caucasians with ocular melanocytosis, a variant that has no cutaneous manifestations, are most at risk. Biopsy is indicated with suspicious changes in the nevus of Ota, and neurologic or ophthalmologic symptoms should initiate immediate referral to appropriate specialists.

   Melanoma may arise in the skin, eye, and the central nervous system in patients with nevus of Ota. Melanoma of the skin and the eye (**choice A**) and melanoma of the skin only (**choice C**) are incomplete and, therefore, incorrect.

   Nonmelanoma skin cancers (basal cell carcinoma and squamous cell carcinoma being by far the most common) do not occur with increased frequency in skin lesions of nevus of Ota. Therefore, melanoma and nonmelanoma skin cancers (**choice D**) and predominantly nonmelanoma skin cancers, although melanoma can also occur (**choice E**), are incorrect.

5. **The correct answer is B.** This patient has *Pseudomonas aeruginosa* bacteremic pneumonia and ecthyma gangrenosum. Bacteremic pneumonia due to *Pseudomonas aeruginosa* begins as a respiratory infection typically associated with neutropenia, subsequent bloodstream invasion, and metastatic spread that produces characteristic lesions in the lungs and other viscera. Alveolar hemorrhage and necrosis are common. Chest roentgenograms characteristically demonstrate a rapid progression from pulmonary vascular congestion to interstitial edema, then to pulmonary edema, and finally to diffuse necrotizing bronchopneumonia with cavity formation. The patient typically dies 3 or 4 days after initial presentation. Ecthyma gangrenosum is a necrotic and bullous skin infection caused by *Pseudomonas aeruginosa*. Clinically, it is characterized by painless red macules that rapidly progress to bullae or pustules followed by development of gangrenous ulcers. Lesions frequently occur in areas with apocrine glands (axillae, breast, groin). Typically, it arises in immunocompromised persons (hematologic malignancy, immunosuppressive treatment, organ transplant, malnutrition, neutropenia, diabetes mellitus) or in persons recently exposed to a hospital environment. The majority of cases are associated with *Pseudomonas* sepsis or bacteremia, but localized lesions without systemic infection have been known to occur. Early recognition of the skin lesions is critical because prognosis is directly dependent on how soon treatment is initiated. The infectious disease service should be contacted and intravenous antibiotic treatment started as soon as skin biopsy specimens for culture and histologic analysis, and blood cultures are secured. Initial treatment is normally a combination of intravenous anti-pseudomonas penicillin such as piperacillin, and aminoglycoside such as gentamycin. If gentamycin-resistant strains are suspected, then a combination of an anti-pseudomonas penicillin and ciprofloxacin can be used. Further adjustments of the antibiotics are made when culture and sensitivity studies are complete. Surgical debridement is not indicated in the treatment of bacteremic ecthyma gangrenosum.

   Intravenous antibiotics and surgical debridement (**choice A**) is incorrect because surgical debridement is not indicated in the treatment of skin infection with *Pseudomonas aeruginosa* secondary to bacteremia.

   Neither oral antibiotics, nor surgical debridement (**choice C**) are indicated in the treatment of *Pseudomonas* bacteremia.

   Oral antibiotics (**choice D**) are used only for the treatment of malignant otitis externa and urinary tract infections caused by *Pseudomonas aeruginosa.*

Surgical debridement (**choice E**) is not indicated in the treatment of bacteremic ecthyma gangrenosum.

6. **The correct answer is C.** PSVT, a dysrhythmia relatively more common in the younger population, is a result of a reentry loop involving the atrioventricular node. Interventions such as carotid massage that will increase vagal tone and short circuit such a reentry loop can therefore, be used as a first-line intervention in the treatment of PSVTs.

   Intravenous heparin (**choice A**) is not needed with PSVTs since this dysrhythmia is not associated with atrial or ventricular blood stasis (as with atrial fibrillation) and risk for thrombosis.

   If vagal maneuvers are unsuccessful, adenosine or verapamil can be used. Digoxin (**choice B**) has a slower onset of action and therefore should not be used for acute therapy.

   Cardioversion (**choice D**) is used for the treatment of PSVTs leading to patient instability (i.e., myocardial ischemia, angina, congestive failure). Cardioversion is not used as a first-line treatment of a patient with a PSVT who is stable.

7. **The correct answer is E.** This patient may be experiencing overwhelming postsplenectomy infection. This is a life-threatening illness that can rapidly lead to sepsis, DIC, and death. Patients without a functioning spleen are at increased risk of sepsis from encapsulated organisms including pneumococcal and meningococcal disease. The lack of other symptoms should not delay treatment, as many patients do not have a localizing sign of infection.

   More than half of patients admitted to the hospital with postsplenectomy infections die within 48 hours. Medical care should not be delayed until the evening (**choice A**).

   Viral syndromes can be treated with symptomatic therapy such as fluids and antipyretics; however, this is not adequate therapy in the splenectomized host. Therefore, drink plenty of fluids and take acetaminophen as needed for fever as she likely has a viral syndrome and her symptoms should resolve in the next few days (**choice B**) is incorrect.

   The patient was likely treated adequately for her urinary tract infection because her symptoms resolved. Therefore, **choice C** is incorrect.

   Medical care of the patient with postsplenectomy infection consists of blood cultures, urine cultures, and chest x-ray with sputum culture. Lumbar puncture may also be considered as well as paracentesis if the patient has ascites. The patient should then receive broad-spectrum antibiotics until the results are available. A urine culture alone (**choice D**) would be inadequate.

8. **The correct answer is D.** The patient has a clinical picture and a CXR consistent with *Pneumocystis carinii* pneumonia (PCP). This is a protozoan organism that causes pneumonia in immunocompromised subjects. It typically has an indolent course and carries a 10% mortality. The treatment is PO or IV trimethoprim-sulfamethoxazole and prednisone if the patient is hypoxic.

   Azithromycin (**choice A**) is inappropriate since this patient is more likely to have PCP than an atypical pneumonia due to his immune status.

   Lactate dehydrogenase (**choice B**) is found to be frequently elevated in patients with PCP. However, it is a very nonspecific marker and cannot be used in deciding management.

   Trimethoprim-sulfamethoxazole alone (**choice C**) in this patient with a PaO_2<70 mm Hg is inappropriate since it has been shown that those patients with PCP and hypoxia also benefit from prednisone treatment initiated 30 minutes prior to trimethoprim-sulfamethoxazole.

   Discharge of the patient on a daily dose of PO trimethoprim-sulfamethoxazole (**choice E**) is indicated for AIDS patients with no pneumonia with a CD4 count less than 200/mm^3. It was shown to reduce the incidence of PCP to less than 5%. It is inappropriate in patients with pneumonia and hypoxia.

9. **The correct answer is C.** The patient is presenting with classic lichen planus (LP). LP typically presents with pruritic, purple, polygonal papules on the following site of predilection; penis, wrists, shins, and buccal mucosa. The real giveaway, however, are the white lacy streaks on the buccal mucosa or Wickham striae as they are called. This is pathognomic for LP and is not candida. Although the exact etiology of LP is unknown, it is often associated with hepatitis C. It is not certain if being infected with the hepatitis C virus allows this yet unknown LP virus to take hold, but there is a definite correlation. Approximately 16% of patients with cutaneous LP and 30% of patients with the oral form of LP have antibodies to hepatitis C. These are not viral warts and they will not respond to typical wart treatment such as liquid nitrogen or imiquimod.

An ANA is ordered (**choice A**) when a connective tissue disease is suspected such as lupus, dermatomyositis, scleroderma, Sjogren syndrome, etc. Patients with LP do not manifest abnormal ANAs.

A complete blood count (**choice B**) should be normal in a patient with LP if there are no other medical problems noted. A CBC is not warranted here as the next most appropriate test.

Patients who have risk factors such as unprotected sex, IV drug abuse, and blood transfusions are at most risk for having HIV (**choice D**). This patient does not have these risk factors. The most common skin manifestations of HIV are seborrheic dermatitis, thrush on the oral mucosa, molluscum on the face, warts, Kaposi sarcoma, and *not* lichen planus. While having the patient consent to an HIV test may be a good idea because of his sexual promiscuity, his current condition is often associated with hepatitis C and so this study (hepatitis panel) is the most appropriate at this time.

Viral load (**choice E**) is only checked in HIV-positive patients, as it is measuring the human immunodeficiency virus' viral load. Since HIV is not a risk factor in patients with LP, one does not need to check the viral load.

10. **The correct answer is D.** The CDC guidelines for the treatment of sexually transmitted diseases, last updated in 1998, recommends offering the hepatitis B vaccine to patients who are treated for any sexually transmitted disease. Hepatitis B is a sexually transmitted disease that can be prevented with administration of the vaccination series of three injections. The CDC also recommends that men having sex with men, patients with more than 1 sexual partner in the last 6 months, prostitutes, illegal drug users, health care workers, all infants, hemodialysis patients, and household contacts of patients with chronic hepatitis B infection be vaccinated. Patients with any exposure to sexually transmitted diseases should be offered screening for other infections such as HIV and syphilis. *Chlamydia* is frequently asymptomatic in both men and women. Given the known exposure this patient should be treated with appropriate therapy, which includes a 1-g single dose of azithromycin. Other options are doxycycline 100 mg orally twice a day for 7 days or erythromycin 500 mg orally 4 times a day for 7 days. This patient should also contact all of his sexual contacts to recommend that they be treated; therefore (**choice E**) is incorrect.

    Ceftriaxone (**choice A**) and ciprofloxacin (**choice B**) are incorrect because these are recommended therapies for gonococcal infection, not *Chlamydia*.

    Metronidazole (**choice C**) is the treatment of *Trichomonas* infection and is therefore incorrect.

11. **The correct answer is A.** This patient most likely has acute gouty arthritis, which is diagnosed by performing arthrocentesis and demonstrating negatively birefringent crystals under a polarizing microscope. Acute gouty arthritis typically presents with the rapid onset of joint pain, swelling, and erythema that wakes the patient from sleep. The patient may be febrile and the joint is usually warm with tense surrounding skin. Gout usually occurs in a peripheral joint, especially the metatarsophalangeal joint of the big toe. It is typically caused by decreased renal excretion of uric acid and is often associated with excessive food and alcohol intake, thiazide usage, starvation, stress, trauma, and infections. Many patients with gout have had or will have kidney stones. The treatment of acute gouty arthritis is an NSAID, such as indomethacin, colchicine, or intraarticular glucocorticoids.

    It may be possible to detect Lyme disease by using PCR to detect spirochetal DNA (**choice B**). Lyme disease is transmitted by a tick bite and typically begins with erythema migrans, which is a well-demarcated, round, red lesion with a central clearing. The next stage is disseminated infection, which involves systemic symptoms such as headache, fever, chills, fatigue, and lethargy. Finally, persistent infection involves intermittent attacks of arthritis. The patient in this case does not have this history, which makes the diagnosis of Lyme disease unlikely. Also, PCR is not used to diagnose gout.

    Cervical, pharyngeal, and rectal cultures (**choice C**) are taken when acute arthritis is thought to be caused by a disseminated gonococcal infection. It may be associated with pain and swelling of other joints and a skin rash. The septic arthritis associated with a disseminated gonococcal infection is typically purulent and destructive. Symptoms of disseminated gonococcal infection often occur during menses. This patient is not the typical patient to have gonococcal arthritis (usually sexually active young adults), and her presentation is almost classic for gout; therefore, cervical, pharyngeal, and rectal cultures should not be performed at this time.

    A technetium radionuclide bone scan (**choice D**) is typically used in the workup for osteomyelitis and is often positive within 24 hours. Appropriate cultures and biopsies should also be performed for a definitive diagnosis.

    An x-ray of the ankle (**choice E**) will not provide a definitive diagnosis of acute gouty arthritis.

12. **The correct answer is D.** This patient most likely has acute gouty arthritis, which is confirmed by finding negatively birefringent crystals under a polarizing microscope. The treatment is an NSAID, such as indomethacin, colchicine, or intraarticular glucocorticoids.

A diffuse increase in technetium uptake around the ankle on the bone scan (**choice A**) would indicate that there is osteoblastic activity and skeletal vascularity. This can be caused by many conditions such as osteomyelitis, fractures, neuropathic osteopathy, tumors, and infarction. It is inappropriate to treat any of these disorders with indomethacin, based on these findings. A more definitive study, such as biopsies or cultures, is necessary to make a definitive diagnosis.

The treatment for a fracture of the head of the fibula and a displaced fracture of the medial malleolus (**choice B**) depends on stability of the ankle mortise, but typically requires closed reduction and casting or open reduction and internal fixation. Indomethacin is not the appropriate treatment.

Intracellular gram-negative diplococci in the cervical, pharyngeal, and rectal cultures (**choice C**) would indicate that the monoarticular arthritis is most likely caused by a gonococcal infection, which requires antibiotic treatment, usually with ceftriaxone, cefotaxime, or ceftizoxime.

If spirochetal DNA is found by PCR (**choice E**), Lyme disease would be the most likely diagnosis. The first-line treatment for Lyme disease is antibiotics, such as doxycycline or amoxicillin. Indomethacin is not an appropriate first-line drug to treat Lyme arthritis.

13. **The correct answer is A.** This patient has herpes zoster and not Kaposi sarcoma. The classic herpes lesions are grouped vesicles on an erythematous base. Herpes zoster is unilateral and can span one or more dermatomes. Kaposi sarcoma is a purplish macule, patch, nodule, or tumor. It usually does not arise in only 1 day. This patient needs oral acyclovir in hopes that when given within 48 hours, there will be a reduced incidence of postherpetic neuralgia.

Topical acyclovir (**choice B**) does not work and is inappropriate treatment for herpes zoster especially in this HIV-positive patient with extension of the outbreak over multiple dermatomes. Topical acyclovir is used, albeit rarely, for patients with recurrent oral or genital lesions. On recognizing the tingle or preview of an outbreak, the ointment is applied every 2 hours while awake in an attempt to prevent or shorten the course. Its efficacy is debatable.

If this rash were described as a purplish macule, patch, nodule, or tumor, then Kaposi sarcoma could be considered in the diagnosis and referral to a dermatologist would then be appropriate (**choice C**). However, Kaposi sarcoma is never described as grouped vesicles on an erythematous base.

If this rash were described as a purplish macule, patch, nodule, or tumor, than Kaposi sarcoma could be considered in the diagnosis and testing for HHV-8 can be done (**choice D**), but a biopsy would be more appropriate to confirm diagnosis. It has been shown that HHV-8 causes Kaposi sarcoma but is not readily performed to confirm the diagnosis.

If this rash were described as a purplish macule, patch, nodule, or tumor, then Kaposi sarcoma could be considered in the diagnosis and you might worry more about the outcome of this patient. It is true that Kaposi sarcoma can be aggressive in untreated AND deeply immunosuppressed AIDS patients, but this patient needs his viral load and CD4 count checked before declaring him severely immunosuppressed (**choice E**). This patient would, however, benefit from a referral to infectious disease to check his immune status and start therapy if appropriate.

14. **The correct answer is A.** Aortic stenosis is characterized by involvement of the aortic valves, which become thickened and immobile, obstructing the flow of blood out of the left ventricle. This condition is usually characterized by a heaving point of maximal impulse, which is often not shifted outward due to the development of concentric left ventricular hypertrophy. Because of the obstruction at the level of the left ventricular outflow tract, one can hear a systolic murmur at the right second intercostal space. The aortic component of the second heart sound is soft from thickening and restricted mobility of the aortic valves.

Mitral regurgitation (**choice B**) is not the correct choice because it is associated with a holosystolic murmur, heard best at the apex and radiating to the axilla. The aortic component of the second heart sound is unaffected.

Mitral stenosis (**choice C**) is not the correct choice because it typically has a middiastolic murmur heard over the apex of the heart. The point of maximal impulse, although not shifted outward, is never heaving in nature.

Pulmonic stenosis (**choice D**) is not the correct choice because it is associated with an ejection systolic murmur, best heard on the left second intercostal space. This usually is accompanied by a right ventricular heave, depending on the severity of the obstruction. The pulmonic component of the second heart sound may be soft.

Ventricular septal defect (**choice E**) is not the correct choice because it is associated with a holosystolic murmur heard along the left sternal border and radiating to the right side of the sternum. The pulmonic component of the second heart sound may be delayed and accentuated due to the increased pulmonic flow.

15. **The correct answer is D.** Multiple myeloma is associated with a number of clinical consequences. One of these is the elaboration of a substance that acts on bone to release calcium. It is very common for patients with multiple myeloma to present with altered mental status from hypercalcemia. Hypercalcemia requires immediate therapy. The most effective way to rapidly eliminate calcium from the body is by diuresis. Since these patients are, however, extremely volume depleted, they first require aggressive hydration with saline. The diuresis alone would only aggravate the hypercalcemia.

    Bisphosphonate therapy (**choice A**) is a very effective intervention for long-term control of hypercalcemia. This therapy requires at least 36 to 48 hours to reach peak effect, however, making it not useful in the acute situation.

    Therapy with calcitonin (**choice B**) is also considered delayed and for long-term use but is much less efficacious than bisphosphonates.

    Glucocorticoid therapy (**choice C**) is considered useful therapy in an acute situation in cases where hydration and forced diuresis have failed.

    Hemodialysis (**choice E**) is indicated once acute medical management has failed or in cases of dramatically elevated calcium in patients with preexisting renal disease where they are not expected to clear the calcium load.

16. **The correct answer is H.** Confidentiality is absolute, unless there is a threat of harm to self or other. There is no manifest or implied threat in this case. Therefore, a physician cannot testify as to any information obtained in his interaction with the patient without the patient's clear consent. The first issue to be established is whether or not the patient will consent. The patient may, for example, be glad about your testimony and wish his health status to be part of the legal debate. For this reason, before deciding how to respond to the court, seek a clear understanding of the patient's wishes, not the American Medical Association's Department of Ethics guidance on the prevailing legal standards (**choice F**).

    Appearing and offering some information about the patient while withholding other information is not an option. Confidentiality covers all information, not just medical information. This is also not a guessing game where the physician will not volunteer information, but will confirm information already known, therefore **choices A, B, C, D, and E** are incorrect.

    Note that one should *always* appear when served with a subpoena. Failure to appear will be considered contempt of court and the physician will be subject to fines and other penalties; therefore, **choices G and I** are incorrect.

17. **The correct answer is D.** This patient has redistributive hyponatremia. He has hyperglycemia, which causes a shift of water from the intracellular compartment to the extracellular compartment with a resultant dilution of sodium. Total body water and sodium are unchanged. The corrected sodium level can be calculated according to the following formula: corrected serum Na (mEq/L) = measured Na (mEq/L) + [1.5 × ([glucose (mg/dL) –150]/100)]. Treatment of hyponatremia is aimed at treating the underlying cause.

    Demeclocycline (**choice A**) is considered when the underlying disease is no longer treatable (metastatic lung cancer) and severe water restriction is not acceptable to the patient.

    Hypertonic 3% saline (**choice B**) is used in patients with severe symptomatic hyponatremia (Na <120) regardless of the cause.

    Providing no treatment is correct, but because the sodium level is normal, not because the patient is asymptomatic (**choice C**).

    Fluid restriction (**choice E**) usually works in patients with euvolemic (SIADH) or hypervolemic (CHF, cirrhosis, and nephritic syndrome) hyponatremia, when the patient is asymptomatic.

18. **The correct answer is D.** Isoniazid given daily for 9 months to persons with positive tuberculin skin test but without active tuberculosis is effective in preventing the subsequent development of tuberculosis; this is called "preventive therapy" or "therapy of latent TB." This is the standard of care according to the latest guidelines of the CDC for patients with positive PPD and no active disease. Explaining that no treatment is indicated, as she does not have tuberculosis (**choice B**), is therefore incorrect.

Respiratory isolation (**choice A**) is indicated for patients with suspected or confirmed pulmonary or laryngeal TB until noninfectious.

This patient doesn't have pulmonary TB and is not coughing so there is no use of sputum stains and cultures for AFB (**choice C**).

The standard treatment of active TB can include a combination of different medications depending on the local resistance pattern: isoniazide, rifampin, and pyrazinamide (**choice E**), or isoniazid, rifampin, pyrazinamide, and ethambutol, or isoniazid, rifampin, pyrazinamide, and streptomycin.

19. **The correct answer is E.** This woman has deep vein thrombosis (DVT) secondary to protein C deficiency (hypercoagulable state). Protein S and protein C are natural anticoagulants, they work by cleaving activated factors V and VIII. When there is a decrease in their levels the patient will have a thrombotic disorder. Patients who have DVT secondary to hypercoagulable states should receive anticoagulation indefinitely. Heparin should be started in hospital and warfarin is started after that with a target INR between 2 and 3. Patients who have no hypercoagulable states and present with their first DVT should be anticoagulated for 3 to 6 months (**choice C**). If the DVT recurs then these patients should be anticoagulated for 1 year (**choice D**).

    Antiplatelet agents such as aspirin (**choice A**) or dipyridamole (**choice B**) are not indicated in venous thrombosis; they are beneficial in lowering the incidence of arterial thrombotic events (MI, stroke).

20. **The correct answer is A.** The primary diagnostic test for diabetes mellitus in asymptomatic patients is fasting plasma glucose according to the guidelines of the American Diabetes Association. Fasting values are a simpler, economically more feasible measure than an oral glucose tolerance test, and yield an earlier diagnosis. Values of 126 mg/dL or higher are suggested as diagnostic because that fasting value predicts a 2-hour postmeal value of 200 mg/dL. The suggested fasting value of 126 mg/dL replaced the older standard of 140 mg/dL and is intended to diagnose diabetes at an earlier stage and afford opportunity for intervention. The new guidelines also include the concept of impaired fasting glucose (values from 110 to 126 mg/dL) to replace the older concept of impaired glucose tolerance. Patients with impaired fasting glucose are at risk for diabetes and its vascular complications. Just repeating the random plasma glucose (**choice E**) is incorrect management.

    Measuring a single fasting plasma glucose and corresponding insulin values (**choice B**) provides no more information than the glucose measurement alone.

    Oral glucose tolerance tests (**choice C**) are often inconvenient and costly, and require a defined protocol so that their use in office practice is not feasible.

    Although HbA1c (**choice D**) measurements have been advocated by some as a criterion for the diagnosis of diabetes, the concept has not received widespread acceptance.

21. **The correct answer is B.** This patient suffers from a common dermatologic problem called tinea cruris, or "jock itch." This is best treated with antifungal creams with activity against *Candida* species as well as against the culprit dermatophyte. Although the dermatophyte has caused the rash, *Candida* is everywhere and should be covered to avoid a candidal superinfection (**choice C**). The clinical clue to help differentiate tinea from *Candida* is the sparing of the testicles, which is seen in tinea. A true candidal rash will often involve the testicles and show satellite lesions consisting of red papules nearby. It is true that patients with diabetes mellitus are more prone to dermatophyte and candidal infections.

    Although it is true that mostly postpubertal males become infected with jock itch, or tinea cruris, age has no correlation to candidal infections (**choice A**). Infants are often infected with candidal rashes (diaper rash) as well as women with pendulous breasts (submammary candidal infections).

    Smokers do not have a higher incidence of bacterial or fungal infections (**choices D and E**). They do, however, heal more slowly. If a smoker has facial surgery, it is usually recommended to cease smoking to allow for proper healing. Topical steroids are not a good choice to treat fungal infections as they may mask the infection temporarily but do not cure it and often exacerbate it. Topical steroid creams can calm down the inflammation and pruritus but an antifungal/anticandidal agent must be used in addition to complete the treatment.

22. **The correct answer is C.** This patient is experiencing a syncopal episode secondary to heart block. The EKG shows a 1:4 block without prolongation of the PR interval, which is consistent with second-degree AV block Mobitz type II. This type of AV block usually reflects significant disease of the conduction system. This block is inherently unstable and can degenerate to complete heart block; therefore, pacemaker implantation is necessary in this case and the patient requires a permanent

pacemaker as opposed to a temporary pacemaker (**choice D**), which will be more appropriate in reversible causes of heart block (e.g., digoxin toxicity).

Atropine (**choice A**) is usually used in the acute management of bradyarrhythmias, symptomatic sinus bradycardia in the setting of acute myocardial infarction, or lesser degrees of AV block (Mobitz type I).

Isoproterenol (**choice B**) can be used in the acute treatment of bradyarrhythmias if atropine fails (but not in the setting of myocardial infarction where it will exacerbate cardiac ischemia).

Simply observing and providing no further treatment at this time (**choice E**) is inappropriate as he can develop complete heart block and therefore requires pacemaker implantation.

23. **The correct answer is E.** This patient has advanced metastatic prostate carcinoma, which is infiltrating his bone marrow (as evidenced by pancytopenia). The patient has symptomatic anemia so a blood transfusion is appropriate. The patient also has thrombocytopenia and is actively bleeding (positive stool guaiac) which is an indication for platelet transfusion regardless of the platelet count in this clinical setting (**choice A**).

DDAVP or desmopressin (**choice C**) is indicated in mild hemophilia, von Willebrand disease, and platelet dysfunction secondary to uremia.

Cryoprecipitate (**choice B**) is derived from FFP and contains factor VIII-C, von Willebrand factor, fibrinogen, and factor XIII. It is indicated in hypofibrinogenemia, von Willebrand disease (when DDAVP is not available), or hemophilia A (only when factor VIII concentrate is not available).

Fresh-frozen plasma (FFP) contains all coagulation factors and fibrinogen (**choice D**) and is indicated in patients who are bleeding secondary to coagulopathy such as liver disease, warfarin overdose, or DIC.

24. **The correct answer is B.** This patient is presenting with a hot, red, and tender joint, in which case septic arthritis needs to be excluded and a knee joint arthrocentesis is warranted, especially in this patient who has a predisposing condition (osteoarthritis); therefore, reassuring him that this is most likely a flare-up of his osteoarthritis and discharging him on pain medications (**choice C**) is incorrect.

Serum uric acid level (**choice A**) is not indicated in the diagnosis of gout because hyperuricemia might be present but is not diagnostic.

Intravenous antibiotics (**choice D**) should be started after the arthrocentesis is done based on the suspected organism (neisserial vs. non-neisserial) and adjusted according to the findings of the joint fluid culture and sensitivity. Monoarticular gouty arthritis can mimic septic arthritis; fortunately aspiration of the synovial fluid and analysis with Gram stain, cultures, and polarized light microscopic examination will distinguish between them.

Intravenous colchicine (**choice E**) is indicated in the treatment of acute gout only as a second-line agent if the patient is unable to tolerate NSAIDs or take oral medications.

25. **The correct answer is E.** This elderly lady has developed asteatotic dermatitis on the parts of her body that are exposed to hydrotherapy several times a week. Asteatotic dermatitis, also known as xerotic eczema or "winter itch," is a mildly inflammatory variant of dermatitis that develops most commonly on the lower legs of elderly individuals during dry times of year. Prolonged soaking of the skin in hot water commonly induces asteatotic dermatitis by destroying the healthy barrier function of the skin. Fine cracks, with or without erythema, characteristically develop on the anterior surface of the lower extremities. Pruritus is variable. Asteatotic eczema responds well to avoidance of irritants, rehydration of the skin, and application of topical emollients.

Normally, asteatotic dermatitis does improve (**choice A**), albeit incompletely, with warmer, more humid weather, but this patient's asteatotic dermatitis was not weather induced (as witnessed by her normal-appearing skin above the waistline). Also, it would be inappropriate not to offer treatment for a symptomatic skin disease that can be resolved significantly faster if treatment is initiated.

If the detergent this woman has been using (**choice B**) for her laundry was causing her skin lesions, they would not be localized to the lower half of the body only but would be widespread and have the clinical appearance of contact dermatitis (red, scaly, crusted patches, and plaques). Changing the detergent will not improve her asteatotic dermatitis. The fact that she does not have dry, itchy skin on her upper body indicates that this is something that she has been coming into contact with (and not an oral medication) that is the culprit of her condition.

Neither ibuprofen (**choice C**) nor valsartan (**choice D**) is known to cause asteatotic dermatitis.

26. **The correct answer is C.** This patient has an acute exacerbation of chronic osteomyelitis. The most appropriate initial treatment for this type of infection is intravenous antibiotics with surgical debridement of the affected bone and surrounding soft tissue. Osteomyelitis, an infection of bone, is caused most commonly by pyogenic bacteria and mycobacteria. Microorganisms enter bone by the hematogenous route, by direct introduction from a contiguous focus of infection, or by a penetrating wound. Trauma, ischemia, and foreign bodies enhance the susceptibility of bone to microbial invasion by exposing sites to which bacteria can bind. Phagocytes attempt to contain the infections and, in the process, release enzymes that lyse bone. Pus spreads into vascular channels, raising intraosseous pressure and impairing the flow of blood; as the untreated infection becomes chronic, ischemic necrosis of bone results in the separation of large devascularized fragments (sequestra). When pus breaks through the cortex, subperiosteal or soft tissue abscesses form, and the elevated periosteum deposits new bone (the involucrum) around the sequestrum. Osteomyelitis secondary to a contiguous focus of infection is a broad category of osteomyelitis that includes infections introduced by penetrating injuries and surgical procedures and by direct extension of infection from adjacent soft tissues. It accounts for the greatest number of cases of osteomyelitis and occurs most commonly in adults. Frequently, the diagnosis is not made until the infection has already become chronic. The pain, fever, and inflammatory signs due to acute osteomyelitis may be attributed to the original injury or soft tissue infection. An indolent infection may become apparent only weeks or months later, when a sinus tract develops, a surgical wound breaks down, or a fracture fails to heal. It may be impossible to distinguish radiographic abnormalities due to osteomyelitis from those due to the precipitating condition. The role of diagnostic imaging in chronic osteomyelitis is to determine the presence of active infection and delineate the extent of debridement necessary to remove necrotic bone and abnormal soft tissues. Although plain films accurately reflect chronic changes, the computerized tomography scan is more sensitive for the detection of sequestra, sinus tracts, and soft tissue abscesses. Magnetic resonance imaging provides detailed information about the activity and the anatomic extent of infection but does not always distinguish osteomyelitis from healing fractures and tumors. Antibiotics are administered only after appropriate specimens have been obtained for culture. The antibiotics selected should be bactericidal and, at least initially, should be given intravenously. The success of therapy for chronic osteomyelitis rests largely on the complete surgical removal of necrotic bone and abnormal soft tissues. Even when diagnosed early, contiguous-focus osteomyelitis usually requires surgery in addition to 4 to 6 weeks of appropriate antibiotic therapy because of underlying soft tissue infection or damage to bone from an injury or surgery.

Amputation of the distal phalanx (**choice A**) is hardly an acceptable initial treatment option for an otherwise healthy 35-year-old person, but if intravenous antibiotics and surgical debridement fail to clear the infection, it may come up as an option later down the road.

Intravenous antibiotics (**choice B**) will achieve adequate levels of medication in the healthy bone, but the necrotic bone and infected soft tissue surrounding it must be surgically removed to provide good conditions for cure of the osteomyelitis.

If initial treatment with intravenous antibiotics and surgical debridement fail to cure the osteomyelitis, oral antibiotics alone (**choice D**) may be elected by the patient as an alternative to multiple surgeries. However, they may eventually have to consider amputation if the infection spreads to involve more proximal structures.

If oral antibiotics do not achieve adequate stable bone levels of the medication and if a patient elects to undergo surgical debridement it would be inappropriate to use oral antibiotics to supplement it (**choice E**); intravenous antibiotics should be administered.

27. **The correct answer is C.** This patient has erysipeloid, an acute bacterial infection of traumatized skin. It is caused by the microorganism *Erysipelothrix rhusiopathiae* (insidiosa), which has long been known to cause animal and human infections. Direct contact between meat infected with *Erysipelothrix rhusiopathiae* and traumatized human skin results in erysipeloid. In animals, the organism causes swine erysipelas and several other diseases in poultry and sheep. Erysipeloid is an occupational disease acquired after direct contact with infected animals. The disease is more common among farmers, butchers, cooks, housewives, and fishermen and more likely to occur during the summer or early fall. The organ most commonly affected other than the skin is the heart. Erysipeloid is usually an acute, self-limited infection of the skin that resolves without consequences. Individuals with the systemic form, in which organs other than the skin are involved, may have neurologic, cardiologic, or other organ involvement. Rarely, death due to sepsis may occur. In the cutaneous form patients present with local burning or pain at the site of injury. They may or may not have fever, malaise, and other constitutional symptoms. The generalized form of infection presents with fever, chills, weight loss, and a variety of other symptoms (e.g., joint pain, cough,

headache), depending on the organ system involved. The most common location of cutaneous infection is on the hands, mainly the webs of the fingers; however, any exposed area of the body may be affected. Well-demarcated, bright red-to-purple, tender, warm plaques with a smooth, shiny surface develop. They leave a brownish discoloration on the skin when resolving. Vesicles may be present. The treatment of choice is oral penicillin. Erythromycin in combination with rifampin may be used if the patient is allergic to penicillin. The cutaneous forms of erysipeloid are self-limited and may remit spontaneously within 2 to 4 weeks; however, treatment with penicillin 250 to 500 mg PO qid for 7 to 10 days hastens the recovery and limits further progression of the disease. Patients should be educated to use care when handling animals and their products.

Intralesional triamcinolone acetonide (**choice A**) is not indicated for the treatment of skin infections of any kind. It is often used for cystic acne lesions, or keloids, where excessive scarring is a concern. Monthly injections of varying strength, anywhere between 5 and 40 mg/mL are injected intralesionally with the goal of preventing exuberant inflammation and fibroblast activity that would result in unsightly scars or keloids.

Local surgical debridement (**choice B**) is not indicated in treating erysipeloid. This method of treatment is utilized when a localized area of necrotic tissue harbors microorganisms that cannot be suppressed solely with antibiotics.

Terbinafine (**choice D**) is an antifungal medication used in the treatment of dermatophyte infections of the skin, hair, and nails. The above given dosage of 250 mg PO qd for 3 months is the standard when treating onychomycosis.

Topical Neosporin ointment (**choice E**) would not affect the natural course of erysipeloid and is not indicated. Even though localized erysipeloid without systemic symptoms may be left to resolve spontaneously, it is recommended that even mild cases receive oral antibiotics to prevent complications.

28. **The correct answer is A.** This patient is experiencing signs and symptoms of acute bronchoconstriction induced by exercise. The first medication to use is an inhaled beta agonist like albuterol or isoproterenol, which can be repeated every 20 min three times and the frequency reduced thereafter. These medications are more potent than intravenous aminophylline (**choice D**), which has no role in exercise-induced asthma.

Inhaled corticosteroids, such as beclomethasone (**choice B**), or intravenous corticosteroids, such as methylprednisolone (**choice E**), will have a delayed onset of action if they are going to be beneficial at all.

Inhaled cromolyn sodium (**choice C**) is usually used for prophylaxis of exercise-induced bronchoconstriction and is not effective in the acute episodes of bronchoconstriction. It is usually taken 15 to 20 min before exercise.

29. **The correct answer is B.** This young, previously healthy woman has a classic syndrome of acute pancreatitis manifested by epigastric pain radiating to the back, vomiting, and elevated pancreatic enzyme levels. The aim is to find a cause that can be treated to prevent subsequent attacks. Abdominal ultrasonography is indicated to look for gallstones, which are the most common cause of acute pancreatitis, and for choledocholithiasis.

An abdominal computed tomographic (CT) scan (**choice A**) will show pancreatic edema but is less sensitive for gallstones.

Endoscopic retrograde cholangiopancreatography (ERCP) (**choice C**) does not visualize the gallbladder well and is not indicated in the acute setting without signs of biliary obstruction or severe pancreatitis.

Oral cholecystography (**choice D**) is not sufficiently accurate to use as a diagnostic test in this situation

A plain abdominal radiographic series (**choice E**) will be of little utility because a perforated viscus has been excluded by the absence of free peritoneal air on the upright chest radiograph. It is uncommon to find gallstones or pancreatic calcifications on plain radiographs.

30. **The correct answer is D.** The available history and exam information is consistent with a diagnosis of inadequately treated hyperthyroidism. Therefore, PTU, an inhibitor of thyroxine biosynthesis, is an appropriate choice.

Ketoconazole (**choice A**), an imidazole antifungal agent that can inhibit steroidal biosynthesis, has no role in the management of hyperthyroidism.

Nitroglycerin (**choice B**), used for blood pressure control and the management of angina, has no role in the management of hyperthyroidism in a patient without hypertension or coronary ischemia.

Nitroprusside (**choice C**), a nitric oxide-liberating agent used in the management of hypertensive urgencies and emergencies, has no role in the management of hyperthyroidism.

Spironolactone (**choice E**), an aldosterone antagonist, has no role in the management of hyperthyroidism.

31. **The correct answer is B.** This patient is presenting with features of atypical pneumonia secondary to *Mycoplasma pneumoniae. Mycoplasma* is the most common cause of pneumonia in school children and young healthy adults. Diagnosis is made based on the clinical setting and confirmed by positive cold agglutinins or complement fixation test. Treatment is usually with oral erythromycin or azithromycin.

Legionella pneumophila, which is usually treated with intravenous erythromycin (**choice A**), causes atypical pneumonia. It is suspected in high-risk patients (smokers, alcoholics, advanced age, renal failure) presenting with symptoms suggestive of multisystem disease. Symptoms include cough, fever, headache, watery diarrhea, nausea and vomiting, and neuropsychiatric symptoms (confusion, disorientation, and hallucinations). Diagnosis is by finding elevated serum aminotransferases and positive urine radioimmunoassay (RIA). Treatment is with a macrolide; if erythromycin is used then a higher dose is needed (i.e., 1000 mg every 6 hours).

Although *Pneumocystis carinii* pneumonia (PCP) will give you a similar picture on the CXR, the clinical picture doesn't correlate with it. PCP usually has an insidious onset with progressive dyspnea on exertion as the main symptom. The patient is usually hypoxemic (decreased O_2 sat on room air). Diagnosis is confirmed by elevated LDH, increased A-a gradient, and low CD4 count in an HIV-infected patient. PCP is treated with trimethoprim-sulfamethoxazole (**choice C**).

This patient is unlikely to have interstitial lung disease, which is a chronic and progressive disease with mainly dyspnea on exertion. Interstitial lung disease shows diffuse interstitial infiltrates on CXR. Diagnosis is confirmed by PFTs (**choice E**), which shows a restrictive pattern, or high-resolution CT scans (**choice D**).

32. **The correct answer is C.** Given the dramatic drop in platelets with the introduction of heparin therapy, this patient most likely has the immune form of heparin-induced thrombocytopenia (HIT). To prevent continued thrombocytopenia and thrombosis, the treatment is immediate discontinuation of heparin.

Cryoprecipitate (**choice A**) is not warranted in this instance since the patient is not coagulopathic, or lacking in any of the factors concentrated in cryoprecipitate (e.g., factor VIII).

Changing the unfractionated heparin to low molecular weight heparin (**choice B**) will not help since low molecular weight heparin is as antigenic as unfractionated heparin in the setting of HIT, and will lead to ongoing platelet clumping and subsequently to thrombosis.

Transfusing platelets (**choice D**) is inappropriate since it will only provide more substrate (i.e., platelets) for clumping while the patient is exposed to heparin.

Transfusing whole blood (**choice E**) will also provide the platelet substrate for ongoing platelet clumping while the patient is receiving heparin. There is also no indication for the other components of whole blood (i.e., red cells) in this patient.

33. **The correct answer is A.** This patient has symptomatic hyperkalemia secondary to a potassium-sparing diuretic (triamterene). Treatment of hyperkalemia depends on the clinical and EKG findings. This patient has EKG changes so the first medication to use is calcium gluconate for its cardioprotective effect.

Dextrose and insulin (**choice B**) should be given after that. They work by temporarily shifting potassium intracellularly. It takes 30 min for the agents to work, but lasts only for a short time.

Beta agonists, such as albuterol (**choice C**), are indicated in the treatment of hyperkalemia and work by shifting the potassium intracellularly. They also work temporarily. As stated above though, this patient has EKG changes and therefore first needs calcium gluconate for its cardioprotective effect.

Potassium-binding resins, such as sodium polystyrene sulfonate (**choice D**), should be given and are effective in 1 to 4 hours. It removes potassium by exchanging sodium ions for potassium ions in the intestines before it is passed with stools and is a definitive treatment for hyperkalemia. It may be repeated every 6 hours.

Hemodialysis (**choice E**) is indicated for the treatment of hyperkalemia in patients with renal failure or if the other measures are ineffective.

34. **The correct answer is C.** Imipenem is a good broad-spectrum antibiotic, which has a known side effect of lowering the seizure threshold and is therefore contraindicated in patients with prior history of seizures (unless absolutely necessary).

Cephalexin (**choice A**) is a cephalosporin that has been known to cause skin hypersensitivity reactions in patients allergic to penicillins or cephalosporins, but it does not typically induce seizures.

Clindamycin (**choice B**) has an excellent coverage for anaerobic and gram-positive bacteria, but it does not cover the gram-negative spectrum. It has been associated with *C. difficile* pseudomembranous colitis.

Levofloxacin (**choice D**) is known to cause an allergic rash and tendonitis.

Ticarcillin/clavulanic acid (**choice E**) is a penicillin class antibiotic with good gram-positive, gram-negative, and anaerobic coverage. At the doses used today, it's not known to cause seizures. Penicillin was known in the 1950s to cause seizure disorder at doses of 60 million and higher when other antibiotics were not available and high doses of penicillin was commonly used. Today this is seldom seen with penicillin antibiotics due to the lower dosages used.

35. **The correct answer is E.** The patient most likely has acute hypersensitivity pneumonia (allergic alveolitis) because of the presence of arthralgia, shortness of breath, bilateral crackles, reticular nodular opacities and patchy infiltrates, and exposure to parakeets for several weeks. Removal of the causative agents is sufficient treatment of patients with mild-to-moderate symptoms.

This patient's findings are also suggestive of sarcoidosis, in which angiotensin-converting enzyme levels (**choice A**) may be helpful, but sarcoidosis is a diagnosis of exclusion. With the bird exposure, hypersensitivity pneumonitis is much more likely and therefore a trial of avoidance of the most likely causative agent is the best next step in management.

Sputum cultures (**choice B**) will not help in the diagnosis of hypersensitivity pneumonias because there is no infectious agent involved.

Lung tissue biopsy (**choice C**) may be needed if there is no relief of the symptoms after removal of the causative agent, but it is not necessary with the clinical characteristics of this patient.

Psittacosis, a pneumonia caused by *Chlamydia psittaci* and transmitted to humans by certain birds, is extremely unlikely without fever or headache. It is usually treated with tetracycline or doxycycline (**choice D**); however, a 10 to 14 day, oral, outpatient therapy is most likely appropriate.

36. **The correct answer is B.** This patient likely has a pulmonary embolus (PE) as evidenced by the proximity to high-risk surgery, tachypnea, tachycardia, and hypoxemia. A ventilation-perfusion scan allows the radiologist to determine if there are any areas of the lung that are being perfused without being ventilated, causing a shunt and hypoxemia. This is a highly specific, but insensitive, method. Thus, a negative result argues against PE, a positive result (especially in the presence of classic symptomatology) supports the diagnosis, but an indeterminate result necessitates further studies.

Extending her hospital stay for oxygen therapy (**choice A**) is not the appropriate next step in management because she needs to be evaluated and treated for a pulmonary embolism. It is likely that her hospital stay will need to be extended, but this decision should be made after diagnostic studies are performed.

Spiral CT scan (**choice C**) can be an alternative to traditional ventilation-perfusion scanning. Its disadvantages include dye exposure and increased incidence of false-positive results. It also has decreased ability to detect peripheral emboli and is more expensive than traditional V/Q scanning.

Venogram (**choice D**) is the gold standard in the diagnosis of DVT. It is currently replaced by lower extremity ultrasound because of decreased cost and decreased number of side effects such as phlebitis, pain, and even DVT.

Pulmonary angiogram (**choice E**) remains the gold standard for diagnosis of pulmonary embolus but it is an invasive procedure with some risk (e.g., allergic dye reaction and acute renal failure [ATN] secondary to dye). It is indicated for patients with high suspicion of pulmonary embolus but with nondiagnostic ventilation-perfusion scan and negative lower extremity ultrasound.

37. **The correct answer is E.** A large proportion of the population will suffer lower back pain at some point in their life and more than 90% of the time the pain resolves within a month. Inappropriate workup of these patients can lead to needless and expensive testing. The appropriate management of a patient who presents with back pain without red flags for infection or cancer and without any neurological deficits is conservative management and a return to activities as tolerated. Red flags are fever, injection drug use, history of cancer, unexplained weight loss, and advanced age. Acetaminophen or nonsteroidal anti-inflammatory agents can be used for pain relief as needed.

Bed rest (**choice A**) is no longer recommended for patients with back pain. Controlled studies have shown that there is no benefit to bed rest and it might even delay the return to normal activities. Patients should be encouraged to resume ambulating as soon as possible.

Most cases of back pain can be managed by the primary care physician and an orthopedic consult is unnecessary (**choice B**). Orthopedic or neurological consultation is required if there is significant neurological deficits, cauda equina syndrome, epidural abscess, or spinal metastasis. Consultation can also be considered for back pain that continues for more than 1 month.

Imaging of the spine with an x-ray (**choice C**) or an MRI (**choice D**) is not required in most patients who present with lower back pain. In a patient who presents with back pain along with signs of the cauda equina syndrome, a stat MRI along with urgent surgical consultation is required. Other instances where an early MRI would be considered are where there is a concern for an epidural abscess or in a patient with cancer and possible spinal metastasis. Likewise routine plain films are unnecessary in young patients without red flags for cancer or infection but are required if there is any concern for fracture or history of trauma.

38. **The correct answer is A.** If there are no contraindications, the first medication to use for diabetic patients with hypertension is an ACE inhibitor. This class of agents has been proven to reduce the incidence of diabetic nephropathy; in fact, if microalbuminuria exists in a diabetic patient, most practitioners would recommend an ACE inhibitor regardless of blood pressure.

Clonidine (**choice B**) is inappropriate as a first- or even second-line agent in this case. This medication may cause severe rebound hypertension and is usually only used if a patient is already at maximum dose of several other antihypertensive agents.

Felodipine (**choice C**) and hydrochlorothiazide (**choice D**) are also inappropriate to begin therapy for this patient since they offer no additional benefits. However, if the patient does not respond sufficiently to an ACE inhibitor, they may be added as second-line drugs.

Losartan (**choice E**) is incorrect since this is an angiotensin receptor blocker. Although some studies show that this class of medications may also offer protection against diabetic nephropathy, they should be reserved for patients who are unable to tolerate or who have failed treatment with ACE inhibitors.

Metoprolol (**choice F**) may be an appropriate second choice if the patient does not achieve adequate control on an ACE inhibitor. However, caution should be used in this particular patient given her history of depression.

39. **The correct answer is E.** Epiglottitis is classically described as a sequelae of *Haemophilus influenzae* type B infection. With the advent of the vaccination for children, this has largely become a disease of adulthood. Symptoms of epiglottitis include sore throat, dyspnea, odynophagia (pain with swallowing), and a change in the character of voice. Signs include tachycardia, a muffled voice, difficulty controlling one's own saliva (secretions), and the so-called sniffing position, in which a patient tilts their head upward and appears to be sniffing a scent in the air (to open their airway). By the time patients demonstrate oxygen desaturation, they may be in the midst of imminent airway collapse. If there is a worrisome level of airway compromise, these patients often require intubation for 1 to 4 days to allow for resolution and safe extubation.

In cases of suspected epiglottitis, it is important not to instrument the airway with a tongue depressor (**choice A**) or other devices. This has the potential to trigger spasm of the larynx and acute airway occlusion.

Because the patient has a muffled voice and has adopted the sniffing position, it is more likely that there is some narrowing of the airway, particularly at the larynx where a moderate amount of swelling can be especially problematic. As such, she has more-worrisome findings than someone with simple tonsillitis (**choice B**) or a viral URI (**choice C**).

Referring her to an otolaryngologist for biopsy of a possible throat lesion within the next several days (**choice D**) is incorrect because the patient has an acute process and airway compromise that requires immediate attention.

40. **The correct answer is D.** This patient has necrobiosis lipoidica (diabeticorum). Lesions of necrobiosis lipoidica are found primarily on the shins (90%), and most patients either have diabetes mellitus or develop it subsequently. Characteristic plaques begin as erythematous papules that enlarge and develop a central yellow color, atrophy, telangiectases, and an erythematous border. Ulcerations can also develop within the plaques. Biopsy specimens show necrobiosis of collagen, granulomatous inflammation, and obliterative endarteritis. Best treatment results are attained using potent topical steroids or intralesional steroids to treat early lesions that have not yet developed the central atrophy, which is permanent. Atrophy, telangiectases, and ulceration are signs of advanced fibrosis and scarring that cannot be reversed. Even though necrobiosis lipoidica diabeticorum more commonly develops in patients with poorly regulated blood glucose levels, getting them under good long-term control does not influence progression of the skin condition.

Montelukast (**choice A**) is a leukotriene receptor antagonist approved by the United States Food and Drug Administration (FDA) for prophylaxis and maintenance treatment of asthma in children 2 years and older and adults. The most common adverse event reported by adults and adolescents receiving montelukast was headache (18.4 versus 18.1% of patients on montelukast and placebo, respectively). Other less common adverse events reported more commonly with montelukast than placebo during clinical trials included dyspepsia, asthenia, rash, gastroenteritis, and fever.

The etiology of necrobiosis lipoidica diabeticorum is not known, but it is highly associated with diabetes mellitus (90% of patients with necrobiosis lipoidica have diabetes), and early lesions may be successfully treated with topical or intralesional steroids. Therefore, it is incorrect that it is an idiopathic skin condition unrelated to his other diseases and medications, and there is no successful treatment available (**choice B**).

Necrobiosis lipoidica is not associated with hypertension (**choice C**), but with diabetes. Sometimes, early lesions can be treated with topical corticosteroids with satisfactory results. Lesions in the atrophic stage leave permanent sequelae on the skin.

Even though necrobiosis lipoidica diabeticorum more commonly develops in patients with poorly regulated blood glucose levels, getting their diabetes under good long-term control does not influence progression of the skin condition (**choice E**).

41. **The correct answer is C.** This patient has arsenical keratoses, "raindrop" hypo- and hyperpigmentation of the trunk, and a superficial basal cell carcinoma, a recognized syndrome known to result from long-term ingestion of arsenic, usually in the inorganic, trivalent form. For a physician, the most critical steps toward recognizing this disorder, and other heavy metal poisonings, is remembering to consider them in the differential diagnosis and taking an appropriate environmental/occupational history as part of the medical workup. The level of detail that is called for depends on the clinical situation. Information should always be obtained on current and major past occupations, and patients should be asked whether they think their health problem is related to their work or to any particular environment or exposure. In the review of systems, patients should be asked if they have been exposed to dusts, fumes, chemicals, radiation, or loud noise. Basal cell and squamous cell carcinomas have been causally related to occupational and environmental exposure to arsenic. In chronic arsenic poisoning, the onset of symptoms is from weeks to years after the exposure. Typical findings are skin and nail changes, such as punctate hyperkeratosis of the palms and soles (especially pressure points), "raindrop" hyperpigmentation, exfoliative dermatitis, and Mees lines (transverse white striae of the fingernails); sensory and motor polyneuritis manifesting as numbness and tingling in a "stocking-glove" distribution, distal weakness, and quadriplegia; and inflammation of the respiratory mucosa. Epidemiological evidence has linked chronic consumption of water containing arsenic at concentrations in the range of 10 to 1820 ppb with diabetes, vasospasm, and peripheral vascular insufficiency culminating in "blackfoot disease," a gangrenous condition affecting the extremities. Chronic arsenic exposure has also been associated with a greatly elevated risk of skin cancer and possibly of cancers of the lung, liver (angiosarcoma), bladder, kidney, and colon. Significant exposure to arsenic occurs through both anthropogenic and natural sources. Arsenic is released into the air by volcanoes and is a natural contaminant of some deep-water wells. Occupational exposure to arsenic is common in the smelting industry (in which arsenic is a byproduct of ores containing lead, gold, zinc, cobalt, and nickel) and is increasing in the microelectronics industry (in which gallium arsenide is responsible). Low-level arsenic exposure continues to take place in the general population (as do some cases of high-dose poisoning) through the commercial use of inorganic arsenic compounds in common products such as wood preservatives, pesticides, herbicides, fungicides, and paints; through the consumption of foods and the smoking of tobacco treated with arsenic-containing pesticides; and through the burning of fossil fuels in which arsenic is a contaminant. Treatment of the arsenical keratoses is not mandatory, but may be useful to palliate tenderness in lesions of the palms and soles. Any destructive method is satisfactory, but the lesions often recur. The skin cancers should be treated accordingly.

The patient's marital history (**choice A**) is irrelevant in establishing a connection of the skin lesions with an occupational or environmental factor.

Wood preservatives, pesticides, herbicides, fungicides, and paints have been known to cause increased exposure to inorganic arsenic, but not cleaning solutions (**choice B**).

Contemporary medications used in the treatment of hypertension and insomnia do not contain arsenic and, in addition to that, this patient has been on medication only for the past 2 years, whereas his skin lesions date back at least 5 years. Therefore inquiring about medications he takes for his blood pressure and sleeping problem (**choice D**) would not solve the quandary of his skin disease.

The question as to when his new house was built (**choice E**) would be relevant if you suspected lead poisoning because, up to the early seventies, lead-containing paints were widely used in the construction business.

42. **The correct answer is D.** This patient exhibits symptoms consistent with acute hepatitis A infection. These typically include fever, anorexia, malaise, vomiting, diarrhea, and jaundice. While jaundice is rare in younger children, in adolescents it is quite common (occurring in >70% of cases of hepatitis A). Hepatitis A is an RNA virus that is spread through the fecal-oral route and has an incubation period between 15 and 30 days. Hepatitis A is a common illness in travelers to endemic areas. Fortunately, there is a safe and effective vaccine for prevention of this disease.

    Although this patient may be at risk for a variety of other diseases from his recent unprotected sexual encounter (**choice A**), including HIV and hepatitis B, hepatitis A is not spread sexually.

    Some of the viral hepatitides (including hepatitis B and C) can cause chronic hepatitis in a substantial proportion of cases, but this is not the case with hepatitis A (**choice B**).

    Hepatitis C, originally called transfusion-associated hepatitis, is one of the major bloodborne pathogens that screening of the blood supply is directed against. Hepatitis A is not transmitted through contact with the blood of an affected patient (**choice C**).

    Ribavirin (**choice E**), an antiviral medication with activity against several pathogenic viruses, including respiratory syncytial virus, has no role in the treatment of hepatitis A infection. Treatment is supportive and, as mentioned above, most cases are self-limited.

43. **The correct answer is C.** Primary hyperparathyroidism and malignancy account for most cases of hyperparathyroidism. Finding elevated calcium with an elevated PTH (or high normal) is diagnostic of primary hyperparathyroidism. Of the patients with primary hyperparathyroidism, adenoma accounts for >80%, while parathyroid carcinoma (**choice D**) accounts for <5%. The remaining patients have parathyroid hyperplasia.

    Multiple myeloma (**choice A**) would be suggested by anemia, fatigue, back pain, renal failure, etc. These findings, along with a *low* PTH level, warrant evaluation with an SPEP and UPEP. High PTH levels are not consistent with malignancy.

    Osteoporosis (**choice B**) is the result of hypercalcemia, not a cause. Osteoporosis is an indication for surgery in primary hyperparathyroidism. Other indications for surgery include urolithiasis, creatinine clearance <70%, serum calcium levels <11.5 mg/dL, age <50 years, or marked hypercalcuria.

    Squamous cell cancers (**choice E**) can cause hypercalcemia via release of parathyroid hormone-related protein. Patients classicly have abrupt, symptomatic onset of their hypercalcemia. Their serum PTH level is low.

44. **The correct answer is C.** The treatment for hypoglycemia is obviously to give glucose; D50 provides a sufficient amount of glucose that should quickly reverse this patient's altered mental status. However, due to the long-acting nature of the NPH insulin that she takes (which can peak 6 to 12 hours after and last for 18 to 24 hours), it would be prudent to observe the patient and continue glucose infusion. For this patient, alcohol may have depressed hepatic glucose production, although other causes should be carefully evaluated. It is not unusual for patients with frequent hypoglycemia to develop "hypoglycemic unawareness," where patients do not develop typical symptoms of hypoglycemia and can instead present in stupor or coma.

    A CT of the head (**choice A**) is not indicated as mental status changes and even focal neurological findings can be due to hypoglycemia, and treatment should not be delayed.

    Given the patient's degree of hypoglycemia, D5W is unlikely to be adequate (**choice B**). Similarly, dextrose 50% followed by NS infusion (**choice D**) will predispose the patient to hypoglycemia after the D50 is given.

    Glucagon (**choice E**) should be available for conditions where IV access is not available, as it can be given IM or SC; however, it can lead to vomiting and especially in a patient with altered mental status with IV access would not be the therapy of choice.

    Normal saline (**choice F**) is the initial fluid of choice in nonketotic hyperosmolar state, where patients often present profoundly volume depleted.

    Even if the patient were fully alert and able to safely drink orange juice (**choice G**), her history of diabetes complications consistent with gastroparesis may indicate gastroparesis, which would delay the absorption of orange juice.

45. **The correct answer is E.** Based on the available history and physical examination, this patient has cardiac tamponade. The electrocardiographic correlate of a pericardial effusion (and tamponade) is pulsus alternans – a phenomenon where the amplitude of the QRS changes from beat to beat. This is believed to be a result of the heart shifting within the fluid-filled pericardium with each beat and thus varying its electrical vector.

Left ventricular hypertrophy (**choice A**) is not associated with pericardial tamponade.

A new left bundle branch block (**choice B**), while being associated with myocardial ischemia, is not associated with pericardial tamponade.

Peaked T waves (**choice C**) can be seen with metabolic abnormalities such as hyperkalemia, but are not associated with pericardial tamponade.

A prolonged QT interval (**choice D**) can be seen with metabolic abnormalities such as hypomagnesemia or hypocalcemia, but is not associated with pericardial tamponade.

46. **The correct answer is A.** Fibromyalgia is a common condition involving mostly women (90% of cases). It is characterized by widespread or diffuse pain with symmetric tender points. No pathological factors can be elicited on physical examination and laboratory test results are often normal. Fatigue is associated with muscle pain in 90% of the affected patients. It tends to relate to lack of prolonged periods of deep restful sleep. The differential diagnosis in these patients includes polymyalgia rheumatica, rheumatoid arthritis, polymyositis, systemic lupus erythematosus, hypothyroidism, paraneoplastic syndrome, and acute HIV infection. Normal physical examination and normal laboratory findings can help to exclude the above diagnoses. Fibromyalgia is a common diagnosis in patients with persistent joint pain. This can be treated with several nonsteroidal anti-inflammatory drugs and low-dose tricyclic antidepressant medication, which has pain-modulating and sedative properties.

Hypothyroidism (**choice B**) is associated with other systemic symptoms and signs and can be diagnosed by thyroid function test.

Polymyalgia rheumatica (**choice C**) can be diagnosed by clinical examination and serological testing.

Polymyositis is also associated with joint pain (**choice D**) but is usually diagnosed from clinical examination and serological testing.

Rheumatoid arthritis (**choice E**) can cause joint pain but is usually associated with several abnormalities on clinical examination and can be detected on serological testing.

47. **The correct answer is B.** This patient is suffering from gonococcal urethritis. This disease is caused by the gram-negative intracellular diplococcus *Neisseria gonorrhoeae*. Diagnosis is based on a history of sexual contact, purulent discharge with dysuria, and a positive Gram stain and/or culture. Culture inoculation uses a calcium alginate urethrogenital swab at least 1 hour after the patient last voided and is placed on a modified Thayer-Martin culture medium. Symptoms in males include urethral discharge and dysuria, and the incubation period is short (from 3 to 10 days). However, up to 60% of men may be asymptomatic. The current recommended treatment of gonococcal urethritis is 125 mg of ceftriaxone IM for one dose. Patients allergic to penicillin may receive a 1 time dose of ciprofloxacin or ofloxacin followed by doxycycline for 7 days. Because concurrent infection with *Chlamydia* is so common, it is recommended to treat for it simultaneously with 1 g of PO azithromycin or a 7-day course of oral doxycycline. It is imperative that all sexual contacts, whether symptomatic or not, should be examined, cultured, and treated. Also, cases of gonorrhea should be reported to the appropriate public health officials.

Azithromycin 1 g (**choice A**) is the treatment recommendation for nongonococcal urethritis (NGU). NGU is caused by *Chlamydia trachomatis, Ureaplasma urealyticum*, *Mycoplasma hominis,* or *Trichomonas vaginalis*. Incubation period is longer, 5 to 21 days, and discharge is watery or mucoid, whitish, and may or may not be associated with dysuria.

Acyclovir (**choice C**) is used for the treatment of genital herpes caused by the herpes simplex virus. Patients complain of painful pustules on the glans and shaft of penis along with constitutional symptoms such as fever, malaise, anorexia, and possibly urinary retention.

IM penicillin G (**choice D**) is the appropriate treatment for patients diagnosed with syphilis. Syphilis is caused by the spirochete *Treponema pallidum*. Incubation is 3 weeks and the primary lesions are painless and located on the glans and penis. The lesions disappear in 1 to 5 weeks.

It would be appropriate to provide the patient with literature on safe sexual practices since this process is a sexually transmitted disease (**choice E**). However, it is imperative that the infection be treated.

In this patient, signs, symptoms, and physical findings are classic for gonorrhea. Therefore, treatment should not be delayed while awaiting culture results (**choice F**).

48. **The correct answer is D.** This patient scenario is perfect for a deep venous thrombosis/pulmonary embolism. The patient had recent hip surgery, which is a significant risk factory in the development of deep venous thromboses. She is on no prophylactic medication to prevent DVTs. The patient has also been rather sedentary after her hip arthroplasty. She will require admission to an acute facility and either a V/Q scan, spiral CT scan, or pulmonary angiography. Due to the extremely high risk for this particular patient, many physicians would immediately heparinize this patient and then obtain a V/Q or CT scan with a duplex scan of the lower extremities to look for the source of the thrombus (likely the deep venous system of the proximal thigh or pelvis).

    The patient has the correct history and physical exam for a DVT/PE. There are no indications of reactive airway disease in this patient's history or physical exam (**choice A**).

    The patient has no fever, chills, or productive cough and no physical findings associated with pneumonia; therefore, there is no indication for cephalosporin (**choice B**).

    Giving warfarin may be the long-term treatment for this patient but in the acute setting warfarin will have no effect on further thrombus formation and embolization (**choice C**).

    This patient may very well have some component of atelectasis but this is usually associated with the first 24 to 48 hours postoperatively. If you send this patient home there is a high chance of further embolization and subsequent cardiopulmonary failure (**choice E**).

49. **The correct answer is C.** Since isotretinoin (Accutane) is teratogenic, before prescribing it to a female patient, the patient must have two negative pregnancy tests, one in the physician's office and one on the second day of her next period or 11 days after her last unprotected intercourse, whichever is later. A prescription for isotretinoin can be given only after these two separate tests. The patient must also be using two types of birth control methods for 1 month before starting treatment and for at least 1 month following discontinuation of the medication. Isotretinoin is only indicated in cases of severe recalcitrant nodular acne.

    It is inappropriate to check her records for previous lipid, CPK, and glucose levels and liver function tests; if normal give her a prescription for isotretinoin (**choice A**). First of all, the most important test is the pregnancy test. And while isotretinoin has been observed to affect lipids, CPK, LFTs, and glucose, it is probably best to obtain current pretreatment values.

    It would be wrong to do a urine pregnancy test and if negative give her a prescription for isotretinoin (**choice B**). Patients must have two negative pregnancy tests before starting isotretinoin.

    You must get two negative pregnancy tests, in addition to obtaining normal lipid, CPK, and glucose levels and liver function tests before giving her a prescription for isotretinoin (**choice D**).

    A pelvic ultrasound (**choice E**) is not performed before starting isotretinoin. Two negative urine pregnancy tests are enough.

50. **The correct answer is B.** Decreased night vision has been reported by patients taking isotretinoin. It is important to tell patients to be cautious when driving or operating any vehicle at night.

    Some patients taking isotretinoin have had elevated CPK levels after vigorous physical activity. Also, up to 16% of patients have experienced musculoskeletal symptoms, such as arthralgia. However, it is not appropriate to tell her to avoid all physical activity (**choice A**). It is best if she informs you of any planned vigorous physical activity, and you can make management decisions based on the specifics.

    Patients must use two separate and effective forms of contraception when taking isotretinoin, therefore it is inappropriate to tell her to make sure to use one form of birth control; it should be an effective one, such as an injectable/implantable contraceptive product (**choice C**).

    Patients taking isotretinoin cannot donate blood during treatment and for 1 month after discontinuing the drug. Telling her that she can donate blood at 3 weeks after discontinuation (**choice D**) is incorrect. This rule is to make sure that if a pregnant woman needs a blood transfusion, her fetus is not exposed to the drug.

    Patients taking isotretinoin should be advised *not* to take vitamin A-containing supplements because of the additive toxic effects that can occur because of the drug's relationship to vitamin A. It is incorrect to tell her to take a multivitamin with vitamin A (**choice E**).

    To avoid scarring, patients taking isotretinoin should be advised *not* to wax or have any skin resurfacing procedures done during and up to 6 months after treatment. Telling her to wax instead of shaving her legs and underarms (**choice F**) is incorrect.

Internal Medicine: **Test Three**

1. A 72-year-old man with coronary artery disease and mild emphysema comes to the clinic because of blood-tinged urine. He states that over the past several weeks he has had intermittent urine that appears slightly bloody. There has been no history of fever or chills. He denies any abdominal or flank pain and there has been no trauma. His temperature is 37.2 C (99.0 F), blood pressure is 130/90 mm Hg, pulse is 78/min, and respirations are 14/min. His lungs are clear and heart examination is remarkable for a 2/6 systolic ejection murmur. Abdomen is soft, nontender, with normal bowel sounds. No masses are palpable. No suprapubic tenderness is present. Rectal examination reveals a normal prostate and guaiac-negative stool. Laboratory studies show a leukocyte count of 7300/mm^3, platelet count of 335,000/mm^3, hematocrit of 48%, BUN of 20 mEq/L, and creatinine of 1.1 mEq/L. Urinalysis reveals >50 red blood cells/HPF, 1 to 2 leukocytes/HPF, and no casts or protein. The most appropriate next diagnostic is

   (A) a followup appointment with repeat urinalysis in 6 months
   (B) an intravenous pyelogram (IVP) and, if negative, a cystoscopy
   (C) a noncontrast CT scan of the abdomen and pelvis
   (D) a retrograde pyelogram
   (E) a testicular ultrasound

2. A 48-year-old man with no past medical or psychiatric history comes to the clinic for a "prescription to help my sexual dysfunction." He is having difficulty attaining an erection while trying to have sex with his wife. There are no physical examination abnormalities noted. The patient states that "I can't relax, even after I have several drinks." The most appropriate next step in management is to

   (A) order a penile nocturnal tumescence test
   (B) prescribe bupropion
   (C) prescribe sildenafil
   (D) recommend that the patient stop drinking prior to sexual intercourse
   (E) recommend that the patient temporarily stop attempting to have sexual intercourse

3. A 68-year-old woman comes to the health center for her annual visit. She states that she has been feeling well over the past year and has no complaints. Her past medical history is significant for pneumonia, for which she was hospitalized 3 years ago. Past surgical history is significant for a total abdominal hysterectomy and bilateral salpingo-oophorectomy that was performed at the age of 40 for fibroids. She takes no medications. She is allergic to penicillin. She smokes 2 packs of cigarettes daily, she does not drink alcohol, and uses no illegal drugs. She lives with her husband of 35 years and their dog. Physical examination, including breast and pelvic examination is unremarkable. The most appropriate next step in the management of this patient is to

   (A) berate her for her tobacco dependence
   (B) offer personalized advice about stopping smoking
   (C) recommend nicotine replacement therapy
   (D) schedule a followup visit in 1 year
   (E) write a prescription for bupropion

4. A 47-year-old woman comes to the emergency department complaining of an acute onset of constant epigastric pain described as 9/10 on a pain scale. She says that it radiates to the back and is associated with severe nausea and vomiting. She occasionally has right upper quadrant pain after eating fatty meals, which she was told was caused by gallstones by her primary care doctor but declined any further workup. Her temperature is 37.0 C (98.6 F), blood pressure is 120/80 mm Hg, pulse is 110/min, and respirations are 18/min. She appears to be in acute distress with an apparent inability to lie still on the table secondary to pain. Her heart is tachycardic and regular, and her lungs are clear. She has epigastric tenderness and voluntary guarding. Turner and Cullen signs are absent. Laboratory studies show:

Sodium	145 mEq/L
Potassium	4.5 mEq/L
Chloride	100 mEq/L
Bicarbonate	24 mEq/L
Glucose	106 mg/dL
Creatinine	1.0 mg/dL
BUN	17 mg/dL
Alkaline phosphatase	143 U/L
AST	30 U/L
ALT	41 U/L
Amylase	1400 U/L
Lipase	425 U/L

An abdominal ultrasound shows:

Numerous stones in the gallbladder
No retained common bile duct stones
No biliary duct dilation

In addition to fluid resuscitation, the most appropriate immediate management includes

(A) H2 blockers
(B) intravenous antibiotics
(C) laparoscopic cholecystectomy
(D) nasogastric suction
(E) pain relief

5. A 37-year-old woman comes to the emergency department in the middle of the night after a severe panic attack. She complains of an overwhelming fear of dying, accompanied with tremulousness and muscle cramps that woke her up from sleep. She also reports having sudden involuntary contractions in her wrist and feet. She has had a few milder attacks but this is the worst one. In the past 4 months she has experienced difficulties concentrating and has been more irritable and argumentative than usual. She had a thyroidectomy secondary to multinodular goiter a few months ago and is now receiving supplemental hormonal therapy. She tells you that she had a recent check of her "thyroid levels" about 2 months ago and everything was fine. Physical examination shows mild alopecia and hyperreactive deep tendon reflexes. An electrocardiogram shows mild QT-interval prolongation. The most appropriate next step in management is to

(A) assure the patient that symptoms are a consequence of panic attack and hyperventilation and tell her to breathe in a sack
(B) call a psychiatry consult
(C) check serum electrolytes and calcium
(D) obtain a CT scan of the brain
(E) order an electroencephalogram

6. A 56-year-old woman with bipolar disorder and arthritis is admitted to the hospital for intravenous antibiotic therapy for pneumonia. Her regular dose of lithium is continued. The intern on the floor orders some medication for her arthritis on an as-needed basis because she complained of worsening of "arthritis pain" in the days before being admitted to the hospital. Over the course of her hospital stay she complains of increased hand tremor, thirst, polyuria, and diarrhea. Initially, the intern thinks it may be related to antibiotics. When you hear about her current complaints, you recommend ordering a lithium level, which comes back elevated even though there was no change in her dose of lithium. The most appropriate next step in management is to

(A) call an endocrinology consult
(B) discontinue the lithium completely
(C) review the list of medications given during her hospital stay
(D) start acetazolamide
(E) stop the antibiotics because of their side effects

7. A highly successful businessman is hospitalized to rule out a myocardial infarction. He is very demanding and has been having conflicts with the usually very kind staff in the coronary care unit. He calls the nurse manager and demands that she take appropriate measures against the nurse who failed to bring him ice in a timely fashion. After talking to the nurse manager, he threatens to leave against medical advice. Because he insists on leaving, you are called to try to talk to him. The most appropriate management is to

   (A) attempt to arrange the transfer to psychiatric ward
   (B) explain that the nurses are responsible for many patients and that he is not the only patient on the floor
   (C) explain to the patient the need to compromise in such a setting
   (D) interpret the patient's threats as the need to avoid dependent position, pointing out that his actions may result in even greater dependency if he ends up very sick
   (E) listen to the patient's complaints and acknowledge the discomfort of a passive position that he is usually not accustomed to

8. An 85-year-old man with diabetes mellitus and emphysema is admitted to the hospital because of shortness of breath. He admits that he failed to fill his prescription for albuterol inhalers, which he uses regularly. The patient is afebrile with normal vital signs. Physical examination is remarkable for diffuse wheezes. A fingerstick glucose is 190 mg/dL. Treatment with aerosolized albuterol, flunisolide, and prednisone is initiated. On the second day of hospitalization, the patient is breathing normally and no longer feels short of breath. You notice that his fingerstick glucose measurements have been in the 400-460 mg/dL range. This patient is most likely experiencing hyperglycemia secondary to

   (A) aerosolized albuterol
   (B) bronchitis
   (C) flunisolide
   (D) pneumonia
   (E) prednisone

9. A 62-year-old woman with type 2 diabetes comes to the clinic because of "fainting spells." She reports having an episode of syncope once a day for the past year. She takes metformin and estrogen. Physical examination is unremarkable. An electrocardiogram shows normal sinus rhythm with a rate of 90/min. A chest x-ray is normal. A fingerstick glucose is 110 mg/dL. Continuous ambulatory cardiac monitoring is carried out during a 2-day period. The patient has two episodes of syncope and both are accompanied by an arrhythmia. One episode occurs with sinus bradycardia with a rate of 40/min and the other episode is associated with supraventricular tachycardia with a rate of 200/min. The most appropriate next step in management is to

   (A) begin atenolol therapy
   (B) begin verapamil therapy
   (C) order an echocardiogram
   (D) recommend pacemaker implantation
   (E) refer her for cardiac catheterization

10. A 30-year-old single mother of a 3-year-old child comes to the clinic for a followup appointment. She was seen 1 month ago for unexplained muscle cramps. She also reported feeling "jittery" at times and "so hot at work even though everyone else was wearing a sweater!" Her thyroid-stimulating hormone level was 0.04 μU/mL. She returns to the clinic after having a thyroid uptake and scan after the administration of I-123. The study demonstrates a diffusely enlarged thyroid gland as well as increased uptake at both 4 and 24 hours. Vital signs today are: blood pressure 130/70 mm Hg and pulse 80/min. She now tells you that she runs a daycare center in her home and is very active in the care of all of the 1 to 4-year-old children. She has no other help in the center and no other source of income. At this time you should

   (A) prescribe low-dose levothyroxine
   (B) prescribe low-dose methimazole
   (C) prescribe low-dose methimazole and refer her for radioiodine therapy
   (D) prescribe low-dose metoprolol
   (E) refer her to a surgeon for a subtotal thyroidectomy

11. A 45-year-old man whom you have been treating for impotence comes to the office with an article describing a research study testing the efficacy of a new drug for impotence and wants to know if the new drug is something he should try. The research described in the article compared erectile failures in 50 men who were given the new drug with 50 men who were given a placebo. The men included in the study were randomly assigned to either the treatment or the placebo group and were blinded as to which group they were in. The study was designed to have a 90% chance of detecting a 50% reduction in erectile dysfunction. Statistical analyses of the resulting data provided a p value of 0.15. Four of the men originally included in the study were dropped from the analyses because of medical complications. The authors of the article concluded that although this new medication looked promising, further research was required to confirm its efficacy. Based on the information presented in this article, you conclude that the new drug does not work and is, therefore, inappropriate for this patient. The chance that you are wrong in your conclusion is best estimated as

(A) 90%
(B) 85%
(C) 50%
(D) 15%
(E) 10%
(F) 5%
(G) cannot be determined from the information provided

12. A 45-year-old man with cirrhosis secondary to hepatitis C and alcohol abuse is in the intensive care unit (ICU) for upper gastrointestinal bleeding. He was admitted from the emergency department 5 days ago with large volumes of bloody emesis. Emergency esophagogastroduodenoscopy (EGD) was performed and revealed multiple gastric varices, which were successfully banded and sclerosed. During his hospitalization, he has been treated with the maximum dose of beta-blockers and vasopressin that his blood pressure could tolerate. The patient was transferred to the ICU when he suddenly started to vomit bright red blood again. His hematocrit after transfusion of 3 units of packed red blood cells was 38%. His hematocrit now is 30%. EGD is repeated at the bedside and demonstrates blood pooling in the stomach. The most appropriate next step in the management is to

(A) consult interventional radiology for emergent transjugular intrahepatic portosystemic shunt (TIPS)
(B) consult surgery for emergency portacaval shunt
(C) increase dosage of beta-blockers
(D) order an emergent CT of the abdomen and pelvis
(E) order an emergent ultrasound of the abdomen

13. A 23-year-old college student comes to the university health center because he has been passing dark red urine. He has no medical problems and takes no medications. He ran his first marathon 3 days ago and has had sore painful muscles in his legs and arms since then. He has run many shorter races in the past and has not experienced this problem before. Vital signs are normal. Physical examination reveals diffusely tender muscles in his lower extremities, but normal strength and reflexes. Urine dipstick is positive for blood. Urinalysis shows

Color	Dark red
Specific gravity	1.030
pH	5.4
Protein	Negative
Glucose	Negative
Ketones	Negative
Bilirubin	Negative
WBC	0-1/HPF
RBC	0/HPF

Microscopic examination of the urine revealed occasional amorphous debris and 3 or 4 granular casts. The most likely explanation for this urinalysis is

(A) hemolyzed blood in the urine
(B) ingestion of food or other material containing red dye
(C) myoglobinuria
(D) trauma to the kidneys
(E) urinary tract infection

Items 14-15

A 58-year-old microchip engineer is admitted to the hospital after a syncopal event. He explains that he felt a sensation of nausea and a strange taste in the mouth and then had an unwitnessed blackout. He recalls being found by his wife after he opened his eyes. He was able to get up and walk to a chair. His wife noted that he had fecal and urinary incontinence and he was bleeding from the mouth. He expressed feeling groggy which soon resolved. He denied chest pain and headache. His history is significant for a myocardial infarction with angioplasty, hypertension, hypercholesterolemia, and his father died at the age of 56 of a myocardial infarction. He is an ex-smoker and drinks 4 pints of beer and 2 shots of "vodka chasers" every evening when he returns from work. His wife discretely tells you that a good friend of his died 6 days ago. His temperature is 36.3 C (97.4 F), blood pressure is 140/94 mm Hg, pulse 86/min with no orthostasis, and respirations are 16/min. He is alert and orientated. He has a ruddy appearance, Duputren contracture of his left hand, and no hepatomegaly. His neurological examination is unremarkable. Laboratory studies show

Hemoglobin	15.9 g/dL
Hematocrit	46.2%
Leukocyte count	9300/mm^3
Platelets	207,000/mm^3
Sodium	137 mEq/L
Potassium	4.0 mEq/L
Chloride	96 mEq/L
Bicarbonate	23 mEq/L
Blood urea nitrogen	11 mg/dL
Creatinine	0.9 mg/dL
ALT	149 U/L
AST	235 U/L

14. The agent that best reduces the likelihood of a further seizure in this patient is

(A) chlordiazepoxide
(B) haloperidol
(C) magnesium
(D) metoprolol
(E) thiamine

15. Later that evening you are paged by the nurse because she thinks that the patient has delirium tremens. You remember that the diagnosis of delirium tremens can be made when the course progresses to include

(A) delusions
(B) diaphoresis
(C) fever
(D) tachycardia
(E) tachypnea

16. A 69-year-old man with metastatic lung cancer and chronic obstructive pulmonary disease (COPD) develops worsening respiratory function secondary to an exacerbation of his COPD. He is treated with doses of morphine adequate to diminish his respiratory hunger and to eradicate the pain he experiences from bony metastases. Both you and the patient are aware of the possibility that the morphine may worsen the respiratory function sufficiently to kill him. As the patient does not wish ventilatory support, intubation with ventilatory support is not an option. Shortly after the injection of intravenous morphine the patient dies from respiratory arrest. This scenario is best described by the phrase

(A) active euthanasia
(B) nonvoluntary euthanasia
(C) palliative care
(D) passive euthanasia
(E) physician-assisted suicide

17. A 48-year-old woman with coronary disease, hypertension, and hyperlipidemia is brought to the emergency department because of chest pain and shortness of breath. A recent coronary catheterization showed significant proximal stenosis of the right coronary artery. She takes aspirin, labetalol, and simvastatin. Her temperature is 37.0 C (98.6 F), blood pressure is 95/60 mm Hg, pulse is 59/min, and respirations are 24/min. Her cardiac rhythm is regular, and her lungs are clear to auscultation bilaterally. Her jugular venous pressure is elevated and her extremities are cold. An echocardiogram shows akinesis of the right ventricle. The most appropriate immediate management is to administer

(A) morphine, intravenously
(B) nitroglycerin, intravenously
(C) nitroglycerin, orally
(D) Ringers lactate, intravenously
(E) streptokinase, intravenously

18. You are reviewing all of the laboratory work that has been sent from your office last week. You notice that one of your partner's patients, a 75-year-old man, came to the office for a routine examination last week and his laboratory studies show

Thyroid-stimulating hormone	0.02 mU/L
Free thyroxine T_4	35 nmol/L

Your partner is on vacation and you cannot find the patient's chart. You have the nurse call him to schedule an appointment to come in to see you. The least likely finding on examination of this patient will be

(A) fatigue
(B) a goiter
(C) tachycardia
(D) a tremor
(E) weight loss

19. You have been treating a 78-year-old woman for diabetes, hypertension, and chronic venous insufficiency. She has often complained of tiredness and achiness in her legs, especially after prolonged standing activities. She has had multiple small venous ulcers develop on her medial malleoli over the past 5 years that have been successfully managed with regular wound care and compression. Her current medications are metformin, pentoxiphylline, and enalapril. You have encouraged her repeatedly to wear supportive stockings and elevate her legs several times a day to reduce the edema, but she says it is very difficult for her to do that because she looks after her three grandchildren during the week. Also, she just prefers using over the counter rubbing creams that give her instant relief of the achiness, albeit for a short while. She comes for an office visit 3 weeks before her scheduled appointment because of severe itching, redness, and weeping of her lower legs that started 2 days ago. She has applied her usual rubbing cream, but it does not seem to be relieving the discomfort. During your examination you note that there is bilateral, symmetrical, well-demarcated erythema and edema from just below the knees to below the ankles. Many translucent thin-roofed vesicles are dispersed throughout the affected areas and there is abundant yellowish crusting. Both medial malleoli have multiple atrophic scars surrounded by rusty brown discoloration. The most likely cause of her acute skin disorder is

(A) enalapril
(B) lanolin
(C) metformin
(D) pentoxiphylline
(E) petrolatum

20. A 72-year-old man living at home comes to this clinic because his sleep pattern has been interrupted by excessive coughing for the past 3 months. He also reports that on awakening in the morning he has a bitter taste in his mouth. He has an intermittent sensation of oral burning and the sensation of a lump in his throat and he sometimes feels that "the air is cut off" in his throat and he can hardly talk. Finally, he experiences strong pressure in his chest unrelated to exercise. On examination, the patient frequently clears his throat and a hoarse vocal quality is apparent. His blood pressure is 142/81 mm Hg. The lungs are clear to auscultation and normal heart sounds are present. The most likely diagnosis is

(A) gastroesophageal reflux disease
(B) panic disorder
(C) Parkinson disease
(D) postnasal drip
(E) sleep apnea

21. A 22-year-old college student comes in to see you because of "fingernail problems." She tells you that over the past year or two, she has noted a slow increase in the number of pits in her fingernails, which has become more problematic for her manicurist. She just completed an alternative medicine class in school where she learned that many internal problems can present on fingernails. She is concerned about cosmetic and medical consequences and would like to find a cure. She denies any significant health issues and is on no medication currently. On examination, there are multiple 1 to 2-mm pits on all fingernails and first toenails of both feet. There are also tan, oval spots ranging in 2 to 4-mm associated with uplifting of the distal portion from the nail bed on some of the fingernails. She has bilateral erythematous round plaques with thick scales on the conchal bowl that she says have been there for about the same amount of time as her nail pits. You should tell her that

(A) she most likely has onychomycosis and ringworm of her ears
(B) she most likely has psoriatic nails and psoriasis of her ears
(C) she most likely has pterygium of her nails and lichen planus of her ears
(D) she most likely has seborrheic dermatitis
(E) the pits of nails are most likely caused from local trauma caused during her manicures

22. Three cases of an unknown virus are detected at a local emergency department. Patients complain of stomach distress, headache, and fever accompanied by periodic delirium and dizziness. Because the causal agent is unknown, the local public health department is notified. To characterize the virus and gain some knowledge about the origins of the outbreak, the type of study that the public health department is most likely to conduct is a

(A) case-control
(B) case series
(C) cohort
(D) community trial
(E) crossover
(F) cross-sectional

23. A 50-year old man comes to the office complaining of continued dyspepsia and "heartburn" despite treatment with over-the-counter H_2 blockers. He reports having similar pain for more than 10 years. He has heard from some of his coworkers that there are new medications that can treat his heartburn. Because of the duration of his symptoms you opt for an upper endoscopic evaluation, which reveals a small, nonbleeding, gastric ulcer. The esophagus is normal. A rapid antibody test performed during the endoscopy is positive for *H. pylori*. At this time the most correct statement about his condition is:

(A) Culture of the gastric biopsy is necessary to confirm the diagnosis.
(B) Infection likely occurred during childhood.
(C) Repeat endoscopy is indicated after treatment to confirm resolution.
(D) The majority of patients with *H. pylori* infection have ulcer disease.
(E) Treatment involves lifelong therapy with proton pump inhibitors.

24. A 47-year-old man comes to the emergency department at 6AM with his wife complaining of severe abdominal pain. He was feeling fine until last night when he felt epigastric pain at 8PM after returning from a cocktail party where he ate and drank heavily. The pain began gradually, and built to full intensity within 30 minutes. It is constant in nature, very severe, radiating to the back, and accompanied by nausea and vomiting. He vomited two cupfuls of greenish material, but later he retched without bringing much up. He has taken no medications. While asking him questions he keeps changing position and he is now lying on his side with his knees drawn up. His temperature is 37.2 C (99.0 F). His skin is pale. Based on this history, his condition is most likely

(A) caused by gastroenteritis
(B) located in the common bile duct
(C) located in the duodenum
(D) located in the pancreas
(E) located in the stomach

25. A 55-year-old woman with hypothyroidism sees you in your clinic for the first time because her regular doctor is away on vacation. She is on L-thyroxine only and has no complaints at this time. You notice in her chart that her father died from myocardial infarction at the age of 45 and her brother recently had a nonfatal myocardial infarction at the age of 50. Her temperature is 37.0 C (98.6 F), blood pressure is 140/90 mm Hg, pulse is 72/min, and respirations are 16/min. Her weight is 280 lb and height is 5 feet and 5 inches. Physical examination is unremarkable. Laboratory studies show

Total cholesterol	242 mg/dL
LDL	169 mg/dL
HDL	32 mg/dL
Triglyceride	180 mg/dL
TSH	0.360 mU/L
Leukocytes	$8000/mm^3$
Hemoglobin	13.2 mg/dL
Hematocrit	40%
Platelets	$153,000/mm^3$
Direct bilirubin	0.1 mg/dL
Total bilirubin	0.4 mg/dL
ALT	14 U/L
AST	17 U/L
Alkaline phosphatase	67 U/L
Albumin	4.0 g/dL
Total protein	7.0 g/dL

She asks you about her cholesterol levels. At this time you should

(A) explain that her cholesterol panel is consistent with the normal range of cholesterol in females of her age group and repeat her cholesterol panel annually
(B) recommend aerobic exercise four times a week and weight control and refer her to a nutritionist for dietary modification and repeating her cholesterol panel in 6 months
(C) reduce the dose of her L-thyroxine for better control of the hypothyroidism since this would explain the current cholesterol panel
(D) start the patient on atorvastatin and repeat the cholesterol and liver panel in 3 months
(E) start the patient on gemfibrozil and repeat her cholesterol and liver panel in 3 months

26. A 65-year-old man with coronary disease, hypertension, and hyperlipidemia is brought to the emergency department complaining of chest pain. He describes the pain as "searing," and radiating from his anterior chest to between his shoulder blades. He takes verapamil, furosemide, and niacin. His temperature is 37.2 C (99.0 F), blood pressure in his right arm is 180/98 mm Hg and 110/56 mm Hg in his left arm. His pulse is 102/min and respirations are 23/min. His cardiac rhythm is regular and his lungs are clear to auscultation bilaterally. An electrocardiogram shows sinus tachycardia. The best study to order to establish a diagnosis is

(A) a cardiac stress test
(B) a chest radiograph
(C) an echocardiogram
(D) a tagged red blood cell scan
(E) a ventilation-perfusion scan

27. A 41-year-old woman comes to the clinic complaining of an itchy rash on her right foot that began 24 hours ago. She thinks it may be as a result of an allergy to nickel from the metal zip of one of her boots that she wore yesterday. She recalls having a nickel allergy in the past. On physical examination she has a well-delineated irregular papular reaction in the skin over the medial malleolus of the right foot. The area coincides with the same contact area of the metal zipper. The rash is limited proximally to the pretibial area and distally to the level of the mid foot. There are some excoriation marks noted. You agree with her diagnosis of contact dermatitis and prescribe a topical corticosteroid cream. You advise her to apply a thin film three times a day to the affected skin. In addition, the most important advice you can provide is to

(A) apply soft bandaging around the ankle after application before going to sleep
(B) apply the cream and then wipe off the cream gently with cotton wool
(C) continue applying the lotion even if the rash is seen to spread
(D) not to apply the cream to the genitalia or face
(E) not to discard the lotion since it could be used to prevent eruptions of contact dermatitis elsewhere on the body

Items 28-29

A 37-year-old African American male factory worker with several recurrences of gout returns to see you for a followup appointment after another "gouty attack." This time the gout was exacerbated in the right foot after jumping off a high step and landing awkwardly at work 2 weeks ago. A 24-hour urinary collection for uric acid shows

Uric acid over 24 hours	120 mg/24 hours (normal range 250-750 mg/24 h)
Total urine volume over 24 hours	1900 mL/24 hours

28. He takes ibuprofen for pain and omeprazole for symptomatic gastroesophageal reflux disease. The most appropriate prophylactic therapy at this time is

(A) allopurinol
(B) colchicine
(C) ibuprofen
(D) indomethacin
(E) probenecid

29. Before beginning the appropriate therapy, you should ask him:

(A) "Are you able to bear weight on the affected foot?"
(B) "Do you have a family history of gout?"
(C) "Do you have a history of gallstones?"
(D) "Do you have a history of renal stone formation?"
(E) "Have you had any fevers recently?"

Items 30-31

A 57-year-old African American woman with hypertension, diabetes, asthma, systemic lupus erythematosus, sarcoidosis, and a benign pituitary adenoma is admitted to the hospital with acute polyarticular joint pain. She is diagnosed with acute inflammatory synovitis and she is started on a course of prednisone. Hydromorphone 2 mg oral every 4 hours is given for pain control. Her medications include albuterol, furosemide, prednisone, quinapril, and torsemide. Laboratory studies show

Sodium	139 mEq/L
Potassium	5.4 mEq/L
Chloride	106 mEq/L
Bicarbonate	22 mEq/L
BUN	54 mg/dL
Creatinine	2.3 mg/dL
Glucose	119 mg/dL
Leukocyte count	$7300/mm^3$
Hemoglobin	12.1 g/dL
Hematocrit	36.2%
Platelets	$208,000/mm^3$
Erythrocyte sedimentation rate	80 mm/h

You are called to see the patient on the ward because she is complaining of a new onset of headache and blurred vision. Her blood pressure is noted to be 220/140 mm Hg and is repeated 20 minutes later to be 225/140 mm Hg. She tells you that her blood pressure normally is 170/80 mm Hg, which is confirmed when you look through her old charts.

30. At this time the most appropriate management for her blood pressure is to

    (A) administer another dose of hydromorphone to reduce the pain and repeat the blood pressure in 2 hours
    (B) administer hydralazine immediately and repeat the blood pressure in 1 hour
    (C) administer labetalol immediately and repeat the blood pressure in 1 hour
    (D) administer normal saline and order another electrolyte panel before starting furosemide and repeat the blood pressure in 1 hour

31. You appropriately stabilize this patient. In the morning you review the repeat electrolyte blood panel

Sodium	135 mEq/L
Potassium	6.7 mEq/L
Chloride	106 mEq/L
Bicarbonate	19 mEq/L
BUN	54 mg/dL
Creatinine	2.2 mg/dL
Glucose	119 mg/dL

An electrocardiogram now shows tented T waves. You administer calcium gluconate, bicarbonate, and sodium polystyrene sulfonate. Of the medications that the patient was previously taking, the one that most likely caused this biochemical abnormality is

(A) albuterol
(B) furosemide
(C) prednisone
(D) quinapril
(E) torsemide

32. A 62-year-old man with hyperlipidemia, gastroesophageal reflux disease, and labile hypertension comes to the clinic complaining of bilateral leg edema. He says it is severe enough to prevent him from putting his shoes on. He is currently receiving physical therapy for a small meniscal tear of his left knee. He has had difficulty ambulating and uses codeine for the pain. A recent echocardiogram demonstrated a normal ejection fraction. He takes atenolol, quinapril, amlodipine, simvastatin, and omeprazole. In the past he was unable to tolerate hydrochloro-thiazide and adamantly refuses to add any new medications to his regimen. His temperature is 38.0 C (98.2 F), blood pressure is 160/90 mm Hg, pulse 72/min, and respirations of 16/min. He has bilateral pitting edema of the legs to the level of the knees. His left knee is swollen and mildly tender over the anteromedial joint line. After much discussion you both agree to pursue nonpharmacological treatment of the leg edema. The approach that would demonstrate the best compliance and efficacy in this patient is advising him to

    (A) continue ambulation with the physical therapy and using a walking aid
    (B) drink plenty of caffeinated drinks such as tea for diuresis
    (C) elevate the legs above the level of the heart while sleeping
    (D) take a cold bath for 45 minutes daily
    (E) use leg compression stockings

33. A 78-year-old man with diabetes mellitus comes to the clinic complaining of scaling and flaking of his skin, mainly from the scalp, the eyebrows, and behind the ear. He also has pruritus around the skin of the eyebrows. The skin is red, greasy, and inflamed bilaterally around the eyebrows. There is flaking and scaling of the skin over the eyebrows, scalp, and ears. The most likely diagnosis is

(A) acne rosacea
(B) alopecia areata
(C) pityriasis rosca
(D) scabies
(E) seborrheic dermatitis

34. A 42-year-old man comes to the employee health clinic with a 2-month history of intermittent, dull epigastric pain that typically occurs several hours after eating. He denies any nausea, vomiting, anorexia, melena, hematemesis, or weight loss. The pain is worse when he skips meals and it is usually improved with eating. On a scale of 1 to 10, the patient rates the pain a 4 at its worst. The patient does not smoke cigarettes or drink alcohol and denies using nonsteroidal anti-inflammatory agents or aspirin on a regular basis. He does not take any prescription medicines. His blood pressure is 130/75 mm Hg and pulse is 72/min. Abdominal examination shows tenderness on palpation in the epigastric region, normal active bowel sounds, and the absence of rebound tenderness or guarding. Rectal examination is negative for occult blood. Laboratory studies show

Hemoglobin	16 g/dL
Hematocrit	48%
Leukocyte count	6000/mm^3
Platelets	250,000/mm^3

You defer an upper gastrointestinal series or upper endoscopy at this time and send serology for *Helicobacter pylori*, which returns positive. At this time, the most appropriate treatment regimen for this patient is

(A) omeprazole alone
(B) omeprazole, clarithromycin, and metronidazole in combination
(C) ranitidine alone
(D) ranitidine and amoxicillin in combination
(E) sucralfate and misoprostol

35. You are staffing a geriatric general medicine outpatient clinic. Your first patient of the morning is an 85-year-old man who has come for advice about his right knee. Over the past 10 years he has noticed increasing pain in his knee that is worsened by prolonged weight-bearing activities. He also notes that his knee is very stiff and painful in the mornings. He denies any history of trauma, notes no episodes of knee instability. His knee is never swollen or warm. He is a former mail carrier who walked his 6-mile route carrying a heavy mailbag. Since his retirement he has gained approximately 100 pounds. The patient denies any fevers, chills, or night sweats and has noted no recent weight loss (rather he continues to gain weight and decrease his activity). He denies any other joint involvement. On examination, the patient is an obese Caucasian male in no distress. His vital signs are within the normal range. The patient's lower extremities are somewhat bow-legged. The patient's right knee is not tender to palpation and no joint effusion is present. The range of motion of the right knee is from 0 to 90 degrees of flexion (normal is generally from 0 to 120 degrees but is variable). The left knee has full motion from 0 to 120 degrees. There is no gross instability noted on ligamentous testing. Radiographs show mild joint space narrowing and osteophyte formation about the knee joint. The most appropriate next step in management is to

(A) admit the patient to the hospital because of a bony tumor (probable osteosarcoma) and begin chemotherapy
(B) tell the patient he has rheumatoid arthritis and he should begin methotrexate and corticosteroid treatment immediately
(C) tell the patient he likely has had an indolent infection of his knee and you will need to do a further infectious disease workup (blood and joint fluid cultures)
(D) tell the patient he likely has moderate osteoarthritis and that his symptoms may improve with activity modification, weight loss, and nonsteroidal anti-inflammatory medication
(E) tell the patient he will require a joint replacement and refer him for emergency orthopedic surgery care

36. A 54-year-old homeless man comes to the emergency department with complaints of a cough for the past 3 weeks productive of yellowish blood-tinged sputum. He denies chest pain, but has had some mild shortness of breath. He also states that he has "felt hot," and has awakened at night several times drenched in sweat. On physical examination he is somewhat emaciated and disheveled. His temperature is 37.8 C (100.0 F), blood pressure is 120/80 mm Hg, pulse is 90/min, and respirations are 18/min. Lung examination is remarkable for coarse breath sounds on the right. A chest x-ray shows a right middle lobe pneumonia. Laboratory studies show a hematocrit of 32%, platelet count of 400,000/mm^3, and a leukocyte count of 13,900/mm^3. The patient should be

(A) admitted and placed on therapy for tuberculosis
(B) admitted, placed on intravenous ceftriaxone, and discharged when afebrile to complete a course of an oral equivalent
(C) admitted, placed on intravenous ceftriaxone, and placed in an isolation room and tuberculosis ruled out with serial sputum samples
(D) discharged on oral levofloxacin and scheduled for a new patient evaluation in 7 to 10 days at the community health clinic
(E) discharged without therapy and scheduled for a new patient evaluation in 7 to 10 days at the community health clinic

37. A 55-year-old man comes to the emergency department because of a 3-day history of pain on urination, fevers, and chills. He also complains of perineal and suprapubic tenderness as well as dysuria and hesitancy. He has no personal physician and has not been to the doctor since childhood. He smokes 2 packs of cigarettes a day and admits to a "hearty meat and potatoes diet." His temperature is 38.5 C (101.3 F), blood pressure is 132/90 mm Hg, pulse is 88/min, and respirations are 18/min. His heart and lungs are normal. Abdominal examination is remarkable for suprapubic tenderness. Digital rectal examination demonstrates a swollen, boggy, and exquisitely painful prostate gland. Laboratory studies show a leukocyte count of 11,500/mm^3, creatinine of 0.9 mg/dL, and blood urea nitrogen of 16 mg/dL. A urinalysis shows too numerous to count white blood cells and gram-negative rods. He is given a prescription for ciprofloxacin, and is advised to followup in the clinic. Appropriate health maintenance for this patient would include

(A) a blood lead level should be obtained
(B) flexible sigmoidoscopy and fecal occult blood testing every 3 years
(C) screening carotid ultrasound biannually
(D) screening chest x-rays annually
(E) screening thyroid ultrasound every 5 years

Items 38-39

A 33-year-old woman comes to the office because of an "itchy rash" on the ring finger of her left hand. She says that she began to notice it about 3 weeks ago, after her son was born and she started washing her hands "every minute" and began pushing the baby carriage. It started out as a "red itchy area" under her wedding band, and it progressed to "scaly bumps that sometimes burst." It is itchy all day long, and not especially worse at night or after a hot shower. She is very upset because she can no longer wear her wedding band. She does not suffer from allergies and has never had any similar episodes in the past. Nobody else in her household has similar symptoms. Physical examination shows an area of localized erythema, vesicles, scales, and thickened skin on the proximal part of her left ring finger. It is difficult for her to stop scratching her finger for long enough for you to examine it. A full-body skin examination does not reveal any other lesions.

38. The most likely mechanism for this reaction is

(A) antibody-mediated cytotoxic reaction to cell surface antigens
(B) antigen-antibody complexes formed in the vessels in response to an antigen
(C) fixation of complement results in osmotic lysis of antibody-coated cell
(D) release of histamine from basophils after antigen interaction with Fc receptor-bound IgE
(E) release of lymphokines from sensitized lymphocytes reacting with antigens

39. The most appropriate treatment at this time is

(A) a high-potency fluorinated topical glucocorticoid
(B) oral prednisone
(C) permethrin cream
(D) a topical coal tar preparation
(E) a topical salicylic acid preparation

40. As part of a nationwide drive focused on accident prevention, you are awarded a $5000 grant. The requirements for the grant are that it be spent so as to have the greatest impact on reducing accidents for the people of your rural community. The five most common types of accidents in this community, along with their annual incidence, are presented in the table below.

Table 1. Leading Cause of Accidents and Incidence Rate for Rural Community

Cause	Incidence rate per 10,000 population
Tractors	49
Falls from heights	41
Truck	25
Automobile	20
Poisonings	15

You decide to spend the grant money on an educational prevention program. The cost of this educational intervention differs for each type of accident, with the preventive intervention cheaper for some and more expensive for others. The following table lays out the estimated cost of intervening with one member of this rural community.

Table 2. Cost of Intervention (Per Person)

Cause	Cost Per Person
Tractors	$4
Falls from heights	$3
Truck	$5
Automobile	$3
Poisonings	$2

If the full $5000 were spent, the most accidents could be prevented if you were to focus on preventing accidents involving

(A) automobiles
(B) falls from heights
(C) poisonings
(D) tractors
(E) trucks

41. A 45-year-old man is admitted to the hospital with shaking chills and a hot, tender erythematous right upper extremity. He has been using intravenous drugs for several years and has lately been "skin popping." He states that earlier this morning he had no redness on his arm, and now it has spread quickly to involve almost the entire upper extremity. His temperature is 38.5 C (101.3 F), blood pressure is 89/52 mm Hg, pulse is 105/min, and respirations are 22/min. There is an area of anesthesia and purple discoloration of the upper extremity. Crepitus is also present. He has a leukocyte count of 33,000/mm^3. The most appropriate immediate management is

(A) broad-spectrum intravenous antibiotics and extensive wound debridement
(B) cephalexin 250 to 500 mg orally 4 times per day for 10 days
(C) nafcillin 1 to 2 g intravenously every 4 hours for 10 days
(D) topical clindamycin applied twice per day for 14 days
(E) an x-ray of the right arm

42. A 55-year-old man is admitted to the hospital for pain control of severe low back pain. Approximately 10 weeks ago he was in a very mild car accident after which he has some mild low back pain. It went away almost completely, but then over the past 3 weeks he has had progressive symptoms. He denies any bowel or bladder incontinence, and has no difficulty with gait apart from the pain. A spine film 3 weeks ago when his symptoms began to worsen showed no significant abnormality. His temperature is 38.5 C (101.3 F), blood pressure is 122/90 mm Hg, pulse 88/min, and respirations are 18/min. His heart, lung, and abdominal examinations are normal. On palpation over the level of thoracic vertebrae 11 and 12 he has significant point tenderness. There are no neurologic deficits. Laboratory studies show a leukocyte count of 17,300/mm^3, an erythrocyte sedimentation rate of 87 seconds, and normal liver function tests, amylase, and urinalysis. Blood cultures are pending. A repeat spine film is negative. The most appropriate next step in management is to

(A) begin therapy with an empiric 4-drug antituberculous medication
(B) obtain a psychiatric consult for possible malingering
(C) order a CT scan of the spine
(D) order an MRI of the spine
(E) start the patient on intravenous narcotics, and when the pain is under control, discharge on a narcotic analgesic taper

43. A 19-year-old woman comes to the clinic because of diarrhea. She states that for the past 6 months, she has had approximately seven loose bowel movements per day, several of which have had blood mixed in with the stool and she often has tenesmus. She has lost approximately 10 pounds. For the past 4 weeks she has had some low-grade fevers. Prior to this, she denies any gastrointestinal symptoms apart from an occasional acute enteritis-type syndrome. She denies any out of town travel within the last year. She states that her aunt may have had a similar problem, but she is not really sure. She denies alcohol use. Her temperature is 37.8 C (100.0 F) and blood pressure is 130/88 mm Hg. Her lungs are clear and cardiac examination is normal. Abdomen is soft, but diffusely tender. She has no peritoneal signs. Rectal examination shows heme-positive brown stool. Laboratory studies show a leukocyte count of 9800/mm^3, hematocrit of 36%, platelet count of 302,000/mm^3, BUN of 18 mEq/L, and creatinine of 0.9 mEq/L. This patient will likely benefit from

(A) cisplatin-based chemotherapy
(B) a course of ciprofloxacin
(C) a gluten-free diet
(D) a lactate-free diet
(E) sulfasalazine therapy

44. A 35-year-old Caucasian woman complaining of irritability, heat intolerance, sweating, and palpitations for the past several days is admitted to the hospital for evaluation. Once on the floor you notice that she has a "rash" on her hands that she claims appeared "months ago." She says that it is getting worse, but she was too busy with a new and very demanding job to go see a dermatologist. On physical examination, the patient has warm, moist skin and a mild lid lag when she blinks. Her pillowcase is covered with hair and she cannot hold her hands out steadily because of a fine tremor. The "rash" on the hands consists of symmetrical, well-demarcated depigmented patches on the fingertips and dorsal hands that have a slightly hyperpigmented border. At this time the most correct statement about her condition is:

(A) Although her skin disease is likely related to the thyroid dysfunction, they will evolve independently of one another and treatment of one would not interfere with the other.
(B) Antithyroid medication will cause progression of her skin disease and she should think well before opting to take it.
(C) Her skin disease will improve spontaneously and treatment is not necessary.
(D) Since the skin disease will evolve to affect her entire skin over the next few months there is no need for treating it at all.
(E) Surgical resection of the thyroid will improve her skin disease so that should be her number one choice of treatment.

45. A 20-year-old man comes to your office complaining of a rash on his chest and back that started 3 weeks ago while he was on vacation. He tells you that it appeared about a week after he arrived in Mexico and comments on how hot and humid the weather was and that spending a lot of time at the beach made it a little easier to tolerate. Although it is unsightly, he remarks that on occasion it does get a little itchy. He recalls seeing a few other people at the beach having "similar spots" on their back. You notice that he is deeply tanned. There are multiple hypopigmented oval macules and small patches covered by fine scale on his upper trunk and extending onto the upper arms. The most appropriate study to confirm the diagnosis is

(A) diascopy
(B) a KOH preparation
(C) patch testing
(D) a skin biopsy
(E) a Tzanck smear

46. A 60-year-old man comes to the office for a routine followup visit. He has a medical history significant for coronary disease, congestive failure, hypertension, and gout. His medications include aspirin, metoprolol, captopril, and allopurinol. He has no allergies to medications, and denies any alcohol or tobacco use. Over the past several months he has had several admissions for congestive heart failure. His temperature is 37.2 C (99.0 F), blood pressure is 110/67 mm Hg, pulse is 62/min, and respirations are 16/min. He is well appearing. His cardiac rhythm is regular, and his lungs are clear to auscultation bilaterally. He has no lower extremity edema. Based on his recent history of congestive heart failure on the current medication regimen, the most appropriate pharmacologic intervention at this time is to

(A) add amiodarone to his current regimen
(B) add furosemide to his current regimen
(C) add propranolol to his current regimen
(D) add spironolactone to his current regimen
(E) discontinue his metoprolol

47. You are called to see a 43-year-old woman who was admitted to the hospital for the management of her pneumonia. She has a medical history significant for hypertension, depression, and rheumatoid arthritis. Her medications at home include metoprolol, sertraline, and prednisone. During her current admission for pneumonia, she is started on cefuroxime and a rapid tapering of her prednisone. On examination, she is sick appearing. Her temperature is 38.1 C (100.6 F), blood pressure is 88/50 mm Hg, pulse is 102/min, and respirations are 24/min. Her cardiac rhythm is regular, and her breath sounds are diminished over the left lower lung field. You note that Ringers lactate is being infused briskly via a peripheral intravenous catheter. The most appropriate next pharmacologic intervention is

(A) administration of hydrocortisone
(B) administration of ketoconazole
(C) administration of propranolol
(D) administration of spironolactone
(E) administration of thyroxine

48. A 24-year-old African American woman comes to the health center complaining of a rash on her left arm that started about 3 weeks ago. She says that it has been slowly enlarging and is only a little itchy. She has no other complaints. With her is her 6-year-old son who she enrolled in kindergarten 3 months ago when she went back to college to finish her MBA degree. On inspection, there is an annular erythematous plaque on the medial aspect of her left upper arm. The central area is clear, but the edge is slightly raised, with tiny vesicles and fine scale. No axillary lymph nodes are palpable. You ask her if she has noticed any skin changes in her son and she admits that he has been having a lot of dandruff lately. The boy's scalp is covered with fine scale and many hairs are broken off at the scalp level leaving the appearance of "black dots." His suboccipital lymph nodes are enlarged and firm, but mobile. You decide to perform a KOH examination and culture of scrapings both from her arm and the child's scalp. The culture is most likely to grow

(A) *Corynebacterium minutissimum*
(B) *Epidermophyton floccosum*
(C) *Microsporum canis*
(D) *Pityrosporum ovale*
(E) *Trichophyton tonsurans*

49. You have been treating a 27-year-old man for anal warts for the past 2 years. During the course of treatment you have prescribed topical applications of imiquimod cream, podophyllotoxin solution, and monthly liquid nitrogen, but despite short periods of clearance, the warts keep recurring to the dismay of both you and your patient. All this time, he has refused to see a proctologist and have anoscopy performed. The factor in this patient's history that would support the existence of intra-anal warts as a reservoir of persistent infection is

(A) intravenous drug abuse
(B) internal and external hemorrhoids
(C) multiple sexual partners
(D) opportunistic infections
(E) receptive anal intercourse

50. A 21-year-old man is brought to the emergency department by the police in handcuffs after assaulting several people in a park. The patient, on mental status examination, is found to be belligerent and threatening. He has psychomotor agitation and is attempting to break free from his handcuffs. He also seems to be responding to internal stimuli and has horizontal nystagmus. Urinary toxicology is positive for phencyclidine. The most appropriate immediate management is to

(A) administer flumazenil intravenously
(B) administer naloxone to reverse the euphoric effects of phencyclidine
(C) obtain consent for HIV testing
(D) perform a lumbar puncture to rule out a chemical meningitis
(E) provide adequate sedation and a low level of environmental stimulation

Internal Medicine Test Three: Answers and Explanations

ANSWER KEY

1. B
2. D
3. B
4. E
5. C
6. C
7. E
8. E
9. D
10. B
11. E
12. A
13. C
14. A
15. A
16. C
17. D
18. D
19. B
20. A
21. B
22. B
23. B
24. D
25. D
26. C
27. D
28. E
29. D
30. C
31. D
32. E
33. E
34. B
35. D
36. C
37. B
38. E
39. A
40. B
41. A
42. D
43. E
44. A
45. B
46. D
47. A
48. E
49. E
50. E

1. **The correct answer is B.** In an elderly patient with hematuria, one of the foremost things to consider is the possibility of malignancy, either renal parenchymal (such as renal cell carcinoma) in the collecting system or the bladder (such as a transitional cell carcinoma). The IVP will diagnose masses of the kidney as well as look at the renal collecting system and ureters. If this is negative then a bladder mass should be ruled out by cystoscopy.

   Simply following up with the patient (**choice A**) in 6 months is not appropriate. This patient needs to have this problem urgently (although not emergently) evaluated.

   CT scans of the abdomen (**choice C**) are often used and are a better test than IVP for renal masses. However, intravenous contrast must be used in order to identify the lesion adequately.

   A retrograde pyelogram (**choice D**) is used to visualize the collecting system by cannulating the ureters via a cystoscopic approach. These diagnostic studies may be preferable to the intravenous pyelogram in the patients with renal insufficiency or in whom poor excretory function precludes adequate visualization of the collecting system.

   A testicular ultrasound (**choice E**) is not indicated in this case.

2. **The correct answer is D.** Alcohol intake/intoxication is one of the most common etiologies of sexual dysfunction. Reversible causes of sexual dysfunction should be ruled out prior to initiation of any sort of pharmacologic treatment for sexual dysfunction.

   A penile nocturnal tumescence test (**choice A**) is premature in this patient. A potentially reversible cause of the patient's sexual dysfunction has been identified, and there are no identifiable medical risks for sexual dysfunction such as diabetes or hypertension.

   Bupropion (**choice B**) is an antidepressant medication with few sexual side effects and has also been used to improve sexual dysfunction in patients treated with selective serotonin reuptake inhibitors. In this patient, however, ceasing alcohol intake would be a more appropriate and potentially definitive first step in management.

   Prior to giving the patient a prescription for sildenafil (**choice C**), the patient should be advised to stop drinking prior to sexual intercourse.

   There is no reason to suggest to the patient that he should stop sexual activity temporarily (**choice E**). It is vague advice to give and also lends to the suggestion that there is nothing that can be attempted to improve his condition.

3. **The correct answer is B.** In the United States, tobacco use is the number one leading preventable cause of death. Each year it leads to more than 400,000 deaths or one out of every five deaths. Estimates are that 70% of smokers see a physician every year: this provides an excellent opportunity for counseling. Many strategies have been developed for providers to approach the problem of smoking with patients. A recommended strategy, as described in the United States Public Health Service's 2000 guidelines, is based on five As: ask, advise, assess, assist, and arrange followup. Each patient should be asked about smoking. If they do smoke, they should be offered personalized advice about stopping. The next step is to assess whether they are interested in quitting. Based on their level of interest, the physician should then assist them in quitting or in becoming ready to quit. Finally, close followup should be arranged to reinforce the efforts. This patient has stated that she smokes 2 packs per day. The next step is to then offer her advice about stopping (e.g., to remind her that quitting is the most important action she can do to stay healthy).

   To berate her for her tobacco dependence (**choice A**) would be inappropriate. Berating the patient is likely to be an ineffective approach and likely risks alienating the patient, which will jeopardize any possible future successes.

   To recommend nicotine replacement therapy (**choice C**) may be appropriate in this patient, but wouldn't be the most appropriate next step. To offer her replacement without counseling her or determining if she even wants to quit is not the most effective approach.

   To schedule a followup visit in 1 year (**choice D**) is incorrect. Cigarette smoking is perhaps the worst threat to her health at this point. To allow her to come to her annual visit and not return for another year with no attempt at a smoking cessation intervention would be a lost opportunity.

   To write a prescription for bupropion (**choice E**) may eventually help this patient, but wouldn't be the most appropriate next step. Bupropion has been shown to be effective in helping patients stop smoking cigarettes, as have the nicotine replacement methods, but to simply write this patient a prescription without first determining if she understands the risks of smoking, or if she even wants to stop smoking, would not be correct.

4. **The correct answer is E.** This patient has acute uncomplicated pancreatitis, most likely secondary to gallstones. The management of these patients includes aggressive hydration and aggressive pain control.

   H2 blockers (**choice A**) have not been conclusively shown to have any benefit in the treatment of acute pancreatitis. That being said, they are often used as an adjuvant therapy because they don't adversely affect the patient and are very well tolerated.

   Intravenous antibiotics (**choice B**) may have some role in the management of necrotizing pancreatitis but do not have a role in uncomplicated pancreatitis.

   Laparoscopic cholecystectomy (**choice C**) is indicated for this patient only after her acute pancreatitis resolves. The surgery can be done electively before discharge from the hospital. This management is appropriate for patients without a large amount of surgical risk.

   Nasogastric suction (**choice D**) has no clear benefit in the management of acute pancreatitis. Patients with symptomatic ileus may benefit, but the decision must be individualized.

5. **The correct answer is C.** Checking calcium and other electrolytes is the first thing that needs to be done in this patient. This patient presents with a clinical picture of hypoparathyroidism, which is seen following thyroidectomy at times. Symptoms may be similar to the ones seen in panic attack. Symptoms also include tetany, carpopedal spasms, hyperactive reflexes, scaly skin and nails, alopecia, seizures, and QT prolongation on EKG. Intracranial calcifications are seen sometimes. Hypoparathyroid myopathy can also be a part of the clinical picture. Vitamin D and calcium supplements are the primary therapy for most forms of hypoparathyroidism.

   Assuring the patient that this is a consequence of hyperventilation (**choice A**) is not appropriate since the patient gives a fairly clear history of symptoms. Each panic attack should be initially ruled out for medical causes.

   Calling a psychiatry consult (**choice B**) without having done a medical workup to rule out medical causes of attack is not an appropriate intervention.

   A CT scan of the brain (**choice D**) can be ordered if other tests have been done because of possible intracranial calcifications seen in hypoparathyroidism. It is certainly not the next diagnostic step.

   Ordering an EEG (**choice E**), even though these patients sometimes may have convulsions, is not helpful. EEG changes are nonspecific in this case and revert to normal with calcium level correction.

6. **The correct answer is C.** Before doing anything else the first step should be to review the medications given during the patient's hospital stay. It is most likely that some of them may have caused the increase of lithium level resulting in signs of lithium toxicity. Given the fact that she was complaining of arthritis pain, she could have been given NSAIDs. NSAIDs given concomitantly with lithium decrease renal clearance of lithium, causing an increase in lithium blood levels.

   Calling an endocrinology consult (**choice A**) is not an appropriate first step. Obvious things should be ruled out first.

   Discontinuing lithium (**choice B**) is a temporary solution in order to let the level go down. However, it should not be done completely and should only be lowered temporarily until the level comes down.

   Starting acetazolamide (**choice D**) has no other justification except to lower the lithium level. This is certainly not the first step since finding the cause of toxicity should be done first.

   Stopping antibiotics (**choice E**) because of the assumption that the symptoms are related to them is not appropriate.

7. **The correct answer is E.** Listening to the patient's complaints and acknowledging his discomfort makes him feel understood and also meets some of his needs for attention. This intervention would most likely make it possible to then try to persuade the patient to finish his examination.

   Arranging transfer to the psychiatric ward (**choice A**) is not an appropriate action. This patient does not meet any criteria for inpatient treatment. Civil commitment based on endangering himself would probably not be possible unless the patient is completely unable to understand the consequences of his actions because of altered mental status.

   Explaining that the nurses are responsible for many patients and that he is not the only patient on the floor (**choice B**) will not help resolve the situation. The patient will most likely feel misunderstood and thus abandon treatment.

   Explaining the need to compromise (**choice C**) in this setting, even though it's correct in some way, doesn't make the patient feel understood. Rather it sends a message that he is a hard one to deal with.

   Pointing out the patient's dependent position and the possibility of getting worse (**choice D**), even though correct, is confrontational. It makes the patient feel patronized and this intervention will worsen the problem.

8. **The correct answer is E.** Steroids such as prednisolone and prednisone are used to decrease airway inflammation in reactive airways disease exacerbations. These drugs are glucocorticoids and hence raise glucose levels. Studies are underway to elucidate in what group of patients with reactive airway disease corticosteroids should be used.

   Albuterol (**choice A**) is a bronchodilator that is frequently used in acute exacerbations of asthma and chronic obstructive disease. It can cause tachycardia as a side effect, but it will not elevate the serum glucose levels. This is true whether albuterol is administered via a metered-dose inhaler or in aerosolized form.

   Bronchitis (**choice B**) is a common finding in patients with chronic obstructive lung disease (COPD). Bronchitis is not associated with hyperglycemia. Patients with COPD, however, are at increased risk of having complications to pneumonia such as sepsis. Serious infections such as sepsis are associated with multiorgan failure and patients may become hyperglycemic. This patient most likely has an acute exacerbation of his underlying COPD and has no signs of sepsis.

   Inhaled steroids such as flunisolide (**choice C**) have little systemic absorption and generally do not cause hyperglycemia the way systemic steroids can.

   Pneumonia (**choice D**) in itself does not cause hyperglycemia. Severe cases of pneumonia may lead to sepsis, which can in turn lead to multiorgan failure and some patients will become hyperglycemic. This patient most likely has an acute exacerbation of his underlying COPD and has no signs of sepsis.

9. **The correct answer is D.** This patient is suffering from tachycardia-bradycardia syndrome, which is causing her syncopal episodes secondary to hypotension as a direct result of her arrhythmias. A pacemaker is necessary to maintain a normal ventricular rate, which is crucial to maintain cerebral perfusion. In this patient with diabetes, hypoglycemia must also be considered as a potential cause of syncope. Her ambulatory cardiac monitoring results, however, clearly demonstrate that her syncopal episodes are caused by arrhythmias.

   Atenolol therapy (**choice A**) is contraindicated in patients with tachycardia-bradycardia syndrome. Treatment with atenolol or any other beta-blocker could exacerbate the bradycardic episodes.

   Verapamil therapy (**choice B**) is contraindicated in patients with tachycardia-bradycardia syndrome. Treatment with verapamil, an AV node blocker, could exacerbate the bradycardic episodes.

   Echocardiography (**choice C**) is not indicated in this patient at this time. It is not a routine part of the workup of syncope in a patient who has no evidence of heart failure.

   Cardiac catheterization (**choice E**) is not indicated in this patient at this time. This patient has no symptoms or EKG evidence of coronary artery disease. Myocardial infarction should be considered as an uncommon etiology of syncope, but is unlikely given this patient's history of having these episodes daily for the past year. Furthermore, her ambulatory cardiac monitoring results clearly demonstrate that her syncopal episodes are caused by arrhythmias.

10. **The correct answer is B.** This patient has signs and symptoms of hyperthyroidism and her thyroid uptake and scan is consistent with Graves disease. Graves disease is the most common cause of hyperthyroidism. It is an autoimmune disorder in which an abnormal immunoglobulin binds to receptors for thyroid-stimulating hormone (TSH) causing diffuse enlargement of the gland and overstimulation of thyroid hormone production. The typical management of Graves disease is either radioiodine therapy or antithyroid medication, such as methimazole or propylthiouracil (PTU). Certain precautions need to be followed after radioiodine therapy, such as the avoidance of close contact with children for several days, which makes this not the best option for this patient, who is a daycare provider and a single mother.

    Levothyroxine (**choice A**) is a synthetic thyroid hormone and is contraindicated in this patient. She most likely has Graves disease, which is manifested by increased production of thyroid hormone. Giving this patient additional exogenous thyroid hormone will only exacerbate her symptoms and is potentially life-threatening.

    Referring this patient for radioiodine therapy (**choice C**) is not the best option at this time because of her job and single mother status. However, it is often recommended as a first-line treatment for Graves disease for adult patients (but it is contraindicated in pregnant women).

    Prescribing metoprolol or any other beta-blocker (**choice D**) is often necessary for patients with Graves disease. This patient, however, has minimal adrenergic manifestations of hyperthyroidism. Patients with tachycardia, excessive sweating, or tremor may benefit from metoprolol. However, many patients can be effectively managed with methimazole and may become euthyroid over time. Her symptoms of feeling jittery and heat intolerance should resolve as her thyroid hormone levels become normal.

Referral to a surgeon for a subtototal thyroidectomy (**choice E**) is not usually the recommended initial treatment of choice. The most appropriate management of this patient is treatment with an antithyroid medication such as methimazole or propylthiouracil (PTU). Many patients can be effectively managed with antithyroid medications and become euthyroid over time. Some patients, however, continue to be clinically hyperthyroid despite the medications. These patients with refractory hyperthyroidism should be referred for more definitive therapy with either radioactive iodine ablation or surgery.

11. **The correct answer is E.** The question asks the chance of a type II or beta error. Recall that type II error is the probability of being wrong if one does not reject the null hypothesis. Assuming the traditional p value criterion of $p<0.05$, we would not reject the null hypothesis for this study. Type II error can be estimated from the formula 1 – power = type II error. Power is the capacity of the study to find a difference if one exists. The study was designed to have a 90% chance of detecting an effect, so power = 90%. 100 – 90% = 10% = chance of type II error. Therefore, this can be determined from the information provided (**choice G**).

    Ninety percent (**choice A**) is the power of the study, not type II error.

    The p value is used for type I error only, not type II error. 1 – 0.15 = 85% (**choice B**) does not yield type II error.

    Fifty percent (**choice C**) is the effect size or the size of the difference the study is looking for. It is related to the estimate of power, but does not tell type II error.

    The computed p value = 0.15 (**choice D**). This is the chance of type I error, but only if the null hypothesis is rejected.

    Five percent (**choice F**) is the traditional p value criterion, but does not tell type II error.

12. **The correct answer is A.** This patient has severe bleeding from gastric varices that is uncontrolled by endoscopic therapy and beta-blockers. The most appropriate management of this patient is a transjugular intrahepatic portosystemic shunt (TIPS). It involves placing a stent between the hepatic vein and the portal vein to allow the high pressure in the portal venous system to decompress systemically. The TIPS procedure is performed in patients with portal hypertension causing severe variceal bleeding or to prevent rebleeding. It may also be performed in an emergency when the bleeding can't be controlled by other means. It is often a successful alternative to surgery when medical management is no longer effective.

    Consulting surgery for emergency portacaval shunt (**choice B**) is not the most appropriate management of this patient. A portacaval shunt allows blood in the portal vein to pass into the inferior vena cava through a surgically placed graft. In theory it works in the same manner as a transjugular intrahepatic portosystemic shunt (TIPS). Surgical portacaval shunts are associated with a higher morbidity and mortality rate than TIPS, and are thus not as frequently performed.

    Increasing the dosage of beta-blockers (**choice C**) is not an option for this patient. He is already on maximum dosage that his blood pressure can tolerate and increasing the dosage is dangerous.

    Ordering an emergent CT of the abdomen and pelvis (**choice D**) is not the most appropriate management of this acutely ill patient. A CT will demonstrate the known diagnosis of cirrhosis and may show his varices. However, this will not contribute to the management of his active variceal bleeding.

    Ordering an emergent ultrasound of the abdomen (**choice E**) is not the most appropriate management of this acutely ill patient. An ultrasound will demonstrate the known diagnosis of cirrhosis and may provide useful information about flow in the portal vein and hepatic veins. However, this will not contribute to the management of his active variceal bleeding.

13. **The correct answer is C.** The finding of dark red urine suggests a number of underlying conditions, most notably hematuria. The absence of red blood cells on microscopic examination of the urine in the setting of a urine dipstick positive for blood suggests the possibility of myoglobinuria. Myoglobin is a pigment that is detected by the orthotoluidine reagent on the dipstick, which causes a false-positive test for blood. In addition, the patient's history of extreme physical exertion also strongly suggests myoglobinuria as the cause of the urine color. Extreme physical activity as in the case of running a marathon leads to muscle cell breakdown and the release of myoglobin into the circulation. The myoglobin is filtered by the kidney and leads to the dark red urine as it is excreted.

Hemolyzed blood in the urine (**choice A**) is a potential cause of dark red urine. In this case, however, one would expect to see a few red blood cells in the urine since it is unlikely that every single red blood cell would be hemolyzed. This is not the case in this urinalysis and it makes hemolyzed blood in the urine less likely.

Ingestion of food or other material containing red dye (**choice B**) is a potential cause of dark red urine. The red dye would not produce a positive urine dipstick test for blood and is not likely the cause of the urine color in this patient.

Trauma to the kidneys (**choice D**) is a potential cause of dark red urine secondary to hematuria. This patient's urinalysis did not demonstrate any red blood cells and as a result hematuria is not the cause of the urine color.

Urinary tract infection (**choice E**) is a potential cause of dark red urine if it is accompanied by hematuria. This patient's urinalysis did not demonstrate any red or white blood cells and as a result this patient does not have a urinary tract infection nor does he have hematuria.

14. **The correct answer is A.** Chlordiazepoxide and other benzodiazepines have documented efficacy of increasing seizure threshold and are recommended as suitable agents for alcohol withdrawal. Trials comparing different benzodiazepines demonstrated that all appear similarly efficacious in reducing signs and symptoms of withdrawal. However, there is some evidence that longer-acting agents (e.g., chlordiazepoxide) may be more effective in preventing seizures. There is also a greater margin of safety and reduced abuse potential.

Neuroleptic agents, including the phenothiazines and haloperidol (**choice B**), demonstrate some effectiveness in reducing signs and symptoms of withdrawal. Phenothiazines are less effective than benzodiazepines in preventing delirium. Both agents increase the incidence of seizures compared with placebo and are much less effective than benzodiazepines in preventing seizures.

Routine administration of magnesium (**choice C**) is generally not recommended. Existing controlled data does not demonstrate improvement in alcohol withdrawal severity, delirium, or seizures. It has long been recognized that magnesium levels are frequently low during alcohol withdrawal. Closer study showed that magnesium levels are usually normal on admission, but then drop during the course of withdrawal before spontaneously returning to normal as symptoms subside.

Beta-blockers like metoprolol (**choice D**) reduce selected signs and symptoms of withdrawal but they have not been shown to reduce delirium or seizures. They may be considered for use in conjunction with benzodiazepines in patients with certain coexisting conditions such as coronary artery disease. Beta-blockers have no known anticonvulsant activity and large enough studies have not been performed to determine whether they reduce or increase seizures during withdrawal. Furthermore, delirium is a known side effect of beta-blockers, particularly those with good central nervous system penetration such as propranolol.

In one large trial thiamine (**choice E**) did not reduce delirium or seizures. However, individuals with alcohol dependence are frequently thiamine deficient with a high risk for Wernicke disease and Wernicke-Korsakoff syndrome. These are sequelae that can be prevented by administration of thiamine.

15. **The correct answer is A.** Delirium tremens or DTs is a complication of chronic alcohol abuse. It is characterized by excessive agitation and confusion. There is an increase in the sympathetic nervous system. The process often begins after sudden deprivation of alcohol. The majority of times the symptoms are self-limited and disappear within 72 hours. However, in a small percentage of people suffering with delirium tremens the symptoms worsen and may be severe enough to lead to death. Risk factors for developing delirium tremens include ethanol withdrawal seizures, prior history of delirium tremens, and higher than usual quantity and frequency of ethanol consumption (so much individual variability exists that the actual answer may not be clinically relevant). The diagnosis of delirium tremens is made when the course progresses beyond the usual symptoms of withdrawal to include severe confusion and disorientation with associated delusions and hallucinations, severe agitation, and generalized seizures.

The features of autonomic nervous system dysfunction include diaphoresis (**choice B**), fever (**choice C**), tachycardia (**choice D**), and tachypnea (**choice E**). These symptoms precede the onset of delirium tremens and are not specific to the diagnosis of delirium tremens.

16. **The correct answer is C.** This scenario is best described by the phrase palliative care. Palliative care is defined by the World Health Organization as the active total care of patients whose disease is not responsive to curative treatment. Control of pain and other symptoms and of psychological, social, and spiritual problems is paramount. The goal of palliative care is achievement of the best possible quality of life for patients and their families. The applied ethical issue of euthanasia or

mercy killing concerns whether it is morally permissible for a third party, such as a physician, to end the life of a terminally ill patient who is in intense pain. For health care workers, the issue of the right to die is most prominent when a patient in their care is terminally ill, is in intense pain, and voluntarily chooses to end his life to escape prolonged suffering. In this case the physician uses morphine for pain relief rather than a means to end the patient's life.

Active euthanasia (**choice A**) is when the health care worker takes active measures to end the patient's life, such as by directly administering a lethal dose of a drug. The health care worker's action is the direct cause of the patient's death. Active euthanasia is the most controversial of the four options and is currently illegal in the United States.

Nonvoluntary euthanasia (**choice B**) refers to the mercy killing of a patient who is unconscious, comatose, or otherwise unable to explicitly make his intentions known. In these cases it is often family members who make the request. It is important not to confuse nonvoluntary mercy killing with involuntary mercy killing. The latter would be done against the wishes of the patient and would clearly count as murder.

Passive euthanasia (**choice D**) is when the worker can discontinue providing life-sustaining treatment to the patient, and thus allow him to die more quickly. This brings on death through nonintervention.

Physician-assisted suicide (**choice E**) is when the health care worker can provide the patient with the means of taking his own life, such as a lethal dose of a drug. This practice is called assisted suicide since it is the patient and not technically the health care worker who administers the drug.

17. **The correct answer is D.** One of the best treatments for the hypotension associated with right ventricular infarction/ischemia is volume loading (in this instance with Ringers lactate). This is because the right ventricle, when ischemic, becomes severely dependent on preload for the maintenance of right-sided output. Thus, by providing augmented right-sided filling with the volume infusion, one can augment right ventricular output, and therefore, left ventricular output and increase the systemic blood pressure.

    Intravenous morphine (**choice A**) can also exacerbate the hypotension with right ventricular infarction/ischemia by causing venodilation. Morphine is also not necessary in this instance since we are not told of ongoing angina.

    Intravenous nitroglycerin (**choice B**) can significantly diminish right ventricular filling by causing venodilation and, therefore, exacerbate the hypotension seen with right ventricular ischemia/infarction.

    Similarly, oral nitroglycerin (**choice C**) can also significantly exacerbate the hypotension seen with right ventricular ischemia/infarction by diminishing right ventricular filling by causing dilation of the venous bed.

    Intravenous streptokinase (**choice E**), an agent used for thrombolytic therapy, is not needed in this instance since we are not told the patient has an ST-segment elevation myocardial infarction. The role of thrombolysis with right ventricular infarction is also controversial.

18. **The correct answer is D.** Hyperthyroidism presents itself in the geriatric population (older than 70 years) differently than in the younger population. Above the age of 70 you may not necessarily find a tremor in patients with hyperthyroidism.

    Fatigue (**choice A**), tachycardia (**choice C**), and weight loss (**choice E**) are the three most common findings in the elderly hyperthyroid patient. In addition, approximately 50% present with a goiter (**choice B**). Fatigue is often misdiagnosed with hypothyroidism in the elderly population sector when it is actually hyperthyroidism. In the younger population up to 90% will present with a goiter. The younger population will also commonly present with hyperreflexia, increased sweating, heat intolerance, tremor, increased appetite, and anxiety.

19. **The correct answer is B.** This patient has allergic contact dermatitis caused by lanolin superimposed on chronic stasis dermatitis. Lanolin is a common compound found in many over the counter moisturizers and rubbing creams for its hygroscopic and emollient properties. It is a well-known sensitizer in patients with stasis dermatitis, a condition known to predispose to contact sensitization. Stasis dermatitis develops on the lower extremities secondary to venous incompetence and chronic edema. Early findings in stasis dermatitis consist of mild erythema and scaling associated with pruritus. The typical initial site of involvement is the medial aspect of the ankle, often over a distended vein. As the disorder progresses, the dermatitis becomes progressively pigmented due to chronic erythrocyte extravasation leading to cutaneous hemosiderin deposition. As with other forms of dermatitis, stasis dermatitis may become acutely inflamed, with crusting and exudate. Chronic stasis dermatitis is often associated with dermal fibrosis that is recognized clinically as brawny edema of the skin.

Stasis dermatitis is often complicated by secondary infection and contact dermatitis. Contact dermatitis presents with well-demarcated edema, erythema, vesiculation, and crusting of the affected skin. Severe stasis dermatitis may precede the development of stasis ulcers. It is prudent to advise patients with stasis dermatitis to read the labels of over the counter products for skin care and rubbing creams and to avoid the ones that contain lanolin, balsam of Peru, and fragrances, as they are frequent contact sensitizers.

Enalapril (**choice A**) is an angiotensin-converting enzyme inhibitor utilized in the treatment of hypertension and heart failure. It does not cause contact dermatitis.

Metformin (**choice C**) is used in the primary treatment of type 2 diabetes. Its side effects are related to gastrointestinal disturbance such as anorexia, nausea, and diarrhea. It is not a contact sensitizer.

Pentoxiphylline (**choice D**) enhances the rheologic characteristics of erythrocytes and is used in the treatment of macrovascular disease. It does not cause contact dermatitis.

Petrolatum (**choice E**) is an inert chemical substance used as a vehicle for many skin care products and topical medications. It has not been known to induce contact sensitization

20. **The correct answer is A.** This patient is most likely suffering from gastroesophageal reflux disease, which can present in the manner described in the question. It is part of the important differential diagnoses of chest pain. The acidic gastric contents may sometimes leave a bitter taste in the mouth and usually do so during the night when the patient is lying supine in bed. Other symptoms include cough, asthma, hoarseness, aphthous ulcers, hiccups, and dental erosions. The pressure in his chest is related to the acid reflux. The patient would benefit from endoscopic evaluation.

Panic disorder (**choice B**) is defined as recurrent episodes of discrete periods of intense fear or discomfort. This is not a part of this patient's symptoms, making a panic disorder unlikely. Other associated symptoms include dyspnea, dizziness, palpitations, feelings of depersonalization, and fear of dying.

Parkinson disease (**choice C**) is also unlikely since there is an absence of tremor, bradykinesia, rigidity, gait disturbance, or "masked face" which all typify Parkinson disease.

Postnasal drip (**choice D**) is defined as a flow of mucus from the back of the nasal cavity onto the pharyngeal surface, usually caused by a cold or seasonal allergies (e.g., hay fever). The patient's symptoms are too severe to fit the nature of a postnasal drip alone.

Sleep apnea (**choice E**) can sometimes be reported prolonged pauses in respiration during sleep. It also requires the presence of loud snoring, daytime hypersomnolence, disturbed nonrefreshing sleep, and weight gain, which are not present in this man. If suspected, a sleep study is warranted to confirm the diagnosis.

21. **The correct answer is B.** She most likely has psoriatic nails and psoriasis of ears because the characteristic psoriatic nail changes include numerous 1-mm pits in addition to "oil spots" consisting of 2 to 4-mm tan, oval spots. Onycholysis (uplifting of distal portion of nail plate from nail bed) as well as heaped up crusts accumulated beneath them is often seen in patients with psoriasis. Some patients may only have manifestation of nails without skin involvement. This patient has a mild amount of skin involvement of her conchal bowl. The well-defined and thickened scales of the ear lesions are more likely psoriasis than seborrheic dermatitis (**choice D**).

Onychomycosis and ringworm (**choice A**) is incorrect because onychomycotic nails are characterized by thickened, dystrophic, discolored nail plates without pits. Onycholysis may occasionally be associated with onychomycosis.

Pterygium and lichen planus (**choice C**) is incorrect because this is a term used to describe destroyed nail matrix secondary to inflammation and replaced by fibrosis. The proximal nail fold fuses with the proximal portion of the nail bed. Involvement of the entire matrix may lead to obliteration of the whole nail.

Seborrheic dermatitis (**choice D**) is incorrect because this disorder is not associated with any nail findings. The skin findings generally consist of greasy, ill-defined, erythematous patches of scale involving bilateral brows, nasolabial fold, external ear canal, and anterior chest, as well as the scalp (most common site).

Pits from trauma during manicure (**choice E**) is incorrect because she has involvement of both finger and toe nails. In addition, common trauma caused by manicure is usually paronychia and longitudinal nail plate changes from damaged proximal nail fold area.

22. **The correct answer is B.** A case series collects cases of the disease and looks for common elements among them. This can be done quickly and yields a good picture of the symptoms, characteristics, and prognosis of

the disease. What a case series does not provide is a clear picture of how diseased people are different from those who do not have the disease.

A case-control study (**choice A**) compares patients with a condition to people without the specified condition and looks retrospectively for risk factors in both groups. Because the disease in this question is not yet well specified and the number of suspected diseased individuals is limited, this study would be difficult to do at this time.

A cohort study (**choice C**) examines segments of the population with specified risk factors and then follows them forward in time looking for the development of disease. Because of the lack of knowledge of precursor factors and the time frame involved, this would not be the study of choice for this question.

A community trial (**choice D**) tests an intervention in a nonmedical setting. Because there is no intervention suggested here, this cannot be the answer.

A crossover study (**choice E**) is a method of balancing the demands of research design with the demands of ethics. Everyone in a crossover study receives the medication at some point. In this question there is no intervention at all, so crossover study is not an option.

A cross-sectional study (**choice F**) assesses the general prevalence of a disease and factors associated with it in the general population.

23. **The correct answer is B.** Colonization with *H. pylori* likely occurs in early childhood. Mechanism for colonization is likely via the fecal-oral or oral-oral route. Without treatment, infection is typically lifelong with only very rare spontaneous remissions. Infection during adulthood is rare.

Gastric biopsy (**choice A**) is not essential for the diagnosis of *H. pylori* infection since there are many noninvasive tests that can be used to document infection. These tests include urea breath tests, antibody test (both rapid testing and qualitative serological testing), and fecal antigen testing. Biopsy with culture can be performed if a biopsy is performed for another reason, but is not necessary to make a diagnosis. If antibiotic resistance were to become a problem in the future, biopsy might be important for antibiotic selection.

Repeat endoscopy (**choice C**) is not always necessary to confirm disease resolution. It is only indicated in those patients with recurrent symptoms or those with complicated ulcer disease.

Many patients are colonized with *H. pylori* and do not have ulcer disease. It is estimated that about 20% of infected patients go on to have ulcer disease in their lifetime. Therefore, (**choice D**) is incorrect. It is probably unnecessary to treat asymptomatic patients with *H. pylori.*

Lifelong treatment with proton pump inhibitors (**choice E**) is not necessary. After treatment of *H. pylori*, patients should have a resolution of their symptoms. If patients have dyspepsia for reasons other than *H. pylori*, treatment regimens can be individualized.

24. **The correct answer is D.** The pattern best fits pancreatitis in view of the gradual flare-up and then constant nature of the pain that is radiating through to the back, which began after a heavy meal and lots of drinking.

In gastroenteritis or food poisoning (**choice A**) you would expect vomiting and diarrhea and the pain would most likely be colicky in nature (intermittent with a crescendo-decrescendo pattern).

A condition located in the common bile duct (**choice B**), such as cholangitis, would be suggested by Charcot triad, which is fever with chills, jaundice, and pain in the right-upper quadrant. Choledocholithiasis, which is also a condition located in the common bile duct, is characterized by jaundice, pale stools, and dark urine.

Pain from the duodenum (**choice C**) could be due to a duodenal ulcer, particularly one that penetrates to the back or even perforates. The pain can be severe but the fact that the pain was gradual in onset and that he is able to move around are small clues against a duodenal ulcer.

The stomach (**choice E**) may be a source of alcoholic gastritis, which should have been somewhat relieved by vomiting and may have produced some bleeding and is therefore unlikely. If vomiting had preceded the pain, one would have considered a perforation of the lower esophagus, but it was the other way around.

25. **The correct answer is D.** The patient has hypercholesterolemia with a high LDL-cholesterol level, which is not consistent with cholesterol panels in females of a comparable age group. She also has significant coronary heart disease risks including being 55 years old, possibly being postmenopausal without estrogen replacement therapy, having borderline hypertension, and a strong cardiac family history. The National Cholesterol Education Program would recommend that patients at higher risk of coronary heart disease receive more intensive interventions for dyslipidemia.

The high LDL level would require that the patient begin drug therapy sooner, because it is unlikely that a patient with an LDL level of 130 mg/dL or greater will be able to achieve the goal of 100 mg/dL with aerobic exercise, weight reduction, and dietary modification alone (**choice B**). Atorvastatin is an HMG-CoA reductase inhibitor, which is the drug category of choice for hypercholesterolemia because they reduce LDL cholesterol most effectively. The patient's liver panel is normal and it would be appropriate to begin atorvastatin while keeping track of the liver panel every 6 months.

Explaining that her cholesterol panel is consistent with the normal range of cholesterol in females of her age group and repeating her cholesterol panel annually (**choice A**) is incorrect because as stated previously, these are not normal cholesterol levels.

Hypothyroidism may be an important cause of the dyslipidemia but reducing the dose of her medication (**choice C**) is incorrect.

Gemfibrozil (**choice E**) is a fibric acid analog and may be a better choice in patients with significant hypertriglyceridemia >1000 mg/dL.

26. **The correct answer is C.** This patient's history and exam are very concerning for a dissection of the thoracic aorta. If the ascending aorta is involved in a dissection, it becomes a surgical emergency. Dissections of the descending aorta can be managed medically. Therefore, whenever an aortic dissection is suspected, it is paramount to determine its presence and extent. The imaging modalities best suited for this include echocardiography, chest CT, and angiography.

A cardiac stress test (**choice A**) is not useful in the diagnosis of an aortic dissection. A patient with a suspected dissection should also not be stressed in any way since increased cardiac contractility and elevated blood pressure can propagate the dissection.

A chest radiograph (**choice B**) is not as useful as an echocardiogram in definitively determining the presence of an aortic dissection and its extent.

A tagged red blood cell scan (**choice D**) used in the diagnosis of areas of small, ongoing bleeding has no role in the diagnosis of an aortic dissection.

A ventilation-perfusion scan (**choice E**) used in the diagnosis of a pulmonary embolus has no utility in the diagnosis of an aortic dissection.

27. **The correct answer is D.** The most important advice to give on using potent topical corticosteroid agents is *not* to apply the cream to the genitalia or face because it causes dermal or epidermal sclerosis which could be disastrous.

Applying a soft bandage (**choice A**) around the foot after application is useful in preventing the cream from sticking to clothes or bed sheets and locks the cream to the skin where it is needed.

Applying the cream and then removing it (**choice B**) defeats the purpose of applying the corticosteroid in the first place.

You should advice her that if the rash continues to spread, she should stop further applications and return to see you because this may be suggestive of a cellulitis. Therefore, telling her to continue (**choice C**) is incorrect.

Medications should always be discarded beyond their expiration date and corticosteroid creams are therapeutic and rarely for prophylactic use (**choice E**).

28. **The correct answer is E.** Current recommendations are to begin prophylactic medication for gout after three attacks of gout. The choice of prophylactic medication is made by determining the 24-hour secretion of uric acid. The patient excreted less than 250 mg/24 hours of uric acid suggesting failure to excrete the uric acid once it was produced. Probenecid would be the best choice since it increases the excretion rate (uricosuric agent).

Allopurinol (**choice A**) would be used if the patient excretes above the normal range of uric acid (750 mg/24 hours), i.e., producing too much uric acid. Allopurinol would then slow the production of uric acid by acting as a xanthine oxidase inhibitor in the synthetic pathway.

Colchicine (**choice B**) and indomethacin (**choice D**) would treat acute flare-ups of gout and would suffice as adjuncts to either of the above two prophylactic agents.

Ibuprofen (**choice C**) can be used to treat the painful symptoms but it is not a prophylactic therapy to prevent gout.

29. **The correct answer is D.** Allopurinol is indicated in patients with uric acid overproduction, history of renal stones, and renal impairment. Probenecid is a uricosuric agent and is contraindicated in patients who have a history of renal stone formation.

Therefore, asking about a history of renal stones is the most relevant question to your management.

Weight-bearing problems (**choice A**) would have been a presenting complaint and does not have much bearing on gout management other than as an indication for symptomatic relief.

There are few studies showing genetic predisposition to gout and family history (**choice B**) would not change your management for this patient.

Gallstones (**choice C**) are mainly cholesterol based and not uric acid based and should not affect your management for gout.

Fever (**choice E**) is may be an associated symptom of gout, but it has no relevance in gout therapy.

30. **The correct answer is C.** The patient has a hypertensive emergency defined as a systolic BP exceeding 210 and a diastolic BP greater than 130 and presenting with blurred vision, headaches, or focal neurological symptoms. This would require immediate blood pressure reduction (not necessarily to normal ranges) to minimize end-organ damage, and an appropriate agent is labetalol.

Pain can be a significant source of acute hypertension, but not to this degree. Treatment of the pain alone with hydromorphone (**choice A**) without attention to reducing the blood pressure to a safer level is wrong.

Hydralazine (**choice B**) is another useful agent except it can cause drug-induced systemic lupus-like syndrome in 10% of patients, which this patient has. Hydralazine works as a direct-acting vasodilator.

Intravenous fluids and furosemide (**choice D**) would not be effective enough in bringing the blood pressure under control in a safe amount of time.

31. **The correct answer is D.** The diagnosis is hyperkalemia, the treatment of which was appropriately given. ACE inhibitors, such as quinapril, can cause hyperkalemia along with cough, fatigue, and tachycardia. It would be prudent to discontinue it. Also remember to monitor the BUN and creatinine (renal function) in severe congestive heart failure, hypertension, and renal artery stenosis (if the latter is diagnosed then stop the ACE inhibitor). Also monitor WCC in renal or collagen vascular disease. All the other medications would cause *hypokalemia*.

Albuterol (**choice A**) can also cause tachycardia and tremor.

Furosemide (**choice B**) can cause excessive diuresis and orthostatic hypotension.

Prednisone (**choice C**) can aggravate glaucoma and cataracts.

Torsemide (**choice E**) can cause hyperuricemia and excessive thirst.

32. **The correct answer is E.** This question deals with patient compliance for therapy once the patient goes home. The best answer would be to wrap compression bandaging as a stocking around each leg, which can be tailor-made for comfort too. This would mean he is more likely to keep them on and benefit from reduction in edema next time he sees you.

He is already ambulating with difficulty and a walking aid (**choice A**) may not be effective. The pain may be a strong deterrent from ambulating in order to reduce the edema.

Caffeinated drink consumption for diuresis (**choice B**) is incorrect as there have been no studies to show efficacy and excess caffeine may cause bladder irritation, palpitations, and erratic blood pressures.

Elevation of the legs (**choice C**) may be a good idea except you cannot guarantee he would do this at home at night especially with the gastroesophageal reflux disease.

Taking cold baths (**choice D**) have no proven benefit in reducing leg edema and are probably unpleasant.

33. **The correct answer is E.** This patient most likely has seborrheic dermatitis, which can present in infants as cradle cap. In adults it affects the scalp, forehead, retroauricular region, eyebrows, cheeks, and nasolabial folds. Pruritus is mild. Treatment with selenium shampoos or tar shampoos to the scalp has been effective.

Acne rosacea (**choice A**) is characterized by papules, erythema, and telangiectasias. It can be exacerbated by sunlight. Treat with doxycycline and sun block.

Alopecia areata (**choice B**) is asymptomatic hair loss commonly involving the scalp and seen as well-defined, single or multiple areas of hair loss.

Pityriasis rosea (**choice C**) is a self-limiting dermatitis of the trunk and extremities typically between the ages of 10 and 35 years. Lesions are 2 cm or less and pink, tan, or light brown.

Scabies (**choice D**) is typically pruritic and usually occurs in areas of the groin, navel, breast, and finger webs. An affected patient and all household members should be treated with lindane.

34. **The correct answer is B.** This patient presents with dyspeptic symptoms likely due to a duodenal ulcer given the positive response to food, lack of nonsteroidal anti-inflammatory use, and absence of nausea and vomiting. The patient does not provide any history that indicates the need for urgent endoscopy such as melena, hematemesis, dysphagia, or weight loss. Thus it is reasonable to attempt to manage his current illness in a noninvasive manner. The majority of ulcers are secondary to either nonsteroidal anti-inflammatory use or *Helicobacter pylori*. The patient does not give any history of nonsteroidal anti-inflammatory use and his serology for *Helicobacter pylori* is positive. Therefore, the most appropriate treatment strategy is to eradicate *Helicobacter pylori* and provide empiric acid suppression with either a histamine blocker or proton pump inhibitor. There are several regimens that can be used to eradicate *Helicobacter pylori*, all of which include a medication to suppress acid production. Eradication of *Helicobacter pylori* is of paramount importance because it has been shown to significantly reduce the recurrence of peptic ulcer disease. Four to six weeks of acid suppression with a histamine blocker such as ranitidine or a proton pump inhibitor such as omeprazole is commonly used to permit healing of active ulcers.

Omeprazole alone (**choice A**) is incorrect because using omeprazole alone does not eradicate *Helicobacter pylori*, which is a likely cause of this patient's peptic ulcer disease. By treating with omeprazole alone the patient's ulcer is likely to heal but also likely to recur.

Ranitidine alone (**choice C**) is incorrect for the same reason stated above. Ranitidine, a histamine blocker, will permit healing of the present ulcer but will not eradicate *Helicobacter pylori*. Thus, the patient is likely to have a recurrent ulcer.

Ranitidine and amoxicillin in combination (**choice D**) is incorrect because amoxicillin alone is not a recommended antibiotic regimen for the eradication of *Helicobacter pylori*. The majority of antibiotic regimens combine two antibiotics (clarithromycin with either amoxicillin or metronidazole) and a proton pump inhibitor. The use of two antibiotics limits the development of resistant organisms.

Sucralfate and misoprostol (**choice E**) is incorrect because sucralfate and misoprostol are used as prophylaxis against the development of ulcers. They are not commonly used in the treatment of active ulcers. Misoprostol, for example, is a prostaglandin analog commonly used to prevent nonsteroidal anti-inflammatory-induced ulcer disease.

35. **The correct answer is D.** This patient has the most common cause for a visit to an orthopedic surgeon: osteoarthritis or degenerative arthritis. It is important to understand the difference between osteoarthritis and the inflammatory arthropathies. Osteoarthritis is typically an arthritis of the large weight-bearing joints: knee, hip, and ankle. It is also seen in the shoulder and less commonly in the hands, wrist, and elbow. Radiographic hallmarks of osteoarthritis include joint space narrowing, osteophyte (extra bone growth) formation, and subchondral sclerosis. Early attempts at treating osteoarthritis include activity modification (less weight-bearing activities), nonsteroidal anti-inflammatory medication, and weight loss. As the patient's symptoms worsen intra-articular steroid injections may be used. As a final option the patient may require joint replacement or other surgical interventions.

The patient has no symptoms or signs of a bone tumor and osteosarcoma is primarily a highly malignant tumor of the childhood years (**choice A**).

This patient has no significant history or physical findings that would suggest rheumatoid arthritis, which is usually a polyarticular process with small joint involvement as well as large joints (**choice B**).

Infections of joints are usually not indolent in nature. Infections within a joint (septic arthritis) are usually acutely painful and accompanied by an elevated erythrocyte sedimentation rate and peripheral white blood cell count (**choice C**).

Although this patient may require a total knee arthroplasty (replacement), surgical intervention is not a first-line treatment. This patient may respond to NSAIDs and activity modification. It would be reasonable to send the patient to an orthopedic surgeon if the patient's symptoms persist (**choice E**).

36. **The correct answer is C.** Although a patient presenting with a right middle lobe pneumonia, in general, will turn out to have an infection with a typical community-acquired organism, tuberculosis continues to grow in prevalence in the homeless and lower socioeconomic classes. Furthermore, the history of subjective fevers with night sweats should further raise your clinical suspicion. Primary tuberculosis can present with infiltrates anywhere within the lungs while reactivation tuberculosis

classicly occurs in the upper lobes. The appropriate treatment in this case is with antibiotics to cover a community-acquired pneumonia (for which ceftriaxone is reasonable), and to isolate the patient in a negative-pressure room and rule out tuberculosis with three serial induced morning sputum samples. If the patient proves to have tuberculosis then treatment should be instituted.

However, in this clinical scenario immediate treatment with antituberculous drugs without confirmation of disease (**choice A**) is not warranted. Similarly not considering TB in this patient and treating him solely for community-acquired pneumonia (**choice B**) is also inappropriate.

Because of the risk of tuberculosis and the fact that the patient is homeless with a high risk of being lost to followup, discharge from the hospital with therapy (**choice D**) or without therapy (**choice E**) is not appropriate.

37. **The correct answer is B.** There is current evidence to suggest that screening for colon cancer every 3 years with guaiac tests and sigmoidoscopy is beneficial.

Blood lead levels (**choice A**) are obtained in 1-year-old children for screening purposes by some physicians.

Screening ultrasound for thyroid nodules (**choice D**) or carotid disease (**choice C**) has not been proven to be beneficial. If however a nodule is felt on physical examination or a bruit heard, then these tests may be appropriate.

Screening chest x-rays (**choice E**) have been shown to not improve survival in lung cancer. There is currently a lot of work being done to evaluate screening low-dose chest CT scan in high-risk patients.

38. **The correct answer is E.** This patient has allergic contact dermatitis, which is a type IV hypersensitivity reaction that is characterized by the release of lymphokines from sensitized lymphocytes reacting with antigens. It is a cell-mediated reaction that does not require antibody formation. The antigen in this case is the nickel in her wedding band. The nickel is typically drawn out of the ring by water, sweating, or detergent. Even good-quality rings may contain nickel.

Antibody-mediated cytotoxic reaction to cell surface antigens (**choice A**) is the mechanism for pernicious anemia, not contact dermatitis.

Antigen-antibody complexes formed in the vessels in response to an antigen (**choice B**) is the mechanism for autoimmune diseases, such as rheumatoid arthritis and lupus, not contact dermatitis.

Fixation of complement resulting in osmotic lysis of antibody-coated cell (**choice C**) is the mechanism for autoimmune-hemolytic anemia, not contact dermatitis.

Release of histamine from basophils after antigen interaction with Fc receptor-bound IgE (**choice D**) is the mechanism for atopy and asthma, not contact dermatitis.

39. **The correct answer is A.** This patient has contact dermatitis, which should be treated with a high-potency fluorinated topical glucocorticoid. Since she already stopped wearing her ring, which is the most likely offending agent, a topical steroid will help to relieve the symptoms.

Oral prednisone (**choice B**) is used for widespread allergic contact dermatitis, or if it involves the face or genitals. It should not be used as a first-line treatment for localized disease.

Permethrin cream (**choice C**) is the treatment for scabies, which is an ectoparasitic infestation that causes a rash and itching that is worse at night and after a hot shower. Burrows are typically present and appear as wavy lines that end in a pearly bleb. Scraping the burrows and examining the scrapings under the microscope reveals the mite, its eggs, or pellets. It is highly contagious and often involves other members of the household.

Topical coal tar (**choice D**) and/or salicylic acid (**choice E**) are used to treat seborrheic dermatitis, not allergic contact dermatitis. Seborrheic dermatitis is characterized by erythema and greasy yellow-brown scales. The scalp and eyebrow are the most common sites.

40. **The correct answer is B.** The best answer is the one that prevents the most accidents for the same money. This question requires the combination of the number needed to treat (NNT) with the cost of prevention. NNT is equal to the inverse of the incidence rate. Thus, if incidence is 50 per 10,000, then NNT = 10,000/50 or 200. This means, concretely, preventive measures with 200 people would prevent one accident. The lowest NNT × cost combination will prevent the most accidents within the cost constraints. That is, the highest incidence combined with the lowest cost of intervention will be the correct answer. We would work out the answer as follows. (Note that for speedy calculations, numbers are rounded before calculations are made.)

Accident Type	Incidence	Rounded	NNT	Cost	NNT × Cost
Tractor	49	50	200	$5	$1000
Falls from heights	41	40	250	$3	$750
Truck	25	25	400	$5	$2000
Automobile	20	20	500	$3	$1500
Poisonings	15	15	667	$2	$1334

This means that spending $750 will prevent one fall, a better prevention rate for the expenditure than any of the other options (**choices A, C, D, and E**).

41. **The correct answer is A.** This patient has a classic profile and presentation for necrotizing fasciitis. This entity can be rapidly fatal and requires aggressive polymicrobial intravenous antibiotic treatment to include group A beta-hemolytic streptococcus and other gram-positive organisms, and also for anaerobic and gram-negative organisms. Culture and extensive wound debridement are necessary. ("Skin popping" is injecting narcotic directly into the skin because of lack of intravenous access).

    Cephalexin (**choice B**) or nafcillin (**choice C**) are appropriate antibiotics for typical gram-positive infections such as an uncomplicated or mildly complicated cellulitis. However, as mentioned above, this patient needs polymicrobial therapy and surgical debridement.

    Topical antibiotics (**choice D**) are generally not effective in cellulitis, and particularly not in this setting.

    An x-ray of the right arm (**choice E**) is important in the general workup of the patient; however, the most important thing at this time is treatment of the patient.

42. **The correct answer is D.** This patient is presenting with worsening back pain and signs of infection in the setting of a normal spine x-ray. This clinical scenario can often be seen in diskitis. His history of trauma in this case is likely not related to the current problem. Oftentimes early in the course of diskitis, the plain films of the spine will be negative. As the disease progresses, one can see loss of disk space height and erosion of the endplates. CT scan (**choice C**) is somewhat more sensitive than the plain film, but MRI is definitely the diagnostic test of choice.

    The most common organism to cause diskitis is *Staphylococcus aureus.* In children or adults, it can also be nonbacterial in nature. Tuberculosis of the spine (also know as Pott disease) is certainly a possibility in this patient, but it is neither the most likely, nor should empiric therapy be begun without a diagnosis (**choice A**).

    There is no reason at this point to think that this patient is malingering (**choice B**).

    The patient may need to be started on narcotic pain medications for pain control (**choice E**); however, a search for the underlying cause of the pain should be undertaken.

43. **The correct answer is E.** The most likely diagnosis in this case is ulcerative colitis. This disease often presents with multiple bowel movements per day over a chronic course and is associated with tenesmus and occasional blood. Patients often will have fevers and chills as well. The main differentiating factor from bacterial dysentery that may benefit from an antibiotic like ciprofloxacin (**choice B**) is the duration of symptoms. Weight loss is also a sign of a more chronic inflammatory process. The treatment of ulcerative colitis depends on severity of the disease. Sulfasalazine-type drugs remain the cornerstone of therapy. Corticosteroids are used for more severe disease or for acute flares. Corticosteroid enemas can also be used for distal disease. Other options in severe disease include immunosuppressants such as Imuran, cyclosporine, or methotrexate.

    Cisplatin-based chemotherapy (**choice A**) is not an appropriate choice as this is used for malignancies and not inflammatory bowel disease.

    A gluten-free diet (**choice C**) is used in patients with celiac sprue. This is due to small bowel inflammation from sensitivity to glutens (found in foods such as bread). It often presents with bloating, foul-smelling stools, and weight loss. Blood should not be present. Lactate sensitivity also will present in a similar fashion but will be associated with lactose products rather than gluten-containing products and will respond to limiting lactate (**choice D**) from the diet.

44. **The correct answer is A.** This patient presents with the classic symptoms and signs of Graves disease associated with vitiligo. Graves disease occurs in up to 2% of

women but is one-tenth as frequent in men. The disorder rarely begins before adolescence and typically occurs between 20 and 50 years of age, though it also occurs in the elderly. The skin is usually warm and moist, and the patient complains of sweating and heat intolerance, particularly during warm weather. Palmar erythema, onycholysis, and, less commonly, pruritus, urticaria, and diffuse hyperpigmentation may be evident. Hair texture may become fine, and a diffuse alopecia occurs in up to 40% of patients, persisting for months after restoration of euthyroidism. Vitiligo is associated with hyperthyroidism in 7% of patients with Graves disease and is also seen with an increased frequency in other autoimmune diseases such as Hashimoto thyroiditis, insulin-dependent diabetes mellitus, pernicious anemia, Addison disease, and alopecia areata. Vitiligo is an acquired pigmentary disorder manifested by depigmented white patches surrounded by a normal or hyperpigmented border. Four types have been described based on the extent and distribution of the involved areas: localized, generalized, universal, and acrofacial. The most commonly affected sites are the face, upper chest, dorsal hands, axillae, and groin.

Spontaneous resolution of vitiligo (**choice C**) is possible but rare, and it has been well established in the literature that early treatment (in the first 3 years) of vitiligo results in a much better chance of resolution than if the lesions are left untreated.

Once vitiligo appears, its clinical course is independent from the course of Graves disease and neither antithyroid medication (**choice B**) nor surgical resection of the thyroid (**choice E**) will have any repeatable influence on the course of the skin lesions.

Universal vitiligo applies to cases where the entire body surface is affected (**choice D**). This is the least common variant of vitiligo and usually very slow to evolve. Even when this is the case, there are often patches of normally pigmented skin interspersed over the body and it is very desirable to treat them with a depigmenting agent so that the patient's entire skin would be of the same color.

45. **The correct answer is B.** This patient most likely has tinea versicolor, a common skin infection in young adults who perspire freely. Tinea versicolor is caused by a nondermatophyte dimorphic fungus that is a normal inhabitant of the skin. As the yeast form *Pityrosporum orbiculare*, it generally does not cause disease (except for folliculitis in certain individuals). However, in some individuals, it converts to the hyphal form (*Malassezia furfur*) and causes characteristic lesions. The expression of infection is promoted by heat and humidity. The typical lesions consist of oval scaly macules, papules, and patches concentrated on the chest, shoulders, and back, but only rarely on the face or distal extremities. On dark skin, they often appear as hypopigmented areas, while on light skin they are slightly hyperpigmented. A potassium hydroxide (KOH) preparation from scaling lesions will demonstrate a confluence of short hyphae and round spores (so-called spaghetti and meatballs). Solutions containing sulfur, salicylic acid, or selenium sulfide will clear the infection if used daily for a week and then intermittently thereafter. It also responds well to topical antifungal creams such as ketoconazole 2% or terfenadine. Treatment with a single 400-mg dose of ketoconazole is also effective. A KOH preparation is performed on scaling skin lesions when a fungal etiology is suspected. The edge of such a lesion is scraped gently with a scalpel blade and the removed scale is collected on a glass microscope slide and treated with 1 to 2 drops of a solution of 10 to 20% KOH. KOH dissolves keratin and allows easier visualization of fungal elements. Brief heating of the slide accelerates dissolution of keratin. When the preparation is viewed under the microscope, the refractile hyphae will be seen more easily when the light intensity is reduced. This technique can be utilized to identify hyphae in dermatophyte infections, pseudohyphae and budding yeast in *Candida* infections, and fragmented hyphae and spores in tinea versicolor. The same sampling technique can be used to obtain scale for culture of selected pathogenic organisms.

Diascopy (**choice A**) is designed to assess whether a skin lesion will blanch with pressure as, for example, in determining whether a red lesion is hemorrhagic or simply blood-filled. For instance, a hemangioma will blanch with pressure, whereas a purpuric lesion caused by necrotizing vasculitis will not. Diascopy is performed by pressing a microscope slide or magnifying lens against a specified lesion and noting the amount of blanching that occurs. Granulomas often have an "apple jelly" appearance on diascopy.

Patch testing (**choice C**) is designed to document sensitivity to a specific antigen. In this procedure a battery of suspected allergens is applied to the patient's back under occlusive dressings and allowed to remain in contact with the skin for 48 h. The dressings are removed, and the area is examined for evidence of delayed hypersensitivity reactions (e.g., erythema, edema, or papulovesicles). This test is best performed by physicians with special expertise in patch testing and is often helpful in the evaluation of patients with chronic dermatitis.

Even though a skin biopsy (**choice D**) is a minor surgical procedure, it is not necessary to perform an invasive procedure that might result in a permanent scar in a straightforward case that can be easily confirmed with a simple KOH preparation of skin scrapings.

A Tzanck smear (**choice E**) is a cytologic technique most often used in the diagnosis of herpesvirus infections (simplex or varicella-zoster). An early vesicle, not a pustule or crusted lesion, is unroofed and the base of the lesion is scraped gently with a scalpel blade. The material is placed on a glass slide, air-dried, and stained with Giemsa or Wright stain. Multinucleated giant cells suggest the presence of herpes, but culture or immunofluorescence testing must be performed to identify the specific virus.

46. **The correct answer is D.** The recent data on congestive failure suggests that aldosterone can play a negative role in patients with heart failure. Therefore, given that the patient has had congestive failure on his current regimen, the institution of an aldosterone antagonist such as spironolactone is reasonable. It should be noted that ACE inhibitors such as captopril are unable to completely inhibit the formation of aldosterone.

Amiodarone (**choice A**) is an antiarrhythmic agent used in dysrhythmias such as atrial fibrillation. It has no role in the management of heart failure.

Starting furosemide (**choice B**), a loop diuretic, is inappropriate since the patient currently has no symptoms of congestive failure.

Starting propranolol (**choice C**), a nonselective beta antagonist, is inappropriate since the patient is already on a beta antagonist (metoprolol) with excellent heart rate and blood pressure control.

Discontinuing his metoprolol (**choice E**) is inappropriate since the patient is not in acute congestive failure, and since beta antagonists have been shown to improve mortality and morbidity in patients with congestive heart disease.

47. **The correct answer is A.** A patient who has been on exogenous steroids long term will have atrophy of their adrenal cortex and be unable to mount an appropriate stress response during periods of physiologic stress such as infection. Since this patient has a history of steroid use, and recently had her steroids rapidly tapered, administering hydrocortisone in this instance is appropriate.

Ketoconazole (**choice B**), a steroidal imidazole antifungal agent, can inhibit steroid hormone biosynthesis overtime and has no role in the management of steroid deficiency-induced hypotension.

Propranolol (**choice C**), a nonselective beta antagonist, is inappropriate in this setting since the patient is hypotensive.

Spironolactone (**choice D**), an aldosterone antagonist, has no role in the treatment of steroid deficiency-induced hypotension.

Thyroxine (**choice E**), used in the treatment of hypothyroidism, has no role in the management of steroid deficiency-induced hypotension.

48. **The correct answer is E.** The young woman has tinea corporis and the child has tinea capitis. Most likely they are caused by the same organism that was initially acquired by the child in kindergarten and then transmitted by close contact to cause ringworm on the arm of this young woman. Ringworm of the scalp is an infectious disease occurring chiefly in schoolchildren and less commonly in infants and adults. Boys have tinea capitis more frequently than girls; however, in epidemics caused by *Trichophyton tonsurans* there is often equal frequency in the sexes. In the United States, the most common cause of tinea capitis (ringworm of the scalp) is *Trichophyton tonsurans* (black-dot ringworm). It begins as a scaly, erythematous eruption with many broken off hairs (leaving black dots on the scalp). In extensive infection fever, pain, and regional lymphadenopathy may be present. Tinea corporis includes all superficial dermatophyte infections of the skin other than those of the scalp, beard, face, hands, feet, and groin. It forms one or more circular, sharply circumscribed, erythematous, dry, scaly, usually hypopigmented patches. They are slightly elevated at the border, where they are scaly and more inflamed than in the center. Progressive central clearing produces annular outlines that give the name "ringworm." Various dermatophytes may cause this type of infection, but *Trichophyton tonsurans* has experienced a dramatic rise as a cause for tinea corporis, as it has for tinea capitis.

Corynebacterium minutissimum (**choice A**) is a bacterium that causes erythrasma in which scaly, erythematous patches are found in the groin or axilla. It is well known for its coral red fluorescence when exposed to Wood light.

Epidermophyton floccosum (**choice B**) is a dermatophyte, too, but it does not cause infection of the hair or nails. It can only cause tinea of glabrous skin, such as athlete's foot.

Microsporum canis (**choice C**) can cause ringworm of the scalp and glabrous skin but has subsided as the leading cause in the United States in the past two decades and now is only third in frequency after *Trichophyton tonsurans* and *Microsporum audouinii*. Also, it more commonly causes a localized inflammatory patch in the scalp covered with gray stubbles of hair broken off at a few millimeters length.

Pityrosporum ovale (**choice D**) is yeast that is commonly found in the scalp of adults and may have a causative role in seborrheic dermatitis. It does not affect children before puberty.

49. **The correct answer is E.** When perianal lesions occur in the course of genital warts (condylomata acuminata), a prior history of receptive anal intercourse will usually predict whether intra-anal warts are present and determine the need for anoscopy. If intra-anal warts are present, they should be treated simultaneously with the genital ones to prevent recurrence (i.e., persistence) by contiguous spread of the infection from the intra-anal area. Genital warts are sexually transmitted, and other sexually transmitted diseases may be found in patients with genital warts. A complete history should be taken and the patient screened for other sexually transmitted diseases as appropriate. Women with genital warts should have a routine cervical cytologic screening (Papanicolaou smear) to detect cervical dysplasia.

History of intravenous drug abuse (**choice A**) would help determine whether your patient is at risk of having contracted one of the hematogenously transmitted diseases, such as hepatitis or human immunodeficiency virus infection, but it would not indicate existence of intra-anal warts.

History of internal and external hemorrhoids (**choice B**) would not prove useful in determining whether this patient has intra-anal warts, but would be another reason to have anoscopy performed and appropriate treatment initiated.

History of multiple sexual partners (**choice C**) would not support the existence of intra-anal warts by itself, but it would underline the need to perform testing for other sexually transmitted diseases (which you should do anyway in a patient who presents with genital warts).

History of multiple opportunistic infections (**choice D**) would indicate that the patient might be having an immune deficiency disease, such as the acquired immune deficiency syndrome. In patients with AIDS, genital warts are frequently resistant to treatment due to the inefficient immune system of the host that normally helps subdue this viral infection. In itself though, they would not indicate that intra-anal warts are present.

50. **The correct answer is E.** Patients with phencyclidine (PCP) intoxication are especially dangerous and unpredictable, even relative to other intoxications. The patients are extremely prone to violence and may have a diminished responsiveness to pain, making them even more difficult to control. Adequate sedation (usually with benzodiazepines) and a low level of environmental stimulation are the safest means of initial management of these patients.

Flumazenil (**choice A**) is used to treat benzodiazepine overdose. It has no indication in the treatment of PCP intoxication.

Naloxone (**choice B**) is an agent used to reverse binding of the opiate receptor by narcotics in overdose. It has no therapeutic use in the management of PCP intoxication.

HIV testing (**choice C**) may later be warranted in this patient because of his impulsive lifestyle. Given the patient's present level of agitation, however, actual HIV testing is not the overriding concern.

Performing a lumbar puncture (**choice D**) on this patient without adequate time for the patient to be sedated would be extremely dangerous. The patient's presentation is classic for PCP intoxication (especially given the positive urine toxicology). There would be a low likelihood of significant and clinically urgent information from a lumbar puncture done in this patient.

Internal Medicine: **Test Four**

1. A 27-year-old woman comes to the clinic because of increased sweating, fatigue, weight loss, loose bowel movements, and irritability for the past few months. She does not drink alcohol or caffeine and she does not smoke cigarettes. Her blood pressure is 120/80 mm Hg and pulse is 88/min. She has a fine resting tremor and warm, moist skin. Physical examination shows mild proptosis with stare and lid lag. The thyroid gland is lobular and asymmetrically enlarged. An electrocardiogram shows sinus tachycardia. Her thyroid-stimulating hormone level is 0.03 μU/mL and thyroxine level is 25 μg/dL. She returns to the clinic and you discuss treatment options for her condition. When discussing radioactive iodine therapy, you should tell her that it is commonly associated with

    (A) arthralgias, agranulocytosis, and a rash
    (B) the improvement of ophthalmopathy
    (C) leukemia
    (D) the need for replacement doses of thyroid hormone within 10 years
    (E) treatment failure requiring repeated doses

2. A 33-year-old woman with no past medical history comes to the clinic for an initial visit. She has not seen a physician in 3 years, offers no specific complaints, has never smoked, rarely drinks alcohol, and denies illicit drug use. She is a graduate student at the nearby university, is sexually active only with her fiancé, and uses the rhythm method for contraception. Her father died of a myocardial infarction at age 72, and her mother is 69 years old and healthy except for arthritis, for which she takes an over-the-counter medication with adequate relief. She denies any other significant family history. She is 163 cm (5 ft 3 in) tall and weighs 46 kg (102 lbs). Her temperature is 37.0 C (98.6 F), blood pressure 100/74 mm Hg, pulse is 76/min, and respirations are 16/min. She appears withdrawn. The rest of the examination is normal, except for the presence of 3 small ecchymoses on her lower extremities, in various stages of healing, that she attributes to bumping into furniture in her apartment. At this time, the least appropriate management is

    (A) checking a fasting serum cholesterol
    (B) counseling her about prevention of sexually transmitted diseases
    (C) inquiring further about her relationship with her fiancé
    (D) instructing her about breast self-examination and asking her to perform this monthly
    (E) performing a Pap smear

3. A 68-year-old man comes to the office for a regular followup appointment. He has a history of hypertension and diabetes mellitus, well controlled on medications. He has an excellent history of compliance, having never missed an appointment. He was seen last 4 months ago for followup. A hemoglobin A1C and three fecal occult blood samples were sent to the laboratory at that time. He returns now without complaints and would like to know the results of his tests. He denies chest pain, shortness of breath, rectal bleeding, dark stools, or melena. Laboratory studies show

Hemoglobin A1C	7.1%
Fecal occult blood	negative
	negative
	positive

Today his temperature is 37.0 C (98.6 F), blood pressure is 138/88 mm Hg, pulse is 64/min, and respirations are 14/min. There is a soft midsystolic murmur, loudest in the aortic region, that he has had for years, and lung examination is normal. Abdominal examination reveals no masses or organomegaly, and he has external hemorrhoids that are nontender. The most appropriate next step in management is to

(A) do colonoscopy
(B) increase his metformin dose from 850 mg tid to 1000 mg tid
(C) inquire about dietary indiscretions and his recent glucose control, and have him follow up as scheduled
(D) repeat the three tests for fecal occult blood
(E) send him to the laboratory for a complete blood count

4. An 82-year-old woman comes to the office for a followup visit. She has a history of osteoarthritis, uncontrolled hypertension, diabetes, severe peripheral vascular disease, and had a myocardial infarction 3 years ago that has been adequately controlled with dietary modification and hydrochlorothiazide, 25 mg daily. She was last seen by you 1 year ago. Today she complains only of occasional fatigue and decreased energy, which she attributes to "getting old." Her temperature is 37.0 C (98.6 F), blood pressure is 138/88 mm Hg, pulse is 64/min, and respirations are 14/min. She has three palpable nontender lymph nodes in the anterior cervical chain, each approximately 1 to 1.5 cm in diameter. The rest of the physical examination is normal. She denies recent symptoms of upper respiratory infection. Laboratory studies show

Hemoglobin	11.7 g/dL
Hematocrit	35.4%
Platelets	540,000/mm^3
Leukocyte count	8600/mm^3
Differential	80% lymphocytes
	15% neutrophils
	3% eosinophils
	2% basophils

Flow cytometry reveals a diagnosis of chronic lymphocytic leukemia. The most appropriate next step in management is to

(A) observe
(B) obtain a CT scan of the chest, abdomen, and pelvis
(C) refer her for a bone marrow biopsy
(D) refer her for chemotherapy
(E) refer her for radiotherapy

5. A 36-year-old woman with insulin-dependent diabetes mellitus is brought to the emergency department because of a fever and cough for 3 days and disorientation since yesterday. She has been feeling excessively thirsty and urinating every 30 minutes since this morning. Her husband is concerned that she "hasn't been herself." Her temperature is 38.5 C (101.3 F), blood pressure is 90/55 mm Hg, pulse is 108/min, and respirations are 20/min. She is oriented to herself only, has dry mucous membranes, and a thready pulse. A Foley catheter is draining clear urine. Blood glucose before receiving 2 L of normal saline was 685 mg/dL. Serum chemistries reveal a sodium of 128 mEq/L, potassium of 4.6 mEq/L, chloride of 96 mEq/L, and bicarbonate of 10 mEq/L. Repeat fingerstick is 522 mg/dL. Chest x-ray shows a left lower lobe infiltrate. Urinalysis reveals glucose >1000, protein 30, 2+ ketones, and no WBCs or RBCs. Blood cultures and urine culture are pending. The most appropriate management is to

(A) admit her to a medical floor after giving intravenous ceftriaxone
(B) admit her to a medical floor after giving intravenous vancomycin
(C) begin aggressive hydration and admit her to the intensive care unit
(D) begin aggressive hydration and an insulin infusion and admit her to the intensive care unit
(E) give regular insulin subcutaneously and observe her in the emergency department

6. A 21-year-old man comes to the office for what he tells the receptionist at the front desk is a "very delicate problem" he will discuss only with you. When you enter the exam room, he tells you that he just disembarked from a freight ship coming from the Far East where he had spent a few nights with the "local girls at the docks." A week ago he noticed a sore on his "private area" that does not hurt but does not seem to be healing either. This was his first trip outside of the country, and he was eager to try something new. He denies any previous sexually transmitted diseases or other medical problems. The aforementioned sexual encounters were unprotected and happened between 3 and 4 weeks ago. He is not taking any medication and denies any known allergies to medications. On physical examination, he is a well-developed, well-nourished young man. On the glans penis, there is a painless, round, superficial, ulcerated papule of 6 mm in diameter with a grayish, moist, indurated base and normal-appearing surrounding skin. There is bilateral, nontender, firm, and mobile inguinal lymphadenopathy. After collecting samples for the necessary diagnostic tests, you suggest immediate initiation of treatment in expectation of results. The most appropriate treatment is

(A) benzathine penicillin G 2.4 mU intramuscularly in a single dose
(B) benzathine penicillin G 2.4 mU intramuscularly, 1 dose weekly for 3 weeks
(C) doxycycline 100 mg PO bid for 2 weeks
(D) procaine penicillin G 2.4 mU IM qd, plus probenecid 500 mg PO qid, both for 10 to 14 days
(E) tetracycline 500 mg PO qid for 30 days

7. A 33-year-old woman comes to the clinic complaining of a 6-month history of weight gain, constipation, and "sluggishness." She denies any fevers, chills, or sweats. She also denies any alcohol, tobacco, or drug use and does not take any medications. Her temperature is 37.0 C (98.6 F), blood pressure is 98/78 mm Hg, pulse is 67/min, and respirations are 18/min. On examination, she has some fullness over her lower anterior neck, without palpable nodules. Her cardiac rhythm is regular, and her lungs are clear to auscultation bilaterally. The most appropriate next diagnostic step is to order

(A) a cervical CT
(B) a radioactive iodine uptake test
(C) a serum glucose level
(D) a serum thyroid-stimulating hormone level
(E) a thyroid ultrasound

8. An 86-year-old woman with severe chronic obstructive pulmonary disease is brought to the emergency department because of a cough and shortness of breath for the last 2 days. She has been intubated several times in the past year for similar presentations of pneumonia complicating end-stage COPD. She is on home oxygen. The patient's daughter states she has been appointed the health care proxy by her mother, and that on the last admission 1 month ago she was intubated and successfully extubated, after which she stated she would not want to be intubated again under any circumstances and signed a do not resuscitate (DNR) order. She did not bring a copy of this with her. Her temperature is 37.0 C (98.6 F), blood pressure is 138/98 mm Hg, pulse is 110/min, and respirations are 38/min. She is oriented and speaking in short sentences but able to answer questions appropriately. She is having labored breathing and using accessory muscles of respiration. The most appropriate next step in management is to

(A) ask the daughter to go home and bring the paperwork to the hospital
(B) ask the patient about her wishes regarding intubation at this time
(C) contact her primary care physician for a copy of the DNR order
(D) intubate the patient with plans to extubate her once her paperwork is obtained
(E) start a morphine infusion to make the patient as comfortable as possible

9. A 35-year-old previously healthy man is admitted to hospital because of a low-grade fever, abdominal discomfort, and watery diarrhea. On physical examination he is noted to have mild distention with no tenderness. Laboratory studies show a total leukocyte count of $5000/mm^3$, hemoglobin of 16 g/dL, blood urea nitrogen of 40 mg/dL, with a normal creatinine value. He is treated with intravenous hydration and antiemetic agents. A repeat complete blood count the next day reveals total leukocyte count of $2300/mm^3$. A CD3, CD4 count done subsequently is suspicious for HIV. You plan to tell the patient of that clinical suspicion and request further diagnostic measures. With this plan, you approach the patient in his room. He is sitting with his brother and a close friend. You inform the patient that you will come back in a couple hours to discuss the results of a blood test. He tells you to go ahead with the discussion, as there are no secrets between him, his brother, and the best friend. You politely inform the patient that you will come back in a couple of hours and it is not of any urgency, and you prepare to leave the room. The patient again says that it is "okay to talk about whatever needs to be discussed," as they are all concerned about his abdominal problems. The most appropriate next step is to

(A) go ahead and discuss with the patient the suspicion of the HIV and further diagnostic measures that are needed
(B) have another health care worker as a witness at the bedside and go ahead and discuss the blood test results with the patient
(C) inform the patient that the blood tests are suspicious of a particular condition and you will come back to discuss with the patient that condition
(D) insist that the matter is of no urgency and you will return in a couple of hours
(E) tell the brother and the family friend that they must leave the room so that you can discuss the matter in confidence with the patient

10. A 70-year-old man comes to the office because he has been unable to sleep for the last 2 days as he has been urinating at least six times per night. He normally wakes up one time per night since you started him on tamsulosin for his obstructive voiding symptoms, but now things are different. Besides waking up at night he has an acute onset of urinary urgency and hesitancy with a feeling of incomplete emptying. He became concerned when he developed a temperature of 38.7 C (100.6 F) today at home. His temperature is 37.9 C (100.2 F) in the office now. He has no abdominal pain or suprapubic discomfort. His genital examination is noncontributory and his prostate is firm and smooth without tenderness. Urine dipstick in the office is positive nitrites and positive leukocyte esterases. At this time the most accurate statement regarding this patient's condition is:

(A) Antibiotics should be given before sending off a urine culture.
(B) He does not require antibiotics at this time.
(C) His tamsulosin dose should be increased.
(D) The most likely causative organism is *E. coli.*
(E) A voiding cystourethrogram is indicated when his condition clears.

11. A 35-year-old woman executive makes an appointment to see you for an incessantly itchy skin lesion that developed on her neck 2 months ago. This is her third rescheduled appointment; her secretary called several times asking to reschedule due to unexpected meetings and trips her boss has had to make. When the patient finally comes she is nervous, constantly looking at her wristwatch, and can't sit still. She tells you she has to leave in "10 minutes tops" to meet her supervisor at the airport. She was appointed to this new and very high position in a big marketing firm only 3 months ago and can't afford to make any mistakes or she will lose the position. She has not had any particular medical problems in the past and the physical examination is within normal parameters except for bilateral, symmetrical lichenified plaques measuring 3 by 5 cm each on the posterolateral aspect of her neck. You gently suggest that she should think about using an oral sedative to relieve the itch, but she vehemently declines, stating that she cannot take anything that will make her sleepy due to her heavy work burden. The most appropriate treatment option for this patient is

(A) intralesional bleomycin monthly until the lesions resolve
(B) oral cephalexin for 10 days
(C) oral steroids for 2 weeks
(D) topical augmented betamethasone cream daily
(E) topical permethrin cream once a week for 2 weeks

12. A 35-year-old man comes to the emergency department complaining of a 24-hour history of sharp retrosternal pain that is most painful when he takes a deep breath. He has no chronic medical conditions but just recovered from an upper respiratory tract infection 1 week ago. His temperature is 37.8 C (100.0 F), blood pressure is 130/60 mm Hg, pulse is 80/min, respirations are 16/min, and oxygen saturation is 98% on room air. There are some scattered crackles in the left base; the rest of the physical examination is normal. A chest x-ray shows no abnormalities. An electrocardiogram shows widespread ST elevation, no Q waves, and PR-segment depression in $V_{5\text{-}6}$. The most appropriate next step in the management is to

    (A) administer intravenous streptokinase
    (B) discharge him and recommend ibuprofen
    (C) order a CT scan of the chest
    (D) order a ventilation-perfusion scan
    (E) perform an emergent cardiac catheterization

13. A 56-year-old man with hypertension and generalized anxiety disorder is brought to the emergency department after his wife found him lethargic and confused with an empty bottle of alprazolam. She tells you that he has been depressed for the past few weeks. He has been taking metoprolol for hypertension and alprazolam for anxiety for 1 year. Vital signs are: temperature 37.2 C (99.0 F), blood pressure 110/60 mm Hg, pulse 62/min, respirations 15/min, and oxygen saturation 98% on room air. He appears lethargic and confused and has diminished reflexes. You insert a nasogastric tube and administer activated charcoal. The most appropriate next step in management is to

    (A) administer flumazenil
    (B) administer N-acetylcysteine
    (C) administer naloxone
    (D) continue with supportive measures
    (E) intubate the patient and start mechanical ventilation

14. A 45-year-old man with Hodgkin disease underwent radiation therapy and is ready to start chemotherapy. An indwelling transthoracic intravenous catheter is placed and chemotherapy is started. Eight days after the initiation of chemotherapy, the patient develops fever and chills. Vital signs are temperature 38.3 C (101.0 F), blood pressure 125/70 mm Hg, and pulse 96/min. He has tenderness and erythema at the catheter insertion site; the rest of the physical examination is unremarkable. A chest x-ray is clear. Gram stain of the blood cultures is negative for microorganisms. Urinalysis is negative. The most appropriate next step in management is to

    (A) change the catheter over a guide wire
    (B) keep the catheter in place and start intravenous vancomycin
    (C) keep the catheter in place and start intravenous gentamicin
    (D) reassure the patient that the fever is caused by his Hodgkin disease
    (E) remove the catheter

15. A 69-year-old man with hypertension comes to the emergency department complaining of dysuria, flank pain, fever, and chills for 2 days. He takes metoprolol and hydrochlorothiazide. Vital signs are: temperature 39.3 C (102.8 F), blood pressure 100/60 mm Hg, pulse 120/min, respirations 28/min, oxygen saturation 98% on room air. He has mild tenderness in the left costovertebral angle. The rest of his physical examination is normal. A chest x-ray is normal. Blood and urine are sent for analysis and cultures. The most appropriate next step in management is to

    (A) call for a urologic consult
    (B) insert a Foley catheter
    (C) obtain an ultrasound of the kidneys
    (D) start a dopamine infusion
    (E) start intravenous antibiotic therapy

16. A 60-year-old man is brought to the emergency department by the paramedics after being found unconscious on the street. You begin treatment, but quite unexpectedly he has a cardiac arrest. You continue resuscitation of the patient, but despite all efforts the heart fails to respond. On your advice, cardiopulmonary resuscitation is discontinued. The patient's family decides to sue for negligence. The most likely outcome would be that the

   (A) courts will hold you liable
   (B) courts will let you off with a warning
   (C) courts will not hold you liable
   (D) courts will recommend that the state board revoke your license
   (E) peer review committee will review your case and advise the court accordingly

17. A 50-year-old woman with diabetes, depression, and metastatic breast cancer is brought to the emergency department with chest pain and shortness of breath. She is status post left radical mastectomy followed by chemotherapy and radiation therapy. She takes NPH insulin, sertraline, and multivitamins. Her temperature is 37.2 C (99.0 F), blood pressure is 90/56 mm Hg, pulse is 112/min, and respirations are 23/min. On examination, she has an elevated jugular venous pressure and a prominent pulsus paradoxus. Her cardiac rhythm is regular and heart sounds are muffled. Her lungs are clear to auscultation bilaterally. The most appropriate next diagnostic step is to order

   (A) bronchoscopy
   (B) a chest x-ray
   (C) a CT scan of the chest
   (D) an echocardiogram
   (E) a ventilation-perfusion scan

18. A 45-year-old woman has an alkaline phosphatase level that is twice normal levels on a chemistry panel ordered for evaluation of pruritis. Other liver tests are within normal limits, including bilirubin and ALT, and repeat testing 2 months later shows no change. A gamma-glutamyltransferase level is also significantly elevated, as is an antimitochondrial antibody titer. Hepatic ultrasonography is unremarkable. The most likely diagnosis is

   (A) choledocholithiasis
   (B) drug-induced cholestasis
   (C) Paget disease of the bone
   (D) primary biliary cirrhosis
   (E) sarcoidosis

19. A 50-year-old hospitalized man with a history of rheumatic aortic and mitral valve disease complains of fever, back pain, and myalgias for the past 3 days. On initial examination, no definite focus of infection is found. His leukocyte count is 24,000/mm^3 with 40% polymorphonuclear leukocytes and 40% band forms. The next day, 2 sets of blood cultures are growing gram-positive cocci. Until specific organism specificity is known, the most appropriate antibiotic treatment regimen at this time is

   (A) ceftriaxone
   (B) ciprofloxacin
   (C) nafcillin
   (D) streptomycin and penicillin
   (E) vancomycin and gentamicin

20. A 27-year-old man comes to the clinic to discuss travel immunizations with you. You learn that he will be getting married in 1 month and that he will be flying to India to get married. You also learn that he will be honeymooning in Thailand. Following this he will then pursue a war correspondence assignment in Afghanistan. He asks, "Are there any shots that I need before I go?" The vaccination that is recommended for nearly all international travelers to developing countries is

   (A) cholera
   (B) hepatitis A
   (C) hepatitis B
   (D) typhoid
   (E) yellow fever

21. A 40-year-old African American man comes to the emergency department complaining of shortness of breath with exertion. Physical examination is unremarkable. A chest x-ray shows marked hilar and peritracheal adenopathy. You think that the patient has sarcoidosis. After admitting the patient, the additional findings that would be most suggestive of this condition are

(A) a 15-pound weight loss and night sweats
(B) a nonspecific granuloma found on liver biopsy
(C) pain, redness, photophobia, and decreased vision of the right eye with pupillary miosis and injections of the conjunctiva
(D) papilledema
(E) a serum calcium level of 6.0 mg/dL

22. A 52-year-old woman with diabetes mellitus comes to the clinic because of urinary frequency, urgency, and dysuria. A urinalysis shows 24 white blood cells/HPF, and a urine culture grew a pan-sensitive *Escherichia coli.* She is given trimethoprim-sulfamethoxazole that is continued after the culture results are available. Over the following week she improves. Shortly thereafter, she developed right-sided flank pain, fever to 39.5 C (103.1 F), nausea, and vomiting. She is hospitalized, blood and urine cultures are sent, and she is started on intravenous ampicillin and gentamicin. A new urine culture grows *E. coli* that is sensitive to the current intravenous antibiotics. She continues to spike to temperatures of 39.5 C (103.1 F). Now it has been 3 days since admission and her condition is unchanged despite antibiotic therapy. The most appropriate next step in management is to

(A) add vancomycin to improve coverage
(B) order an abdominal CT scan
(C) order an intravenous pyelogram to rule out an obstructive uropathy
(D) order a radionuclide renal scan
(E) order a urine culture for tuberculosis

23. A 49-year-old man comes to the clinic with acute erythema and pain in the first metatarsal-phalangeal joint. Apparently this is the second such "attack" in the past 5 months. On physical examination there is no joint effusion. A radiograph of the foot is normal. Laboratory studies show

Hemoglobin	11.3 g/dL
Hematocrit	33.2%
Leukocyte count	$6800/mm^3$
Platelets	$262,000/mm^3$
MCV	$92\ \mu m^3$
Erythrocyte sedimentation rate	7 mm/h
BUN	8 mg/dL
Creatinine	0.5 mg/dL
Glucose	78 mg/dL
Calcium	9.0 mg/dL
Magnesium	2.2 mEq/L
Phosphate	3.2 mg/dL
Uric acid	5.0 mg/dL
Direct bilirubin	0.1 mg/dL
Total bilirubin	0.3 mg/dL
Alanine transaminase (ALT)	10 units/L
Aspartate transaminase (AST)	10 units/L
Alkaline phosphatase	80 units/L

The most likely diagnosis is

(A) acute gouty arthritis
(B) Morton neuroma
(C) osteoarthritis
(D) septic arthritis
(E) systemic lupus erythematosus

24. A 38-year-old man comes to the clinic because of coughing at night that is nonproductive and usually wakes him up from sleep. He also complains of chest pain (at which time he points to his sternum and moves his hand up and down). He describes the pain as a "burn" that can also be felt in the throat. He drinks 2 cups of coffee every evening that he thinks might be worsening his symptoms. Physical examination is unremarkable. At this time the most appropriate advice for this patient is

(A) antacids should be avoided as they may cause rebound symptoms
(B) consumption of coffee has nothing to do with his symptoms
(C) elevating the head of the bed should be used as a last resort
(D) high-fat foods should be avoided because they may increase the severity of his symptoms
(E) a histamine receptor blocker should be used for a maximum of 6 weeks

25. A 76-year-old woman from Portugal is admitted to the hospital because of a poor appetite and weight loss. She has a past medical history of hypertension, hypercholesterolemia, and a background of "strokes" in her family. While hospitalized she begins to experience feelings of palpitations and shortness of breath. An electrocardiogram shows atrial fibrillation, and when you compare this electrocardiogram with previous ones in her charts you note that this is her first episode of atrial fibrillation. Appropriate rate control is achieved with diltiazem. Echocardiography reveals no cardiomegaly and a normal left atrial dimension. The therapy that would give this patient the highest likelihood of conversion from atrial fibrillation to sinus rhythm is

(A) amiodarone
(B) direct-current cardioversion
(C) propafenone
(D) quinidine
(E) sotalol

26. A 36-year-old woman comes to the clinic after doing some gardening earlier last week. She has intense pruritis, erythema, and vesiculation, involving extensive areas of her arms, neck, and face. She had been exposed to some poison ivy and approximately 48 hours later developed a pruritic, erythematous, papulovesicular eruption on her arms and neck. She initially began treating herself with over-the-counter low-dose topical hydrocortisone cream that did not result in an improvement within 24 hours of treatment. She then went to the emergency department where she was given oral methylprednisolone. Over 4 days there was temporary improvement but this was followed by the immediate exacerbation of the eruption as seen by you today. The most appropriate management at this time is

(A) beginning high-dose oral prednisone
(B) beginning oral diphenhydramine
(C) discontinuing the systemic and topical medications and recommending tepid baths and cool compresses with astringent solutions
(D) discontinuing the topical hydrocortisone and switching to a superpotent topical steroid
(E) repeating the oral methylprednisolone treatment

27. A 65-year-old man is brought to the clinic from a skilled nursing home by his caregiver. This patient is normally of a quiet disposition but has been very agitated over the past 2 days. His appetite apparently has also waned. He has had some watery bowel movements and fecal incontinence but no fever, vomiting, or urinary incontinence. He takes risperidone 4 mg oral twice daily that was prescribed by his community psychiatrist for schizophreniform disorder. Otherwise he has no relevant past medical history. His physical examination confirms fecal incontinence. Laboratory studies show

Hemoglobin	13 g/dL
Hematocrit	38%
Leukocyte count	$5000/mm^3$
Platelets	$100,000/mm^3$
MCV	$80\ \mu m^3$
Sodium	141 mEq/L
Potassium	4.7 mEq/L
Chloride	102 mEq/L
Bicarbonate	26 mEq/L
Urea nitrogen (BUN)	12 mg/dL
Creatinine	0.9 mg/dL
Glucose	88 mg/dL
Calcium	9.0 g/dL
Magnesium	2.1 mEq/L
Phosphate	4.0 mg/dL

An upright plain abdominal x-ray shows plenty of stool in the descending colon. Appropriate management is to

(A) order a head CT scan
(B) prescribe fiber supplements
(C) prescribe magnesium hydroxide
(D) prescribe mineral oil
(E) reduce the risperidone dose to 2 mg oral twice daily

28. A 30-year-old woman comes to the clinic in late July because of a red, raised rash on her face and scalp. It has also been particularly evident in areas of her body that have been exposed to the sun. She explains that these "raised areas" have become scaly and thick. In the past they have lasted for a few days, notably in the summer, before disappearing, and had a tendency to recur. They are not itchy. She has had no other systemic complaints and her past medical history is completely normal. When you examine her you note that the rash is indeed red and raised, covering the nose and cheeks beneath the eyes in a symmetrical pattern. The rash is also on her scalp, thighs, back, and arms in an atypical distribution over the sun-exposed areas. It is scaly in places. Her elbows and knees are spared and her fingernails appear normal. There are no excoriation marks. There is no paresthesia noted. The most likely cause of her rash is

(A) acne vulgaris
(B) acute intermittent porphyria
(C) discoid lupus erythematosus
(D) psoriasis
(E) systemic lupus erythematosus

29. A 75-year-old African-American woman with asthma, type 2 diabetes mellitus, hypertension, a triple cardiac bypass operation, and chronic renal failure is seen in the emergency department for melena. She also complains of left flank pain over the past 24 hours. Her review of symptoms is otherwise normal. Vital signs are: temperature of 37.0 C (98.6 F), blood pressure 135/72 mm Hg, pulse 70/min, and respirations 18/min. Her abdomen is soft and nontender. There is tenderness over the left costovertebral angle. Laboratory studies show

Hemoglobin	8.4 g/dL
Hematocrit	25.6%
Leukocyte count	12,000/mm^3
Platelets	463×10^9/L
MCV	90 μm^3
Sodium	131 mEq/L
Potassium	6.7 mEq/L
Chloride	101 mEq/L
Bicarbonate	26 mEq/L
Urea nitrogen (BUN)	50 mg/dL
Creatinine	2.5 mg/dL
Glucose	228 mg/dL
Calcium	9.0 mg/dL
Magnesium	2.2 mEq/L
Phosphate	3.1 mg/dL

The therapy that would allow for the most effective excretion of potassium in this patient is

(A) inhaled beta agonists
(B) intravenous calcium (10 mL of a 10% solution of calcium gluconate)
(C) intravenous insulin and glucose
(D) intravenously administered sodium bicarbonate
(E) oral sodium polystyrene sulfonate

30. A 79-year-old man has been living independently and has no health problems. One day he has a cardiopulmonary arrest while mowing his lawn. His heart rhythm is restored after 8 minutes of cardiopulmonary resuscitation by a neighbor. He is now a patient in the coronary care unit on a ventilator. He has severe hypoxic encephalopathy and an ejection fraction of 15%, secondary to a massive anterior myocardial infarction. A neurology consultation confirms that the patient will be ventilator-dependent and will never be able to communicate meaningfully. He has no living relatives, and his attorney confirms that he has no written advance directives. The neighbor, who knew him well, tells you that on several occasions recently he and the neighbor had discussed such a scenario, and the patient had said, "I don't want to be on life support if I'm going to become a vegetable." The most appropriate decision by the hospital ethics committee is to

(A) ask a court to appoint a guardian to make the medical decisions
(B) ask the patient's attorney to decide whether to terminate life support
(C) defer the decision regarding life support to the hospital attorney
(D) transfer the care of the patient to another physician
(E) withdraw life support

31. A 40-year-old nurse comes to the emergency department with a headache, palpitations, and a tremor. She says that she has a history of hypoglycemic episodes. She denies any history of chest pain, shortness of breath, or drug abuse. She has no history of hyperthyroidism or psychiatric problems. Her blood pressure is 110/80 mm Hg, pulse is 80/min, and respirations are 19/min. Physical examination is normal. She is orientated to time, place, and person. Her serum glucose level is 38 mg/dL. She is hospitalized and prescribed a high sugar diet and a dextrose infusion. After the hospitalization she has frequent episodes when her glucose level is between 40 and 100 mg/dL. Her insulin level is 12 μU/mL (normal is <6 μU/mL) and her C peptide level is 0.05 ng/mL (normal is 0.8 to 4.0 ng/mL). The most likely cause of her problem is

(A) exogenous insulin administration
(B) an insulinoma
(C) a pituitary tumor
(D) small cell carcinoma of the lung
(E) a sulfonylurea overdose

32. An 81-year-old woman comes to the clinic complaining of "feeling depressed." She also has recurrent muscle cramping and tingling of her fingers. On physical examination there is no evidence of carpal spasm when a blood pressure cuff is inflated above systolic pressure on the arm for 3 minutes. There is no twitching of the facial muscle when the facial nerve is tapped anterior to the ear. Her serum calcium level is 6.8 mg/dL and her serum phosphorus level is 5.6 mg/dL. An additional finding(s) that would be most consistent with the diagnosis of primary hypoparathyroidism is

(A) normal renal function and decreased parathyroid hormone level
(B) papilledema
(C) polyuria
(D) prolongation of the QT interval on an electrocardiogram
(E) renal failure and a normal parathyroid level
(F) shortening of the QT interval on an electrocardiogram

33. A 35-year-old man comes to the office because of a rash on his penis that he has had on and off for the past 2 years. It typically starts with a "tingling sensation" and then "little blisters" form, which are painful for the first day. This happens every month and the blisters last for about 1 week. He initially tried over the counter antifungal treatments because he thought this could be "jock-itch" but is unsure if it has helped. He denies any urethral discharge or dysuria. He reports having four sexual partners in the past year. He remembers that a physician gave him a pill with the first outbreak. He does not think that it helped, because the rash came back. He is interested in taking a medication to "make it go away." The most appropriate recommendation is

(A) acyclovir for the remainder of his life for continuous suppression
(B) that he and his sexual partners are treated with acyclovir as he is likely being reinfected
(C) that he take acyclovir for 1 year and then stop the medication to reassess the frequency of outbreaks
(D) treatment with acyclovir for a longer course during the next outbreak, as he may have a resistant infection
(E) treatment with imiquimod cream for 8 weeks

34. A previously healthy 29-year-old pediatric nurse comes to the clinic because of a 3-day history of malaise, arthralgias, and a nonpruritic rash. Her temperature is 37.0 C (98.6 F). She has a faint, maculopapular, irregular, reticulate exanthem that covers her thighs and the inner aspects of her arms. There are no excoriation marks noted. There is symmetrical synovitis in the distal and proximal interphalangeal joints and in her metacarpophalangeal joints. In addition, small effusions, warmth, and tenderness are noted in her left wrist and right elbow. No other joints are affected. Her abdominal examination is negative for organomegaly. The most likely viral etiology causing her rash is

(A) adenovirus
(B) human immunodeficiency virus (HIV)
(C) measles (rubeola)
(D) parvovirus B19
(E) varicella-zoster

35. A 43-year-old man has spent the past 3 months working extensively in a 19th-century farmhouse. He comes to the office complaining of headache, fatigue, and muscle pain. He denies difficulty swallowing, photophobia, and limb weakness. He is not on any medications and has no remarkable personal or family history. Physical examination is normal. At this time, the most appropriate study to help establish a diagnosis is

(A) a complete blood count with a peripheral smear
(B) an erythrocyte sedimentation rate
(C) a fasting blood glucose level
(D) liver function tests
(E) long bone x-rays

36. A 25-year-old man comes to the clinic concerned about a painless ulcer on his penis. He specifically says, "My last sexual encounter was heterosexual and about 4 weeks ago." On physical examination you notice 2 painless, indurated superficial ulcerations over the glans of the penis. You diagnose him with primary syphilis. He has no drug allergies and you treat him with 2.4 million units of benzathine penicillin intramuscularly in a single dose. About 9 hours later during the evening clinic he returns complaining of a temperature of 38.1 C (100.6 F), a bad headache, and generalized "aching all over." At this time the most appropriate action is to

(A) give him a prescription for oral doxycycline 100 mg twice daily for 14 days
(B) obtain 3 blood cultures from different sites at 30-minute intervals
(C) order a head CT scan with contrast
(D) perform a lumbar puncture
(E) provide reassurance and administer antipyretics

Items 37-39

A 79-year-old woman with type 2 diabetes mellitus, stroke with residual right-sided hemiparesis, atrial fibrillation, and a colostomy is brought to the emergency department because of a 7-day history of reduced oral intake, fatigue, and fever. She has a rectal fistula that her caregiver states is "open" and is now draining a thin, clear, yellow discharge. She has urinary incontinence and normally wears diapers. Two weeks ago she visited the emergency room for an assessment of the fistula. She had a Foley catheter inserted to control the urinary incontinence and to prevent infection exposure to the fistula. She was discharged home with the catheter in place. Three days later her family doctor visited her at home and noted that she had a temperature of 38.9 C (102.0 F) and that the urine in the catheter bag was cloudy. The doctor decided to replace the catheter and treat with ciprofloxacin 500 mg oral twice daily. Now in the emergency department the patient appears comfortable and obeys verbal commands. Her temperature is 36.6 F (97.9 F), blood pressure is 140/75 mm Hg, pulse is 72/min and irregular, and respirations are 16/min. Her skin turgor is poor and her mucous membranes are dry. She has mild basal crepitations in the right lung field only. You note cellulitic changes of the rectal fistula that is located in the right part of the perianal area. She has a urethral catheter in place that appears to have drained 300 mL over 17 hours. There is no peripheral edema. Laboratory studies show

Hemoglobin	10.6 g/dL
Hematocrit	31.0%
Leukocyte count	12,500/mm^3
Platelets	383,000/mm^3
Sodium	134 mEq/L
Potassium	2.9 mEq/L
Blood urea nitrogen	44 mg/dL
Creatinine	2.0 mg/dL
Glucose	150 mg/dL

Urinalysis shows a specific gravity of 1.030. It is positive for nitrites and leukocyte esterase. A chest x-ray shows cardiomegaly but no infiltrates. An electrocardiogram shows rate-controlled atrial fibrillation.

37. This patient's blood urea nitrogen and creatinine levels can best be explained by

(A) acute renal failure
(B) dehydration
(C) nephritic syndrome
(D) ureteral obstruction at the trigone of the urinary bladder caused by neoplasia
(E) ureteral obstruction caused by urolithiasis

38. You suspect that this patient may have an aspiration pneumonia based on her history of being bed-bound, the residual paresis of the stroke, and the coarse basal crepitations on auscultation of the right lung field. You note that the admission chest x-ray is negative for infiltrates. The most appropriate next step to establish the diagnosis of an aspiration pneumonia in this patient is to

(A) obtain a sputum culture
(B) order bedside pulmonary function tests
(C) order a blood gas while the patient is breathing oxygen at 4 L/min
(D) order a blood gas while the patient is breathing room air
(E) order a CT of the chest
(F) repeat the chest x-ray after administration of intravenous fluid

39. You want to start maintenance intravenous fluids for her. The most appropriate intravenous fluid is

(A) 0.9% normal saline at a rate of 125 mL/hour
(B) 0.9% normal saline at a rate of 75 mL/hour with 20 mmol/L of potassium chloride
(C) 0.45% normal saline at a rate of 75 mL/hour
(D) 0.45% normal saline at a rate of 75 mL/hour with 20 mmol/L of potassium chloride
(E) 0.45% normal saline with 5% dextrose at a rate of 75 mL/hour with 20 mmol/L of potassium chloride
(F) 0.45% normal saline with 5% dextrose at a rate of 125 mL/hour with 20 mmol/L of potassium chloride

Items 40-41

A 24-year-old woman comes to the emergency department because of a dry mouth and blurred vision associated with nausea, malaise, and the recent onset of diplopia. You find out that 2 days ago she had been eating home-canned foods at her brother's house in the woods of Connecticut. Before this she had been healthy with no medical problems. On physical examination, you note slight ptosis and a disconjugate gaze. Laboratory studies show

Sodium	139 mEq/L
Potassium	5.0 mEq/L
Chloride	99 mEq/L
Bicarbonate	24 mEq/L
Blood urea nitrogen	7 mg/dL
Creatinine	0.7 mg/dL
Calcium	7.7 mg/dL

40. The diagnostic evaluation that is most likely to establish the diagnosis is

(A) detection of toxin of *Clostridium botulism* in the patient's serum
(B) a doxycycline challenge for tick paralysis
(C) a lumbar puncture to rule out a cerebrovascular event
(D) an MRI to rule out Guillain-Barré syndrome
(E) a psychiatric consult to evaluate for hysteria

41. The patient complains that she is getting weaker and notes a feeling of dyspnea. The most appropriate next step in management is to

(A) admit the patient to the intensive care unit to monitor respiratory status closely
(B) begin therapy with ciprofloxacin, intravenously
(C) begin treatment with a steroid inhaler
(D) get a psychiatric consult
(E) notify the Centers for Disease Control and Prevention or the public health department

42. A 39-year-old man with hypertension comes to the office for a followup visit. He has been taking captopril for 2 years and his blood pressure is not well controlled. He asks if you know about the new antihypertensive agents that are being studied. You tell him that you will get back to him after doing some research. Later that day while flipping through a new journal you come across an article about a Phase II clinical trial that was conducted as part of a procedure to gather evidence for the efficacy of a new hypertension drug. In this study, 49 patients were given 50-mg doses of the drug and 36 other patients were given 25-mg doses. The table below displays systolic blood pressure reduction data from the study.

	N	Mean	Median	Mode	Standard deviation
50-mg group	49	–23.8	–17.3	–15.5	7.8
25-mg group	36	–16.4	–16.2	–16.1	6.6

Based on these results, if you follow the protocol for administering a 50-mg dose to a hypertensive patient, you should expect that the patient would have a 95% chance of experiencing a reduction in blood pressure between

(A) –17.0 and –31.6
(B) –9.2 and –39.4
(C) –9.5 and –25.1
(D) –1.7 and –32.9
(E) –7.7 and –23.3
(F) +0.01 and –31.1
(G) cannot be adequately determined from the information given

Items 43-44

A 32-year-old woman is brought to the emergency department by her husband because, as her husband states, "it feels as though her heart is leaping out of her chest and she is having difficulty catching her breath." This episode came on abruptly as they were finishing dinner. She has had similar episodes in the past that usually resolve by breath holding; however, this was not effective in "breaking this attack." She is generally healthy and does not take any medications. There are no carotid bruits present. Her blood pressure is 120/80 mm Hg and pulse is 210/min. An electrocardiogram shows supraventricular tachycardia. She remains electrocardiographically monitored.

43. The most appropriate immediate management is to

(A) administer digitalis glycoside, orally
(B) administer verapamil, orally
(C) insert a temporary pacemaker, pervenously
(D) perform gentle massage over the right carotid sinus
(E) wait 2 hours for the "attack" to subside spontaneously

44. The appropriate step is taken, however the attack does not cease. The most appropriate next step in management is to

(A) administer adenosine, intravenously
(B) administer lidocaine, intravenously
(C) administer procainamide, intravenously
(D) insert a permanent pacemaker
(E) perform a direct-current cardioversion

45. A 20-year-old woman comes to the office for a followup visit for atopic dermatitis/eczema that was diagnosed by your partner. She tells you that the rash has spread to the back of her hands, notably over the knuckles. She also complains of "feeling weak." She had gone to another physician 1 year ago with a purplish swollen eyelid rash, which in haste, secondary to the doctor's busy schedule, was diagnosed as atopic dermatitis/eczema on that visit. The rash improved with mild topical steroids but never fully cleared. A few months later the patient came to your partner complaining of a worsening eyelid rash but denied other associated complaints. She was prescribed the newest topical eczema drug called tacrolimus. Physical examination now shows that the rash on her knuckles consists of flat-topped papules that precisely spare the skin over the phalanges. Upon questioning after seeing the rash, she admits to having difficulty rising from a seated position and combing her hair at night. The most appropriate next step in management is to

(A) begin allergy testing as patients with recalcitrant eczema need to be allergy tested to rule out important offending agents that may be overlooked

(B) check CPK and refer to a dermatologist for skin and muscle biopsy

(C) continue the tacrolimus for her severe atopic dermatitis despite her muscle weakness, which is an expected side effect of both atopic dermatitis and tacrolimus

(D) perform patch testing, be sure to include the eyeshadow and hand cream she uses on a daily basis

(E) stop the tacrolimus and increase the strength of the topical corticosteroids; eczema on the eyelids and dorsal hands is stubborn and requires the strongest class of topical corticosteroids

46. A 45-year-old Caucasian woman comes to the clinic stating that when "I wake up in the morning my hands and feet feel stiff and painful. I haven't fallen or injured my hands or feet, but I have noticed some bumps around my elbows. Can you give me some medicine to make the pain tolerable?" After taking an appropriate history you discover that she has had this stiffness for several years. She has fatigue, myalgias, and dry eyes. She denies any recent fevers, chills, or night sweats. Her social and occupational history includes being a teacher who has never used tobacco products and drinks a glass of red wine every night. On physical examination the patient's wrists are swollen and slightly ulnarly deviated. Her metacarpal-phalangeal joints appear swollen as well. Over the olecranon process there are palpable subcutaneous nodules that are soft and not fixed. The patient now asks "what is causing all of these changes?" Preliminary laboratory results include a leukocyte count of $8300/mm^3$, negative blood cultures, a normal serum uric acid level, and normal prothrombin time (PT), INR, and partial thromboplastin time (PTT). The most likely underlying cause of her condition is

(A) an acute bacterial infection involving multiple joints

(B) a chronic infection with an acid-fast bacterium

(C) a decrease in the levels of a clotting factor

(D) an immune process characterized by a destructive immune reaction

(E) a neoplastic process, likely malignant

47. A 40-year-old African American woman that you have been treating for gluten-sensitive enteropathy over the past 2 years develops crops of itchy blisters on her elbows. A skin biopsy shows microabscesses of neutrophils in the tips of dermal papillae. You want to initiate dapsone treatment to control the gastrointestinal and skin lesions with 1 medication. Before initiating treatment you should send laboratory studies to determine levels of

(A) alpha-galactosidase
(B) glucose-6-phosphate dehydrogenase
(C) lactate dehydrogenase
(D) steroid sulfatase
(E) thiomethyltransferase

48. A 70-year-old woman with a history of recurrent ventricular tachycardia comes to the office with joint and muscle pain, fatigue, and a rash of 4 weeks' duration. She tells you that she takes several "heart pills." On reviewing her chart, you note that no new medications have been started in the previous 6 months. Your physical examination finds her to be in no acute distress but with some discomfort in the joints of her hands and feet and muscle tenderness. On her nose and cheeks there is a confluent erythema and edema. Laboratory studies indicate a low hemoglobin and hematocrit level with elevated reticulocyte count. The medication that is the most likely cause of her condition is

(A) digoxin
(B) disopyramide
(C) minoxidil
(D) procainamide
(E) quinidine

49. A 50-year-old man comes to the emergency department with a 24-hour history of fever, abdominal pain, and bloody stool. He had extensive oral surgery 2 weeks earlier that resolved without complications. At the time, he was given a 10-day course of oral antibiotics, a tapering dose of steroids, and an antiseptic mouthwash. He does not recall the name of the antibiotic, but is quite sure that his son had the same medication for his acne, only in the form of a gel. Otherwise, he is healthy and takes no medication on a regular basis. He has not traveled recently and has no sick contacts. Vital signs are: temperature 38.3 C (101.0 F), pulse 95/min, and respirations 21/min. His abdomen is slightly distended and moderately tender to palpation. A rectal examination shows watery, greenish, mucoid stool that tests positive for occult blood. The most appropriate pharmacotherapy for this patient is

(A) chloramphenicol
(B) ciprofloxacin
(C) clindamycin
(D) erythromycin
(E) metronidazole

50. You have been treating a 67-year-old man for diabetes with a regimen of medication, dietary modifications, and daily exercise. During a routine followup visit, the patient shows you a research article on lifestyle factors associated with diabetes that he discovered during several days searching through a local medical library. The article was recently published in a medical journal with a national reputation. The patient does not understand some of the technical aspects of the article and asks you to help him understand the implications of what he has found. The main table in the article shows a series of correlation coefficients between assessed glucose levels and lifestyle factors within a diabetic population. The table is presented below:

Table 1. Pearson Correlation Coefficients Among Glucose Levels and Selected Lifestyle Factors in a Diabetic Patient Population (N = 125)

	Glucose levels	Number of desserts/week	Minutes of exercise/week	Hours of TV/week
Desserts	+0.57*	+1.00	–0.55*	–0.44*
Exercise	–0.35*	–0.55*	+1.00	–0.68*
TV hours	+0.28*	–0.44*	–0.68*	+1.00

*$p \leq 0.01$

Based on the results of this research article, you should tell the patient that

(A) eating desserts and watching TV will produce a dangerous increase in glucose levels

(B) general research articles are of little use in deciding clinical interventions

(C) increased exercise and eliminating desserts from one's diet are sufficient to reduce glucose levels in most patients

(D) increased exercise is associated with decreased consumption of sweets, less TV watching, and lower glucose levels

(E) it is essential to avoid eating when watching TV

(F) the article does not apply to his particular situation

(G) watching more TV will increase glucose levels and reduce time for exercise

Internal Medicine Test Four: **Answers and Explanations**

ANSWER KEY

1. D
2. D
3. A
4. A
5. D
6. A
7. D
8. B
9. D
10. D
11. D
12. B
13. D
14. E
15. E
16. C
17. D
18. D
19. E
20. B
21. C
22. B
23. A
24. D
25. B
26. A
27. B
28. C
29. E
30. E
31. A
32. A
33. C
34. D
35. A
36. E
37. B
38. F
39. D
40. A
41. A
42. G
43. D
44. A
45. B
46. D
47. B
48. D
49. E
50. D

1. **The correct answer is D.** This patient has Graves disease, which is a common cause of hyperthyroidism, and it is important to discuss the advantages and disadvantages of the treatment options. The major disadvantage of radioiodine therapy is that 40 to 70% of patients develop hypothyroidism and require thyroid hormone replacement within 10 years. Graves disease is characterized by diffuse goiter, dermopathy, and ophthalmopathy. The clinical manifestations are those of hyperthyroidism and include palpitations, tremors, weakness, weight loss despite an increased appetite, frequent, loose bowel movements, heat intolerance, and oligomenorrhea or amenorrhea. Proptosis, lid lag, and stare may be present. The dermopathy, which is called pretibial myxedema, is usually characterized by waxy, infiltrated plaques over the dorsum of the legs and a *peau d'orange* appearance. Laboratory studies show low or undetectable levels of TSH and elevated levels of T_4, T_3, and the RAIU and RT3U. Radioactive iodine therapy is a good choice for treating hyperthyroidism in adult patients, patients with previous thyroid surgery, and patients who cannot undergo surgery. Long-term antithyroid therapy with methimazole or propylthiouracil is usually used in children. Radioiodine therapy should never be given to pregnant women because fetal radiation is harmful. Antithyroid drugs are usually used during pregnancy.

   Arthralgias, agranulocytosis, and a rash are not common side effects of radioiodine therapy (**choice A**). These complications are associated with antithyroid drugs, not radioiodine therapy.

   Radioiodine therapy typically does not improve the ophthalmopathy (**choice B**). It actually worsens it in some patients, but most are unchanged.

   There is no evidence to support that radioiodine therapy is associated with leukemia (**choice C**) in adults.

   Repeated doses of radioiodine usually are not necessary (**choice E**). Continuous or repeated therapy with antithyroid drugs (methimazole or propylthiouracil) is often necessary.

2. **The correct answer is D.** Self-breast examination, although commonly advised and used in the outpatient setting for breast cancer screening, has never been shown to be of any mortality benefit. An annual screening examination by a physician is currently the standard of care, in conjunction with annual mammography beginning at age 40 or 50, depending on whether you ask the American College of Physicians or the American Cancer Society.

   Minimum screening age for hypercholesterolemia was recently changed to 18 by the NCEP (National Cholesterol Education Panel) and is recommended at age 30 by most other professional panels. They have also recently changed their recommendation from a screening cholesterol to a full fasting lipid panel (with measurements of HDL, LDL, and triglyceride level) in everyone (**choice A**), not just those with a family history of early coronary artery disease or hyperlipidemia.

   Counseling her on the prevention of gonorrhea, *Chlamydia* (even actually screening for them, say some), and HIV (**choice B**) is clearly indicated in this patient not using any effective prophylactic measure.

   This patient has some evidence that should alert the clinician to possible domestic abuse, including her affect and the lesions on her legs, so inquiring further about her relationship with her fiancé (**choice C**) is appropriate.

   A Pap smear (**choice E**) is indicated in a young, sexually active woman such as this, because it is effective in reducing mortality from cervical cancer, and should commence once the patient is sexually active, or at 18 years of age.

3. **The correct answer is A.** The hemoccult has a high false-positive rate and an even higher false-negative rate, but a single positive value should still ring alarm bells in a patient his age, and prompt evaluation by colonoscopy. This is true even in the presence of hemorrhoids, as many patients with hemorrhoids have coincident colonic polyps and should be evaluated thoroughly for the presence of occult malignancy.

   Increasing his metformin dose (**choice B**) is incorrect. He is essentially asymptomatic, and his diabetes is reasonably well controlled over the last 3 to 4 months, as evidenced by the glycohemoglobin (target is <7, but 7.1 is nothing to get crazy about, immediately anyway). Also, 850 mg tid is the maximum dose of metformin.

   Although it is important to inquire about dietary indiscretions and recent glucose control (**choice C**) for a patient with diabetes at any followup visit, it isn't the thing that's most concerning about this case, and he should not be followed as scheduled. He needs to be evaluated for an occult malignancy at this time.

   A single positive fecal occult blood test necessitates thorough evaluation. There is no need to repeat the test (**choice D**)–once it's positive it should be treated as blood in the stool.

   A complete blood count (**choice E**) can be done but should not preclude immediate evaluation by colonoscopy.

4. **The correct answer is A.** A diagnosis of CLL does not automatically warrant treatment, especially when symptoms are few and there isn't evidence of bone marrow compromise (i.e., all the cell lines in this patient are okay, quantitatively). The natural history of this disease in this patient is likely not to be the cause of her demise. Early stage CLL has a median survival on the order of 15 years. She should be monitored probably no more than annually for worsening adenopathy, hepatosplenomegaly, anemia, and thrombocytopenia.

   A CT scan of the chest, abdomen, and pelvis **(choice B)** would be useful for staging in a patient with lymphoma (it used to be staging laparotomy, and some places still do this). There is no role for this in CLL.

   A bone marrow biopsy **(choice C)** would be appropriate if she was symptomatically anemic, thrombocytopenic with evidence of bleeding, pancytopenic, or if there was a dramatic change in her cell counts on followup (annually) CBCs. That is, if treatment of her CLL were contemplated, a bone marrow examination would be appropriate. From the information given here, however, treatment is not necessary at this point.

   Chemotherapy **(choice D)** would not be indicated here, and generally for Step 3 you wouldn't need to know when someone needs chemotherapy, but rather you should know when to refer the patient to an oncologist.

   Radiotherapy **(choice E)** also has no role here; if treatment were indicated, limited-field radiotherapy might be part of the overall treatment regimen, but Step 3 wouldn't expect you to know that.

5. **The correct answer is D.** This patient has diabetic ketoacidosis (DKA), most likely set off by her pneumonia. She is diabetic and therefore immunosuppressed, and has a typical and common presentation of polyuria, polydipsia, hyperglycemia, and an elevated anion gap (calculated as [Na-Cl-HCO_3], with 18 being the upper limit of normal). Other triggers for DKA include other infections, especially urosepsis and skin infections, and myocardial ischemia/infarction. She needs an insulin drip because her liver is producing ketoacids, as evidenced by her urinalysis and her elevated anion gap. She should be monitored in the ICU with an insulin drip and measurement of serum chemistries every 4 hours (remember to replace potassium as the insulin will drive it intracellularly) until her anion gap normalizes, and then she can be started on long-acting insulin and sent to a regular medical floor. Managed inappropriately, this diagnosis carries a high mortality.

   Admitting her to a medical floor after giving intravenous ceftriaxone **(choice A)** is wrong because even though you will be treating her pneumonia, she absolutely should be monitored in the ICU to avoid shock and worsening acidosis, and to permit frequent monitoring of serum chemistries.

   Admitting her to a medical floor after giving intravenous vancomycin **(choice B)** is wrong because vancomycin is not the drug of choice for community-acquired pneumonia, and board-examination writers in general are obsessed with avoiding the overuse of "big-gun" antibiotics, rightly so. Also, she needs intensive care, as outlined above.

   Beginning aggressive hydration and admitting her to the intensive care unit **(choice C)** is wrong because she has an elevated anion gap and therefore requires an insulin drip until it normalizes.

   Giving regular insulin 10 units subcutaneously and observing her in the emergency department **(choice E)** is wrong on several levels. Although she definitely needs admission to an ICU nonetheless, subcutaneous insulin is ineffective in the volume-depleted patient because skin perfusion is decreased. She should be getting intravenous insulin in a continuous fashion.

6. **The correct answer is A.** This patient has primary syphilis of less than 1 year's duration. Penicillin is still the drug of choice for treatment of all stages of syphilis. Patients with primary, secondary, or early latent syphilis known to be of less than 1 years' duration can be treated with a single intramuscular injection of 2.4 million units (mU) of benzathine penicillin G. In nonpregnant, penicillin-allergic, HIV-negative patients, tetracycline 500 mg orally four times a day or doxycycline 100 mg orally bid for 2 weeks is recommended. Syphilis is a sexually transmitted disease caused by the spirochete *Treponema pallidum.* When untreated, the infection evolves through a primary, secondary, latent, and late stage. The chancre is usually the first cutaneous lesion. A crusted, superficial erosion evolves into a round or oval, indurated, slightly elevated papule with an eroded, moist surface. It has a firm, cartilagelike consistency on palpation. It is most often painless. The regional lymph nodes on both sides become enlarged, firm, and nontender within a week or two of the appearance of the chancre. They do not suppurate or drain. Untreated, the chancre tends to heal spontaneously in 1 to 4 months, at which time signs of the secondary stages start to appear. The diagnosis of primary syphilis is confirmed by performing dark-field microscopy of exudate collected from the base of the chancre and by doing usually two serologic tests (a rapid

plasma reagin test is commonly done first, and it's positivity confirmed with a specific treponemal test, such as the microhemagglutination assay for *Treponema pallidum*). All patients with diagnosed syphilis should be questioned and examined for signs and symptoms of other sexually transmitted diseases and should also be tested for HIV.

Benzathine penicillin G 2.4 mU intramuscularly, 1 dose weekly for 3 weeks (**choice B**) is the recommended treatment for late or late–latent syphilis of more than 1 years' duration in an HIV-negative patient.

Doxycycline 100 mg PO bid for 2 weeks (**choice C**) is used for the treatment of primary, secondary, or early latent syphilis known to be of less than 1 years' duration in patients who are allergic to penicillin, are nonpregnant, and are HIV negative.

Procaine penicillin G 2.4 mU IM qd, plus probenecid 500 mg PO qid for 10 to 14 days (**choice D**) is the recommended treatment regimen for neurosyphilis.

Tetracycline 500 mg PO qid for 30 days (**choice E**) is the recommended treatment in penicillin-allergic, nonpregnant, HIV-negative patients with late or late–latent syphilis of more than 1 years' duration.

7. **The correct answer is D.** The available history and physical examination is consistent with a diagnosis of hypothyroidism. Therefore, the appropriate test is the thyroid-stimulating hormone level assay, which is the most sensitive screen for thyroid dysfunction.

A cervical CT (**choice A**) is not used in the routine evaluation of hypothyroidism.

A radioactive iodine uptake assay (**choice B**) is typically used in the differential diagnosis of hyperthyroidism rather than hypothyroidism.

The history and physical examination are not consistent with a diagnosis of impaired glucose homeostasis. Therefore, a serum glucose level (**choice C**) would not provide any useful information.

Since no nodules or masses were evident on exam, a thyroid ultrasound (**choice E**) would not be appropriate at this juncture.

8. **The correct answer is B.** In the stem of the question it clearly says that the patient appropriately answers questions and is oriented. A prior DNR order is irrelevant in this situation, as is her health care proxy, both of which take effect (with the patient's own written advance directive taking priority) when the patient becomes too incapacitated to state her own decisions reliably. Even if the paperwork were in hand, the patient can always rescind it, and should be asked if she wants to in this setting.

Asking the daughter to go home and bring the paperwork to the hospital (**choice A**) doesn't make sense, as this patient is in impending respiratory failure but, as stated above, still appears able to relate her own wishes regarding intubation.

Contacting her primary care physician for a copy of the DNR order (**choice C**) is equally nonsensical, from a timing standpoint and that of patient autonomy.

Intubating the patient with plans to extubate her once her paperwork is obtained (**choice D**) is wrong, as you wouldn't have a competent patient intubated without asking them first if that's what they'd want.

Starting a morphine infusion to make the patient as comfortable as possible (**choice E**) also is wrong, at the other extreme. You wouldn't make a decision not to intubate without again addressing the issue with the patient, if she is competent. This is regardless of what the daughter/proxy says, even if she shows you a prior valid DNR order.

9. **The correct answer is D.** It is correct to insist that the matter is not of urgency and that you will return in a couple of hours to discuss the blood tests. Although the patient insisted that the blood test should be discussed in the presence of his brother and the best friend, the nature of the discussion is not known to the patient at this point in time. A sensitive matter like diagnostic measures for HIV especially should be discussed alone with the patient before disclosing it to family or friends. Even though in this case the patient insisted that the matter should be discussed in front of the visitors, as the patient had no idea regarding the nature of the discussion it is not appropriate to go ahead and discuss it in front of the visitors.

For the reasons explained above, disclosing the blood test results and discussing the clinical suspicion (**choice A**) is not appropriate.

Even in the presence of another health care worker (**choice B**), confidential matters should not be discussed in public or even in the presence of family members or best friends. These matters should first be discussed with the patient. Once the nature of the discussion is known to the patient, if he or she requests further discussion in the presence of the family, further discussions may be carried out.

To tell the patient that the blood test was suspicious (**choice C**) but you cannot discuss the results in the presence of the family will only make the patient more uncomfortable and anxious.

To tell the family and friends that they must leave the room (**choice E**) is incorrect because you cannot force them to leave because the patient strongly requested their presence.

10. **The correct answer is D.** This patient is suffering from an acute urinary tract infection. One must not confuse his urinary complaints with a worsening of his BPH symptoms. Patients may have similar complaints with these two conditions. This patient has an acute worsening of his symptoms, however; he has developed fever and his urine dipstick is suggestive of urinary tract infection. Approximately 90% of all first-time occurrences of urinary tract infections are caused by *E. coli. E. coli* has the ability to produce pili that are able to interact with urothelial receptors that allow for adherence of the bacteria in the urinary system. The patient requires appropriate diagnosis and treatment. This is best accomplished by first obtaining a urine sample for culture and sensitivity before giving antibiotics (**choice A**). Getting a culture specimen before therapy is crucial, as the results will allow you to tailor antibiotic treatment accordingly.

    By not giving antibiotics (**choice B**) or increasing his tamsulosin dose (**choice C**) his infection may worsen and make him septic.

    Voiding cystourethrograms, or VCUG, is used to evaluate for vesicoureteral reflux. They are done in the pediatric population for recurrent UTI (**choice E**). This study does not play a role in the evaluation of an elderly man with UTI.

11. **The correct answer is D.** This patient has developed lichen simplex chronicus secondary to continuous habitual scratching of the back of her neck. The most appropriate treatment option at this time is topical betamethasone cream daily until the lesions resolve. Lichen simplex chronicus may represent the end stage of a variety of pruritic and eczematous disorders. It consists of a well-circumscribed plaque or plaques with lichenified or thickened skin due to chronic scratching or rubbing. Common areas involved include the posterior nuchal region, dorsum of the feet, or ankles. Treatment of lichen simplex chronicus centers on breaking the cycle of chronic itching and scratching, which often occur during sleep. High-potency topical glucocorticoids are helpful in alleviating pruritus in most cases, but in recalcitrant cases, application of topical glucocorticoids under occlusion or intralesional injection of glucocorticoids may be required. Oral antihistamines such as hydroxyzine (10 to 50 mg every 6 h) or tricyclic antidepressants with antihistaminic activity such as doxepin (10 to 25 mg at bedtime) are useful as antipruritics primarily due to their sedating action, and are particularly useful at bedtime. Patients need to be counseled regarding driving or operating heavy equipment after taking these medications due to their potentially potent sedative activity.

    Intralesional injections of bleomycin (**choice A**) are used in the treatment of recalcitrant viral warts that have failed all other treatment modalities.

    This patient's skin condition is not the result of a bacterial infection, so oral cephalexin for 10 days (**choice B**) is not indicated.

    Oral steroids for 2 weeks (**choice C**) would probably bring temporary relief but their side effect profile and rebound phenomenon associated do not justify utilization for such a limited case of lichen simplex chronicus.

    Topical permethrin cream (**choice E**) is used to treat infestations with lice and scabies. Liberal application over the affected areas is performed twice, with a 7-day interval in between.

12. **The correct answer is B.** This patient has acute pericarditis. Most patients with acute pericarditis have either viral (echovirus and coxsackievirus are most common) or idiopathic pericarditis. Clinical manifestations include chest pain that is pleuritic and sharp in nature, a pericardial friction rub, and a widespread ST elevation on the EKG. Therapy is targeted at relieving the pain and decreasing the inflammation, which can be achieved by aspirin or any other NSAID. It is important to distinguish acute pericarditis from acute myocardial infarction, which is achieved through the history, physical examination, and the EKG. EKG features distinguishing acute pericarditis from acute MI are: diffuse ST elevations that are concave upward, PR-segment abnormalities, and the absence of Q waves.

    Thrombolytics, such as intravenous streptokinase (**choice A**), are indicated in the treatment of ST-segment elevation MI.

    An aortic dissection can manifest with acute sharp chest pain, but usually in elderly patients who have predisposing factors (mainly HTN). It is usually diagnosed with a CT scan of the chest (**choice C**).

    A pulmonary embolism, which can be diagnosed with a ventilation-perfusion scan (**choice D**), can also produce sharp pleuritic chest pain. It usually occurs in patients with predisposing factors like immobilization, surgery, stroke, malignancy, and DVT. Patients usually present with dyspnea. They are usually tachypneic, tachycardic, and hypoxemic.

Emergent cardiac catheterization (**choice E**) with PTCA is done in patients who have a contraindication to thrombolytics or who fail to respond to thrombolytics. Cardiac catheterization with PTCA is as effective as thrombolytics in acute MI.

13. **The correct answer is D.** This patient is presenting with benzodiazepine overdose and suicidal attempt. Clinical features of sedative intoxication include slurred speech, unsteady gait, and impaired memory and attention; severe overdose can cause coma and respiratory depression. Management includes supportive measures including maintenance of airways, ventilation, and cardiovascular function. Activated charcoal should be given to patients who ingested the benzodiazepine orally.

Flumazenil (**choice A**), which is a benzodiazepine antagonist, can be given in patients with acute intoxication, but is contraindicated in patients with physical dependence because it will precipitate seizures. It might not reverse the respiratory depression associated with benzodiazepine overdose.

N-acetylcysteine (**choice B**), a glutathione precursor, is used for an acetaminophen overdose.

Naloxone (**choice C**) is an opiate antagonist and is given when an opiate overdose is suspected.

Intubation and mechanical ventilation (**choice E**) is indicated if the degree of respiratory depression is severe and the patient is becoming hypoxemic or hypercapnic.

14. **The correct answer is E.** This patient has an infection of a central venous catheter (CVC). He is manifesting local signs of infection (swelling, tenderness, and erythema) that mandate removal of the line. The most common organisms causing CVC infections are *Staphylococcus* sp., *Candida* sp., and enterococci. Intravenous antibiotics with vancomycin and gentamicin should be used after the catheter is removed.

Changing the catheter over a guide wire (**choice A**) in the presence of insertion site infection may result in bacteremia and septic emboli and is not recommended; on top of that the new catheter will be contaminated.

Gentamicin (**choice C**) should be empirically added to vancomycin therapy if the patient is immunocompromised or showing signs of sepsis.

Because most infections are typically caused by *Staphylococcus*, intravenous vancomycin (**choice B**) should be started pending culture results; however, this patient should also receive gentamicin.

Although fever is a common manifestation of Hodgkin disease, it shouldn't be attributed to it (**choice D**) in this patient with signs of line infection.

15. **The correct answer is E.** This patient is experiencing signs and symptoms of gram-negative sepsis stemming from a urinary tract infection. The most important intervention is early antibiotic therapy. The choice of antibiotic depends on the history and Gram stain of the urine. The most common pathogens are gram-negative rods (*E. coli*), so initial antibiotic coverage should include gram-negative coverage and be adjusted depending on the culture sensitivity. Urinary tract infection in men is less common than in women, owing to anatomic difference, and is usually caused by obstruction because of benign prostatic hyperplasia (BPH), especially in elderly men.

A urologic consultation (**choice A**) is indicated if the patient remains febrile or shows no signs of clinical improvement after 72 hours of treatment to rule out obstruction, renal or perinephric abscess, or other complications of pyelonephritis.

Bladder catheterization with a Foley (**choice B**) may be necessary if there is an obstruction.

An imaging procedure like ultrasound (**choice C**) probably should be obtained in all men with acute pyelonephritis because it is usually associated with anatomic abnormality such as obstruction or prostatic disease; however, antibiotics should be started immediately.

Although this patient is somewhat hypotensive, he is maintaining his mental function, so pressors like dopamine (**choice D**) are not indicated at this time. This patient should be challenged with fluid boluses. If he does not respond or deteriorates then he should be started on pressors.

16. **The correct answer is C.** The decision of the physician to stop further cardiopulmonary resuscitation is correct. Although the legal definition of death is brain death, failure on the part of the myocardium to respond despite all therapeutic measures would constitute a valid reason for discontinuing CPR on the grounds of futility. The courts would decide the matter on the grounds of

futility as determined by the judgment of the physician. In medical ethics, futility is defined as the unilateral decision by the physician to withhold or revoke medical interventions if in the opinion of the physician the intercession has no pathophysiologic rationale, has failed previously, has failed despite maximal therapeutic efforts, or will not attain the therapeutic goal. Futility forms part of beneficence and there are two components to it—physiologic and medical.

Although physiologic futility is determined by the physician, medical futility is decided by the patient or his surrogate

Physiologic futility is determined by the physician who decides whether continuity of therapeutic intervention would achieve the physiologic goal, which in this particular patient was clearly not the case. Under the concept of physiologic futility, a physician has the right to deny CPR to a patient, as would be the case in a patient who is terminally ill from widespread metastasis, but in certain extenuating circumstances he may institute or prolong futile therapy for a short period of time at the request of the patient or family (e.g., if relatives have to travel and would arrive in a day or two, and whom the patient would like to see before treatment is discontinued). The courts would bestow great significance to the judgment of the physician as to the physiologic futility in continuing therapeutic measures.

In all situations, a physician should exercise reasonable medical judgment. This means that the physician has considered all the facts of the case and has come to a logical medical conclusion after paying scrupulous attention and care during diagnosis and therapy. The physician should never permit other factors to come into play in making a decision. Thus, moral, ethical, sociologic, religious, or philosophic factors should not cloud his medical judgment, as the decision should rest on medical facts alone so as to be able to withstand the scrutiny of his peers. This is because ethics committees and lay persons involved in the decision-making process have to rely on the physician's analysis as the primary source for their verdict to withdraw or terminate life support systems. It is important to note that brain death is not a necessary requirement for withdrawing or withholding life support. And, withdrawing or withholding life support does not come into conflict with the principles of beneficence, nonmaleficence, or autonomy. Thus, even if the plaintiff were to suggest that brain death should have been confirmed before discontinuing CPR, the courts would hold this untenable.

Medical futility is the understanding by the patient or surrogate about the quality of life that would accrue during or after treatment. In this situation, the physician should provide all the information to the patient or surrogate for them to make the appropriate decision. Once again, the physician should not be swayed by his own beliefs, but lay it out threadbare. **Choices A, B, D, and E** are incorrect.

17. **The correct answer is D.** Based on the available history and physical examination, this patient has a pericardial tamponade. The best modality from which this can be confirmed is a cardiac echocardiogram looking for evidence of a pericardial effusion with tamponade physiology.

    A bronchoscopy (**choice A**) cannot help in the diagnosis of a possible pericardial tamponade.

    A chest x-ray (**choice B**), while sometimes showing evidence of a pericardial effusion (a globular appearance of the heart), should not be used as a screen for a pericardial effusion with possible tamponade physiology.

    A chest CT (**choice C**), while often able to show a pericardial effusion, is not recommended as the screening test for the evaluation of a possible effusion with tamponade physiology.

    A ventilation-perfusion scan (**choice E**), used in the diagnosis of a pulmonary embolus, does not help in the diagnosis of a pericardial effusion.

18. **The correct answer is D.** This middle-aged woman with elevated levels of alkaline phosphatase, antimitochondrial antibody titer, and gamma-glutamyltransferase is likely to have primary biliary cirrhosis.

    Patients with choledocholithiasis (**choice A**) usually have dilated hepatic ducts on ultrasound evaluation. In addition, infiltrative liver disease, as seen with choledocholithiasis is not associated with increases in antimitochondrial antibody levels. The same is true of drug-induced cholestasis (**choice B**), and sarcoidosis (**choice E**).

    Levels of 5′-nucleotidase or gamma-glutamyltransferase are usually elevated in parallel with those of alkaline phosphatase in patients with liver disease, but not in patients with bone disorders (**choice C**).

19. **The correct answer is E.** The diagnostic criteria for endocarditis include evidence for continuous bacteremia, a new murmur, and echocardiographic evidence of valvular lesions. This man has endocarditis caused by gram-positive coccus. Until sensitivities of the organisms

are known, treatment involves antibiotic coverage for *Enterococcus, Streptococcus,* and methicillin-resistant or resistant *Staphylococcus.* A patient without a prosthetic valve should be started on vancomycin and gentamicin, with monitoring of serum levels.

Cephalosporins like ceftriaxone (**choice A**) are not a good initial choice because *Enterococcus* and methicillin-resistant *Staphylococcus* are not resistant to cephalosporins.

There is no cited evidence for a fluoroquinolone (**choice B**) as an indication for endocarditis management.

If the organism proves to be sensitive to nafcillin (**choice C**), the patient can then be switched to a regimen of nafcillin and gentamicin, but it is not the best initial therapy when the exact organism and sensitivity are unknown.

Streptomycin (**choice D**) is not typically used for endocarditis management. It can cause ototoxicity and skin rash. It is currently being used in conjunction with other drugs for tuberculosis treatment and gonorrhea.

20. **The correct answer is B.** There are several vaccines available for diseases with a high prevalence in developing countries. The primary care physician should make sure that international travelers are up to date in their routine immunizations, given that vaccine-based immunity to tetanus, diphtheria, polio, and measles decreases over time, and these diseases are highly prevalent abroad. Although location-specific situations require specific immunizations such as cholera, typhoid, yellow fever, and hepatitis B vaccinations, hepatitis A vaccine is recommended for nearly all international travelers. Hepatitis A is common in all areas of the world except Canada, Western Europe and Scandinavia, Japan, New Zealand, and Australia.

Cholera (**choice A**) is an uncommon disease in travelers. The injected vaccine was of poor efficacy. Immunization against cholera is not appropriate for most travelers, unless it is known that border officials may demand a cholera certificate.

Hepatitis B (**choice C**) is a viral disease of the liver that is endemic in many tropical countries. It is transmitted by sexual activity and through contaminated needles and syringes. Travelers at particular risk should consider being in date for this immunization. The course comprises 2 injections separated by 1 month and a further injection at 6 months. An accelerated schedule is available for those who do not have time to complete the recommended course.

Typhoid (**choice D**) is a disease contracted from contaminated food and water that leads to high fever and septicemia. There are now three vaccines for protection against typhoid. These are the older monovalent vaccine, a new injected single to dose vaccine, and a live oral vaccine.

Yellow fever immunization (**choice E**) is usually advised for those going to areas where the standards of food and water hygiene are low. Vaccines are available that provide protection for 10 years.

21. **The correct answer is C.** Sarcoidosis is an idiopathic, multisystemic granulomatous disease occurring most frequently in individuals between the ages of 20 to 40 years. It is usually asymptomatic but it may present with pulmonary abnormalities (e.g., diffusion capacity defects). Airway obstruction may also be present. Patients with sarcoidosis typically present with hilar and peritracheal lymphadenopathy. There is also association with acute peripheral arthritis, uveitis, and erythema nodosum. Pain, redness, and conjunctival injection are consistent with a uveitis and would be the most suggestive of sarcoidosis.

Constitutional symptoms other than fatigue are unusual for sarcoidosis. Indeed, when anorexia, weight loss, and fever are present (**choice A**), other diseases should be strongly considered.

Sarcoid granulomas are whorls of epithelioid cells showing multinucleated giant cells. Fibrosis and hyalinization are present to a variable degree. True caseation is unusual. Nonspecific granules are usually present. Transbronchial biopsies are done for tissue biopsies and they reveal positive results in 60 to 90% of people with sarcoidosis. This is in contrast to liver or lymph node biopsies (**choice B**) in which nonspecific granulomas may be seen.

Apart from uveitis, no other ophthalmologic signs are typically seen in sarcoidosis and there are no space-occupying lesions noted in the brain; therefore, papilledema (**choice D**) is not suggestive of sarcoidosis and other diagnoses would need working up (e.g., tumor).

Biochemical changes in sarcoidosis include hypercalcemia and elevation in angiotensin-converting enzyme. A serum calcium level of 6.0 mg/dL (**choice E**) is hypocalcemic and is not suggestive of sarcoidosis.

22. **The correct answer is B.** Whenever a patient continues to spike fevers despite adequate antimicrobial coverage over an adequate time frame one should consider an

abscess as a potential cause. In this case the useful predictive factor in distinguishing uncomplicated pyelonephritis from a (perinephric) abscess is flank pain and persistent fever for more than 3 to 4 days after beginning antibiotic therapy. A perinephric abscess is a collection of pus in the Gerota fascia surrounding the kidney. A CT scan of the abdomen would be the next step to take. It would detect the presence of perirenal fluid, enlargement of the psoas muscle, and the presence of perirenal gas.

The antibiotic coverage of ampicillin and gentamycin are adequately covering the likeliest organisms for pyelonephritis. These are *E. coli* (commonest), enterococci (second most common), and *Pseudomonas aeruginosa*. Adding another antibiotic like vancomycin (**choice A**) probably will not help.

The CT scan would have much greater sensitivity and specificity than ultrasonography or an intravenous pyelogram (**choice C**).

A radionuclide renal scan (**choice D**) (e.g., a Mag3 or a DTPA scan) gives information about the blood flow to the kidneys and how well each kidney is functioning for the production of urine. The test also shows if there are any obstructions in urine output. The patient is given radioactive isotopes orally or intravenously while a gamma camera is positioned overhead for a series of images of the kidneys.

A "sterile pyuria" with WBCs present in urine but a *negative* routine bacterial culture may suggest the diagnosis of renal tuberculosis (**choice E**). This patient has grown *E. coli* twice.

23. **The correct answer is A.** This patient most likely has acute gout. Typical symptoms of gout include erythema, redness, and pain in the first metatarsal-phalangeal joint. The uric acid levels can be normal at various times in gout.

Morton neuroma (**choice B**) is an entrapment neuropathy of the interdigital nerve, usually occurring between the third and fourth toes, not associated with erythema and redness.

Osteoarthritis (**choice C**) typically involves the larger joints in a bilateral manner such as the knees, hips, and shoulders. Radiologic findings include loss of joint space, osteophytic changes, osteosclerosis, and cystic changes in the bone.

Septic arthritis (**choice D**) is unlikely because there is no effusion on physical examination and the white cell count and erythrocyte sedimentation rate are normal. Had there been an effusion present, the next thing would be to aspirate the effusion and send it off for crystal and cell content, culture, and sensitivity.

Acute arthritis in systemic lupus erythematosus (**choice E**) typically involves the small joints of the hands, wrists, and knees.

24. **The correct answer is D.** This patient has symptoms consistent with gastroesophageal reflux disease or GERD. It is secondary to esophageal relaxation leading to acid reflux. Fat in the duodenum has been shown to increase the frequency of episodes of esophageal relaxation of the lower esophageal sphincter, allowing reflux to occur. Reduction of fat intake is a logical treatment modality.

Antacids and prolonged use of histamine blockers are appropriate therapies for GERD, unlike **choices A and E**.

Other basic lifestyle modifications that should be encouraged early on include eating small meals, refraining from eating for 2 to 3 hours before lying down, decreasing the intake of chocolate, caffeine (**choice B**), cola, and alcohol, and elevating the head about 6 inches (**choice C**). Elevation of the head has been found to result in subjective and objective improvement in reflux—the degree of improvement approaches that associated with therapy with histamine receptor blockers.

25. **The correct answer is B.** Atrial fibrillation is the most common sustained arrhythmia encountered in primary care practice and hospitalized care. Although many patients with atrial fibrillation experience relief of symptoms with control of the heart rate, some patients require restoration of sinus rhythm. External direct-current (DC) cardioversion has a higher rate of success than medical cardioversion for converting atrial fibrillation to sinus rhythm. Pharmacologic cardioversion, although less effective, offers an alternative to DC cardioversion.

Sotalol and amiodarone slow conduction and prolong refractoriness in the atrioventricular node and thus can control ventricular response to atrial fibrillation. Amiodarone (**choice A**) does not appear to be more effective than placebo in converting recent-onset atrial fibrillation to sinus rhythm, although patients who are treated with amiodarone tend to have a more controlled heart rate. It is believed that intravenous amiodarone has little effect in atrial tissue. Side effects of intravenous amiodarone include hypotension and bradyarrhythmias. On the other hand, oral amiodarone, which prolongs atrial refractoriness, may be effective in cardioversion, either alone or as an adjunct to DC cardioversion. Unfortunately, it is not useful for acute cardioversion. Sotalol (**choice E**) also is not useful for the acute termination of atrial fibrillation, probably because it tends to prolong atrial refractoriness more at a slow rate than during tachycardia.

High-dose oral propafenone (**choice C**) has been shown to be effective for cardioversion of atrial fibrillation, with conversion rates of up to 76% at 8 hours after treatment.

Oral quinidine (**choice D**) may be used for the acute termination of atrial fibrillation. The conversion rate is reported to be up to 60%. Torsades de pointes is a major side effect in patients who undergo therapy with quinidine. It appears that episodes of torsades de pointes are most likely to occur after reversion to sinus rhythm.

26. **The correct answer is A.** The patient has poison ivy dermatitis and systemic corticosteroids are recognized for their high efficacy on the subjective and objective course of poison ivy dermatitis, in which case, oral prednisone tapered over 2 to 3 weeks is a typical regimen.

    Antihistamines, such as diphenhydramine (**choice B**), and cool compresses (**choice C**) offer symptomatic relief only and do not alter the course of the established disease.

    Over-the-counter topical hydrocortisone is typically ineffective for all but the mildest cases, and once the disease is established, superpotent topical corticosteroids (**choice D**) do little to alter the overall course and natural history. Generally speaking one should prescribe topical steroids to the face and genitalia with extreme caution because of the risk of dermal sclerosis.

    Methylprednisolone (**choice E**) is a shorter prepackaged course. Such products begin with an initial dose about one-half that of the commonly recommended dose with a very rapid taper. Repeating the methylprednisolone can result in complications such as significant rebound flares.

27. **The correct answer is B.** This patient's change in behavior can be explained by the chronic fecal impaction that is evident on the abdominal x-ray as a side effect of the antipsychotic medication (risperidone). It would also explain the watery bowel movements as fecal overflow. Otherwise, the patient's history, physical examination, and blood results appear normal. The patient could now benefit from treatment of constipation, for which the best first-line treatment is fiber supplements. In the ambulatory elderly patient, they have a good safety profile and low cost. Bran is the most inexpensive and natural fiber supplement.

    A head CT scan (**choice A**) would be a useful component of a delirium workup, except that there is a low suspicion of delirium in this patient based on the benign history, physical examination, and blood work.

    Magnesium hydroxide (**choice C**) is useful for intermittent use but may be harsh in the elderly and can cause excess fluid shifts.

    Mineral oil (**choice D**) if aspirated can cause lipid pneumonia, and it can cause rectal leakage as well as affect drug and vitamin absorption.

    Risperidone (**choice E**) may be the ultimate cause of the constipation and fecal incontinence. It would not be appropriate to halve the dose of this antipsychotic simply because of the constipation side effect, particularly if the patient's psychiatrist had finally controlled the patient's positive or negative symptoms of the schizophreniform disorder.

28. **The correct answer is C.** The skin features are suggestive of a lupus rash and because only the skin is affected without multisystem involvement, a discoid lupus erythematosus is the most likely cause. Discoid lupus erythematosus refers to a skin disorder in which a red, raised rash appears on the face, scalp, or elsewhere. The raised areas may become thick and scaly and may cause scarring. The rash may last for days or years and may recur. A small percentage of people with discoid lupus have or develop systemic lupus erythematosus.

    Acne vulgaris (**choice A**) is inflammation of the pilosebaceous glands. The incidence is greatest in women ages 16 to 18 years (40% have clinical acne) and in men ages 17 to 19 years (35% have clinical acne). Androgens and genetic disposition can cause plug formation and increased sebum production; bacterial infection drawing white blood cells to the gland weakens and ruptures the gland wall. Clinically it is composed of comedones and a papulopustular rash.

    Acute intermittent porphyria (**choice B**) is an autosomal dominant disorder caused by a defect in porphobilinogen deaminase activity. Dermatologic manifestations are rare. Its acute attack involves neurologic dysfunction that can involve any portion of the nervous system. It is believed that an imbalance in the autonomic innervation of the gut leads to abdominal pain that is commonly associated with the attack and precedes peripheral neuropathy, such as pain in the back and legs.

    Psoriasis (**choice D**) typically presents as well-delineated silver or salmon pink rashes on the elbows and knees with nail pitting of the fingers and toes and scaling (hyperkeratosis) beneath the nails.

Skin rashes are common with systemic lupus erythematosus or SLE (**choice E**). The most characteristic rash is seen across the malar region of the face, the so-called "butterfly rash" that is accentuated by sun exposure. SLE must be distinguished from discoid lupus erythematosus that affects the skin (but only in sun-exposed regions) and is unlikely to be associated with systemic illness, such as renal disease. A biopsy of sun-exposed skin that is not involved with a rash will demonstrate immune complex deposition with SLE, but not with DLE.

29. **The correct answer is E.** This patient has a complex medical picture and is probably going into acute *prerenal* failure secondary to hypovolemia. The hyperkalemia is the most important priority and needs to be corrected immediately to alleviate the occurrence of potentially fatal arrhythmias. Treatment depends on the degree of hyperkalemia and the changes seen on the electrocardiogram. All of the above options are actually management steps in the treatment of hyperkalemia. Of these options, potassium *excretion* is achieved with oral consumption of sodium polystyrene sulfonate. It basically exacerbates fecal bowel movement, thereby excreting potassium through the gut. Diuretics like furosemide, although not listed here, will also aid in potassium excretion.

    Inhaled beta agonists (**choice A**), intravenously administered sodium bicarbonate (**choice D**), and intravenous insulin and glucose (**choice C**) shift the potassium intracellularly and do not actually end up in excretion of potassium.

    Intravenous calcium (10 mL of a 10% solution of calcium gluconate) (**choice B**) is cardioprotective and temporarily reverses the neuromuscular effects of hyperkalemia.

    If the above pharmacotherapy fails in alleviating the hyperkalemia, then dialysis should be started.

30. **The correct answer is E.** A patient's conversation with relatives and friends is the commonest form of advance directive and it carries the same ethical and legal weight as those in writing. Thus, withdrawing life support complies best with the patient's earlier wishes and is the correct answer.

    Because the patient has previously expressed his wishes it is unnecessary to have the court appoint a surrogate decision-maker (**choice A**).

    Neither the patient's (**choice B**) nor the hospital's attorney (**choice C**), in the absence of a previous discussion with the patient, has the ethical or legal authority to make the decision.

    Care would be transferred to another physician (**choice D**) only if the original physician had a philosophical or religious objection to carrying out the patient's wishes.

31. **The correct answer is A.** The insulin level and C peptide levels help distinguish different types of hypoglycemia. This patient's condition is most likely caused by exogenous insulin administration because it causes insulin levels to be elevated and C peptide levels to be low or undetectable. The nurse may also have easy access to exogenous insulin through her occupation. Fictitious hypoglycemia is a serious psychiatric illness in which the patient deliberately lowers their serum blood glucose with exogenous insulin or sulfonylureas. This may lead to coma or death if untreated.

    An insulinoma (**choice B**) is commonly seen in the islet cells of the pancreas and corresponds to the following triad: attacks of hypoglycemia with serum glucose less than 50 mg/dL, attacks consisting of mental status changes such as stupor, confusion, and even loss of consciousness, and prompt relief with feeding or parenteral administration of glucose. Typically the insulin and C peptide levels are elevated and in this case it is not the correct answer.

    A pituitary tumor (**choice C**) is incorrect because it can present in a myriad of additional ways through abnormal secretions of ACTH, TSH, gonadotrophins, LH, and FSH from the anterior gland alone. It may present as bilateral temporal hemianopia.

    A small cell carcinoma (**choice D**) would typically cause hypercalcemia as its commonest metabolic paraneoplastic syndrome. In addition, the syndrome of inappropriate antidiuretic hormone secretion (SIADH) may also occur to present a different clinical picture from the one in this question.

    Sulfonylurea overdoses (**choice E**) would also cause C peptide and insulin levels to be elevated.

32. **The correct answer is A.** A low parathyroid hormone level, hypocalcemia, and hyperphosphatemia with normal renal function are pathognomic of primary hypoparathyroidism. In hypoparathyroidism, mobilization of calcium from bone, renal reabsorption of calcium, phosphaturia, and 1,25$(OH)_2$ vitamin D formation are all reduced, which results in a decrease in intestinal calcium absorption. The end results are hypocalcemia and hyperphosphatemia.

    Papilledema (**choice B**) is not a finding associated with hypoparathyroidism. Usually cataracts may be associated with hypocalcemia.

Polyuria (**choice C**) and polydipsia are typical findings of *hyper*calcemia and probably would not be seen in hypoparathyroidism.

Prolongation of the QT interval (**choice D**) is an electrocardiogram finding associated with hypocalcemia but is not specific to hypoparathyroidism (hypocalcemia may be from other causes).

Renal failure (**choice E**) may cause hypocalcemia and hyperphosphatemia but when the parathyroid hormone level is normal it is not pathognomonic of hypoparathyroidism!

Shortening of the QT interval (**choice F**) is an electrocardiogram finding associated with *hyper*calcemia and again does not reflect hypoparathyroidism.

33. **The correct answer is C.** This patient has herpes simplex infection, and based on the frequency of outbreaks and the patient's desire to prevent outbreaks, suppressive therapy should be offered. Because the frequency of outbreaks usually decreases over time, it is advisable to stop therapy at some time to reassess the frequency of outbreaks.

Herpes simplex infection does last for the patient's lifetime and suppression for longer than a year may be needed. However, the safety of acyclovir has only been studied for up to 6 years and the frequency of outbreaks may become so infrequent that the patient may no longer wish to take medication daily for them. Therefore, having him take acyclovir for the remainder of his life (**choice A**) is incorrect.

Treating the patient and his sexual partners with acyclovir, as he is likely being reinfected (**choice B**), is incorrect. Herpes simplex infection is one of frequent recurrences and these do not represent recurrent infection. The virus remains dormant in nerve roots and can flare at any time. This patient, however, should be counseled that he can transmit this infection to his sexual partners and prevention with the use of condoms is recommended.

Treatment with acyclovir for a longer course during the next outbreak as he may have a resistant infection (**choice D**) is incorrect. Treatment with acyclovir during acute outbreaks may slightly decrease the duration of symptoms, but will not have an affect on recurrences. This infection is not resistant, but is the typical course of herpes simplex infection with frequent recurrences.

Imiquimod is a medication approved for the treatment of symptomatic genital warts. Patients apply this medication themselves over an 8-week period with usually good results. This patient's symptoms are not suggestive of this infection (**choice E**).

34. **The correct answer is D.** Parvovirus B19 or erythema infectiosum or fifth disease can be a fairly common cause of exanthematous rashes and arthritis in young women. A high suspicion is indicated in health care workers who have frequent contact with children. The rash may last from a few days to several weeks. The rash in children is also maculopapular in nature, affecting the trunks and extremities, and is pruritic.

Adenovirus (**choice A**) rarely causes arthritis and its defining characteristic is conjunctivitis.

Human immunodeficiency virus (**choice B**) can cause a musculoskeletal syndrome later on the disease; however, it rarely causes arthritis. Its most frequent skin eruption is a papulopruritic eruption or "itchy folliculitis."

Measles (**choice C**), like HIV, rarely causes an arthritis.

Varicella-zoster (**choice E**) may cause a large-joint arthritis, but the rash is distinctively vesicular and pruritic.

35. **The correct answer is A.** This patient most likely has lead poisoning. Lead is toxic to enzymes and works by bonding to sulfhydryl groups of proteins. It is accompanied by anemia and basophilic stippling of red blood cells that would best be seen on a CBC and peripheral smear.

An erythrocyte sedimentation rate (**choice B**) is a cheap and nonspecific parameter of inflammation, and even when elevated would not be specific to lead poisoning.

A fasting blood glucose test (**choice C**) is inappropriate mainly because it is not pathognomonic to lead poisoning in any way. In addition, there is not enough information in the history to back a diagnosis of type 2 diabetes mellitus.

The main organ affected by lead poisoning is the kidney. This may be backed up by proteinuria and pyuria on urinalysis reflecting renal abnormalities. In addition, the BUN climbs as the toxicity increases. Liver function tests are not typically useful (**choice D**).

Long bone films (**choice E**) may be useful in children where lead lines develop in their metaphyseal plate, but this is not a useful test in adults.

36. **The correct answer is E.** Syphilis is caused by *Treponema pallidum* and may develop within several weeks of exposure. It involves painless indurated, superficial ulcerations or chancres. The patient is

experiencing the Jarisch-Herxheimer reaction—an acute, transient febrile reaction that occurs within the first few hours after treatment for syphilis. The pathogenesis is probably caused by the liberation of antigens from the spirochetes. The illness peaks at 6 to 8 hours and disappears within 12 to 24 hours after therapy. Temperature is low grade and there is often associated myalgia, headache, and malaise. It is usually of no clinical significance and may be treated with antipyretics in most cases.

Doxycycline is the alternative treatment choice for primary syphilis and is chosen when the patient has a documented allergy to penicillin. The patient has no drug allergies and therefore the addition of doxycycline (**choice A**) would be incorrect.

The onset of the symptoms immediately after the administration of the antibiotic should suggest that a drug reaction is a likelier cause than a superimposed infection. A temperature of 100.6 F is low grade and would not require an immediate need for blood cultures (**choice B**). Therefore, this choice is incorrect.

A head CT scan (**choice C**) is inappropriate because there is nothing to suggest that the patient has a change in mental status. A complete history and physical examination (the latter of which has not been done yet) is the first step in the evaluation of a headache, not a head CT scan.

Meningitis should be considered in any patient with fever and neurologic symptoms, especially with a history of other infections or head trauma. In the absence of focal neurologic signs, a cerebrospinal fluid specimen should be obtained. Going by the above history at this stage, however, a drug reaction is a likelier cause, undermining the suspicion of meningitis. A lumbar puncture (**choice D**) is not the best choice.

37. **The correct answer is B.** This patient has mild to moderate dehydration probably caused by the urinary tract infection, causing the fevers and decreased oral intake. The dehydration signs in this patient include poor skin turgor and dry mucous membranes. Dehydration leading to a decreased glomerular filtration rate is indicated by the decreased urine output (300 mL divided by 17 hours gives a urine output of only 17 mL/hour) and leads to the resultant prerenal azotemia. The urine specific gravity being greater than 1.030 is another useful indicator of prerenal azotemia. Finally, when the ratio of BUN to creatinine is greater than 20, this is another indicator of the prerenal azotemia, of which the most common cause is dehydration.

Acute renal failure (**choice A**) is unlikely because the clinical signs would typically occur in less than 1 week (usually hours to days), the patient would appear very ill, the body condition is normally less dehydrated, and the kidneys are sometimes painful. Hyperkalemia may occur and the urine sediment may show casts, proteinuria, or glucosuria caused by tubular necrosis. Based on the history and physical exam, this patient's oliguria is likely to be caused by dehydration.

Nephritic syndrome (**choice C**) would present with hematuria, red blood cell casts, hypertension, and edema superimposed on a deteriorating renal function (we only have one BUN and creatinine in the question and not a series of BUN and creatinines). The large blood in the patient's urine analysis may be from microtrauma from the urethral catheter.

Ureteral obstruction either by neoplasia at the trigone of the bladder (**choice D**) or by urolithiasis (**choice E**) would be uncommon causes of postrenal azotemia (postrenal azotemia most often results from *urethral* obstruction). In any case there is not enough information in this patient's history to back up either of these two possibilities (e.g., sharp loin-to-groin pain for stones or weight loss for a neoplasia). Also, in order for ureteral disease to cause azotemia, it must be bilateral or must occur with concomitant renal disease.

38. **The correct answer is F.** When suspecting a potential pneumonia that is not immediately evident on the initial chest x-ray, hydration with an intravenous bolus and then maintenance fluids intravenously will show up as pneumonia on a subsequent chest x-ray.

A sputum culture (**choice A**) may be difficult to obtain in this patient, will take several days to grow (if it's positive in the first place!), and may be contaminated by other microorganisms.

Blood gases, whether they be on oxygen (**choice C**) or room air (**choice D**), will only inform you about the ability of gas transfer in the lungs and the extent of oxygenation in the bloodstream. They will not directly inform you about the presence of a pneumonia.

A CT of the chest (**choice E**) exposes the patient to excessive radiation. The quality of the CT scan sometimes benefits from the patient getting adequate fluid hydration before the scan.

Pulmonary function tests (**choice B**) like the blood gas will not directly indicate the presence or absence of a pneumonia in the way that a chest x-ray can. A single pulmonary function test will help establish whether the patient has restrictive or obstructive lung disease.

39. **The correct answer is D.** This patient requires maintenance fluids to improve her urine output and for general hydration. (This would typically be started *after* a bolus of 1 L to "catch up" with her insensible losses.) Maintenance fluid can usually be provided by the administration of 0.45% normal saline with 5% dextrose at a rate of 125 mL/hour with 20 mmol/L of potassium chloride. She is diabetic, however, and therefore no dextrose should be added. In addition, because she is elderly with coronary artery disease she is easily at risk for fluid overload in her lungs (pulmonary edema) and therefore her rate of infusion should be reduced to 75 mL/hour. Based on this, the correct choice of maintenance fluids would be 0.45% normal saline at a rate of 75 mL/hour with 20 mmol/L of potassium chloride.

0.9% normal saline (**choices A and B**) would be reserved initially for patients with hypotension or shock.

0.45% normal saline without the potassium chloride (**choice C**) would not treat the patient's hypokalemia (potassium = 2.9 mmol/L), which then causes a risk for arrhythmia.

0.45% normal saline with 5% dextrose (**choices E and F**) may significantly increase the hyperglycemia (serum glucose = 150 mg/dL) in this diabetic patient.

40. **The correct answer is A.** The patient describes a classic history of botulism that is caused by *Clostridium botulism* (a common anaerobic, gram-positive bacillus that produces several types of neurotoxins). Initial symptoms may be nonspecific, but food-borne botulism frequently begins with nausea, vomiting, abdominal cramps, and diarrhea. Dry mouth, blurred vision, and diplopia are usually the earliest neurologic signs. This is followed quickly by dysphonia, dysphagia, and peripheral muscle weakness. A symmetric descending paralysis is characteristic of botulism. Paralysis begins with the cranial nerves, then the upper extremities, and then the respiratory muscles. Onset is usually 18 to 36 hours after exposure. The diagnosis can be confirmed by detection of the toxin in the serum, stool, or a sample of the food consumed before the illness.

A doxycycline challenge test for tick paralysis does not exist (**choice B**).

Stroke syndromes are part of the differential for botulism but the patient is in her mid-twenties and of good previous health. A stroke is of low suspicion and a lumbar puncture would be futile (**choice C**).

Guillain-Barré syndrome (GBS) (**choice D**) is also on the differential along with myasthenia gravis and Eaton-Lambert syndrome. GBS is an ascending symmetric paralysis with proximal weakness. It is usually diagnosed by the history and with a lumbar puncture in which the protein is elevated. It is not diagnosed with an MRI.

A psychiatric consult is unnecessary (**choice E**) in view of the definite neurologic findings.

41. **The correct answer is A.** Admission to an intensive care unit for intensive monitoring would be appropriate. The mainstay of treatment of botulism is supportive therapy with mechanical ventilation. Notifying the Centers for Disease Control and Prevention (**choice E**) is part of the management, as the botulism antitoxin is only available from the CDC; however, immediate management of her "feeling of dyspnea" is indicated at this time.

Antibiotics like ciprofloxacin (**choice B**) are not useful. The only specific treatment available for botulism is the antitoxin. Antitoxin administration without mechanical ventilation, however, is hardly useful.

A steroid inhaler (**choice C**) has no efficacy in this particular situation.

The presence of hard neurologic findings clearly indicates this is not a psychiatric illness and a psychiatric consult (**choice D**) is unwarranted.

42. **The correct answer is G.** The comparison of the mean and the median for the 50-mg group shows that the mean is substantially different from the median. This indicates that the distribution is skewed and does not approximate a Gaussian, or normal curve. Therefore, the constant percentage of cases within 1, 2, and 3 standard deviations of the mean (68%, 95.5%, and 99.7%, respectively) cannot be used to answer this question. **Choices A, B, C, D, E,** and **F** give the range of plus or minus 1 and 2 standard deviations around the mean, median, and mode. Because the distribution is not normal, none of these calculations are valid.

43. **The correct answer is D.** This patient has paroxysmal supraventricular tachycardia, which is the most common cause of paroxysmal arrhythmias with a rapid heart rate. Patients typically experience the sudden onset of palpitations, shortness of breath, and chest pain. The pulse is usually between 160 to 220/min. Patients may be able to interrupt these attacks with breath holding, the Valsalva maneuver, or body and arm stretching. Gentle massage over the right carotid sinus can terminate the arrhythmia in the majority of cases.

Therefore, this should be tried before moving on to antiarrhythmic agents. It should only be performed while the patient is electrocardiographically monitored (to assess for other arrhythmias) and should not be performed in a person with carotid bruits.

Digitalis (**choice A**) should not be used for acute therapy because of the slow onset.

Verapamil (**choice B**) may be given if the carotid sinus pressure does not break the arrhythmia. Adenosine is typically preferred over verapamil because of the shorter half-life (less side effects); however, both should be administered intravenously.

A temporary pacemaker (**choice C**) is only placed after vagal maneuvers (carotid sinus pressure) and antiarrhythmic agents fail.

Waiting for the arrhythmia to subside spontaneously (**choice E**) is inappropriate because something must be done to terminate the tachycardia and return her to normal sinus rhythm.

44. **The correct answer is A.** If vagal maneuvers fail to terminate the tachycardia, adenosine should be administered intravenously.

Lidocaine (**choice B**) is used to treat ventricular tachyarrhythmias, especially in the setting of an acute myocardial infarction. It is not used to treat paroxysmal supraventricular tachycardia.

Procainamide (**choice C**) may be used to prevent an attack of paroxysmal supraventricular tachycardia, but it is not used as a treatment during an acute episode.

The insertion of a permanent pacemaker (**choice D**) is the treatment for symptomatic sinus node dysfunction or AV block. This patient most likely has paroxysmal supraventricular tachycardia, which can usually be treated symptomatically or prevented with antiarrhythmic drugs, and rarely requires a permanent pacemaker.

Direct-current cardioversion (**choice E**) is only used if severe hypotension and/or ischemia is caused by the supraventricular tachycardia. The patient is normotensive and does not have evidence of ischemia.

45. **The correct answer is B.** This patient has dermatomyositis and not atopic dermatitis. Dermatomyositis is a systemic inflammatory muscle disease with skin manifestations such as the classic heliotrope eyelid rash (a violet-colored, swollen rash of the eyelids), Gottron papules (hypertrophic plaques on the knuckles which characteristically spare the skin in between the knuckles), photosensitive violaceous eruptions, calcium deposits in the skin and muscles, telangiectasias on a face, chest, and the proximal nail folds, and pitting edema over shoulders, arms, and neck. Systemic findings include fever, malaise, anorexia, weight loss, arthralgias, and severe muscle weakness and pain. It is common for the skin findings to occur 2 to 3 months before the muscle symptoms. Adults in their fifth and sixth decades with dermatomyositis have an increased association with internal malignancies compared to children and younger adults with dermatomyositis. The next best action to take for a young patient you suspect has dermatomyositis is to measure their serum CPK (creatine phosphokinase) and refer to a dermatologist for a skin and muscle biopsy. Most dermatologists will do a muscle biopsy and if not, they will refer the patient to a surgeon. The complete workup should also include checking for elevation of other muscle enzymes in the serum such as transaminases, lactic dehydrogenase, and aldolase, which indicate active muscle disease. If the patient is older (fifth or sixth decade) a search for malignancy is imperative.

Allergy testing (**choice A**) is of no use for a patient with dermatomyositis and is debatable whether it is beneficial in an eczema patient as well. Patients with atopic dermatitis do tend to have allergies to environmental objects such as pollen, dust, mold, and animals, but allergy testing will not change their management, as "allergy shots" are not the standard of care according to most dermatologists.

Tacrolimus is a new class of topical medicines, which has been shown to be extremely safe in the treatment of atopic dermatitis with virtually no side effects (**choice C**). It is a topical immune response mediator (TIMS), which, in brief, inhibits cytokine release through calcineurin-mediated mechanism. (Tacrolimus was originally used systemically for transplant patients to inhibit transplant rejection.) Tacrolimus has not been reported to cause muscle weakness. Muscle weakness is not a common complaint in eczema patients either. Asthma, hay fever, and allergies often coincide with eczema.

Patch testing (**choice D**) is a diagnostic tool for a patient with suspected contact dermatitis. This patient does not have any stated reason for suspecting a contact allergy. Contact dermatitis will often be seen in gardeners (to poison ivy), clothing workers (to leather tanning accelerators, dyes and rubbers), or in regular citizens most commonly to nickel, fragrances, and cosmetics. The important clinical feature of contact or eczematous dermatitis is the presence of scale. Erythema, vesicles, and fissuring can also be seen but swelling and hypertrophic papules are rare.

Tacrolimus was invented because topical corticosteroids have side effects. Strong topical corticosteroids (class I-II) are rarely used on the face or groin (**choice E**). If they are prescribed, it is usually for a very short period of time (less than 1 week) and patients are warned about the potential side effects (atrophy, striae, telangiectases, and rebound phenomenon).

46. **The correct answer is D.** This patient likely suffers from rheumatoid arthritis (RA). RA is a self-perpetuating inflammatory process. It is characterized by joint swelling and stiffness lasting several weeks. Serologic studies such as the rheumatoid factor, erythrocyte sedimentation factor, and acute phase reactants may be elevated in patients with RA but *none* are pathognomonic. The diagnosis rests on clinical and radiographic findings. Although the true etiology of RA is unknown, it is characterized by a striking and destructive immune reaction. Polymorphonuclear leukocytes (PMNs) are found in synovial fluid, and when the PMNs degranulate they produce reactive oxidants, arachidonic acid, and other metabolites, which breakdown articular cartilage.

This patient has no historical factors that would lead one to believe she has an acute infectious process. Septic arthritis is typically found in immunocompromised patients and is usually localized to one large joint (knee/hip/shoulder). An acute infectious process would also likely generate a peripheral leukocytosis and if from a hematogenous source one would expect positive blood cultures (**choice A**).

Tuberculous arthritis generally does not involve the small joints of the hands and feet and is more typically associated with a destructive process in the spine (**choice B**).

Hemophilia or other clotting disorders may cause frequent large joint hemarthroses; however, this patient had normal clotting studies (**choice C**).

There is no known neoplastic process (**choice E**) that would present like this patient. Rheumatoid nodules are subcutaneous in nature. Most malignant soft tissue lesions will present as deep, firm, and fixed masses.

47. **The correct answer is B.** This patient has developed dermatitis herpetiformis in association with gluten-sensitive enteropathy. This disease is commonly treated with dapsone (diaminodiphenylsulfone), a sulfone drug with potent antineutrophilic and anti-inflammatory properties. It is well known that patients with abnormal glucoso-6-phosphate dehydrogenase levels in erythrocytes develop hemolytic anemia and methemoglobinemia when challenged with dapsone. Even low doses used to initially treat dermatitis herpetiformis can induce high methemoglobin levels with resultant cyanosis. The first sign is often a bluish discoloration of the lips, tongue, and fingernail beds. Prompt discontinuation of dapsone is advised if such signs develop. Glucoso-6-phosphate dehydrogenase levels are routinely determined in laboratories and should be tested in any patient who is being considered for dapsone treatment. Genetically low levels of this enzyme are more commonly found in African Americans.

Alpha-galactosidase deficiency (**choice A**) is found in patients with Fabry disease, an X-linked recessive disorder in which an accumulation of glycolipids causes skin lesions in the form of diffuse angiokeratomas, as well as multiple other systemic lesions secondary to deposition of the unmetabolized glycolipids. Deposits are present in endothelial cells, smooth muscle, blood vessels, and erector pili muscles. They are birefringent when viewed with polarized light.

Lactate dehydrogenase (**choice C**) does not participate in the metabolism of drugs and levels are not used to determine a possible adverse reaction to medication. Nevertheless, drugs that are metabolized by way of the liver should be used judiciously in patients with elevated lactate dehydrogenase levels.

Steroid sulfatase (**choice D**) is deficient in patients with X-linked recessive ichthyosis, a retention hyperkeratosis. Onset is at birth or early infancy, and corneal opacities detectable by slit-lamp examination are commonly present. Diagnosis is established by performing serum lipoprotein electrophoresis.

Thiomethyltransferase (**choice E**) is necessary for the adequate metabolism of azathioprine, an antimetabolite used in the treatment of some autoimmune and myeloproliferative disorders. Routine determination of this enzyme's level is available in most laboratories.

48. **The correct answer is D.** This patient has developed lupus-like syndrome, a drug reaction that is most commonly caused by the drugs procainamide and hydralazine, and resembles systemic lupus erythematosus. It will develop in as many as 30% of patients taking procainamide for long periods, and up to 70% develop positive antinuclear antibody tests. The latter occurs more rapidly in slow acetylators. Antihistone antibodies are closely associated with symptomatic disease that may be mild and innocuous or more severe and disabling. Skin changes (in the form of malar erythema or discoid lesions), oral ulcers, arthralgias, myalgias, and

laboratory changes (hemolytic anemia, white blood cell count <4000/mm^3) are similar to those encountered in systemic lupus erythematosus. The syndrome is reversible on discontinuation of procainamide in most cases and resolves promptly. Still, rare patients experience prolonged symptoms or persistent systemic disease despite cessation of the offending drug.

Digoxin (**choice A**) is used in the treatment of low-output cardiac failure, atrial fibrillation and flutter, and paroxysmal atrial tachycardia. Adverse side effects are related to toxicity and manifest with anorexia, nausea, vomiting, diarrhea, headache, fatigue, malaise, vision changes, gynecomastia, and cardiac effects.

Disopyramide (**choice B**) is similar to quinidine in its action on the heart, inhibiting rapid inward current and prolonging repolarization. The major side effects of this drug are conduction disturbances, congestive heart failure, hypotension, and anticholinergic effects.

Minoxidil (**choice C**) is used to treat severe hypertension, especially when coupled with renal failure. Side effects are related to increased reflex sympathetic stimulation and to salt and water retention. A pericardial effusion may ensue. Hypertrichosis occurs in some patients. This side effect has been used in the treatment of androgenetic alopecia.

Quinidine (**choice E**) is believed to block sodium channels and decrease conduction velocity while increasing the effective refractory period. It is used for supraventricular and arrhythmias. Major side effects are proarrhythmia and diarrhea. Quinidine is not known to induce lupus-like drug eruptions.

49. **The correct answer is E.** This patient has developed pseudomembranous colitis after receiving clindamycin for antibiotic prophylaxis of anaerobic infection associated with dental surgery. This potentially fatal condition, caused by *Clostridium difficile*, is treated with metronidazole or vancomycin. Pseudomembranous colitis is believed to result from an inflammatory reaction of the bowel wall to luminal toxins produced by *Clostridium difficile.* Disease-producing *Clostridium difficile* may be newly acquired or may represent endogenous overgrowth, following disruption of the normal flora, usually by antibiotic therapy. Presence of pseudomembranes highly suggests a toxin-mediated process secondary to *Clostridium difficile.* These pseudomembranes represent a mixture of inflammatory cells, fibrin, and bacterial and cellular components that exude from the bowel mucosa. Infection with toxigenic *Clostridium difficile* is a potentially life-threatening disease process; however, when properly treated, patient mortality is low. Patients who are not treated or who have a treatment delay may develop fulminant toxic megacolon. These patients may suffer multiple colonic perforations and have mortality rates reported as high as 30%. Symptoms can develop as early as 1 day after exposure, although symptoms typically develop at approximately 5 to 10 days after the initiation of antibiotic therapy. Symptoms can occur as late as 10 weeks after cessation of antibiotic therapy. Commonly implicated antibiotics include clindamycin, ampicillin and other penicillins, and third-generation cephalosporins. The clinical presentation of *Clostridium difficile*-associated disease can range from diarrhea to severe colitis with pseudomembrane formation complicated by development of toxic megacolon or colonic perforation. The most common presentation is cramping abdominal pain with profuse, mucoid, greenish-colored, foul-smelling, watery stools.

Chloramphenicol (**choice A**) is potentially severely toxic, so its use is limited to infections that cannot be treated effectively with other antibiotic agents. It is the drug of choice for typhoid fever, and is effective for bacterial meningitis caused by *Haemophilus influenzae*, rickettsial diseases, and brucellosis.

Ciprofloxacin (**choice B**) is a fluoroquinolone antibiotic used for the treatment of complicated and uncomplicated urinary tract infections, soft tissue infections, and infections of the bones, joints, skin, and respiratory tract.

Clindamycin (**choice C**) is used in the treatment of infections with Bacteroides, especially *Bacteroides fragilis*, which is often the cause of anaerobic abdominal infections. It is also used for prophylaxis of dental complications after oral surgery. Topically it is used for the treatment of acne. Use of clindamycin is associated with pseudomembranous colitis, resulting in diarrhea, abdominal pain, fever, and mucus and blood in the stool.

Erythromycin (**choice D**) is useful in the treatment of patients allergic to penicillin, as long as the organism is susceptible. Its therapeutic uses include infection with group A *Streptococcus pyogenes*, *Streptococcus pneumoniae*, *Mycoplasma pneumoniae*, and topically in the treatment of acne.

50. **The correct answer is D.** All of the correlations presented in this table are indicated as statistically significant, so all may be interpreted. The key to this question is understanding how to correctly interpret the data presented. Correlation coefficients describe observed linear relationships, but do not by themselves tell us causality. A positive correlation indicates a proportional relationship

(high with high and low with low). A negative correlation indicates an inverse relationship (high with low and low with high). In this table, minutes of exercise per week has a negative correlation with each of the other three variables, meaning that lower levels of each of these variables are associated with higher rates of exercise.

Eating desserts and watching TV will produce a dangerous increase in glucose levels (**choice A**) is a causal statement. Eating desserts and watching TV are positively correlated with higher glucose levels, but we cannot leap to the conclusion that one causes the other based on the data presented here.

It is incorrect to tell the patient that general research articles are of little use in deciding clinical interventions (**choice B**). Research articles are how we assure ourselves that our recommendations to our patients are grounded on empirical data, not personal opinion. Treatment closely linked to research is called "evidenced-based medicine" and is becoming the standard for deciding among competing treatment options.

Just because something has a significant association with glucose levels (**choice C**) does not mean that control of those factors is *sufficient* to treat the diabetic patient.

This general instruction is good behavior modification (**choice E**). To control eating, avoid situations in which it is most likely to occur, such as snacking while watching TV. There is no direct evidence for this issue presented in the findings of this article, however.

Telling the patient that the article does not apply to his particular situation (**choice F**) is incorrect because the article certainly seems relevant. It examines how lifestyle factors are related to the patient's underlying condition. In fact, the article the patient presents provides the physician with an excellent opportunity to emphasize how these lifestyle factors are important in the control of diabetes.

While this may be true (**choice G**), telling the patient that watching more TV will increase glucose levels and reduce time for exercise is a casual statement and should not be inferred from this correlational data.

Neurology: Test One

1. A 71-year-old man with benign prostatic hyperplasia is brought to the emergency department because of repeated falls. His daughter explains that for the past 4 weeks, he has had an unsteady gait, memory disturbances, concentration impairment, and urinary incontinence. Serum chemistries, complete blood count, and thyroid function tests are all within normal limits. A CT scan of the head shows slightly enlarged ventricles and slightly compressed cerebral gyri. This patient is most likely suffering from

    (A) benign intracranial hypertension
    (B) normal pressure hydrocephalus
    (C) Paget disease of bone
    (D) senile dementia, Alzheimer type
    (E) vascular dementia

2. A previously healthy 40-year-old man comes to the clinic because of dizziness. The patient states that 1 week ago at 5 AM he started to get out of bed to the left and had the acute onset of "feeling the room move." He denies any tinnitus, hearing loss, double vision, dysphagia, or dysarthria. He got up and went to the couch feeling somewhat unsteady and his legs felt weak. He returned to normal within 1 hour. Similar episodes have occurred three to four times since then. He denies any alcohol or drug use, but does take vitamin B complex, ginseng, and ginkgo biloba. During your evaluation particular attention should be given to

    (A) cardiac examination
    (B) cranial nerve examination
    (C) joint position sense
    (D) mental status testing
    (E) Romberg sign

3. A 37-year-old previously healthy woman who was involved in a motor vehicle accident 6 months ago comes to your office with several "odd" symptoms. She has had poor visual acuity and significant changes in her cognitive function since the accident. Specifically, she says that she easily went through law school at the same time she worked a full-time job and then had been a successful corporate lawyer. Presently, she is still employed as a lawyer but has a lot of trouble paying attention and "multitasking." She also sometimes has trouble "finding words." Since the accident she has experienced olfactory hallucinations of "bad smells" that occur several times per week and are often clustered within 1 to 2 hours. During the accident she hit a truck head-on and there was loss of consciousness for an unclear period following the accident, though she does have some memory of getting into the ambulance. She stayed in the hospital for 3 to 4 days following the accident. A head CT scan done at the time of the accident was normal. Today, a complete physical and neurologic examination is normal. The most appropriate next step in management is to

    (A) immediately send the patient to the emergency department
    (B) obtain a neurologic consult
    (C) obtain a psychiatric consult
    (D) order a brain MRI
    (E) start the patient on phenytoin and see her back in 6 months

4. A 23-year-old woman comes into the emergency department complaining of sudden loss of vision in her right eye that occurred earlier in the evening while she was out in a restaurant with her friends. She reports a subjective fever as well as a sense that "colors seem to be a little faded." She has no past medical or surgical history. Her only medication is injections of medroxyprogesterone for contraception. She has no allergies. She denies tobacco use and only drinks socially. There is no illicit drug use. She works as a graphic designer and is very distressed about the sudden decrease in her vision. Her family history is positive only for type II diabetes in her father. Her temperature is 37.0 C (98.6 F), blood pressure is 126/78 mm Hg, pulse is 89/min, and respirations are 16/min. Her pupils are equal, round, and reactive to light and accommodation. However, when you swing your penlight from eye to eye, it appears that the right pupil constricts more slowly and dilates more rapidly than the left pupil. Conjunctiva are clear and sclera are anicteric bilaterally. Extraocular movements are intact. The fundi and optic discs appear normal bilaterally. Upon visual field testing, a central defect is noted on the right eye. The remainder of the examination, including neurologic examination, is normal. Based on these findings, this patient is most at risk for developing

(A) acute lymphocytic leukemia
(B) amyotrophic lateral sclerosis
(C) Behçet syndrome
(D) Hodgkin disease
(E) multiple sclerosis
(F) systemic lupus erythematosus

5. A 57-year-old man comes to the clinic complaining of neck stiffness that began 1 month ago after lifting weights for 2 consecutive days. He has been using acetaminophen, but it has continued to get worse. He feels "sore" in his left shoulder and explains that the pain radiates down his left neck to his upper back. Sometimes he feels tingling along the radial aspect of his left forearm. His neck is stiffest in the morning. Cold packs and hot showers help "a little." Physical examination shows severe tenderness and spasm of paracervical muscles and restricted neck range of motion. Motor and sensory examination is normal. A cervical spine MRI shows degenerative disk disease at multiple levels without foraminal or spinal canal compromise. The treatment most likely to help this patient is

(A) aggressive physical therapy and neck manipulations
(B) C5-C6 laminectomy and fusion
(C) electromyography
(D) oxycodone 10 mg 3 times per day
(E) soft cervical collar and diazepam 2 mg 3 times per day

6. A 34-year-old man comes to the clinic because of intermittent numbness and pain in his left upper arm and "shooting" back pains. The pain began after he had been shoveling snow outside his house last winter. He recently has been "having trouble seeing," which he attributes to "reading in dim lights." He occasionally has urinary accidents where he cannot make it to the bathroom in time. He denies shortness of breath, fatigue, or chest pain, but does complain of some itching and redness of the abdomen and constipation. He tells you that his previous doctor ordered an electrocardiogram and cardiac stress test that were negative. He does not smoke cigarettes and has an occasional glass of wine. He also complains that he is "weak, tired, and anxious" on the weekends when he has to run around with his 3-year-old daughter. The factor in this patient's history that is most consistent with his condition is

(A) anxiety
(B) constipation
(C) incontinence
(D) pruritus
(E) tiredness

7. A 13-year-old girl comes to the office because she has been feeling unusually tired, especially at the end of the day. Review of systems also reveals she has noticed some blurred vision and now that she thinks about it, she has found it difficult to swallow her food lately. Her physical examination reveals findings of bilateral ptosis and normal deep tendon reflexes. The strength that it takes for her to squeeze your fingers seems normal, but repeated efforts lead to noticeable weakness. Her sensorium, memory, and intelligence seem normal. The best test to perform to help arrive at the diagnosis is

   (A) botulism titer
   (B) CPK
   (C) a CT scan of the head
   (D) ELISA for Lyme disease
   (E) a Tensilon test

8. A 54-year-old woman with hyperlipidemia and polyarticular pain comes to the office because of lightheadedness and a feeling the room is spinning to the point that she needs to hold onto a piece of furniture in order to steady herself. In addition, the spinning is noted to occur when lying supine and made worse with rapid turning of the head. She denies vomiting, ear pain, or fever. She takes simvastatin and diclofenac. On physical examination the tympanic membranes appear normal. The presence of hearing loss in this patient would suggest

   (A) acute unilateral vestibulopathy
   (B) benign positional vertigo
   (C) classic migraine
   (D) Ménière disease
   (E) otitis media

9. A 40-year-old woman with atrial fibrillation is brought to the emergency department following a fall down a flight of stairs. She takes warfarin and an oral contraceptive agent. She has no known allergies to medications, and has no history of tobacco or alcohol use. Her temperature is 37.2 C (99.0 F), blood pressure is 98/67 mm Hg, pulse is 102/min, and respirations are 99/min. She is slightly confused, but has a non-focal neurologic examination. Her cardiac rhythm is regular and her breath sounds are clear bilaterally. A head CT shows a region of enhancement that is concerning for a small subdural hematoma. Routine laboratory studies show a prothrombin time of 15.5 seconds. The most appropriate immediate intervention is to administer

   (A) aprotinin
   (B) cryoprecipitate
   (C) fresh frozen plasma
   (D) low molecular weight heparin
   (E) vitamin K

10. A 74-year-old man who lives with his sister is brought to the clinic because of behavioral changes and increasing "forgetfulness" over the past year. He often forgets to lock the bathroom door or change his underwear after he takes a shower. He does some things twice because he has forgotten that he has already done them. Sometimes he accuses his nephew of stealing his money because he cannot find his wallet. He wanted to come to the doctor because he wanted to prove that he was "fine." He has no history of major medical problems in the past. Mini-Mental Status examination reveals cognitive deficits with the Folstein score of 21. Additional testing is ordered and the findings indicate the diagnosis of dementia of Alzheimer type. He is brought back to the clinic for re-evaluation and discussion. His Folstein score on this visit is 20. Further steps are discussed in a family meeting with the patient and his family. Given the present clinical picture of dementia, Alzheimer type, the most appropriate next step in management is to

   (A) admit him to the geriatric psychiatry unit
   (B) begin a trial of donepezil and keep the patient at home
   (C) reassure the family that the addition of vitamins B and E will be sufficient to control the symptoms
   (D) recommend a brain biopsy
   (E) recommend a residential facility with close supervision

11. You are in the middle of a busy emergency department shift when a man is brought in by an agitated co-worker. He was working down the hall on a plumbing problem and was splashed in the eyes about 2 minutes ago by a lye-containing solution. At the time he was not using protective eyewear. He appears to be in great pain, with both eyes tightly shut and copious tearing. After taking the brief history above, the most appropriate immediate course of action is to

(A) administer a mydriatic agent to assess the fundi
(B) begin copious irrigation with sterile water
(C) call for ophthalmologic consultation
(D) perform a rapid assessment of visual acuity
(E) perform a slit lamp examination

12. A friend of yours is a high-school basketball coach and he invites you to watch his team's playoff game. In the last minute of the first half of the game a player jumps for the rebound but collides with the elbow of another player and falls to the floor, striking the back of his head. Upon questioning the boy and his surrounding teammates, the boy claims to have been dizzy and confused for a minute or two, but apparently there was no loss of consciousness and he denies any amnesia. His head hurts, especially in the "back region" where it struck the floor. The boy's parents tell you that he has not had significant head trauma before. You inform your coach friend that the boy has had a mild concussion and that the medical guidelines would advise that:

(A) He can return to play in 30 minutes if he is asymptomatic and has a normal exam
(B) He cannot return to play during this game because he was dizzy and confused for a few minutes
(C) He should not play for the rest of the season
(D) If he vomits tonight he should be taken to the ER for further evaluation
(E) If his headache persists over the next few hours he should go to the ER

13. A 14-year-old previously healthy boy is brought to the office because of a 1-month history of headaches. The headaches usually occur when he is tying his shoes or picking up something on the floor. They are sometimes accompanied by nausea and vomiting and are most intense in the morning. They occasionally wake him up from sleep. He often experiences "tunnel vision" when they are most intense. There are no other neurologic symptoms associated with his headaches. The most likely underlying cause of his condition is

(A) intracranial hypertension
(B) intracranial hypotension
(C) psychologic tension
(D) vascular hypertension
(E) vascular hypotension

14. A 32-year-old previously healthy woman comes to the office because of a 1-month history of dizziness and "the spins." The events usually occur when she is lying down in bed. She will roll over onto her side and all of the sudden the whole room is spinning and she becomes nauseated and vomits. She denies any tinnitus, hearing loss, double vision, dysphagia, or dysarthria. She tells you that the symptoms resolve if she lies still. They happen about three times per week, but have been increasing in frequency this past week. The primary elements of the neurologic examination are normal, however during Dix-Hallpike maneuver with the right ear down she had 1 to 2 beats of rotational nystagmus without symptoms. With the left ear down, her symptoms are replicated and she has marked rotational right-beating nystagmus, which dampens after a few minutes. As she sits up she has rebound nystagmus that fatigues as well. The most correct statement about her condition is:

(A) She may benefit from vestibular rehabilitation
(B) She should be sent to the emergency department for further evaluation
(C) She should have a brain MRI
(D) She will benefit from diazepam
(E) She will benefit from meclizine

15. A 41-year-old single Caucasian man comes to the clinic asking for disability on the basis of low back pain. He has been a maintenance worker for a large office building for approximately 18 years. He tells you that he has had low back pain for "years" that he has been treating with nonsteroidal anti-inflammatory medication and he is currently unable to work due to his pain. He asks for "stronger medicine" for the pain that he describes vaguely as "achy and sharp." Physical examination reveals subtle decreases in range of motion of the back and hips and no focal neurologic findings. An MRI is pending. The most predictive determinant of whether the patient will return to work is

    (A) job satisfaction
    (B) marital status
    (C) presence of disc herniation on MRI
    (D) preserved passive range of motion
    (E) use of narcotic analgesics to treat pain

16. An 81-year-old woman with gastroesophageal reflux disease and mild dementia is brought to the emergency department for new onset left-sided weakness. She has a long history of coronary artery disease and hypertension and has been hospitalized two times prior for a myocardial infarction and a transient ischemic episode. She is given intravenous fluids and treatment with aspirin after a head CT. She is transferred to the floor to finish the "stroke workup" and receive heparinization. On the floor, she is felt to be "sundowning" and given chloral hydrate for sleep, with good results. Two days later, she shows no evidence of progression of the stroke and her lower limb strength is slightly improved. Laboratory studies, electrocardiogram, and carotid Doppler ultrasounds are all within normal limits. An echocardiogram shows some long-standing ventricular dilatation with a mural thrombus. She is started on warfarin for long-term anticoagulation. The patient is at greatest risk for

    (A) agitation and combativeness from the interaction of chloral hydrate and warfarin
    (B) sedation from the interaction of chloral hydrate and warfarin
    (C) hypercoagulation from the interaction of chloral hydrate and warfarin
    (D) hypocoagulation from the interaction of chloral hydrate and warfarin
    (E) decreased gastrointestinal motility from the interaction of chloral hydrate and warfarin
    (F) nausea, vomiting, and diarrhea from the interaction of chloral hydrate and warfarin

17. A 35-year-old pregnant woman requests an amniocentesis. She is healthy and her pregnancy so far has been unremarkable. She is asked about family history of disease. Her father had Duchenne muscular dystrophy and died when he was 25 years old. She has one brother and two sisters who are all healthy. She is very concerned that her child will have Duchenne muscular dystrophy. You should tell her that if her infant turns out to be a boy, the chance that he will have the Duchenne muscular dystrophy is

    (A) 25%
    (B) 50%
    (C) 75%
    (D) 100%
    (E) a random chance of a new mutation

18. A 67-year-old man comes to see you in clinic to "get to the bottom of his problem." Two months ago he was lifting something and "threw out his back." He initially developed some back pain, and then bilateral leg weakness and difficulties with balance. Ibuprofen did not help. At about the same time he had difficulty holding his head up, so that he now has to hold his head manually with his hands or else it rests on his chest. He has to "throw" his head back to see because he has bilateral eyelid drooping. He needs a walker because of worsening leg weakness. In addition to all of this, he has difficulty swallowing and has been short of breath after exertion. He went to the hospital a month ago and had MRIs of his brain, cervical spine, and lumbar spine, all of which had no abnormalities that were inconclusive. He was discharged without being given a clear diagnosis. Today he presents with worsening of all of these symptoms. Physical examination shows severe neck extensor weakness, severe bilateral ptosis, dysarthria, proximal extremity weakness with preserved reflexes, downgoing toes, and intact sensation. The diagnosis will most likely be established with

    (A) a CT scan of his head
    (B) an electroencephalogram
    (C) an electromyogram and nerve conduction study
    (D) a lumbar puncture
    (E) an MRI of his thoracic spine

19. A 34-year-old woman with progressive multiple sclerosis is being admitted to the hospital for pulse methylprednisolone therapy. She was diagnosed with multiple sclerosis 10 years ago after presenting with bilateral decreased visual acuity and an MRI was abnormal at that time. She has been hospitalized approximately 10 times since presentation, with her flare-ups consisting of increasing bilateral lower extremity weakness and decreased sensation manifest as a "heavy" feeling, waxing and waning generalized fatigue, and bilateral hand "tingling." She has also had bilateral optic neuritis and one transient episode of aphasia in the past. For the past 2 years she has been on cyclophosphamide and methylprednisolone, originally every 4 weeks and now every 6 weeks, with the last treatment 1 month ago. She has tried and failed interferon beta therapy. For the 2 months prior to admission, she has had worsening bilateral lower extremity weakness/"heaviness," increased fatigue, and mild low back "numbness," as well as intermittent and alternating decreased hearing in both ears while at work. She has also noticed mild unsteadiness walking. Included among her admission orders should be

(A) a heart-healthy diet
(B) an insulin sliding scale
(C) neurologic checks every hour for the first 48 hours
(D) placement of a central venous line
(E) a stat head CT for change in mental status

Items 20-21

A 79-year-old woman is brought to the office because of increasing forgetfulness and personality changes over the past few months. She lived alone up until 6 months ago when she moved in with her daughter because she could no longer bathe and dress herself. The family is concerned because she has become suspicious and aggressive. The son says that her thinking is "off" and that she often gives the "strangest" responses to questions. For example, when they ask her if she wants "to go to dinner," she says that she can't "go to dinner because dinner is not a place." She frequently wanders around the house, disoriented to time and place. She does not remember the names of her grandchildren and she has difficulty "finding her words." He says that she always appears "a bit unsteady," but nobody has ever seen her fall. She asks you your name five different times during the history. She takes no medications, has had no major illnesses over the years, and never drank alcohol or smoked cigarettes. Physical examination shows two well-healed scars on her forehead. Laboratory studies show:

Sodium	139 mEq/L	Hemoglobin	13.5 g/dL
Potassium	4.4 mEq/L	Hematocrit	43%
Chloride	103 mEq/L	Platelets	360,000/mm^3
Bicarbonate	25 mEq/L	Leukocyte count	6000/mm^3
Creatinine	0.9 mg/dL		
Glucose	95 mg/dL		
Calcium	9.2 mg/dL		
Thyroid-stimulating hormone	4.3 μU/mL		

20. The most appropriate next step is to

(A) admit her to the hospital and prepare her for immediate neurosurgery
(B) perform a lumbar puncture
(C) prescribe a trial of phenelzine
(D) schedule her for a cerebral angiogram
(E) schedule her for an MRI of the head

21. The appropriate steps are taken and either no abnormalities are found or she did not respond to the treatment. The most likely diagnosis is

(A) Alzheimer disease
(B) chronic subdural hematoma
(C) depression
(D) multi-infarct dementia
(E) schizoaffective disorder

22. An 82-year-old woman with Alzheimer disease, hypertension, and "a cardiac arrhythmia" is admitted to the hospital from a nursing home because of an altered mental status. She takes digoxin, calcium channel blocker, and warfarin. Her warfarin levels are monitored regularly at the nursing home by way of checking INR. The nursing aide who accompanied her reports that her mental status has been waxing and waning for the past 1 month and she has sustained falls because of her unsteady gait. She has been admitted to the hospital twice before, after falling, but further investigation was inconclusive. Now she has an altered mental status, waxing and waning in nature, without any focal neurologic deficit. Physical examination is normal and there is no evidence of any external trauma. The most likely finding on the CT scan of the head is

(A) a cerebral contusion
(B) a cerebral tumor
(C) chronic subdural hematomas
(D) skull fracture
(E) subarachnoid hemorrhage

23. A 54-year-old woman is brought to the emergency department because of the sudden onset of recent memory loss. She was last seen by her husband around 4 PM yesterday in her usual state of health before taking off for a business meeting on her own by car. When she returned around 7 PM, she could not remember her trip back home. She did know whom she had met but not the specifics of the meeting. She had profound loss of recent memory and could not recall what had happened on the last few previous days. There does not appear to be any history of trauma or illicit drugs. On further questioning, she notes that she remembers patches of events over the last couple of weeks. Her remote memory is intact. She recalls in detail stories from her childhood and English lit class in college. During your examination she repeatedly asks the same questions over and over again. Memory testing reveals immediate retention of 3/3 words, but 0/3 recall at 1 minute. She is admitted to the hospital and when you go to examine her 17 hours later, her symptoms have completely resolved. The treatment most likely to prevent this from happening again is

(A) electroconvulsive therapy
(B) gabapentin
(C) sumatriptan
(D) there is no treatment likely to prevent this
(E) tissue plasminogen activator

24. A 40-year-old HIV-positive man comes to the office with a 3-week history of nausea, vomiting, and difficulty walking. Besides being very stressed about his business, he was in his usual state of health until 3 weeks ago when he had onset of the above symptoms. He specifies that he thinks his difficulty walking is due to being tired. His partner died a year ago from AIDS. On examination, he is afebrile, pleasant, interactive, and in no apparent distress. Cranial nerve examination is normal. He has normal tone and bulk, and no tremors or fasciculations. Strength is full in all major muscles of the upper and lower extremities bilaterally. Normal light touch, cold touch, vibration, and proprioception is present in all extremities. Reflexes are 2+ and symmetric at triceps and 1+ at biceps and brachioradialis bilaterally in upper extremities 1+ at patellar bilaterally. Toes are downgoing bilaterally. He has normal rapid alternating movement, finger-nose-finger and heel-to-shin bilaterally. His gait is wildly ataxic, he tends to grab onto furniture and walls, but does not fall when these are not available. Romberg sign is not present. A brain MRI is normal. The underlying problem causing this patient's gait disorder is most likely to be

(A) autoimmune
(B) infectious
(C) multifactorial
(D) psychogenic
(E) vascular

25. A 24-year-old woman with insulin-dependent diabetes mellitus is admitted to the hospital for intravenous management of a Crohn disease flare-up. You are called to see her because she is complaining of pain in her left eye for the last 5 days and left eyelid swelling for 3 days. She also notes that the eyelid appears reddened as well. There is mild irritation and tearing of the eye, especially today. You note in her chart that her blood glucose levels have been well controlled recently. On physical examination, there is a 4 × 4-mm nodule on the lower margin of the left upper eyelid. It is erythematous, firm, and very tender to palpation. Slight conjunctival injection is present on the left. The right eye is normal. The most appropriate management is

(A) application of a warm compress
(B) immediate consultation with an ophthalmologist
(C) incision and drainage of the nodule
(D) ophthalmic steroid solution
(E) oral erythromycin

26. A 55-year-old right-handed man with no known medical history comes to the clinic after being involved in three motor-vehicle accidents today. However, he seems to be unconcerned about his problem today. The first accident (12:30) was caused by not being able to see out of his left eye. A car hit him on the left. The patient got back into his car after the first accident and then got into another accident when he ran into a mirror from a truck on the left side of his car. He was then told by a police officer not to drive, but continued to drive nevertheless. He got into a third accident when he did not see a car on his left side. He claims that he did not remember what he was doing while he was driving but now remembers it. He also had some transient left arm numbness and a right-sided headache between the second and third accidents. All accidents occurred at a low speed. His blood pressure is 170/90 mm Hg. He is alert and oriented to person, place, and time. He has full visual fields with left-sided visual extinction during double simultaneous stimulation and normal visual acuity. The examination is otherwise normal. You should tell this patient that he

(A) can go home, but cannot drive for 6 months
(B) can go home if he does not drive for the rest of today
(C) needs to be admitted to the hospital for evaluation and testing
(D) needs to be seen emergently by an ophthalmologist
(E) will need to be evaluated urgently by a psychiatrist

27. A 68-year-old man with diabetes mellitus and poorly controlled hypertension comes to the emergency department because of right-sided weakness for approximately 7 hours. The weakness began acutely that morning and has remained unchanged since he first noticed it. He denies any sensory complaints, visual field deficits, or language difficulties. He has had clumsiness in his right hand and mild dragging of his right leg. The weakness is proportional in the face, arm, and leg. He has never had any similar previous episodes. His blood pressure is 190/105 mm Hg. He is awake and alert and his speech is fluent. Visual fields are full to confrontation. He has some mild drooping of his right lower face, but otherwise cranial nerve examination is normal. There is some drift in his right upper extremity and slow finger movements. He is able to lift his right leg against gravity and some resistance. Sensory examination is normal to all modalities bilaterally. He has some circumduction of his right leg on ambulation. Other than blood glucose of 210 mg/dL, his chemistries, coagulation studies, and complete blood count are normal. The most appropriate initial step in management is to

(A) check a urine drug screen
(B) give an enteric coated aspirin
(C) give intravenous tPA for acute ischemic stroke
(D) obtain an MRI/A of the brain
(E) obtain a non-contrast head CT scan

28. A 37-year-old man comes to the emergency department with a 1-day history of headaches, fevers, and neck pain. His family reports that he has been "more sleepy" today and while you are talking to them, the patient has a witnessed seizure. His temperature is 40.1 C (104.2 F). He is lethargic, but otherwise the rest of the examination is non-focal. His leukocyte count is 27,000/mm^3 with 23% bands and a leftward shift. Chemistries are normal. The most appropriate initial step in management is to

(A) begin antibiotic therapy
(B) begin carbamazepine therapy
(C) obtain a non-contrast CT of the head
(D) order an electroencephalogram
(E) perform a lumbar puncture

29. A 66-year-old man with diabetes is brought to the emergency department because of a "change in mental status" over the past 3 days. His wife explains that he has "just not been himself." He is normally a "jovial man" who derives an enormous amount of joy from being a grandfather of three. However, over the past 3 days he has been apathetic to his grandchildren, with mostly sad or flat affect. He has stated that he "doesn't feel like doing anything because he's tired and sad." He has no known past psychiatric or neurologic history. On physical examination, there is no aphasia, gross motor or sensory deficits, or cranial nerve signs. An MRI will most likely reveal a lesion in the

(A) left frontal lobe
(B) left parietal lobe
(C) right parietal lobe
(D) right pons
(E) vermis of the cerebellum

30. A 55-year-old man comes to the emergency department with a severe headache. You examine the patient and find nothing unusual, and his wife insists that he had been healthy until now. Nevertheless, you decide to consult with a neurologist. The neurologist listens to you over the phone, and advises you that the patient can be discharged, with analgesics and an appointment to return in a week. He also talks to the patient. The patient departs, but 24 hours later, clutches his head and collapses and dies while in the bathroom, according to the wife, who witnessed the event. The family decides to sue not only the hospital and you, but also the neurologist who was consulted. In this event, the neurologist would

(A) be held liable by the courts
(B) be let off with a warning
(C) be suspended from the neurology service
(D) have his license revoked
(E) not be held liable by the courts

31. You are taking care of an 82-year-old man after coronary artery bypass surgery. Following surgery yesterday he was transferred to the intensive care unit with an episode of hypotension that improved with pressors and fluids. Today sedation was tapered and he is not moving his left side. His blood pressure is 122/55 mm Hg, central venous pressure is 12 mm Hg, and oxygen saturation is 96%. He is intubated with little spontaneous movement and a right gaze deviation. He is arousable by voice, opens his eyes for approximately 15 seconds, and follows simple commands such as showing two fingers, thumb, raising hand, and moving toes. He can raise his right arm and bend his right leg against gravity. He has no left arm/leg movement and his left lower extremity is externally rotated. He grimaces to pinch in all extremities and withdrew right arm/leg. There is triple flexion on the left foot. The pathophysiology of this patient's neurological deficits is most likely

(A) autoimmune
(B) mechanical
(C) neoplastic
(D) toxic
(E) vascular

32. A 55-year-old woman with labile hypertension comes to the clinic because of a transient visual disturbance. She tells you that she recently got a new pair of glasses and that the lower half is slightly thicker, and she has not become accustomed to using them yet. However, two nights ago, as she was driving home, she noticed that she was not seeing the left half of her visual field. For example, when she drove by a sign saying "Wellesley" she was not able to see the letters "W-e-l." She also noticed that she could not see the left headlight of the car in front of her. This persisted for approximately 20 minutes. By the time she arrived home, her vision was back to normal. She felt a bit nauseous when she arrived home, but did not vomit. The following day she spoke to her ophthalmologist, who mentioned optic migraine as the possible etiology of her symptoms the night before; however, an eye examination was not performed. Yesterday she mentioned her symptoms to her employer at work, who recommended she contact her primary care doctor for further evaluation. She tells you that she takes aspirin 81 mg per day and labetalol. Examination now is completely normal. The most appropriate next step in management is

(A) a dilated fundus examination
(B) brain magnetic resonance spectroscopy
(C) an echocardiogram and carotid ultrasound
(D) an electroencephalogram
(E) visual evoked potentials

33. A 12-year-old boy is brought to the clinic because of "eye fluttering" episodes that last several seconds. Also, there are times that he will lose track of his thoughts in the middle of a sentence. There are no other associated symptoms, and the "eye fluttering" may occur up to 20 or more times per day. His development and health have been normal up until this point. The parents recall that their son had two head injuries as a young child. The first was when he fell off a low-to-the-ground tricycle and the second was when he fell off of a play set onto his head. Both episodes resulted in a brief loss of consciousness and he was not thinking clearly for part of the day afterwards, but had no medical intervention. The test most likely to confirm this patient's diagnosis is

(A) a brain CT scan
(B) a brain MRI
(C) an electroencephalogram
(D) a lumbar puncture
(E) a nerve conduction study

34. A 27-year-old African American woman comes to the clinic because of progressive weakness and difficulty walking. She also notes that her fingers have been feeing "numb and tingly" in the last 2 days. She tells you that she is generally very healthy except for a "bout of gastroenteritis" 2 weeks ago that lasted for 4 days. Her temperature is 37.0 C (98.6 F), blood pressure is 130/80 mm Hg, pulse is 70/min, and respirations are 14/min. On physical examination, there is weakness of her lower extremities with absent ankle jerk reflex and 1+ patellar tendon reflexes. The remainder of the examination is unremarkable. The most likely diagnosis is

    (A) Guillain Barré syndrome
    (B) myasthenia gravis
    (C) poliomyelitis
    (D) reflex sympathetic dystrophy
    (E) transverse myelitis

35. You are seeing a 43-year-old obese woman for headaches. She reports that she has had holoacranial headaches for several months, which are present throughout most of the day but often worse in the morning and when she strains. She also notes a "whooshing" sound in her ears, and reports seeing black spots in her vision when she bends over or strains. She denies any nausea or photophobia, but has had some blurry vision. On physical examination there is most likely to be

    (A) bilateral optic disc edema
    (B) generalized weakness
    (C) hyperactive reflexes
    (D) hypoactive reflexes
    (E) normal findings

36. A 57-year-old man comes to the clinic because of a worsening tremor in both of his arms that began several years ago. It is worse when he is doing certain tasks, such as writing or drinking a cup of coffee. He does not drink alcohol often, but he notices that the tremor "somewhat subsides" when he does have a drink. His father had a history of a similar tremor. On physical examination there is an action and postural tremor noted, as well as a mild head tremor. Otherwise, the examination is normal. The most likely diagnosis is

    (A) alcohol withdrawal tremor
    (B) essential tremor
    (C) multiple sclerosis
    (D) Parkinson disease
    (E) physiologic tremor

37. A 77-year-old woman is brought to the emergency department by her family because of a change in her mental status. They report a 3-day history of gradually increasing confusion, tiredness, and combative behavior. The patient sometimes has more lucid periods, but overall her symptoms have been getting worse. On physical examination, the patient is somewhat somnolent but arousable and is oriented to name only. Otherwise, there are no focal findings. Her urine is noted to be foul-smelling. The most likely diagnosis is

    (A) acute stroke
    (B) delirium
    (C) dementia
    (D) partial seizure
    (E) psychotic episode

38. A 74-year-old woman with a history of senile dementia, Alzheimer type, is brought to the office by her family for a regular appointment. The patient's dementia is moderate, and her last Mini-Mental status exam score was 16/30. The patient has begun to evidence delusions of persecution. Specifically, she makes accusations against home health aides of stealing money and belongings from her. She is not physically assaultive, but has made loud verbal threats directed against her home care attendants. She becomes especially confused and more prone to agitation when she is in unfamiliar surroundings, when changes of shift occur for her home health aides, or when family members whom she still recognizes leave after a visit. She has no physical complaints and her physical examination is unremarkable. The only medication that the patient takes is donepezil. The most appropriate recommendation to the family that can aid in minimizing the patient's agitation is

(A) keeping the patient in bed most of the time
(B) prescribing scheduled sedating medication for the patient to keep her awake but drowsy
(C) reprimanding the patient anytime she makes an accusation of stealing against a home health aide
(D) stopping the patient's home health services and observing her level of adaptation
(E) suggesting that the patient's family not rearrange the patient's apartment

39. A 22-year-old woman is brought to the emergency department after being found by a friend unresponsive at a park. She has no known medical history or medication history. While she is in an examination room, she begins to seize. Her temperature is 37.2 C (99.1 F), blood pressure is 108/78 mmHg, pulse is 98/min, and respirations are 30/min. A quick examination reveals that her cardiac rhythm is regular, and that her lung fields are clear to auscultation bilaterally. You rapidly secure her airway and insert a bite block. An assistant places a peripheral intravenous access line. The next appropriate intervention is

(A) administration of acetaminophen, orally
(B) administration of flumazenil, intravenously
(C) administration of glucose, intravenously
(D) administration of metoprolol, intravenously
(E) administration of naloxone, intravenously

40. A 7-year-old boy is brought to the office because of "brown spots" on his trunk. The patient's mother just saw a television special on skin cancer and thinks her son's brown spots may be melanoma because of their large diameter. Family history is unknown since the patient's mother is adopted and the patient's father is not involved in his care. The mother thinks the spots have been there since birth but have increased in size. On exam, the boy has nine uniformly pigmented light brown macules and patches ranging from 0.5 to 5 cm in diameter on his trunk. In addition, there are multiple light brown small macules in bilateral axillae. On his left upper arm, there are two small, pendulous, flabby masses that can be pushed down into the panniculus and spring back when released. You should tell the mother that:

(A) Her son most likely has McCune-Albright syndrome
(B) Her son most likely has neurofibromatosis type I
(C) Her son most likely has neurofibromatosis type II
(D) Her son most likely has Watson syndrome
(E) The large size of these brown macules and patches is suspicious for atypical nevi and a biopsy is indicated of the largest lesion

41. A 19-year-old college student comes to the clinic because of "sleeping attacks" that began in early adolescence. He explains that he suddenly falls asleep and often has "odd" hallucinations of "people walking around" him when he is about to wake up from sleep. He also has had periods of sudden loss of muscular tone when he is having an emotional discussion with his parents or an argument with his girlfriend. Appropriate therapy for this patient is

(A) calcium supplementation
(B) continuous positive airway pressure while asleep
(C) haloperidol for hallucinations
(D) methylphenidate
(E) valproic acid

42. A 77-year-old woman has had gradual memory loss and her family is concerned that she has Alzheimer dementia. She also seems very confused, often wandering "aimlessly" around the house and neighborhood. She is moody, gets angry easily, and starts laughing or crying for no reason. The family does not know of any serious medical problems in the past because she recently came to live with them after her husband died in a car accident. After a complete physical and neurologic examination, the first diagnostic step in the dementia work up of this patient is to

(A) draw blood for HIV testing
(B) obtain a CT scan of the brain
(C) order B_{12}, calcium, and TSH levels
(D) order neuropsychologic testing
(E) perform a lumbar puncture

43. A mother brings her previously healthy 6-year-old boy to the emergency department because of a 4-week history of headaches. The headaches wake him up in the middle of the night from sleep and the pain is primarily over his forehead. She says that he has also come down with some kind of "stomach bug" because he has been vomiting every morning when he wakes up for the past week. He does not have fever or diarrhea. There is a family history of migraine headaches. His vital signs are stable. Physical examination shows blurring of the optic discs. His examination is otherwise normal. The most appropriate next step in management is to

(A) admit him to the hospital for observation
(B) admit him to the hospital and obtain imaging of the brain
(C) discharge him home and ask the mother to keep a headache diary
(D) discharge him home with a prescription for acetaminophen
(E) reassure the mother that these are migraine headaches

44. A 15-year-old comes to the office complaining of a "bad headache" for the past year. The onset of the headache was preceded by an inability to clearly visualize an area of his right outer visual field and eventually his left eye, too. It was associated with some difficulty speaking and walking, and his hands and mouth felt "weird." The pain is on both sides of his head and it is not the worst headache in his life. He is on the wrestling team at school and has had two concussions over the past 2 years. He has never had to lose weight in order to meet his weight class on the wrestling team and denies any recreational drug use. When assessing the presence of raised intracranial pressure, the most specific question to ask would be which of the following:

(A) "Are your headaches similar from attack to attack?"
(B) "Do you get headaches when you wake up in the morning?"
(C) "Do you have any neck pain?"
(D) "Do you have any problems with bright light with these headaches?"
(E) "Have you ever been told that you have an unpredictable personality?"
(F) "Have you ever had any seizures or loss of consciousness?"

45. A 12-year-old girl is brought to the emergency department 2 hours after a sudden loss of consciousness that occurred while watching television. This episode was witnessed by her father, who tells you that she regained consciousness after 1 minute. She was drowsy for 30 minutes afterwards but she is now back to her normal self. Her temperature is 37.0 C (98.6 F), blood pressure is 115/70 mm Hg, pulse is 72/min, and respirations are 16/min. Her tongue has bite marks and dried blood. Physical examination is unremarkable. Funduscopic examination of the right eye is normal. The left eye demonstrates blunting of the optic disc, disc swelling, and edema as you focus in and out of the eye. The rest of the retinal field is normal. The funduscopic findings in the left eye are highly suspicious of

(A) a cerebral tumor
(B) child abuse
(C) a migraine
(D) a subarachnoid hemorrhage
(E) viral meningitis

46. A 19-year-old man has probable migraine headaches that you decide to treat with a combination of butalbital, acetaminophen, and caffeine and a trial of sumatriptan nasal spray 20 mg once daily. You ask him to return in 1 week for follow-up. Before leaving the office he says, "Before I shove anything up my nose I want to know how this thing can help me." You explain that sumatriptan's method of action in the treatment of migraine headaches is most likely by

    (A) antagonizing certain peripheral actions of serotonin
    (B) causing vasoconstriction by acting as an agonist to dopamine receptors in the central nervous system
    (C) initiating platelet aggregation in the central nervous system
    (D) inhibiting the reuptake of serotonin
    (E) selectively activating a particular subpopulation of serotonin receptors, thereby rectifying serotonin depletion

47. A 68-year-old tax attorney is brought to the clinic by his daughter. He suffered head trauma during an armed robbery at his home 6 months ago and has never been the same since. His daughter tells you that recently he has been "slowing down and having a lot of urinary accidents." The patient is expressionless and his speech is monotonous. You notice that he has difficulty starting to walk and that he shuffles his feet, and does not swing his arms. He has lead-pipe rigidity at the elbow, cogwheel rigidity at the wrist, and a positive glabellar tap. There is a mild tremor of the eyelids when the eyes are gently closed. A CT scan of the head shows:

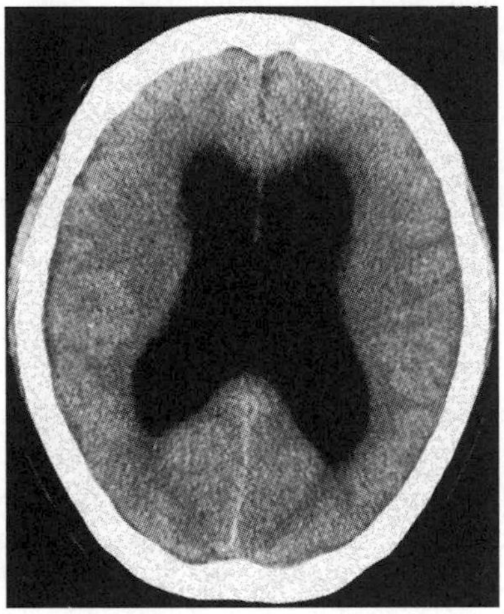

The most appropriate next step in management is to

    (A) prescribe benztropine
    (B) prescribe bromocriptine
    (C) prescribe donepezil
    (D) prescribe fluoxetine
    (E) refer him to a neurosurgeon for possible ventriculosystemic shunting

Items 48-49

A 77-year-old man who was recently diagnosed with Alzheimer disease is brought to the clinic by his wife and daughter for followup examination. The patient takes lisinopril, cimetidine, a nitroglycerin patch, simvastatin, and aspirin. He and his wife live alone in a two-story house. His wife supervises his dressing, bathing, and toileting and provides constant reassurance for her husband. She tells you that he often asks her the same questions several times a day, which is very frustrating. The patient's Mini-Mental Status examination score has declined from 18/30 to 16/30 over the past year.

48. The most effective intervention to promote continued caring for this patient in his home is to

    (A) prescribe a benzodiazepine agent
    (B) prescribe a neuroleptic
    (C) prescribe diphenhydramine
    (D) prescribe donepezil
    (E) recommend the use of respite services

49. The following year this same patient is admitted to a nursing home because his wife and daughter are having difficulty caring for him at home, due to increased confusion, incontinence, and combativeness. For the last week he has been having visual hallucinations. On admission to the nursing home he remains combative, striking staff and other residents. He is inattentive and distractible, and resists attempts at physical examination. His vital signs are stable and a physical examination and laboratory workup fail to reveal any acute infections or other significant changes. The medication that is likely to be contributing to his altered mental state is

    (A) aspirin
    (B) cimetidine
    (C) lisinopril
    (D) a nitroglycerin patch
    (E) simvastatin

50. A 65-year-old man with the recent diagnosis of mild dementia, Alzheimer type, has been followed by you for several years. The laboratory evaluation together with a several-year history of symptoms is consistent with this diagnosis. Although this patient can no longer work as a physicist, he is still able to visit family and friends, play tennis and golf, enjoy church, and travel with his wife. He has lost the ability to keep track of the family finances, and his wife has taken over that responsibility. Two months ago, after obtaining a baseline Mini-Mental Status examination score, you start him on donepezil 5 mg oral once daily, which you subsequently increase to 10 mg daily without side effects. You also prescribe vitamin E 400 IU twice daily. The family notes some improvement and they are encouraging the patient to stop taking the donepezil as they do not believe in long-term medication usage. At this time the most correct statement about his condition and management is:

    (A) Increasing the dosage of donepezil to 20 mg daily may lead to more noticeable improvement and would be appropriate
    (B) Plasma levels of donepezil may be above therapeutic range; decreasing the dosage to 5 mg daily is appropriate
    (C) These medications are not expected to lead to major improvement but may enhance cognitive functioning; continuing current treatment is appropriate
    (D) These medications do not always work; tapering and then stopping them is appropriate
    (E) Vitamin E may be adversely influencing the efficacy of the donepezil; discontinuing the vitamin E while maintaining the donepezil would be appropriate

Neurology Test One: **Answers and Explanations**

ANSWER KEY

1. B
2. B
3. B
4. E
5. E
6. C
7. E
8. D
9. C
10. B
11. B
12. A
13. A
14. A
15. A
16. D
17. B
18. C
19. B
20. E
21. A
22. C
23. D
24. D
25. A
26. C
27. E
28. A
29. A
30. A
31. E
32. C
33. C
34. A
35. A
36. B
37. B
38. E
39. C
40. B
41. D
42. C
43. B
44. B
45. A
46. E
47. E
48. E
49. B

50 C

1. **The correct answer is B.** The patient presents with the classic clinical triad of gait disturbance, dementia, and urinary incontinence that characterizes normal pressure hydrocephalus. The patient's CT scan results demonstrating enlargement of the cerebral ventricles and compressed gyri are the result of expansion of cerebrospinal fluid.

   Benign intracranial hypertension (**choice A**), or pseudotumor cerebri, typically presents in obese or pregnant women. The classic clinical signs of this disorder include headache and visual loss.

   Paget disease of bone (**choice C**) does not typically present with dementia or neurologic signs. Additionally, a CT scan of the patient's head would be able to detect cranial lesions of Paget disease of bone.

   The patient's rapidly progressive course and CT scan not demonstrating cerebral atrophy do not suggest a diagnosis of senile dementia, Alzheimer type (**choice D**).

   Vascular dementia (**choice E**) is manifested by a dementing illness with a "step-wise" rather than a progressive course accompanied by focal neurologic signs. The rapidly progressive course of this patient's illness and the patient's CT scan done distantly from the onset of symptoms not showing vascular lesions make this diagnosis unlikely.

2. **The correct answer is B.** This patient gives a history of vertigo. The most likely etiology is benign positional paroxysmal vertigo. This is because he has no vascular risk factors, no other symptoms, and the events are positional. Although this is most likely, a good cranial nerve examination is essential to make sure that there is no brainstem involvement.

   "Dizziness" due to cardiac etiologies (**choice A**) most commonly is not vertiginous. That is, there is not an abnormal sensation of movement. Additionally, he has no cardiovascular risk factors.

   Mental status testing (**choice D**) is unlikely to be critical in making the diagnosis in this case. Vertigo may be caused by a problem in the cervical spinal cord, brainstem, cerebellum, or peripheral vestibular structures. Except in very severe cases, the mental status exam primarily gives information about supratentorial function.

   Joint position sense (**choice C**) and Romberg sign (**choice E**) are tests of dorsal column function. Dorsal column dysfunction results in gait unsteadiness, but not true vertigo.

3. **The correct answer is B.** This patient gives a typical history for a post-concussive syndrome. Additionally, she has olfactory hallucinations, which are a classic presentation of temporal lobe epilepsy. Temporal lobe epilepsy is very common following traumatic brain injury. The neurological examination, including mental status exam, is often normal in these cases. These are complicated issues, which should be managed by a neurologist.

   There is no acute issue which would warrant sending this patient to the emergency department (**choice A**).

   There is no history suggestive of mental illness. Isolated olfactory hallucinations would be a very unusual presentation of psychiatric disease, so a psychiatric consult is not necessary (**choice C**).

   There is no reason to think that she has had additional brain injury since the CT was done after the accident. It is true that a brain MRI (**choice D**) might detect some subtle brain changes not seen on the CT. However, this is unlikely to influence your treatment and should wait until a proper neurologic evaluation has been done.

   Olfactory hallucinations following a brain injury are highly suggestive of temporal lobe epilepsy. However, further evaluation should be done before starting phenytoin (**choice E**). Additionally, she will need to be closely followed and phenytoin is often a poor first-choice anti-seizure medication for a young woman.

4. **The correct answer is E.** This patient is presenting with retrobulbar optic neuritis. The main feature is that of sudden loss of vision, typically with a central scotoma as described in this case. Other symptoms may include pain that increases with extremes of gaze motion and decreased perception of color brightness. On examination, an afferent papillary defect may be noted. Optic neuritis may occur within the globe (papillitis) or posterior to the globe of the eye (retrobulbar optic neuritis.) In papillitis, edema and hyperemia cause the optic disk to look abnormal. In retrobulbar optic neuritis, the fundus appears normal. Treatment of retrobulbar optic neuritis may include high-dose steroids, however this only serves to hasten return of vision and does not affect the final visual acuity. In 20 to 40% of all cases of optic neuritis, patients will go on to develop multiple sclerosis. In these cases (those that are related to MS), the patient usually experiences improvement in vision within 4 weeks, although decreased color intensity and a pale optic disk will always remain in the affected eye.

   Acute lymphocytic leukemia (**choice A**), amyotrophic lateral sclerosis (**choice B**), Behçet syndrome (**choice C**), and Hodgkin disease (**choice D**) are incorrect because there is no additional risk for developing these conditions in a patient with optic neuritis.

Systemic lupus erythematosus (SLE) (**choice F**) is incorrect because this patient is at a much higher risk of developing multiple sclerosis than SLE. However, it should be noted that papillitis is sometimes caused by autoimmune disorders, including SLE.

5. **The correct answer is E.** This patient has cervical muscle spasm secondary to a recent injury superimposed on chronic arthritic changes. A soft cervical collar and muscle relaxant such as low-dose diazepam is an excellent way to manage this case. Aggressive physical therapy and neck manipulations (**choice A**) are likely to just make things worse, although very gentle massage and heat may provide some relief.

   A C5-C6 laminectomy and fusion (**choice B**) might be indicated if there was a disk herniation at that level seen on MRI and there were clinical sensory or motor findings which correlated.

   Electromyography (**choice C**) is a diagnostic test for nerve and muscle diseases. It has no therapeutic uses.

   Use of a narcotic such as oxycodone (**choice D**) may provide some pain relief, but will not work as well as a soft cervical collar and diazepam.

6. **The correct answer is C.** This patient most likely has multiple sclerosis, which is often associated with bladder incontinence. Other symptoms that would back up a diagnosis of multiple sclerosis are sensory loss, paresthesia, and diplopia. To make a diagnosis of multiple sclerosis based on history you need two separate episodes of the symptoms involving two different areas of the central nervous system.

   Pruritus (**choice D**), constipation (**choice B**), anxiety (**choice A**), and tiredness (**choice E**) are not specific to the classic symptoms of multiple sclerosis.

7. **The correct answer is E.** This patient has the findings consistent with myasthenia gravis. Myasthenia gravis may typically occur during early adolescence. It classically presents with bilateral ptosis, facial weakness, and hypotonia. Other complaints may include dysphagia, dysarthria, and problem chewing foods. After a test dose of Tensilon or edrophonium there is usually improvement in the eye muscles or increased strength in the extremities. Edrophonium is an anticholinesterase drug that acts by inhibiting the breakdown of Ach and increases the concentration of Ach at the neuromuscular junction.

   Botulism can give weakness and ptosis, but typically has other signs on physical examination such as pupillary changes (dilated pupils that react slowly) and decreased deep tendon reflexes. Infant botulism may present with symptoms of poor feeding, drooling, and even obstructive apnea (**choice A**).

   CPK would be abnormal in muscle diseases such as myositis and muscular dystrophy, not myasthenia gravis (**choice B**).

   The best next test would not be a CT scan of the head (**choice C**) to rule out a brain tumor. Brain tumors in children typically present with symptoms of increased intracranial pressure including headache, vomiting, lethargy, and papilledema. They might present with oculomotor palsy, but not with all of the findings in this vignette.

   Lyme disease may be associated with neurologic symptoms, notably Bell palsy, but not the pattern described above (**choice D**).

8. **The correct answer is D.** The presence of hearing loss in this situation should alert you to Ménière disease, which is also characterized by tinnitus or a roaring sound. Some patients experience a pressure sensation in the ear. Episodes occur at regular intervals for years, with periods of remission. The cause is an increase in the volume of endolymph.

   Acute unilateral vestibulopathy (**choice A**) typically presents as acute onset of vertigo, nausea, and vomiting lasting for several days and preceded by an upper respiratory tract infection.

   Benign positional vertigo (**choice B**) is the most common cause of vertigo but is not typically associated with hearing loss. Patients have brief episodes of vertigo with positional changes, typically when turning over in bed.

   A classic migraine (**choice C**) usually presents as visual or olfactory aura followed by severe headaches and photophobia. Vertigo is not a typical finding.

   Otitis media (**choice E**) typically presents with a mild fever, ear pain, and injected or inflamed tympanic membranes on physical exam.

9. **The correct answer is C.** A coagulopathy in the presence of a possible subdural hematoma should always be treated. Since the coagulopathy is likely related to warfarin use, the most appropriate intervention is the administration of fresh frozen plasma, which will provide the clotting factors needed to return the coagulation cascade to normal.

Aprotinin (**choice A**), a serine protease with anti-plasmin activity used as an anti-fibrinolytic, has no role in the treatment of warfarin-induced coagulopathy.

Cryoprecipitate (**choice B**) is most often used to treat a coagulopathy related to hypofibrinogenemia. It has no role in the management of warfarin-induced coagulopathy.

An anticoagulant such as low molecular weight heparin (**choice D**) is contraindicated in the presence of a subdural hematoma.

Vitamin K (**choice E**) is used as an antidote for warfarin-induced coagulopathy. However, it is inappropriate in this case since its onset is too slow to immediately reverse the coagulopathy.

10. **The correct answer is B.** The best management is to keep the patient at home in a familiar environment and under the supervision of his family. He is not displaying severe behavioral problems that his family wouldn't be able to manage. Starting donepezil should help the cognitive deficits. His family needs to be educated about the need for closer supervision and safety issues. The focus is initially on the attempt to preserve quality of life.

Admitting him to the geriatric psychiatry unit (**choice A**) is currently not justified. The workup for dementia has been done and current symptoms are not severe enough to justify inpatient treatment.

Starting the patient on vitamins E and B (**choice C**) could be useful; however, it won't change the course of illness or significantly impact cognition or behavior. The family should be educated about the course and prognosis of illness. Available treatment possibilities should be presented instead of misleading reassurance that vitamins-only will produce miracles.

Ordering a brain biopsy (**choice D**) is not a standard diagnostic procedure. In case of dementia of Alzheimer type it would provide patho-histologic proof. Brain biopsy is done in cases of unclear pathology, rather than for the purpose of diagnosing dementia of Alzheimer type.

Residential facility with close supervision (**choice E**) is recommended for patients with no family or in a progressed stage of disease when the danger of leaving them unsupervised can lead to tragic consequences and the families are not able to provide sufficient care. It is certainly not the appropriate next step in this patient's case.

11. **The correct answer is B.** In chemical eye injuries, the first few minutes after the injury occurs will determine the final outcome. It is extremely important to apply first-aid measures immediately, preferably at the scene of the accident. Both acid and alkali injuries can cause severe injury, but in general alkali burns are much more dangerous. Acids cause immediate damage to the superficial tissues in the eye, but usually do not penetrate deeply. Loss of vision usually occurs immediately. Alkalis, however, are able to penetrate the eye by dissolving superficial tissues and then causing intraocular damage. Loss of visual acuity often occurs several days after an alkali injury. In this case, the lye involved (which is sodium hydroxide) is a very powerful alkaline agent. Appropriate treatment at the scene by family, friends, or coworkers involves immediate and copious irrigation of the eye with any available neutral pH liquid including, water, soda, tea, coffee, etc. A second person should hold the eye open, which can be difficult due to the severe blepharospasm induced by pain. Then and only then should any other intervention take place. In an emergency room setting, such as in this case, a topical anesthetic could be used to assist in irrigation.

A mydriatic agent (**choice A**) is incorrect because fundal visualization is clearly of secondary concern.

Ophthalmologic consultation (**choice C**) is an appropriate action but should be done after irrigation is performed. Ideally, another person is calling while you are irrigating.

Similarly, a rapid assessment of visual acuity (**choice D**) and performing a slit lamp examination (**choice E**) should be deferred until after emergent treatment has been completed. Indeed, further evaluation should probably be left to the ophthalmologist.

12. **The correct answer is A.** The boy suffered a mild concussion. The definition of "concussion" is "a transiently induced alteration in mental status." The boy was dazed, but there is no history that he had loss of consciousness or any amnesia after his trauma. If he has a normal exam and is without symptoms he may return to play in the game after 30 minutes; it is not necessary for him to sit out the rest of the season (**choice C**).

The dizziness and confusion from striking the back of one's head on the basketball court floor is not surprising. But there is no history of amnesia or loss of consciousness (**choice B**). If the player had any loss of consciousness then it would be appropriate to take him out for the entire game.

Vomiting once after head trauma, in and of itself, is not a reason to make a trip to the ER (**choice D**). It is more important to know if the symptoms are improving and how the person is acting.

A headache following a mild concussion is not necessarily a concern (**choice E**). Most important is to know if there was loss of consciousness or amnesia.

13. **The correct answer is A.** The history is typical for headache of intracranial hypertension. Causes include intracranial masses and idiopathic intracranial hypertension. (Note, however, that most cases of idiopathic intracranial hypertension are females.)

Intracranial hypotension (**choice B**)-type headache is worse with standing up and alleviated by lying down. Causes include post-lumbar puncture and spontaneous cerebrospinal fluid leaks.

Psychologic tension (**choice C**) may contribute to migraine or muscle tension-type headaches.

Vascular hypertension (**choice D**) only causes headache in very rare extreme cases and is generally asymptomatic, which is why anti-hypertensive medication compliance is often poor.

Vascular hypotension (**choice E**) can cause syncope or presyncope.

14. **The correct answer is A.** This patient gives a history of vertigo. The most likely etiology is benign positional paroxysmal vertigo. This is because she has no vascular risk factors and no other symptoms, and the events are positional. Additionally, the positive Dix-Hallpike maneuver is highly suggestive of this diagnosis. Vestibular rehabilitation has been shown to be helpful in some of these cases.

There is no need for an emergency department evaluation (**choice B**), as you have made the diagnosis and this condition requires no further testing.

Had there been other neurologic findings, a brain MRI (**choice C**) might have been indicated to look for lesions in the posterior fossa. These include strokes, tumors, and hemorrhages.

Diazepam (**choice D**) and meclizine (**choice E**) are sometimes used to treat benign positional paroxysmal vertigo, however they have never been adequately proven to benefit these patients. There is empirical evidence that they help symptoms. However, they may actually prolong the disease course by prolonging the body's adaptation period.

15. **The correct answer is A.** Even more than objective findings on imaging or physical exam, the most predictive factor in return to work for patients with low back pain is job satisfaction.

Marital status (**choice B**) is not as predictive of the patient's return to work concomitant with low back pain as the individual's job satisfaction.

Evidence of disc herniation on MRI (**choice C**) is not as predictive of return to work for patients with low back pain as job satisfaction. A significant proportion of the general population on autopsy have some degree of disc herniation, with most of the population of patients with disc herniation having no history of seeking treatment for disability.

Findings on physical exam such as passive range of motion (**choice D**) do not correlate as highly as job satisfaction in determining whether a patient with low back pain will return to work.

The use of narcotic analgesics for pain treatment (**choice E**) is not as predictive of return to work as job satisfaction for patients with low back pain.

16. **The correct answer is D.** Chloral hydrate is greater than 95% protein-bound, and can cause a significant increase in the effect of warfarin by displacing it from protein binding sites. Warfarin has a low therapeutic index and this interaction is potentially serious. Protein binding is a pharmacokinetic interaction that is very important when using drugs with a low therapeutic index.

Agitation and combativeness (**choice A**) and decreased GI motility (**choice E**) are not associated with chloral hydrate. Chloral hydrate is often chosen in the demented or depressed elderly for mild sleep problems because it does not have the unwanted anticholinergic side effects (delirium, ileus) common to antipsychotics and tricyclic agents.

Warfarin does not potentiate chloral hydrate and therefore we do not expect the common side effects of chloral hydrate, which are sedation (**choice B**) or GI irritation (**choice F**).

Since chloral hydrate can cause a significant increase in the effect of warfarin, which is an anticoagulant, this patient is at risk of hypocoagulation, not hypercoagulation (**choice C**).

17. **The correct answer is B.** Duchenne muscular dystrophy is an X-linked recessive disorder. The disease of the affected grandfather that did not appear in his own children has a 50% chance of appearing in any son of his daughter. This is because his daughters would be carriers. The muscular dystrophy will not be evident in any offspring of his sons, because they would either have the disease or not. Also, a daughter of a carrier will have a 50% chance of being a carrier. There is not a 25% chance of the disease. A son will have an equal chance of having the disease or not (**choice A**).

    Seventy-five percent is incorrect (**choice C**).

    All the grandfather's daughters will be obligate carriers, and the sons will have a 50% chance of having the disease (**choice D**).

    The chance of a new mutation for X-linked disorders such as Duchenne muscular dystrophy is very rare. This is not the correct answer (**choice E**).

18. **The correct answer is C.** The most likely diagnosis in this case is a neuromuscular junction problem such as myasthenia gravis. Less likely possibilities include Guillain Barré, motor neuron disease, or myopathy. Electromyography and a nerve conduction study will most likely distinguish between these possibilities.

    A CT scan of his head (**choice A**) would be useful to look for a brain anatomical problem, such as hemorrhage or hydrocephalus.

    An electroencephalogram (**choice B**) is useful in evaluating patients with seizures or encephalopathy.

    A lumbar puncture (**choice D**) may show an elevated protein, particularly if the diagnosis were Guillain Barré. However, it will not give as much useful information as the electromyogram and nerve conduction study in this case.

    An MRI of his thoracic spine (**choice E**) is extremely unlikely to explain cranial nerve findings. It would show thoracic spine anatomical problems such as cord compression.

19. **The correct answer is B.** Blood sugar must be watched carefully and treated appropriately when a patient is given high-dose corticosteroids. Insulin sliding scale and a diabetic diet should be used.

    Patients with high cholesterol should be given a heart-healthy diet (**choice A**).

    Neurologic checks every hour (**choice C**), central venous line placement (**choice D**), and a stat head CT for change in mental status (**choice E**) are all things that should be done for unstable trauma patients with a cranial component and are not indicated for this patient.

20. **The correct answer is E.** Even though this patient's clinical history is most consistent with Alzheimer disease (the slow and insidious onset of memory loss, language impairment, visuospatial impairment, delusions, hallucinations, and the loss of interest in activities), an MRI may rule out other conditions that may mimic this common dementing disorder, such as a chronic subdural hematoma. This should be ruled out because the son says that she is "unsteady" and there are well-healed scars on her forehead that may indicate falls in the past. This may present with a headache, confusion, slowed thinking, and personality and behavioral changes. It can be caused by a very minor injury. An MRI can also be useful in differentiating between Alzheimer disease and multi-infarct dementia.

    It is inappropriate to admit her to the hospital and prepare her for immediate neurosurgery (**choice A**) at this time. This patient has dementia, which is most likely due to Alzheimer disease, and neurosurgery is not part of the treatment. A chronic subdural hematoma should be ruled out with an MRI. If a chronic subdural hematoma is present, corticosteroids or surgical evacuation may be necessary.

    A lumbar puncture (**choice B**) is uninformative in most cases of dementia. Also, it is not recommended if a chronic subdural hematoma is suspected because of the possibility of shifting the tissues.

    A trial of phenelzine (**choice C**) is not appropriate at this time because even though it is sometimes difficult to distinguish Alzheimer disease from depression, there are signs and symptoms that may be consistent with a subdural hematoma (unsteadiness and scars on her forehead) and therefore, an MRI should be performed. Sometimes a trial of antidepressants is appropriate in cases where depression may be present; however the most appropriate agents are tricyclics or SSRIs. Phenelzine is an MAOI, which should only be used after the others have failed.

    A cerebral angiogram (**choice D**) is useful in evaluating the morphology of the cerebral vasculature and to detect the location and degree of atherosclerotic stenosis, as well as aneurysms and malformations.

21. **The correct answer is A.** This patient most likely has Alzheimer disease, which is a diagnosis of exclusion that is characterized by the slow and insidious onset of memory loss, language impairment, visuospatial impairment, delusions and hallucinations, and the loss of interest in activities. This patient has most of these symptoms, and most other causes of dementia were ruled out with the laboratory studies and MRI.

    A chronic subdural hematoma (**choice B**) would most likely have shown up on the MRI and since the MRI was normal and these symptoms are consistent with Alzheimer disease, this (Alzheimer disease) is the most likely diagnosis.

    It is unlikely that she has depression (**choice C**), because the history is almost classical for Alzheimer disease. She does not have weight loss, insomnia, feelings of guilt, worthlessness, or suicidal ideation, which are all symptoms of depression. This patient has cognitive impairment that she does not complain about. A depressed individual with cognitive impairment often complains about his/her deficits.

    Multi-infarct dementia (**choice D**) typically has a stepwise progression. This patient's course is slow and insidious, which is more consistent with Alzheimer disease than multi-infarct dementia. Also, the MRI would have most likely shown evidence of this disease if it were present.

    Schizoaffective disorder (**choice E**) is characterized by the presence of psychosis and a mood disorder. This patient does not have the psychotic or depressive symptoms that are characteristic of this disorder, such as bizarre hallucinations or delusions, weight loss, insomnia, feelings of guilt, worthlessness, or suicidal ideation.

22. **The correct answer is C.** Chronic subdural hematomas may occur in infants and the elderly without a clear history of incident trauma. They can present months to years after the initial injury and should be suspected in patients with a decreasing or a fluctuating mental status out of proportion to the focal neurologic deficit. The hematoma is liquid and drainage by way of burr holes is usually all that is necessary for treatment. Chronic subdural hematomas frequently reoccur when they are associated with multiple subdural membranes. In these cases, craniotomy to strip the membranes is necessary.

    Cerebral contusion (**choice A**) usually starts with severe headache and may progress to alteration in mental status. Cerebral contusion by itself rarely causes chronic symptoms.

    Cerebral tumor (**choice B**) incidence is less in this age group and the presentation is usually progressive deterioration rather than waxing and waning nature.

    Skull fractures (**choice D**) may be found on investigation but are unlikely to be the cause of the waxing and waning nature of deterioration in consciousness in this woman, unless associated with other pathologic findings.

    Subarachnoid hemorrhage (**choice E**) is usually of sudden onset associated with altered consciousness. Focal neurologic deficits may occur but they are less common in these patients with prolonged history.

23. **The correct answer is D.** This patient has transient global amnesia. The etiology of transient global amnesia in most cases is cryptogenic and there is no treatment.

    Electroconvulsive therapy (**choice A**) is used to treat depression. A common side effect of electroconvulsive therapy is transient short-term memory problems.

    Gabapentin (**choice B**) is an anticonvulsant, which is also used to treat neuropathic pain. It is possible, but very unlikely, that she had a seizure.

    Sumatriptan (**choice C**) is a treatment for acute migraine. Migraine has been proposed as the etiology of transient global amnesia, but there is no good evidence

    Tissue plasminogen activator (**choice E**) is used for the acute treatment of stroke or heart attack. Isolated memory problems would be an extremely unlikely presentation for stroke.

24. **The correct answer is D.** This is a typical presentation for psychogenic gait disorder. The patient has significant psychological stressors (HIV, death of partner, business problems) and an entirely normal elemental neurologic exam.

    There is no evidence of an autoimmune (**choice A**) process in this patient. Multiple sclerosis plaques are an autoimmune process, which could cause a gait disorder.

    Since he is HIV-positive he is at risk for infections (**choice B**). However, we have no evidence of infection in this case. An infection such as toxoplasmosis would also probably cause a focal neurologic deficit in association with gait dysfunction.

    Multifactorial gait disorder (**choice C**) is a common cause of gait dysfunction in the elderly.

    Peripheral vascular (**choice E**) gait dysfunction is characterized by claudication during exercise.

25. **The correct answer is A.** This patient has a hordeolum, otherwise known as a "sty." It is the result of an acute bacterial infection of one or more glands of the eyelid. The most common etiologic agent is *Staphylococcus aureus.* It usually presents as a painful nodule that contains a core of pus. External hordeolum are located on the margin of the eyelid such as in this case. An internal hordeolum can usually only be seen by everting the eyelid; however, it often causes local irritation of the conjunctiva. Treatment includes topical antibiotic ointments and application of heat (a red heat lamp is recommended, but most patients find it easier to apply a warm compress). After the nodule erupts and drainage of the pus occurs, the hordeolum rapidly resolves. It is more common in diabetics, patients with GI disorders, and those with acne.

Referral to an ophthalmologist (**choice B**) is incorrect because a primary care provider can very easily treat a hordeolum.

Incision and drainage (**choice C**) is incorrect because a hordeolum will usually resolve without surgical intervention. A related entity, called a chalazion, also presents as a firm nodule in the eyelid. It is caused by chronic inflammation and buildup of material from a meibomian gland of the eyelid. It usually develops over several months and is not usually painful. Incision and drainage are often necessary to treat this lesion.

Ophthalmic steroids (**choice D**) is incorrect. Steroids are not indicated in an acute bacterial infection such as this.

Oral erythromycin (**choice E**) is not correct since systemic antibiotics are not necessary for treatment.

26. **The correct answer is C.** This man has a typical history and exam for a right parietal syndrome. Pertinent findings include neglect and anosognosia. He may have had a stroke or hemorrhage, and must be evaluated promptly.

If this had been a first seizure, then a reasonable plan might be to resume driving in 6 months if there was no seizure recurrence (**choice A**).

There is no reason to think that he will be safe to drive tomorrow (**choice B**). Additionally, he should get an evaluation including brain CT or MRI and a diagnosis made.

This is not an ophthalmologic problem (**choice D**). The problem localizes to the right cerebral hemisphere or perhaps thalamus. If there was a problem which localized anterior to the optic chiasm an ophthalmic evaluation might be useful.

A specific brain lesion causes this patient's problem. At some point therapy may be useful in coping, but he does not have a condition requiring urgent psychiatric evaluation (**choice E**).

27. **The correct answer is E.** This patient is presenting with a pure motor hemiparesis, which is most likely secondary to a subcortical ischemic stroke. There are no other symptoms which would localize the patient's stroke to the cortex (i.e., aphasia, visual field cut, face and arm weakness more than leg weakness). The syndrome of pure motor hemiparesis is one of the classic lacunar syndromes described, and typically localizes to the contralateral internal capsule or contralateral basis pontis. Small vessel strokes (lacunes) are usually secondary to long-standing hypertension and diabetes mellitus. The first step in this patient's management is to obtain a non-contrast head CT scan.

A urine drug screen (**choice A**) may be a helpful laboratory test to order, and may help elucidate the etiology of stroke in certain patients. It should be checked in any patient in whom drug abuse, particularly cocaine and amphetamines, is suspected. However, it will not help with the acute management of a patient presenting with acute stroke.

An aspirin a day (**choice B**) helps prevent recurrent stroke. However, it is important to rule out the presence of an intracranial hemorrhage with a non-contrast head CT scan before any therapeutic decisions are made.

The duration of symptoms would preclude the patient from being considered for IV tPA (**choice C**), which must be administered within 3 hours of symptom onset, provided that there is no hemorrhage on CT scan. There are other contraindications for using IV tPA as well.

An MRI and MRA of the brain (**choice D**) would be an appropriate test to order, but not as a first diagnostic step in a patient presenting acutely.

28. **The correct answer is A.** This patient has a history that is suggestive of acute bacterial meningitis, the triad of meningismus, fever, and altered sensorium. However, other possible etiologies that must be considered include non-bacterial causes of meningitis (i.e., TB, fungus, viruses), encephalitis, and abscess.

Antibiotics are the first step in the management of this patient, especially when bacterial meningitis is suspected. In a patient such as this, a head CT (**choice C**) should be obtained as soon as possible, and should be obtained before performing a lumbar puncture because of the possibility of a mass lesion such as abscess. If a focal lesion, such as an abscess, is found on imaging, a lumbar puncture would likely be contraindicated. If no mass lesion is found, a lumbar puncture (**choice E**) to look for bacterial meningitis can be performed. However, antibiotics should not be withheld until these tests can be completed. Bacterial cultures of the CSF remain positive for several hours after the first dose of antibiotics.

Carbamazepine (**choice B**) is not used in the acute treatment of seizures. Benzodiazepines, such as lorazepam or diazepam, are used in the acute setting, as well as phenytoin, all of which can be given intravenously.

An electroencephalogram (**choice D**) would not be appropriate to order in the acute setting; however, if the patient's mental status did not improve after the seizure, an EEG may help to rule out subclinical seizures or nonconvulsive status epilepticus. An EEG would also be helpful to look for herpes encephalitis, as most cases have nonspecific temporal lobe EEG abnormalities.

29. **The correct answer is A.** Lesions of the left frontal lobe may present with a clinical syndrome that is indistinguishable from a depressive illness. The clinical key to this presentation is that this depressive presentation is secondary to a medical disorder and the abrupt clinical deterioration being over 3 days. This would be highly atypical of a primary psychiatric disorder.

Left parietal lesions (**choice B**) may present largely with language and speech difficulties that are absent in this patient's presentation.

Right parietal lesions (**choice C**) may present largely with visuospatial integration problems and neglect syndromes that were not delineated in the patient's presentation.

Pontine lesions (**choice D**) would be manifested by cranial nerve signs and multiple motor and sensory deficiencies.

Cerebellar lesions (**choice E**) present largely with coordination difficulties and would likely have accompanying cranial nerve signs depending on the location and the nature of the lesion (mass versus bleed versus infarct).

30. **The correct answer is A.** In this situation, the neurologist would be sued because he had established a physician/patient relationship when he spoke directly to the patient, after he had discussed the case with you, the primary physician, and had also advised him to go home. The lesson learned from this question is that one should be careful not to talk to patients on the telephone while covering the emergency room, and especially those who are totally unknown. Proffering therapeutic or other advice exposes one to the possibility of a lawsuit. Even if the patient is known, one has to be careful and decide whether this course should be taken, for in doing so, one has established a physician/patient relationship. Had the neurologist spoken only to you, the physician, and not to the patient, litigation would not have succeeded.

The neurologist will be held liable; however, it is unlikely that he will be let off with only a warning (**choice B**).

It is unlikely that he will be suspended from the neurology service (**choice C**) or have his license revoked (**choice D**).

The neurologist established a physician/patient relationship and therefore it is incorrect to say that he will not be held liable by the courts (**choice E**).

31. **The correct answer is E.** This patient probably had a stroke. Stroke is a well-known complication of coronary artery bypass surgery. Typically, it is caused either by emboli produced during aortic cross clamping or by hypoperfusion related to perioperative hypotension.

Acute disseminated encephalomyelitis is an autoimmune (**choice A**) disease that can produce focal neurologic deficits.

Mechanical (**choice B**) causes of focal neurological dysfunction include trauma, neurosurgic instrumentation, and chiropractic neck manipulations.

Neoplastic (**choice C**) causes of neurologic dysfunction include primary central nervous system tumors such as astrocytomas and oligodendrogliomas, as well as malignancies that are metastatic from elsewhere.

Toxic (**choice D**) causes of neurologic dysfunction, such as sedating medications, usually do not produce focal deficits but rather a diffuse encephalopathy.

32. **The correct answer is C.** This patient gives a typical story for a transient ischemic attack involving the visual pathway. The acute onset and negative phenomena are characteristic. Since cortical function was involved, an embolic etiology is likely. An echocardiogram and carotid ultrasound should be performed to evaluate for a source.

Since there seems to have been an entire hemifield loss, the problem must be posterior to the optic chiasm. It is true that since the patient did not do a cover/uncover test we cannot be positive. However, it is still more important to search for an embolic source before doing a dilated fundus examination (**choice A**).

Brain magnetic resonance spectroscopy (**choice B**) is useful for the non-invasive characterization of brain lesions; for example, to distinguish an abscess from a tumor.

An electroencephalogram (**choice D**) can confirm the diagnosis of a seizure. Seizures usually have a march of symptoms lasting for a few seconds and positive phenomena.

Visual evoked potentials (**choice E**) do not generally have a role in the evaluation of transient ischemic attacks. They can be used to help confirm a diagnosis of optic neuritis.

33. **The correct answer is C.** This is a common presentation for primary generalized epilepsy of childhood. An electroencephalogram showing the classic 3-Hz spike-and-wave pattern would confirm this diagnosis.

A brain CT scan (**choice A**) and a brain MRI (**choice B**) are useful for evaluating brain anatomy. Anatomic problems can cause seizures, but these tests will not tell anything about brain electrical activity.

Lumbar puncture (**choice D**) is useful for measuring cerebrospinal fluid pressure and looking for central nervous system inflammation or infection. Central nervous system inflammation or infection may cause seizures.

Nerve conduction study (**choice E**) is useful to evaluate peripheral nerve injuries, such as nerve entrapment.

34. **The correct answer is A.** Guillain Barré syndrome (GBS) is a postinfectious polyneuropathy that causes demyelination in mostly motor nerves. It can affect people of all ages and there is no family history. Paralysis follows a URI or gastroenteritis by 10 days. (GI infection may have been caused by *Campylobacter* species.) Weakness and paralysis is ascending. Onset is gradual over days or weeks. Bulbar involvement may occur with dysphagia and respiratory distress.

Myasthenia gravis (**choice B**) is characterized by weakness of muscles innervated by the brainstem, usually worsening with increasing activity and use of those muscles. It is caused by antibodies to acetylcholine receptors. Clinical signs and symptoms include difficulty chewing, proximal limb weakness, ptosis, and nasal voice.

Poliomyelitis (**choice C**) has a very low incidence (1:10 million to 1:1 million due to vaccination) and can cause aseptic meningitis or brief febrile illness. One to 2% of children will have a more severe illness progressing to myalgia, loss of reflexes, and flaccid paralysis. Patients may also have bulbar involvement. Usually proximal limb muscles are more often involved than distal.

Reflex sympathetic dystrophy (**choice D**) is usually in one extremity and demonstrates autonomic dysfunction such as dyshidrosis and color and temperature changes. There is also marked hyperesthesia of the affected limb.

Transverse myelitis (**choice E**) is often postviral, but unlike GBS there is root and back pain with sensory loss below the level of the lesion. There is also rapidly developing paralysis.

35. **The correct answer is A.** This patient's history is consistent with pseudotumor cerebri, or idiopathic intracranial hypertension. It occurs most commonly in obese females, and typically presents with headaches. Pulsatile tinnitus and transient visual obscurations, secondary to increased intracranial pressure, are common associated historical findings. Patients may also complain of diplopia, which is secondary to transient sixth nerve palsies as a result of the increased intracranial pressure. Some medications and endocrinologic conditions are associated with the disease. Exam findings are usually limited, but bilateral optic disc edema secondary to increased intracranial pressure (papilledema) is common; therefore normal findings (**choice E**) is incorrect. Other than papilledema, occasionally sixth nerve palsies, and possible visual field deficits, the neurologic exam is usually normal. Visual loss is the most serious complication. There are no specific correlations with increased (**choice C**) or decreased (**choice D**) reflexes, and generalized weakness (**choice B**) should not be seen. Diagnosis is made with normal neuro-imaging, followed by a lumbar puncture documenting increased opening pressures and normal CSF contents. The treatment is usually acetazolamide, and patients should have serial visual field testing to follow any visual complaints.

36. **The correct answer is B.** This patient's history is consistent with essential tremor, which is the most common movement disorder in adults. The positive family history and the improvement of tremor with alcohol are both typical historic features of essential tremor. Typically, the tremor is more pronounced with action or postures; rest tremor is usually not seen.

The patient does not give a history suggestive of alcoholism; therefore, alcohol withdrawal (**choice A**) is unlikely to be the etiology of his tremor.

The patient's history is not consistent with multiple sclerosis (**choice C**), which is a demyelinating illness. Tremor can be a symptom associated with multiple sclerosis, but other historical and physical exam clues would be needed to make that diagnosis.

Parkinson disease (**choice D**) typically begins asymmetrically, and has a characteristic resting tremor. Rigidity, bradykinesia, and postural instability are other common features seen in Parkinson disease.

The patient's family history and response to alcohol make physiologic tremor (**choice E**) unlikely. Hyperthyroid disease and medications (valproate, lithium) may cause an enhanced physiologic tremor.

37. **The correct answer is B.** This patient is presenting with delirium, which is characterized by fluctuating mental status and a relatively acute onset. Frequently, there are signs of global cerebral dysfunction. Delirium has a long list of possible causes; frequently, infections, metabolic derangements, and medications are the culprits, especially in elderly patients. In this patient's case, a urinary tract infection as the cause of her delirium is probable.

    Acute stroke (**choice A**) can present with acute confusional states; however, these symptoms are of abrupt onset and usually have other associated symptoms pointing to the diagnosis of stroke.

    Dementia (**choice C**) is a common underlying condition in patients presenting with delirium; however, dementia is a chronic condition and fluctuations are not characteristic.

    Partial seizures (**choice D**) may cause confusional states, either as a direct symptom of the seizure itself or secondary to a postictal state. However, there is often a history of similar episodes, and symptoms are abrupt in onset.

    A psychotic episode (**choice E**) in an elderly patient with no history of psychosis would be unlikely.

38. **The correct answer is E.** The patient seems to have some decompensation with environmental changes such as changes in the people surrounding her and changes in location. These changes may appear confusing and frustrating to a patient with dementia and can contribute to agitated behavior and paranoia. A physically consistent home environment may help decrease the amount of confusion that the patient feels.

    Keeping the patient bed bound (**choice A**) is an absolutely contraindicated intervention. The risk of illness such as aspiration pneumonia, deconditioning, and decubitus ulcer make this choice particularly unacceptable.

    Sedating the patient (**choice B**) would leave the patient at risk for falls and aspiration.

    Reprimanding the patient when she accuses people of stealing from her (**choice C**) is likely to further agitate the patient and will not likely help a memory-impaired patient because of deficits in the acquisition of new knowledge.

    Leaving the patient in charge of her own care (**choice D**) is also incorrect. The patient's level of mentation leaves her vulnerable to danger if not supervised.

39. **The correct answer is C.** One of the major items in the differential diagnosis of seizures is hypoglycemia, especially in a younger patient without other obvious etiologies. Therefore, the administration of a glucose bolus following obtaining intravenous access is reasonable.

    Acetaminophen (**choice A**) has no role in the management of a non-febrile patient with seizures.

    Flumazenil (**choice B**) is used in the treatment of benzodiazepine overdose and has no role in the management of seizures.

    Metoprolol (**choice D**), a beta-1 selective antagonist, has no role in the management of seizures.

    Naloxone (**choice E**), an opioid antagonist used in the treatment of opioid overdose, has no role in the management of seizures.

40. **The correct answer is B.** Neurofibromatosis type I is correct. Also known as von Recklinghausen disease, it is characterized by café-au-lait macules, neurofibromas, Lisch nodules, optic gliomas, bony dysplasia, intertriginous freckling (Crow sign), and autosomal dominant inheritance. Fifty percent of cases appear to be spontaneous mutations. The cutaneous neurofibromas are dermal tumors that vary from pinhead sized to large, soft, flabby masses. Many show "buttonholing" character (can be pushed down into the pannus). Café-au-lait macule is a hallmark of this disease. Usually they are uniformly pigmented, light brown macules that are unevenly round or oval and range in size from 1.5 to 15 cm in diameter. They most often present at birth and almost always present by the time the patient is 1 year of age. Diagnosis of neurofibromatosis type I requires two or more of the following criteria: *1*) six or more café-au-lait macules of more than 5 mm in greatest diameter in prepubertal individuals and more than 15 mm in greatest diameter in postpubertal individuals; *2*) two or more neurofibromas of any type or one plexiform neurofibroma; *3*) freckling in the axillary or inguinal regions; *4*) optic glioma; *5*) two or more Lisch nodules; *6*) distinctive osseous lesion; *7*) first-degree relative.

McCune-Albright syndrome (**choice A**) is incorrect. This is characterized by polyostotic fibrous dysplasia, irregular skin pigmentation, and sexual precocity.

Neurofibromatosis type II (**choice C**) is incorrect because this type is characterized by bilateral acoustic neuromas. The characteristic cutaneous features include neurofibromas and schwannomas, but not café-au-lait macules or freckling.

Watson syndrome (**choice D**) is incorrect. This syndrome is characterized by café-au-lait macules, dull intelligence, and pulmonary stenosis; no neurofibromas or freckling of intertriginous areas.

Biopsy (**choice E**) is incorrect. The uniform pigmentation with even borders is not consistent with atypical nevi. The criteria for atypical nevi include: *1*) asymmetry; *2*) scalloped border; *3*) uneven pigmentation; *4*) greater than 6 mm in diameter.

41. **The correct answer is D.** The patient presents with a classic case of narcolepsy. Treatments that have shown efficacy in patients with narcolepsy include methylphenidate and amphetamine, as well as some antidepressant medications when cataplexy (sudden loss of muscular tone) is present.

    There is no evidence to support the use of calcium supplementation (**choice A**) for patients with narcolepsy.

    Continuous positive airway pressure (**choice B**) is a treatment used for obstructive sleep apnea to keep the patient's airway patent. It does not have a use in narcolepsy, a condition where airway status while asleep remains essentially unaffected.

    Haloperidol (**choice C**) is not a recommended treatment for narcolepsy, even for the hypnagogic or hypnopompic hallucinations that are experienced as part of the clinical picture for many narcoleptic patients. The sedative effects of haloperidol are definitely not desired in this population of patients.

    Valproic acid (**choice E**) is not a recommended treatment for narcolepsy. Like haloperidol, the sedative effects of valproic acid are not desired in this population of patients.

42. **The correct answer is C.** The first thing to do apart from physical and neurologic exam is to determine the reversibility of this condition. Checking B_{12}, calcium, and TSH levels along with other routine blood work should help determine if the symptoms are caused by any deficiencies or treatable infections. If this is the case, mere treatment of the underlying condition should result in improvement of symptoms of dementia.

    Drawing blood for HIV testing (**choice A**) should be done if everything else is excluded or if there is significant suspicion that the symptoms are related to HIV infection. The patient needs to consent to the test. It is certainly not the first step to be taken in the case presented above.

    Ordering a CT scan of the brain (**choice B**) can be considered; however, it is not the first diagnostic step in this case. Even though pathologic changes may be found, the better way to detect the possible changes is by ordering MRI and MRA. A CT of the brain may not contribute to the etiology and thus possible treatment in the way that MRI does. However, these methods increase the cost of the workup and are not routinely recommended by all authorities except in uncertain cases.

    Ordering neuropsychologic testing (**choice D**) can be done as a part of a further workup to detect specific cognitive deficits. It won't resolve the question of reversibility of the condition, though.

    Performing a lumbar puncture (**choice E**) can be done after all the non-invasive methods have been exhausted. It is not the first step in a dementia workup.

43. **The correct answer is B.** The child in this vignette is showing the classic signs of increased intracranial pressure: headaches that wake him up from sleep, early morning vomiting, and papilledema. Visual disturbances, changes in personality/behavior, and altered levels of consciousness can also be seen in increased intracranial pressure. He should be admitted to the hospital and imaging of the brain must be done to evaluate for the cause of his increased intracranial pressure, which include cerebral edema, mass lesions, trauma, infection, pseudotumor cerebri, and hydrocephalus.

    Admitting him to the hospital for observation (**choice A**) is not aggressive enough in this situation. Because this child is manifesting signs of increased intracranial pressure, he needs to have imaging studies performed to look for the cause.

    Discharging this patient home with a prescription for acetaminophen (**choice D**) or asking the mother to keep a headache diary (**choice C**) are inappropriate. The symptoms of the child in this vignette indicate increased intracranial pressure which requires further evaluation.

    Reassuring the mother that these are migraine headaches (**choice E**) is not appropriate given the child's symptoms.

Migraine headaches are more likely if there is a positive family history; however, an organic cause for this child's headaches needs to be ruled out with these symptoms before reassurance can be given to the mother.

44. **The correct answer is B.** This illustrates the importance of a good history in the evaluation of headaches. The question most specific to raised intracranial pressure would be if the patient had headaches on rising in the morning. The presence of vomiting on rising would be specific, too. These symptoms may suggest a tumor as a likely cause.

Headaches that are similar from attack to attack (**choice A**) are suggestive of chronicity and associated with migraine.

The presence of neck pain (**choice C**) or neck stiffness along with an aversion to bright light (**choice D**) leads one to suspect meningitis.

Personality changes (**choice E**), seizures, and alteration of consciousness (**choice F**), particularly before puberty, point to a tumor but are less specific to raised intracranial pressure.

45. **The correct answer is A.** The funduscopic exam of the left eye demonstrates papilledema, which is observed in intracranial lesions producing increased intracranial pressure (e.g., a tumor). The loss of consciousness, the drowsiness shortly after this, the bite marks of the tongue and oral mucosa, and the papilledema could conceivably be due to a seizure secondary to a cerebral tumor.

Child abuse (**choice B**) is unlikely here considering how quickly the father brought the patient to the emergency room. You would typically see retinal hemorrhages if it were a child-abuse scenario. More history is needed.

Migraine (**choice C**) typically has no obvious signs on physical exam with no signs of toxicity, normal vital signs, and a normal neurological exam.

A subarachnoid hemorrhage (**choice D**) may present with a hypertension physical exam along with a classically severe headache. They are not typically associated with papilledema. Papilledema in the presence of an isolated high blood pressure is called malignant hypertension and the blood pressure warrants urgent normalization.

Viral meningitis (**choice E**) would present with signs of "meningismus," including neck stiffness, fever, and altered mental status. Papilledema is not a classic sign of this.

46. **The correct answer is E.** The exact pathophysiology of migraine headaches is unknown but it is thought to relate to serotonin. Sumatriptan is a serotonin receptor agonist that selectively activates a particular subpopulation of serotonin receptors (namely, 1A and 1D receptors) and is an effective treatment in many patients.

Sumatriptan itself does not initiate platelet aggregation (**choice C**) and it works as a serotonin agonist, not antagonist (**choice A**).

Sumatriptan has no direct effect on dopamine receptors when treating migraine (**choice B**).

Sumatriptan is not a serotonin reuptake inhibitor (**choice D**). This describes the mechanism of fluoxetine or paroxetine (serotonin specific reuptake inhibitors) that work effectively as antidepressants.

47. **The correct answer is E.** This patient exhibits parkinsonian features including the bradykinesia, rigidity, tremor, gait apraxia, and dementia. His head CT shows dilated ventricles and, combined with his "urinary accidents" (indicative of urinary incontinence), he most likely has normal pressure hydrocephalus. He should be referred to a neurosurgeon for possible ventriculosystemic shunting.

Benztropine (**choice A**) is an anticholinergic agent that is an effective adjunctive treatment for parkinsonism and drug-induced extrapyramidal symptoms. It will treat the symptoms of parkinsonism but not the cause of this patient's symptoms, and is not the best answer.

Bromocriptine (**choice B**) is a dopamine agonist agent for parkinsonian syndrome. It may not be effective in treating this patient's extrapyramidal symptoms for the same reason as choice A. Its side-effect profile includes involuntary movements and hallucinations.

Donepezil (**choice C**) is a reversible acetylcholinesterase inhibitor recently being used in the treatment of Alzheimer dementia by preventing further deterioration in dementia. It would not do the same to this patient's dementia, which is parkinsonianlike.

Fluoxetine (**choice D**) is a serotonin specific reuptake inhibitor that is effective against depression. This patient may have a component of depression. However, more time with the patient is needed than given to find sleep disturbance, appetite/weight changes, attention problems, depressed moods, guilt feelings, and suicidal thoughts, etc., before beginning fluoxetine.

48. **The correct answer is E.** The question asks which is the best intervention to allow the patient to stay at home without the need for a long-term facility. The primary reason for nursing home placement is stress on the primary caregiver, in this case, the patient's wife. By offering the caregiver respite care (a "break" from taking care of the patient) this may delay placement by up to 1 year.

Benzodiazepines and any medication that affects cognition should generally be avoided in the elderly, particularly outside of the hospital setting (**choice A**). There is also an increased incidence of falls if a short-acting benzodiazepine is used.

One could try a neuroleptic (**choice B**), but this is usually reserved for certain symptoms such as "sundowning," paranoia, and psychosis. In addition, prescribing a medication is not an effective means of allowing the caregiver to cope.

Diphendydramine (**choice C**) has sedative effects and should not be used in patients with Alzheimer dementia because the anticholinergic effects of Alzheimer will be potentiated.

Donepezil (**choice D**) may be useful in preserving the current mental function at baseline for a number of months. It has been shown to delay the transfer of the patient to a long-term facility for 3 months.

49. **The correct answer is B.** The patient has a delirium picture superimposed on underlying dementia. As part of any delirium workup (ruling out sepsis, electrolyte imbalance, endocrinologic abnormalities, cancer, etc.) a detailed account of the patient's drug list and any recent changes would also be useful. Cimetidine is a drug that can cause CNS disturbances and somnolence that may be contributing to this patient's delirium. It is a commonly prescribed H_2 blocker and an awareness of this particular side effect is paramount when prescribing it in the elderly. Its other side effects include diarrhea, arrhythmias, headache, arthralgia and myalgia, nephritis, and pancreatitis.

Aspirin (**choice A**) does not cause impairment of mental cognition. It has been shown to have cardioprotective properties in patients with coronary artery disease. Its side effects include gastric upset, prolonged bleeding time, asthma, and trinities.

Lisinopril (**choice C**) is an ACE-inhibitor and does not cause impairment of mental cognition. Its use requires caution in elderly patients, who are more easily predisposed to renal impairment. Obtain a baseline blood urea nitrogen level (BUN) and cretonne before starting ACE-inhibitors. Its other side effects include postural hypotension, fatigue, and diarrhea.

Nitroglycerin patches (**choice D**) mainly cause postural hypotension, headache, flushing, and nausea as their main side effects in the elderly. They do not cause mental impairment.

Simvastatin (**choice E**), as with all HMG-CoA reductase inhibitors, mainly cause myopathy, rhabdomyolysis, and gastrointestinal upset as their main side effects. They have not been found to cause mental cognitive impairment.

50. **The correct answer is C.** Donepezil works in the brain as a cholinesterase inhibitor at the neuronal synapse. By inhibiting the cholinesterase enzyme it increases the level of acetylcholine neurotransmitter and aids in maintaining mental function. It does not stop the decrease in cells that produce the acetylcholine component. The goal of donepezil is to enhance cognitive function. This can be monitored using a Mini-Mental Status exam. If there is no change or an improvement in the Mini-Mental Status exam then donepezil should be continued. If there is deterioration in the Mini-Mental Status exam one should then consider stopping the donepezil. Once stopped, a precipitous drop in the patient's mental function may occur.

Increasing the dosage of donepezil (**choice A**) at this time is inappropriate because increasing doses have not been shown to cause statistically significant greater clinical benefit. Also, the recommended doses are 5 and 10 mg, not 20 mg.

Plasma levels of donepezil (**choice B**) are not used to determine the dosage of the drug. If the patient's cognitive function does not deteriorate and if no side effects are noted then continue the drug at the current dosage.

Tapering donepezil is not required (**choice D**), as the drug may be discontinued safely when there is documented deterioration in cognitive function while donepezil is being used.

The mechanism by which vitamin E (**choice E**) produces this benefit is not known for sure, but it is believed that it may be related to the vitamin's ability to protect nerve cell membranes from oxidative damage. Because it is less expensive and readily available, high-dose vitamin E is often recommended. No evidence of interactions between vitamin E and donepezil have been noted.

Neurology: Test Two

1. A 30-year-old woman comes to the office complaining of "visual hallucinations." She has recurrent episodes of flashing, zigzagging lights, which typically last for 30 minutes. After the lights "go away" she gets a throbbing pain behind one of her eyes as well as nausea, vomiting, photophobia, and phonophobia. She has been getting these episodes for the past year. Ibuprofen provides no relief. She has no other medical problems and takes no medications. She had severe motion sickness as a child. A complete physical examination, including neurologic and ophthalmologic examination, is normal. The most appropriate next step in management is to

   (A) obtain neuroimaging studies to rule out an intracranial process
   (B) prescribe haloperidol for hallucinations
   (C) prescribe sumatriptan (or another triptan)
   (D) recommend that she return to the office during one of the episodes so that you can perform an examination at that time
   (E) start therapy with acetaminophen as needed

2. A 75-year-old otherwise healthy woman comes to the office with new onset frontotemporal right-sided headaches for the last 10 days and an acute onset of painless decreased vision in her right eye yesterday. She has tenderness and pain in her frontotemporal region when combing her hair. She has lost 10 pounds in the last month, which she suggests is because she is unable to chew her food normally. She reports that she has had more "aches and pains" in her shoulder. Physical examination reveals tenderness over her right frontotemporal region of her scalp. Her vision in her right eye is 20/100 and her left eye is 20/20. She has an afferent papillary defect in her right eye. Funduscopy shows a swollen optic nerve on the right side and a normal optic nerve on the left side. The rest of her examination is normal. The most appropriate next step in management is to

   (A) begin systemic steroids immediately and then arrange for ancillary testing
   (B) call the local ophthalmologist for possible ophthalmic surgical intervention
   (C) observe the patient and reassure the patient that the vision will improve in the right eye and the left eye will remain 20/20
   (D) obtain immediate neuroimaging
   (E) order an immediate erythrocyte sedimentation rate

3. A 68-year-old woman comes to the clinic because of a history of severe headaches for the last few months. She has also been having progressive trouble writing and speaking and occasional urinary incontinence. Over the past 2 days she has been having problems with balance and has been "walking like a drunk." She has a history of chronic low back pain, heart palpitations, gallbladder surgery, a hysterectomy 20 years ago for uterine cancer, and polio and rheumatic fever as a child. The most appropriate management of this patient is to

(A) order a brain MRI next month if symptoms persist
(B) order a head CT today
(C) prescribe oxybutynin and re-examine her in 1 week
(D) send her for electromyography and nerve conduction studies tomorrow
(E) send her to a urologist

4. A 73-year-old man who has been a patient of yours for many years comes to the office for a family meeting to discuss the possibility of Alzheimer disease. He has a long history of drinking and now has a moderate to severe hepatic impairment. In recent years, the family has noted the gradual onset of personality and cognitive changes. Overall, the patient articulates well and seems orientated to time and place. No behavioral issues such as depression, anxiety, paranoia, and psychosis are evident. On further testing, he seems lacking in his ability to name objects. He is also found to have brittle mood swings, poor judgment, and his written language is a mess. His wife reports that she has had to take over most of his activities of daily living, as he seems unable to complete them on his own. The wife is most worried that he is now starting to forget who she is, on occasion referring to her as "the nurse." After an extensive medical history, thorough physical examination, and appropriate laboratory testing, you diagnose him with Alzheimer disease. The wife asks you about medications specifically for Alzheimer and requests one that is lowest in side affects. You tell her the most appropriate medication for her husband is

(A) donepezil
(B) galantamine
(C) nothing, as there is no cure for Alzheimer
(D) rivastigmine
(E) tacrine

5. An 80-year-old man with prostate cancer, coronary artery disease, diabetes, and hypertension comes to the office because of vertigo. His symptoms started 1 week ago when he had suddenly felt like he was on a merry-go-around as he stood up, which apparently lasted 5 minutes and dissipated. At that time he did not have any nausea, vomiting, or focal neurological symptoms. Since then he has continued to have brief episodes of dizziness ("as if I was going to pass out"), roughly one episode a day. The dizziness would come about mostly when he would stand up fast and would last 30 seconds to 1 minute and would be alleviated by sitting down. Two days ago he thought that he was feeling better, but then yesterday as he was going upstairs he had another dizzy feeling and he does not remember what happened next. According to his wife, the patient sustained a two to three-stair fall with a loss of consciousness. He came around quickly but was noted to be dysarthric. Immediately afterwards the patient denied any feeling of weakness in any of his extremities, but did realize he was dysarthric. He was a little unsteady when he got up. He spent most of yesterday in bed and came to his scheduled appointment today. He is not dysarthric today and feels well. The most correct statement about his condition is

(A) A cardiac pacemaker will likely prevent this problem in the future
(B) An electroencephalogram will likely be diagnostic in this case
(C) This patient has a peripheral nervous system problem
(D) This patient should be treated with meclizine
(E) This patient's problem is likely be related to vascular disease

6. A 64-year-old man comes to the office for a followup visit. A year ago he was diagnosed with normal pressure hydrocephalus and had a ventriculoperitoneal shunt placed. Most of his symptoms have improved since the shunt placement. He is no longer incontinent of urine; however, he is still using a cane for walking outside of the house. He now tells you that about once every week or two, for a few moments, he gets the sensation that his body is spinning. He has no history of cerebral aneurysm, meningitis, or significant trauma. The most pertinent part of the neurologic examination at this time is

(A) deep tendon reflexes
(B) gait evaluation
(C) looking for nystagmus
(D) pinprick sensation
(E) testing of cranial nerve I

7. A 19-year-old sociology student with epilepsy comes to the student health service after having a witnessed generalized tonic-clonic seizure this morning. He had about 2 hours of sleep last night because he was studying for a final exam that he just missed because of this seizure. He had been healthy until age 12 but then after a fall off a ladder, he began to have "eye fluttering" episodes. He has been treated with valproic acid. At one point he was off all medications, but the seizures returned, and so he restarted to the medication. He asks what you think is going on. At this time, the most appropriate response is:

(A) "I think that you faked this seizure to avoid taking a test."

(B) "Lack of sleep may have triggered this seizure."

(C) "You can expect to have tonic-clonic seizures on a regular basis from now on."

(D) "Your seizures are getting worse and there is not much we can do about it."

(E) "You should consider taking the next semester off to recover."

8. The wife and child of one of your patients known to have end-stage Huntington disease come to the clinic for counseling. The patient is a 42-year-old man whose father was affected with Huntington disease and whose mother was not. The patient, at present, requires 24-hour nursing care in a skilled facility because of frequent violent psychotic outbursts and cognitive and coordination difficulties that make it impossible for the patient to tend to his own activities of daily living. There is no history of Huntington disease on the patient's wife's side of the family. She asks you directly of the chances that the son will be affected with Huntington disease. Given the available history, and disregarding rates of mutation and crossing-over, the correct response is

(A) 0%

(B) 25%

(C) 50%

(D) 75%

(E) 100%

9. A 50-year-old woman comes to the clinic because of a 1-month history of stiffness in her neck that began after lifting weights for 2 consecutive days. She has been treating it with ibuprofen, but it has continued to get worse. It is most stiff in the morning and more severe when she is sitting or lying down than when standing up. She feels "sore" in her left shoulder and tells you that the pain radiates down her left neck to her upper back. Sometimes she feels "tingling" along the radial aspect of her left forearm and her left hand feels weak. Cold packs and hot showers provide some relief. She has also been taking hydrocodone and rofecoxib daily. In addition, a chiropractor has been treating her with ultrasound. Ten years ago she had neck pain, which was caused by lifting luggage into overhead bins when she worked as a flight attendant. She was on disability leave for 6 weeks, but has been doing better since then. She had chiropractic neck adjustments at that time and frequently since then, but her last chiropractic neck adjustment was over 6 months ago. She also reports that she was in a couple of motor-vehicle accidents many years ago and had some transient neck discomfort following them. Examination shows tenderness at the left superior trapezius, minimally restricted neck range of motion, and weakness of the left deltoid and biceps. Light touch, pinprick, and joint proprioception are all normal. Vibration is minimally decreased in the toes. Deep tendon reflex is absent at the left bicep. This patient's lesion is best described as

(A) an autonomic nervous system lesion

(B) a central nervous system lesion

(C) a paraneoplastic process

(D) a peripheral nervous system lesion

(E) a vascular process

10. A 44-year-old woman with multiple sclerosis comes to the office concerned that she is having a "flare." Two days ago she began to notice decreased sensation in the palm of the left hand that has gotten a little worse, especially when she exercises. Yesterday she noticed diminished sensation along the lower left trunk in the front and back. She has no pain, tingling, exacerbation of symptoms with neck movement, neck injury, incontinence, gait disturbance, diplopia, fever, chills, nausea, or vomiting. She initially presented 4 years ago with left-eye optic neuritis. She did not receive steroids at that time. Three years ago she had loss of sensation in her hands that progressed over weeks to motor involvement, limiting her ability to write with her right hand. She received steroids at that time. She began interferon beta-1A 4 years ago. One year ago she developed right-leg weakness, constipation, and urinary urgency. She received steroids at that time as well. Examination shows full visual fields with a left afferent pupillary defect as well as normal bulk, strength, and tone. Light touch is decreased over the left trunk and back, roughly at T8-T12 dermatomes. She has normal finger tapping, rapid alternating movements, finger-nose-finger, and heel tapping to shin. At this time the most appropriate pharmacologic treatment is

(A) interferon beta-1B
(B) corticosteroids
(C) gabapentin
(D) glatiramer
(E) pramipexole

11. A 42-year-old African American man comes to the emergency department with severe right-eye pain that came on suddenly as he was leaving his daughter's school play. He tells you that the pain is worse upon looking at light. He also reports blurred vision in that same eye as well as a severe headache in the frontal part of his head. His blood pressure is 130/90 mm Hg. Examination of his right eye reveals corneal edema and a fixed mid-dilated pupil. Intraocular pressure in the right eye is 40 mm Hg. The left eye is completely normal. Appropriate pharmacotherapy for this condition is

(A) intravenous acetazolamide
(B) gentamycin eye drops
(C) tetracaine eye drops
(D) topical prednisone
(E) tropicamide eye drops

12. You are working in a busy emergency department located near a well-known ski resort. A 30-year-old woman comes in complaining of decreased vision, bilateral eye pain, a sensation of "something in my eyes," and photophobia. She notes that her eyes are watering a great deal. She had been out skiing for several hours earlier that day. She has no prior history of ocular disorders and does not use contact lenses. Her only medical history is fibrocystic breast disease and she had an appendectomy as a child. She takes no medications and reports that she is allergic to penicillin. Her temperature is 37.0 C (98.6 F), blood pressure is 130/70 mm Hg, and pulse is 75/min. You note that she has first-degree sunburn over her entire face. Due to severe blepharospasm, which makes it difficult for her to cooperate with the slit lamp examination, you administer a topical anesthetic. About 10 seconds after placing the anesthetic drops, she blinks her eyes several times and remarks that her pain has completely resolved and that her vision seems more clear. Slit lamp examination with fluorescein dye reveals superficial punctate lesions. The most likely etiologic agent of her condition is

(A) herpes simplex virus
(B) particles of dust embedded in the cornea
(C) *Staphylococcus aureus*
(D) ultraviolet radiation
(E) varicella-zoster virus

13. A 20-year-old previously healthy woman comes to the urgent care clinic because of a 1-month history of headaches, nausea, and vomiting. The headaches are positional, particularly when she tries to bend forward, and are intense in the morning and at times wake her up at night. There are no other neurologic symptoms. A head CT scan is normal. During physical examination, particular attention should be paid to

(A) coordination examination
(B) deep tendon reflexes
(C) motor examination
(D) sensory examination
(E) visual field testing and funduscopy

14. A 57-year-old man comes to the clinic with complaints of weakness and tingling in his legs for 1 week. The symptoms began gradually over a couple of days and initially began in his feet. Over the next several days the weakness progressed to involve more proximal leg muscles to the point that the patient had some difficulty walking. He has had tingling as well. There are no complaints of bowel or bladder dysfunction. He had a gastrointestinal illness a few weeks prior to his current symptoms, but has otherwise been healthy. On physical examination, there is most likely to be

(A) absent reflexes
(B) homonymous hemianopia
(C) hyperactive reflexes
(D) normal motor findings
(E) a thoracic sensory level

15. A 60-year-old homeless man with hypertension and gout is brought to the emergency department by another homeless man after being found unresponsive. He does not take any medications. The patient begins to seize and you immediately secure his airway. His temperature is 37.2 C (99.1 F), blood pressure is 120/67 mm Hg, pulse is 105/min, and respirations are 32/min. A quick physical examination is unremarkable. A urine toxicology screen is negative. A serum toxicology screen is pending. You begin to administer thiamine, glucose, lorazepam, and phenytoin. Laboratory tests you sent earlier show a serum magnesium level of 1.5 mmol/L. You begin to administer magnesium sulfate intravenously and suddenly notice that the patient's blood pressure has fallen to 89/56 mm Hg. The most appropriate immediate intervention is to

(A) discontinue the glucose infusion
(B) discontinue the lorazepam load
(C) discontinue the magnesium infusion
(D) discontinue the phenytoin infusion
(E) discontinue the thiamine infusion

16. A 23-year-old woman is brought to the emergency department after she collapsed while standing in a line, laughing and joking with friends. She denies any loss of consciousness and is able to state in her own words a detailed account of what happened. She denies any pain or any other symptoms, and except for being scared, she feels fine. She is worried that she has "epilepsy or something," even though she has never had a similar "attack" in the past. Her grandmother had a similar problem. Physical and neurologic examination is unremarkable. Routine laboratory studies and a pregnancy test are negative. An electrocardiogram is normal. On further questioning you learn that she has had difficulties at work in the past several weeks because she felt "so sleepy" during the day, but she did not pay much attention to it until now. At this time you should

(A) assure her that this was most likely a vasovagal syncope and she will be fine
(B) call a neurology consult to evaluate for narcolepsy
(C) call psychiatry because the woman may have conversion disorder
(D) order a standard electroencephalogram
(E) release her home because this was most likely an episode of transitory weakness because of exhaustion

17. A 2-year-old girl is brought to the emergency department following a generalized seizure that lasted 2 minutes. Her mother states that she had had a fever for the preceding 2 days and has been pulling on her right ear. She also tells you that she herself had seizures when she had a fever as a child but she "outgrew them." The child's rectal temperature is 39.7 C (103.4 F). She is now alert with a normal neurologic examination. Physical examination is significant for a right otitis media. The most appropriate next step in management is to

(A) order a head CT
(B) order a neurologic consultation
(C) perform EEG
(D) perform tympanocentesis
(E) prescribe antibiotics and antipyretics and provide reassurance

18. A 9-year-old boy from Hong Kong is brought to the emergency department, very ill with symptoms of fever, vomiting, and lethargy. Mild nuchal rigidity is noted on examination, so a sepsis workup is initiated and a lumbar puncture is performed. The cerebrospinal fluid findings include an elevated opening pressure, 250 white cells/μL (predominantly lymphocytes), decreased glucose, and elevated protein. A CT scan of the head shows hydrocephalus. These results suggest that the best management for this child should include

(A) ampicillin and cefotaxime
(B) ceftriaxone and vancomycin
(C) isoniazid, rifampin, pyrazinamide, and streptomycin
(D) observation in the hospital without therapy
(E) surgery

19. A 67-year-old man with diabetes mellitus, congestive heart failure, and hypertension comes to the emergency department because of a severe headache. His wife explains that he fell yesterday while getting out of the bathtub and he was able to stand up on his own after 2 minutes but complained of severe headache. There was no external injury noted at the time. He is compliant with his medications, which include digoxin, a calcium channel blocker, and warfarin. Physical and neurologic examinations are unremarkable. A CT scan of the head is normal. The patient continues to complain of a headache without any neurologic deficit and is admitted to the medical floor for observation. On admission to the floor, he is noted to have a blood pressure of 180/100 mm Hg and blood glucose of 150 mg/dL. He is started on intravenous hydration and advised to continue his regular medications. You are called to the floor by the nurse because the patient is complaining of a severe, worsening headache. His vital signs have been stable since arrival on the floor. On approaching the patient, you notice that his mental status has significantly altered. He is less responsive and is not able to follow commands. His pupils are equal bilaterally and reactive to light. He is actively moving his four extremities, although there seems to be decrease in the motor power in the upper extremities. The most likely explanation for the worsening of the patient's symptoms is a

(A) cerebral contusion
(B) diabetic coma
(C) hypertensive crisis
(D) subarachnoid hemorrhage
(E) subdural hematoma

20. A 42-year-old African American man is brought to the emergency department because of a severe, "bursting" headache. He has a history of well-controlled hypertension and is being treated with a calcium channel blocker. His blood pressure is 130/90 mm Hg and pulse is 75/min. No focal neurologic deficits are noted at this time. While waiting for initial evaluation and laboratory studies, his consciousness rapidly deteriorates. Initial laboratory studies are unremarkable. A CT scan of the head is inconclusive and does not show signs of a subarachnoid hemorrhage or subdural hematoma. The most appropriate next step in management is to

(A) admit him to the hospital for neurologic observation
(B) order cerebral angiography
(C) perform a lumbar puncture
(D) send him for a magnetic resonance angiogram
(E) repeat the CT scan of the head in 24 hours

21. A 76-year-old man with hypertension is brought to the emergency department because of a 4-hour history of left-sided weakness and difficulty speaking. He routinely takes nifedipine and hydrochlorothiazide. Vital signs are: temperature 37.0 C (98.6 F), blood pressure 180/95 mm Hg, pulse 78/min, respirations 16/min, and oxygen saturation 98% on room air. Physical examination shows a left facial droop and left upper and lower extremity weakness. There are no audible carotid bruits. The rest of the examination is unremarkable. A CT scan of the head shows an ischemic stroke in the right internal capsule. An electrocardiogram shows normal sinus rhythm with no other abnormalities. The most appropriate next step in the management is to

(A) administer intravenous heparin
(B) administer intravenous labetalol to lower blood pressure
(C) administer intravenous tPA
(D) give oral aspirin
(E) give oral warfarin

22. As you are driving to the hospital, you notice a young man suddenly fall to the ground convulsing. You stop your car and rush to his assistance while a passerby goes to summon emergency services. Unfortunately, he has aspirated during the convulsion, and despite your best efforts, you are unable to clear the airway and he succumbs before help arrives. This act would make you

(A) liable for disciplinary action by the American Medical Association
(B) liable for disciplinary action by the state medical board
(C) liable for a lawsuit, as you were grossly negligent while trying to secure the airway
(D) liable for a lawsuit, as you were responsible for his death
(E) not liable for a lawsuit, as it would have happened anyway

23. A 70-year-old man comes to the emergency department with a sudden onset of speech difficulty that started 6 hours ago. He has hypertension and coronary artery disease, and smokes a pack of cigarettes a day. When you talk to him he appears very frustrated because he understands everything that you say but has great difficulty speaking back to you. This patient's condition is most likely located in the region of the brain supplied by the

(A) basilar artery
(B) left middle cerebral artery
(C) left vertebral artery
(D) right anterior cerebral artery
(E) right posterior cerebral artery

24. A 30-year-old man comes to the clinic complaining of "episodes" of severe, right-sided headaches. He tells you that his headaches have been occurring for the past 7 years and are periodic in nature. During the most recent episode, the headaches occurred on most days over a 2-month period and usually lasted for about an hour. The most likely diagnosis is

(A) cluster headache
(B) migraine headache
(C) temporal arteritis
(D) tension headache
(E) trigeminal neuralgia

25. A 6-month-old little boy is brought into your office for a well-child checkup. His family recently moved to this city and this is your first encounter with him. His mother says that his birth history was unremarkable; he was full-term and born via normal spontaneous vaginal delivery. However, at 3 months of age he began having seizurelike activity and was diagnosed with infantile spasms by a neurologist. His mother states that there is a maternal uncle in the family with tuberous sclerosis. The cutaneous finding that you are most likely to discover on your initial physical examination is

(A) ash leaf macules
(B) axillary freckling
(C) café-au-lait spots
(D) Lisch nodules
(E) a port wine stain

26. A 62-year-old right-handed man with hypertension comes to the emergency department with symptoms and signs consistent with a stroke. He admits to smoking a pack of cigarettes a day for 30 years. His brother had a stroke at the age of 56 years. On physical examination he is alert and orientated to place and person only. His temperature is 37.0 C (98.6 F), blood pressure is 192/95 mm Hg, pulse is 100/min, and respirations are 20/min. He has right-sided hemiparesis and is aphasic. There are no other significant signs. At this time, the most immediate management in the emergency department would include

(A) beginning an intravenous heparin infusion
(B) giving parenteral corticosteroids
(C) monitoring oxygenation status with pulse oximetry
(D) prompt lowering of systolic blood pressure to less than 140 mm Hg
(E) restricting oral fluid intake to 75 cc/hr

27. A 70-year-old man with a long-standing progressive multiple sclerosis is now only able to move his little toe. He is not interested in "continuing like this" any longer, and has been informed that his illness is progressive and terminal. His wife and adult children agree with his decision. In fact, on one occasion, he managed to get disconnected from the life support systems, but was reconnected soon after by the nurses, who rushed in upon hearing the alarms go off. He pleaded with them to let him die with dignity. He petitions the court to end his reliance on the life support systems. The most likely outcome would be that the courts would

    (A) accede to his request
    (B) refer the matter to an expert panel for deliberation
    (C) seek the opinion of the clergy
    (D) seek the opinion of human rights groups
    (E) turn down his request

28. A 42-year-old woman comes to the office because of a tremor that has become more bothersome. She thinks it originally began as a very mild tremor 12 years ago. It typically affects her hands and head and usually occurs when she moves her extremities. She tells you that she makes sure to drink one or two alcoholic beverages every day because alcohol seems to lessen the tremor. Her mother suffered from a similar disorder. Neurologic examination is essentially normal other than the tremor. The movement disorder that this patient most likely has is

    (A) alcoholic withdrawal tremor
    (B) cerebellar tremor
    (C) essential tremor
    (D) parkinsonian tremor
    (E) psychogenic tremor

29. A 35-year-old woman had a brief loss of consciousness that prompted a recent visit to the emergency room. She now comes to the clinic 2 days later for followup. When reading the discharge summary report from the emergency room you note that no tonic-clonic activity was observed, nor did the patient experience urinary or fecal incontinence. She does recall that 10 seconds before "blacking out" she felt nauseated, began sweating, and became pale. She had no memory loss or confusion on recovery. Her vital signs at the time were: temperature 37.0 C (98.6 F), blood pressure 135/75 mm Hg, pulse 72/min, and respirations 16/min. Her neurologic examination was normal. Laboratory studies including a complete blood count and an electrocardiogram were all within normal limits. At this time, the most appropriate next step in management is to

    (A) order a CT scan of the head
    (B) order an echocardiogram
    (C) order an electroencephalogram
    (D) provide reassurance
    (E) recommend 24-hour Holter monitoring

Items 30-31

A 52-year-old Japanese woman business executive comes to the clinic complaining of painful, burning dysesthesias in her hands and feet for the past 2 years. She has a past medical history of ovarian cancer successfully treated with chemotherapy. She denies a history of diabetes mellitus and a hemoglobin A1c from 6 months ago was normal. She is currently on no medications. Physical examination shows diffuse sensory peripheral neuropathy. Her strength, tone, and reflexes are otherwise normal.

30. In trying to establish a cause of her symptoms, a useful question to ask at this time is:

    (A) "Do you drink alcohol?"
    (B) "Have you been feeling tired recently?"
    (C) "Have you been very thirsty recently?"
    (D) "Have you injured yourself recently?"
    (E) "What do you take for the pain?"

31. She then asks you, "Are there any medications that I might try to help out with the numbness?" A useful medication for the treatment of chronic neuropathy in this patient is

    (A) amiloride
    (B) amiodarone
    (C) amitriptyline
    (D) amlodipine
    (E) gabapentin

32. While examining an 88-year-old woman at a local large nursing home facility you encounter the medical director of the facility, who tells you that she wishes to identify which elderly patients are at risk for developing Alzheimer dementia. She explains that historically about half of the patients in this particular facility develop Alzheimer dementia. She says that after searching the recent medical literature she was able to identify five screening tests. The characteristics of the five identified tests are presented below:

	Sensitivity	Specificity	Positive Predictive Value	Negative Predictive Value
Test A:	0.80	0.71	0.73	0.78
Test B:	0.93	0.65	0.73	0.90
Test C:	0.72	0.94	0.92	0.77
Test D:	0.85	0.85	0.85	0.85
Test E:	0.89	0.99	0.99	0.90

If the medical director wants to be most certain of identifying all of the patients who are at risk for developing Alzheimer dementia, the test that she should use is

(A) Test A
(B) Test B
(C) Test C
(D) Test D
(E) Test E

---

33. You are seeing a 32-year-old woman in the emergency department after she suffered a "spell." Witnesses describe that the patient began to talk gibberish, and then was staring with a blank look on her face for 2 minutes. She was unresponsive during this time, and witnesses reported some right facial twitching. Afterwards, the patient was noted to be somewhat sleepy and confused, and had complaints of a mild headache. This resolved over 30 to 45 minutes. The patient has no recollection of the events. Physical examination is normal. The most likely diagnosis is

(A) complex partial seizure
(B) hypoglycemic episode
(C) migraine headache
(D) simple partial seizure
(E) transient ischemic attack

34. A 16-year-old golfer comes to see you for a sports examination before an upcoming tournament. He is of good health and there have been no new problems to report since his last visit 2 years ago. He has not been sexually active recently and denies any substance abuse. An updated family history reveals that his mother has some kind of medical problem and is seeing a neurologist. His mother's older sister has some problem with her legs and is in a wheelchair. When asked about his golf game the boy says he is fairly good and enjoys golf because he does not have to run. He tells you that for some reason in the last year or so it has been more difficult for him to run than it is for his friends. Golf is much more leisurely and practice makes perfect. Occasionally if he overdoes the golf swing he notices that his hands feel weak and tingly, but this does not happen very often. On physical examination, his deep tendon reflexes are noticeably decreased in the ankles compared with the knees. Mild decrease in muscle bulk of the anterior calf muscles is apparent and there is atrophy of the muscles in both hands. The remainder of the examination is unremarkable. An electromyogram shows slowed nerve conduction. The best test to confirm the diagnosis of this patient's condition is

(A) a biopsy of the sural nerve
(B) CPK levels
(C) drug screening
(D) lead levels
(E) Tensilon testing

35. A 63-year-old man is admitted to the hospital at 2 AM with left-eye pain and the acute onset of decreased vision. He states that he is seeing halos around lights. On physical examination he has conjunctival injection of the left eye, fluorescein stain is negative, and funduscopic examination is difficult because of some clouding of the cornea. His visual acuity, which is usually 20/20, is now 20/100 in the left eye and normal in the right. The intraocular pressure on the left is elevated by tonometric examination. At this time the most appropriate statement about his condition is:

(A) Enucleation will likely be required
(B) No treatment is necessary
(C) Ophthalmology consultation first thing in the morning is indicated
(D) Topical erythromycin four times per day to the left eye should be applied
(E) Topical pilocarpine, beta-blocker, and alpha-2-agonist to the left eye should be applied and intravenous acetazolamide administered

36. A 9-month-old infant has been failing to achieve the expected developmental motor milestones over the past several months. On examination he appears to have some decreased tone and both lower extremities reveal hyperreflexia and ankle clonus. There is persistence of the Moro and asymmetric tonic neck reflex (ATNR). You decide he most likely has cerebral palsy. As you make a referral to the neurologist, you discuss the probable diagnosis with the parents. They want to understand why. At this time you should tell them that

(A) cerebral palsy correlates with low APGAR scores
(B) cerebral palsy is probably a genetic disorder
(C) cerebral palsy is usually associated with perinatal asphyxia
(D) children with cerebral palsy are usually born premature and small for gestational age
(E) children with cerebral palsy are usually full-term infants and appropriate for gestational age

37. You are called to see a 67-year-old woman who was admitted to the hospital with unstable angina because of acute right-sided visual disturbance. She underwent cardiac catherization earlier in the day, which showed severe 3-vessel coronary artery disease and an ejection fraction of 40%. A recommendation was made for bypass grafting. She states that approximately 10 minutes ago she had the abrupt loss of vision in her right eye, which felt like a "shade coming down over her eye." She has no pain or discomfort in the eye and she denies any "floaters" or flashing lights. Her temperature is 37.0 C (98.6 F), blood pressure is 120/80 mm Hg, pulse rate is 80/min, and respirations are 20/min. Visual acuity in the left eye is 20/20, and she can only see fingers 3 inches in front of her right eye. Extraocular movements are intact, there is very minimal pupillary reaction on the right, and there is no conjunctival irritation noted. On fundoscopic examination the arteries appear thin and attenuated, and some whitening of the retina is present. Cardiac examination reveals a regular rate, with no murmurs, rubs, or gallops. Lungs are clear to auscultation. Just as you are finishing her examination, her symptoms completely resolve. The most appropriate management of this patient is to

(A) administer systemic thrombolytics
(B) perform carotid ultrasound prior to surgery
(C) perform coronary artery bypass grafting as scheduled in the morning
(D) perform emergent carotid angiogram
(E) perform emergent MRI of the brain

38. A 47-year-old man comes to the clinic because he has been "having problems walking" for 4 months. His symptoms began after a fall, in which he injured his neck and had significant neck pain. The pain still persists, but has improved with over-the-counter pain medications. Physical examination shows increased tone in his lower extremities and absent bicep reflexes bilaterally. There is some patchy sensory loss up to the patient's nipple line. He has a spastic gait. The most appropriate next step in evaluation is to order

(A) an electromyogram (EMG) and nerve conduction studies
(B) a lumbar puncture
(C) an MRI of the brain
(D) an MRI of the cervical spine
(E) an MRI of the lumbar spine

39. You have been taking care of a 25-year-old Caucasian woman with neurofibromatosis type I for the past 5 years. Her mother and grandfather have also been diagnosed with neurofibromatosis, albeit expressed to a very mild degree in all three family members. Neither one of them has had any serious complications from the disorder. She is very happy with your care and calls to ask if you would see a relative visiting from abroad and examine him to determine whether he has the same disorder. Their families had been separated during World War II and it seems that only the ones who have settled in the United States have the disease. You agree to see this patient and several days later a 45-year-old man with no significant medical history comes for an office visit. On physical examination, you notice that he has freckling of the axillary and inguinal regions and a 3×5 cm café-au-lait macule on the lower back. The diagnosis of neurofibromatosis type I in this patient can be confirmed by finding

(A) ash leaf macules
(B) bamboo hair
(C) skin and retinal angiomas
(D) subtle, faint, hypochromic or atrophic Blaschko-linear lesions on the extremities
(E) two or more Lisch nodules

40. A 36-year-old man with Down syndrome is brought to the clinic by his social worker because of a "decrement in functioning." He has been able to live semi-independently in a supportive group setting for most of his adult life. He has also worked in an assisted vocational program for the past 6 years. For the past few months he has become increasingly forgetful at his job, has been wandering off of the grounds of the residence and getting lost, and has demonstrated a noticeably more limited vocabulary when he speaks. The patient has no past medical history and the results of chemistries, complete blood count, thyroid function tests, vitamin B_{12}, and folate levels are all within normal limits. This patient's dementing process is most consistent with

(A) dementia secondary to renal failure
(B) Huntington dementia
(C) Parkinson dementia
(D) senile dementia, Alzheimer type
(E) vascular dementia

41. A 32-year-old woman comes to the office complaining of a 24-hour history of numbness on the medial side of the left leg and foot. She denies any history of trauma. Recently she has been having some mild discomfort and backache in the lower part of the spine but she thought that it is related to her new mattress and so she ignored it. No pain is reported in any other joints or extremities. On palpation, there is mild tenderness in the lower spine. No associated neurologic deficit is elicited in the right lower extremity. Examination of the left lower extremity demonstrated no patellar tendon reflex and weakness of the tibialis anterior muscle. At this time the most appropriate diagnostic test is

(A) a bone scan
(B) a CT scan of the lumbar spine
(C) an electromyogram
(D) an MRI of the lumbar spine
(E) x-rays of the lumbar spine

42. A 54-year-old chronic smoker comes to the clinic with a 3-week history of a drooping right eyelid. The onset of the "drooping" was gradual and first noticed by his wife. He also notes decreased sweating on the right side of his face. He suffered a stroke 2 years ago but did not have any residual paresis or symptoms. On physical examination he has ptosis of the right upper lid and miosis of the right pupil; extraocular muscle movements are intact. The remainder of the physical and neurologic examination is normal. The most appropriate next step in management is to

(A) determine acetylcholine receptor antibody level
(B) determine fasting blood glucose level
(C) order a chest x-ray
(D) order a [^{131}I] thyroid scan
(E) order an MRI scan of the brain and orbits

43. A 20-year-old woman comes to the student health center after collapsing at the local coffee shop. She was hanging out with friends and they were laughing at a joke when she suddenly collapsed. She describes losing muscle tone when she fell but was otherwise fully aware of what happened. She denies any loss of consciousness. She has had a 3-month history of increased daytime sleepiness and several times a few of her professors caught her asleep in class. She thinks that the daytime sleeping episodes are due to poor night sleep secondary to vivid dreams she has upon falling asleep. Her medical and developmental history is unremarkable. Her father has had similar symptoms in the past. Physical and neurological examination is normal. Laboratory studies are unremarkable. To diagnose this disorder you should

    (A) obtain electromyography
    (B) obtain a multiple sleep latency study
    (C) order a CT scan of the brain
    (D) order electrocardiography
    (E) order HLA testing

44. You are seeing a 48-year-old obese woman with complaints of numbness and tingling in her right hand and arm. She has a history of fairly controlled diabetes mellitus but is otherwise healthy. She reports that she has had these symptoms for several months now and that they are worse at night. Over the past few weeks, she has had some clumsiness of her right hand as well. Her current symptoms have begun to affect her job as a computer programmer, which she has done for 10 years. The examination is significant for decreased sensation to pinprick in the first three digits of her right hand. No atrophy is seen. All reflexes are present, normal, and symmetric. The most likely diagnosis is

    (A) brachial plexopathy
    (B) carpal tunnel syndrome
    (C) cervical spondylosis
    (D) diabetic peripheral neuropathy
    (E) stroke

45. A 34-year-old woman has visual loss and pain in her right eye. Her symptoms began approximately 2 weeks ago as eye discomfort and blurry vision and have progressed over several days to significant visual loss. She describes eye pain and pain with movement of her eyes. She wears glasses normally, but they have not helped with her complaints. On examination, she has normal vision in her left eye, but 20/200 in her right eye. There is a relative, afferent, papillary defect on the right. On funduscopic exam, the optic disc appears swollen on the right. The next most appropriate question to ask to help establish the diagnosis is:

    (A) "Does anyone in the family have similar symptoms?"
    (B) "Do you smoke?"
    (C) "Have you had any head trauma?"
    (D) "Have you had any previous episodes of visual loss or other neurologic symptoms?"
    (E) "How long have you worn glasses?"

46. An 80-year-old woman has a 2-week history of a headache. She states that her headache is over her left temple area. She has also noticed pain when she eats and when she combs her hair. Upon further questioning, she admits that she has had some blurring of her vision over the past several days. Her symptoms have been continuous since onset and do not seem to get better with over-the-counter pain medications. On review of systems, she reports some low-grade fevers and a 5 to 7-lb. weight loss over the past several weeks. The most likely diagnosis is

    (A) a brain tumor
    (B) giant-cell arteritis
    (C) a migraine headache
    (D) a pseudotumor cerebri
    (E) a subarachnoid hemorrhage

47. A 57-year-old woman with diabetes mellitus and hypothyroidism comes to the office because of left-hand numbness, tingling, and weakness. She reports that the symptoms have been going on for several months and have been getting progressively more severe. Her symptoms are worse in the evening. She has no other known medical problems, does not smoke or drink, and has worked as a switchboard operator for the past 23 years. Physical examination shows weakness in her left thumb abduction and atrophy of the thenar eminence. There is diminished sensation over the first three digits of her left hand. All reflexes are present and symmetric. Otherwise, her neurologic and physical examination is normal. The most appropriate next step in diagnosis is to order

(A) a CT scan of the brain
(B) an electromyogram (EMG) and nerve conduction studies
(C) a lumbar puncture
(D) an MRI of the brain
(E) an MRI of the cervical spine

48. You are visited in your clinic by a 47-year-old woman who has a 25-year history of headaches. The first headache that she remembers occurred about 1 week after an automobile accident during which she hit her head on the windshield. The headaches are characterized by a throbbing pain behind one eye and they are usually accompanied by nausea and sensitivity to light, smells, and sounds. They are sometimes severe enough to keep her in bed up to 3 days. She has no sensory, motor, or visual auras. She gets 8 to 10 headaches per month, which all occur during the same week. Her last headache was 2 to 3 weeks ago. She treats them with sumatriptan injection, which works over 80% of the time. If she feels some initial pressure behind her eye, she may be able to abort the headache with diphenhydramine. In the past she had done well with only aspirin, but developed a gastric ulcer. Amitriptyline and verapamil were not effective prophylactically. She believes that the headaches are triggered by lack of sleep, smoke-filled rooms, weather changes, and wine, and that they are not related to menstruation. Her past history includes high cholesterol, and peptic ulcer disease. Her only medication is atorvastatin daily. She has had worsening problems with daytime sleepiness over the past 5 years and she is now taking afternoon naps. She snores at night and has gained weight over that time. She has no known drug allergies, works as a kindergarten teacher, and lives with her husband and twin 14-year-old daughters. She does not smoke or use alcohol or drugs. Her mother has high cholesterol, father has lung cancer, and sister suffers from headaches with a visual aura. The pharmacologic treatment that will most help this patient is

(A) daily propranolol
(B) metaxalone daily
(C) oral corticosteroids
(D) oxycodone as needed
(E) propranolol at headache onset

49. A 26-year-old college student comes to the emergency department after 2 days of fevers, night sweats, light sensitivity, and a mild headache. He has no past medical history. Vital signs are: temperature 39.1 C (102.4 F), blood pressure 120/50 mm Hg, pulse 120/min, and respirations 12/min. He is drowsy, but alert and oriented to person, place, and time. The oropharynx is clear, extraocular movements are intact, and the pupils are equal and reactive. There is no cervical lymphadenopathy. The heart, lung, and abdominal examinations are normal. The neurologic examination reveals 4/5 weakness in the upper extremities bilaterally with normal strength in the lower extremities. Cranial nerves are intact and sensation is normal. Reflexes are 2+ in both upper and lower extremities. Ophthalmologic examination is normal. Laboratory studies show:

Blood	
Leukocyte count	39,200/mm^3
Bands	25%
Hematocrit	46%
Platelets	213,000/mm^3
Serum	
Sodium	136 mEq/L
Potassium	4.5 mEq/L
Chloride	98 mEq/L
Bicarbonate	24 mEq/L
Creatinine	0.5 mg/dL

The most appropriate next step in managing this patient is to

(A) administer antibiotics, intravenously
(B) send spinal fluid for analysis and culture and await results
(C) order an MRI of the brain
(D) order an x-ray of the abdomen
(E) order an x-ray of the chest

50. Emergency medical services (EMS) rushes a 17-year-old football player to the emergency department after he took a "helmet-to-helmet hit" and fell backwards onto his head. The patient lost consciousness for approximately 1 to 2 minutes. EMS states that from the field to the hospital the patient's vital signs were completely normal and that they noted only confusion. The patient is still confused and is unable to recall any of the events of the evening. On examination, he is sitting up on a stretcher rubbing his neck. His vital signs are normal. There is no backboard or cervical collar noted on examination. He is alert and oriented to person, place, and time; however, he cannot recall the events of the football game. His neck is tender to palpation in the midline, and flexion and extension are not checked. With the exception of some mild weakness of the patient's right biceps and lateral arm numbness there are no other findings. The most appropriate next step in management is to

(A) admit the patient to the hospital for observation because he has sustained a severe concussion
(B) inform the patient and his family that the patient has sustained a very mild concussion and that when his family takes him home they should watch him closely for any headaches, nausea, or vomiting
(C) obtain stabilization of the patient's cervical spine (place a c-collar on), obtain radiographs of the cervical spine, and inform all caregivers not to move the patient without using spine precautions
(D) schedule a CT scan of the patient's head for Monday morning at the radiology center
(E) send him home but tell him he is not allowed to play football for 1 week

Neurology Test Two: **Answers and Explanations**

ANSWER KEY

1. C
2. A
3. B
4. A
5. E
6. B
7. B
8. C
9. D
10. B
11. A
12. D
13. E
14. A
15. D
16. B
17. E
18. C
19 E
20. C
21. D
22. E
23. B
24. A
25. A
26. C
27. A
28. C
29. D
30. A
31. C
32. B
33. A
34. A
35. E
36. E
37. B
38 D
39. E
40. D
41. D
42. C
43. B
44. B
45. D
46. B
47. B
48. A
49. A
50. C

1. **The correct answer is C.** Migraines are commonly preceded by visual phenomena, which can include flashing lights, visual blurring, or visual field cuts. First-line therapy for migraines is a nonsteroidal antiinflammatory agent. These agents may or may not be effective and if not, then the patient can try sumatriptan (or another triptan) or ergotamine.

   When a patient gives a classic history for migraine headaches, neuroimaging studies do not need to be performed (**choice A**). If the headache is atypical or if the usual treatments fail, then the clinician can consider neuroimaging studies.

   These are not psychiatric phenomena and will not respond to anti-psychotic medications, such as haloperidol (**choice B**).

   Since the patient has a classic history, she does not need to return for a repeat examination during the episode (**choice D**).

   Acetaminophen usually does not alleviate the pain of a migraine headache (**choice E**).

2. **The correct answer is A.** According to the American College of Rheumatology, criteria for classification of temporal arteritis includes meeting three of the following five criteria: age over 50, new onset headache, temporal artery abnormality (tenderness or reduced pulsation), ESR over 50 mm/hour, and a positive temporal artery biopsy. This patient meets the first three criteria and a diagnosis of temporal artery diagnosis can be made clinically. A frequent and devastating manifestation of temporal arteritis is anterior ischemic optic neuropathy, which presents as unilateral vision loss, a swollen optic nerve, and an afferent papillary defect. This entity can quickly involve the other eye within a few hours to days; therefore observation (**choice C**) would be grounds for a malpractice suit. Once a diagnosis of temporal arteritis is obtained (or possibly even considered) systemic steroids should be instituted immediately to prevent anterior ischemic optic neuropathy as well as other complications of temporal arteritis.

   There is no available ophthalmic surgical intervention for anterior ischemic optic neuropathy (**choice B**).

   For the routine patient with temporal arteritis, neuroimaging is not indicated (**choice D**). If both optic nerves were swollen, stat neuroimaging would be obtained to rule out an intracranial mass.

   An erythrocyte sedimentation rate (ESR) (**choice E**) is indicated, but even if it were normal the provider still must start the patient on systemic steroids. A normal ESR does not rule out the diagnosis. The most appropriate next step in management would be to treat the patient and then obtain studies including ESR, a complete blood count, and a temporal artery biopsy.

3. **The correct answer is B.** This patient needs a brain CT or MRI urgently. She is presenting with a typical presentation for hydrocephalus, although other intracranial pathology such as brain tumor is also possible. By next month (**choice A**) there may be irreversible damage done or she may be dead.

   Oxybutynin (**choice C**) inhibits the muscarinic action of acetylcholine on smooth muscle. It will probably improve her incontinence, but will not treat the problem with her brain.

   Electromyography and nerve conduction studies (**choice D**) are used to diagnose peripheral nerve, neuromuscular junction, and muscle disease.

   A urologic consultation (**choice E**) will not be helpful as there is most likely a brain problem that must be addressed.

4. **The correct answer is A.** Donepezil would be the best choice for this patient. There is no hepatotoxic potential. The GI side effects are appreciably lower with donepezil than either galantamine and especially compared with rivastigmine. Another advantage is once-a-day dosing compared to the BID dosing schedule of galantamine and rivastigmine.

   Galantamine (**choice B**) is also contraindicated in patients with severe hepatic and renal impairment. As with tacrine, the patient is not an appropriate candidate.

   Although there is no cure for Alzheimer disease, recent clinical trials have shown that cholinesterase inhibitors have been proven most effective for symptomatic treatment of mild to moderate Alzheimer disease. They seem to stabilize the condition overall, reduce caregiver burden, and delay nursing-home placement. As such, doing nothing (**choice C**) is not appropriate.

   Rivastigmine (**choice D**) does not carry the warning for hepatotoxicity as the medicines above. However, there are now warnings about the potential for GI side effects included in the package since reports of severe vomiting and esophageal rupture have appeared in case reports. Compared to donepezil or galantamine, the rate of discontinuation of rivastigmine is nearly three times higher than placebo (15%) versus 5% and 7%, respectively, of the first two mentioned medications.

Tacrine (**choice E**) was the first approved treatment for Alzheimer disease, in 1993. It is rarely prescribed today due to the potential for serious hepatotoxicity. Regular liver function test monitoring is warranted if this medicine is initiated. With the patient already having moderate to severe hepatic impairment from his past drinking, this medicine would not be a great choice.

5. **The correct answer is E.** This patient has multiple vascular risk factors and gives a good history for posterior circulation transient ischemic attacks. This is a typical presentation. A full cerebrovascular evaluation should be performed.

   He does not give a history suggestive of a cardiac etiology (**choice A**). Had he mentioned chest pain or palpitations this would be more suspicious. It is possible that a cardiac arrhythmia in conjunction with a posterior circulation stenosis may cause this presentation. However, this is not the best choice.

   If you suspected seizures, an electroencephalogram may be diagnostic (**choice B**). He did not have any loss of consciousness, personality changes, hallucinations, or rhythmic movements suggestive of seizures.

   Since there are other neurologic features (dysarthria) to this case and he has vascular risk factors, it is unlikely that this patient's symptoms are due to a peripheral nervous system problem (**choice C**).

   Meclizine (**choice D**) is indicated for the prophylaxis of motion sickness. It has a limited role in the treatment of peripheral vertigo. However, this patient should receive a full cerebrovascular evaluation and should not be prescribed meclizine.

6. **The correct answer is B.** The triad of normal pressure hydrocephalus is urinary incontinence, mental status changes, and gait disturbance. These are all due to stretching of frontal lobe tracts.

   Deep tendon reflexes (**choice A**) may be useful to distinguish an upper motor neuron from a lower motor neuron lesion.

   Nystagmus (**choice C**) on end gaze is present in many normal individuals. There are pathologic types of nystagmus associated with vestibular or brainstem lesions.

   Pinprick sensation (**choice D**) should be evaluated particularly carefully if you suspect a peripheral neuropathy, peripheral sensory nerve lesion, or central lesion to the spinal-thalamic-cortical system.

   Cranial nerve I (**choice E**) should be carefully tested if the patient reports any smell abnormality or if damage along the olfactory pathway is suspected.

7. **The correct answer is B.** Lack of sleep is a common seizure trigger. There is no reason to believe that he faked the seizure (**choice A**). It is impossible to predict his future seizure course (**choice C**) based on this one event. Just because he had one seizure we don't know for sure that his seizures are getting worse, and if they are there are many treatments available (**choice D**). There is no reason for him to take a prolonged leave of absence from school because of one seizure (**choice E**). This may even have detrimental psychological consequences.

8. **The correct answer is C.** Huntington disease is a terribly disabling neuropsychiatric condition that is characterized by a choreiform movement disorder and a myriad of psychiatric manifestations that may include depression, dementia, anxiety, and psychosis. Transmission of this disease is autosomal dominant, so the patient's son inherits a 50/50 chance of inheriting Huntington disease from his father, not a 75% chance (**choice D**).

   There would be a 0% (**choice A**) chance of the patient's son inheriting Huntington disease if the condition were X-linked dominant, meaning that the patient's son would have inherited a healthy gene from his unaffected mother.

   Autosomal recessive conditions with both parents being unaffected carriers confer a 25% risk (**choice B**) of transmission to offspring.

   If the patient were homozygous for the gene causing Huntington disease (meaning that both of the parents would have to have been affected with Huntington and both passed their Huntington gene to the patient), then the patient's son would have a 100% (**choice E**) chance of acquiring Huntington disease.

9. **The correct answer is D.** This patient has a typical presentation for a C5 radiculopathy, probably from a herniated disk related to the weight-lifting. Since nerve root and not cord pathology causes these symptoms, it is a peripheral nervous system lesion. A central nervous system lesion (**choice B**) such as at the spinal cord would be expected to increase reflexes and cause weakness primarily of extensor muscles in the upper extremities (biceps would be relatively spared).

Autonomic nervous system lesions (**choice A**) cause problems with blood pressure, sweating, and gastrointestinal mobility. These include diabetic gastroparesis.

Paraneoplastic processes (**choice C**) include limbic encephalitis and cerebellar degeneration. They are caused by malignancy-associated antibodies.

Vascular processes (**choice E**) include vasculitis which can appear to present as multiple radiculopathies. However, with one radiculopathy and a clear antecedent event it is very unlikely to be the diagnosis in this case.

10. **The correct answer is B.** Corticosteroids are an appropriate treatment for a multiple sclerosis flare-up. They will reduce the length and severity of the flare-up in most cases, although they are not likely to change the long-term disease outcome.

Interferon beta-1B (**choice A**) and glatiramer (**choice D**) are appropriate treatments to reduce the frequency of multiple sclerosis flares; however, they are not useful for the acute treatment of a flare.

Gabapentin (**choice C**) is an anticonvulsant medication which is also useful for the treatment of "neuropathic" pain, such as burning and allodynia. It will not help a multiple sclerosis flare.

Pramipexole (**choice E**) is a dopamine agonist used to treat parkinsonism. It has no role in the treatment of multiple sclerosis.

11. **The correct answer is A.** This patient has acute angle closure glaucoma which occurs secondary to blockage of aqueous humor outflow. This crowding is caused by the interaction of a shallow anterior chamber and a mid dilated pupil. Intravenous acetazolamide and topical timolol (beta-blocker) will decrease aqueous humor production and decrease the intraocular pressure. Pilocarpine eye drops (cholinergic agent) cause pupil constriction and decrease the outflow obstruction. An ophthalmology consult should be sought as soon as possible.

Gentamycin eye drops (**choice B**) are not indicated, as infection is not related to glaucoma nor is it a complication.

Tetracaine (**choice C**) is a local anesthetic that is used when examining a patient with a corneal abrasion. It has no role in the treatment of acute angle closure glaucoma.

Topical prednisone (**choice D**) is not indicated in the treatment of acute angle closure glaucoma. It is used in acute iritis, which is differentiated by normal intraocular pressure and cell and flare on slit lamp exam of the anterior chamber.

Tropicamide (**choice E**) is an anticholinergic agent that will dilate the pupil and worsen the pupillary block and the glaucoma.

12. **The correct answer is D.** Her condition, ultraviolet keratoconjunctivitis, is one of the most common eye injuries. It usually results in persons who are exposed to high-altitude sunlight without adequate UV eye protection, skiers who are exposed to light reflected off snow at high altitudes, or welders who do not use correct protection. The injury is caused by ultraviolet radiation damaging the superficial corneal epithelium. The damaged cells slough off in a few days. Symptoms usually are noticed about 6 hours after injury, much like a sunburn on the skin. Patients then complain of severe pain, foreign body sensation, photophobia, and loss of visual acuity. Application of topical anesthetic relieves these sensations almost immediately. However, it is very important that patients do not have access to anesthetic agents for continual use because the loss of protective sensation can lead to serious corneal damage. This condition is treated with topical antibiotic ointment and usually resolves completely within 24 to 48 hours.

Herpes (**choice A**) is incorrect. Although HSV can cause an infectious keratitis and presents with severe pain and photophobia, the lesions usually seen under slit lamp examination are dendritic in form. Also, the patient's history of skiing and lack of eye protection are more consistent with a non-infectious etiology.

Dust particles (**choice B**) is also incorrect based on the slit lamp examination and history.

Staphylococcus aureus (**choice C**) is not correct because there is no indication of bacterial infection.

Varicella infection (**choice E**) is also incorrect. Like HSV, the varicella-zoster virus can also cause a keratitis. This occurs when the ophthalmic division of the trigeminal nerve is involved. In addition, it would be expected that the tip of the nose would also be affected with vesicular lesions (this is called Hutchinson sign). Again, this patient's history and physical exam are most consistent with ultraviolet keratoconjunctivitis.

13. **The correct answer is E.** This patient gives a typical history for headache of intracranial hypertension. The normal CT makes a diagnosis of idiopathic intracranial hypertension likely. Careful visual field mapping and viewing the optic disk for signs of papilledema should be done. Coordination (**choice A**), deep tendon reflexes (**choice B**), motor system (**choice C**), and sensory systems (**choice D**) should all be tested as part of a complete neu-

rologic examination. However, with the above history and normal CT scan, they do not have to be done in the same amount of detail as visual field testing and funduscopy.

14. **The correct answer is A.** This patient's history is suggestive of Guillain Barré syndrome, which is an acquired demyelinating polyneuropathy. It usually has an acute onset, and progresses over several days to weeks. Precipitating factors include viral illnesses (both respiratory and gastrointestinal), as well as immunizations and surgery. The exact etiology is unknown, but is thought to be immune-mediated. Tests to support the diagnosis include electromyography and nerve conduction studies, as well as a lumbar puncture looking for elevated protein. Treatment is with intravenous immunoglobulin or plasmapheresis. Characteristic exam findings include both motor and sensory findings, though sensory findings can be quite variable. Other findings may include cranial nerve involvement and autonomic dysfunction. Respiratory compromise can be a serious consequence, and patients must be monitored closely for this. Reflexes are consistently lost; an alternative diagnosis should be considered if the patient has hyperactive reflexes (**choice C**).

    A homonymous hemianopia (**choice B**) would suggest a central lesion involving the visual pathways, while Guillain Barré is a peripheral disorder.

    Motor exam (**choice D**) typically shows a pattern of ascending weakness.

    A discernible thoracic sensory level (**choice E**) would be more consistent with a spinal cord process, rather than a disease involving the peripheral nerves.

15. **The correct answer is D.** Phenytoin, a sodium channel antagonist, is frequently used as a first-line anti-seizure medication. However, if infused too fast, phenytoin can cause profound hypotension. The maximum recommended infusion rate is 50 mg/min. Note that fosphenytoin is often used now, and it does not cause significant hypotension.

    As with thiamine, glucose is often administered in the setting of seizures of unknown etiology. Glucose administration is not associated with hypotension. Therefore, discontinuing the glucose infusion (**choice A**) is inappropriate.

    Lorazepam, a benzodiazepine, is used in the treatment of seizure in order to increase the seizure threshold. It is not associated with hypotension. Therefore, discontinuing the lorazepam infusion (**choice B**) is inappropriate.

    While extreme hypermagnesemia may cause cardiovascular collapse, it is unlikely that a brief infusion of magnesium in the setting of hypomagnesemia is responsible for this patient's hypotension. Therefore, discontinuing the magnesium (**choice C**) is inappropriate.

    Thiamine is often administered in the setting of seizures of unknown etiology. Thiamine is not associated with hypotension. Therefore, discontinuing thiamine (**choice E**) is inappropriate.

16. **The correct answer is B.** The clinical symptoms may well indicate the possibility of narcolepsy. She needs to be evaluated and eventually treated. Neurology consult can provide adequate appointment and followup with sleep studies.

    Vasovagal syncope (**choice A**) is not typically associated with daytime sleepiness.

    Conversion disorder (**choice C**) can be diagnosed after other medical causes are ruled out and criteria for it are met. In this case that may not be correct.

    Ordering an electroencephalogram (**choice D**) can be done, but in order to evaluate for narcolepsy, a sleep electroencephalogram is better than a standard electroencephalogram. However, a sleep EEG is not the best way to diagnose narcolepsy, as it might show REM onset, but that can also be sleep deprivation. A multiple sleep latency study is better.

    Blaming it on exhaustion (**choice E**) in the presence of other possible symptoms indicating something else is not adequate. One should take a good history and consider all diagnostic categories possible.

17. **The correct answer is E.** The scenario demonstrates a simple febrile seizure. The child should be treated for otitis media and fever control and discharged home. There is no indication to evaluate her for anything else.

    This seizure was generalized and brief (less than 5 minutes), and there is a return to complete neurologic function afterwards. Febrile seizures occur in children 6 mo to 6 years old, are brief (less than 5 minutes), and involve no CNS infection. There is often a family history. A CT (**choice A**), neurological consultation (**choice B**), or EEG (**choice C**) is not indicated provided the seizure was not complex (more than 1 in a 24-hour period or focality) and the child has returned to baseline.

    Tympanocentesis (**choice D**) is not indicated for OM unless there is antibiotic failure and the physician is in need of a specimen for culture.

18. **The correct answer is C.** The CSF findings of increased pressure, protein, decreased glucose, and lymphocytosis suggest a diagnosis of tuberculosis meningitis. Therefore, anti-tuberculosis therapy with isoniazid, rifampin, pyrazinamide, and streptomycin is indicated.

Ampicillin and cefotaxime or ampicillin and gentamicin are appropriate therapies for bacterial meningitis for the first 3 months of life. They would provide adequate coverage for such organisms as group B streptococcus, *Enterobacteriaceae, Listeria monocytogenes, Streptococcus pneumoniae, Haemophilus influenzae*, and *Neisseria meningitidis*. They would not, however, be effective against tuberculosis (**choice A**).

In children older than 3 months of age the addition of vancomycin is advised for better coverage against penicillin-resistant *Streptococcus pneumoniae*. This is not anti-tuberculosis therapy (**choice B**).

Observation in the hospital without therapy might be appropriate if this child was thought to have aseptic or viral meningitis. The high number of WBCs in the spinal fluid along with the decreased glucose and elevated protein, however, do not support this diagnosis (**choice D**).

Shunt surgery may be indicated in this case of tuberculosis meningitis with hydrocephalus if signs and symptoms of increased intracranial pressure persist despite adequate medical therapy (**choice E**). Surgery would not be the first step in management.

19. **The correct answer is E.** Subdural hematomas are caused by rupture of the veins traversing the subdural space or by arterial bleeding from parenchymal laceration. The presentation of subdural hematoma and the treatment depends on the rapidity of hematoma formation. Subdural hematomas can present as acute, subacute, or chronic. They are characterized by the presence of a decreased level of consciousness out of proportion to the observed focal neurologic deficit. Acute subdural hematomas, such as in this patient, are those that cause progressive neurologic deficit within 48 hours of injury. They usually follow severe head trauma, are unilateral, have arterial and venous sources of bleeding, and can progress rapidly. The diagnosis should be considered in any patient with a severe head injury who shows deteriorated neurologic status or who is unresponsive with a focal neurologic deficit. The hematomas may be visualized by a CT scan. They can be bilateral, and adjacent intracerebral hematomas are often present. Treatment typically involves craniotomy with removal of solid clot and control of bleeding points.

In cerebral contusion (**choice A**), the CT scan usually shows evidence of cerebral edema. This patient may complain of headache but deterioration of the neurologic symptoms is unlikely, unless the patient has an associated subarachnoid subdural hematoma.

A diabetic coma (**choice B**) is unlikely in this patient as he is compliant with his medications. Also he has been in the hospital, being monitored with clinical examination and laboratory examination.

A hypertensive crisis (**choice C**) can manifest with subarachnoid hemorrhage, if it is associated with a rupture of one of the intracranial arteries. Hypertensive crisis, however, is usually associated with elevated blood pressure.

Subarachnoid hemorrhages (**choice D**) usually present as sudden headache followed by altered consciousness. Focal neurologic deficits may occur but are less common than those seen after occlusion of major intracranial arteries. The sequelae vary, depending on the size of hemorrhage and ranging from headache to death. A CT scan is usually diagnostic in greater than 90% of patients.

20. **The correct answer is C.** A sudden headache followed by altered consciousness is suspicious for a subarachnoid hemorrhage. Focal neurologic deficits may occur but are less common than those seen after occlusion of major intracranial arteries. The sequelae of subarachnoid hemorrhage depend on the size and the rapidity of the hemorrhage. The presentation can manifest in outcomes ranging from headache to death. A CT scan often confirms a subarachnoid hemorrhage in greater than 90% of patients. Approximately 10% of patients with a documented hemorrhage, however, have a normal CT scan within 24 hours of the subarachnoid hemorrhage. It is important, therefore, to perform a lumbar puncture when a subarachnoid hemorrhage is suspected and the CT scan is negative.

In the absence of positive findings on investigation, admission to the medical floor and further observation (**choice A**) are necessary but further investigation should be carried out to determine the cause of this deterioration.

Cerebral angiography (**choice B**) is required to confirm the presence of an aneurysm. The further treatment of subarachnoid hemorrhage depends on the presence or absence of aneurysm, and whether rupture of the aneurysm has occurred or not. The presence of subarachnoid hemorrhage, however, should be diagnosed initially by lumbar puncture to be followed by cerebral angiogram in the presence of a negative CT scan.

A magnetic resonance angiogram (MRA) **(choice D)** is useful in delineating any intracranial aneurysms. This is to be done as an elective investigation rather than in an emergency situation. Elective MRA of the head can reveal vascular abnormalities, malformations, or aneurysm of intracranial arteries. In this case, however, an immediate lumbar puncture needs to be performed for evaluation of a subarachnoid hemorrhage.

Subdural hematomas in the initial stage may not show on the CT scan of the head but might be diagnosed on the repeat CT scan **(choice E)**, providing the patient's clinical condition did not improve or deteriorated. In this patient with sudden loss of consciousness, further investigation is necessary to evaluate for a subarachnoid hemorrhage instead of just repeating the CT scan in 24 hours.

21. **The correct answer is D.** This patient is presenting with an ischemic stroke but he is out of the thrombolytic therapy window. Thrombolytic therapy **(choice C)** with tPA has shown to improve functional outcome when give within 3 hours of symptom onset.

Aspirin therapy is recommended for patients with ischemic stroke who are not receiving tPA, intravenous heparin, or anticoagulation therapy. Aspirin should be started within 48 hours of stroke onset.

Intravenous heparin **(choice A)** in the acute management of stroke is warranted in patients who are ineligible for tPA and who have a cardioembolic stroke or progressive stroke (waxing and waning symptoms).

Treatment of hypertension **(choice B)** following an ischemic stroke is indicated if systolic BP is >200 mm Hg or diastolic BP is >120 mm Hg, and in patients with heart failure or aortic dissection.

Warfarin **(choice E)** has no role in the acute management of ischemic stroke. It is indicated for long-term anticoagulation in patients with cardioembolic stroke (atrial fibrillation).

22. **The correct answer is E.** The rescuer would not be liable for a lawsuit, as the patient would have aspirated and obstructed his airway as a consequence of the convulsions and not from the negligence of the physician. Even if a lawsuit were brought to bear, the defendant would triumph. This is because under the Good Samaritan statute, the defense's argument that the patient would have died in any event, despite the physician maintaining the accepted standard of care, would be upheld by the courts, and the case would be dismissed. In a similar vein, if a lawsuit were brought in a case wherein a patient who sustained injuries that would prove lethal (such as torrential hemorrhage) developed quadriplegia as a result of the rescuing physician inadvertently moving his neck, the courts would dismiss the plaintiff's plea of gross negligence or even ordinary negligence on the grounds that the patient would have died in any event because of the gross nature of the hemorrhage and not as a result of quadriplegia. Therefore, **choices A, B, C, and D** are incorrect.

23. **The correct answer is B.** This patient has an expressive aphasia. The capacity for language resides in the left hemisphere (Broca area) in most people. Therefore, even without any localizing signs, if aphasia is present one can predict with reasonable certainty that the lesion is *left*-sided and involves the left carotid system, and is usually the left middle cerebral artery.

Vertebral-basilar strokes **(choices A and C)** affect the posterior circulation of the brainstem and brain. They often produce unilateral or bilateral motor/sensory deficits and may be accompanied by cranial nerve and brainstem signs (e.g., vertigo, difficulty with balance); speech is rarely affected.

Because it is a left-sided lesion it would rule out the right-sided cerebral artery system **(choices D and E)**.

24. **The correct answer is A.** Cluster headaches are predominantly a male disorder with a mean age of onset of 27 to 30 years. The "attacks" occur in cycles and are unilateral. Oftentimes they are associated with lacrimation of the ipsilateral eye, conjunctival injection, and with the complaint of pain behind that eye.

Migraines **(choice B)** can occur in both sexes but are more commonly seen in women and start between the ages of 20 to 30 years. They typically last 4 to 24 hours and are associated with an aversion to loud sounds and bright lights and may include vomiting. They can be initiated by fatigue, hunger, sleep deprivation, and certain foods such as wine, cheese, and chocolate.

Temporal arteritis **(choice C)** typically presents in patients over the age of 50 years and is associated with a tender temporal artery, a unilateral headache, and other systemic complaints such as fatigue.

Tension headaches **(choice D)** are chronic, bandlike, non-pulsatile, and usually associated with neck pain. Look for stressors in the patient's social life (e.g., job loss, family problems). They occur daily and are variable in intensity.

Trigeminal neuralgia (**choice E**) is a disorder of the trigeminal nerve that causes episodes of intense, stabbing, electric shock-like pain in the areas of the face where the branches of the nerve are distributed: lips, eyes, nose, scalp, forehead, upper jaw, and lower jaw. Onset of symptoms occurs most often after age 50, but cases are known in children and even infants. Something as simple and routine as brushing the teeth, putting on makeup, or even a slight breeze can trigger an attack, resulting in sheer agony for the individual.

25. **The correct answer is A.** Tuberous sclerosis is an autosomal dominant neurocutaneous disorder. It is associated with seizures, mental retardation, intracranial calcifications, and cutaneous findings. Ash leaf macules are hypopigmented areas with irregular borders. They may be present at birth and the majority of patients with tuberous sclerosis will have ash leaf macules visible on exam by age 2.

    Axillary freckling (**choice B**) and café-au-lait spots (**choice C**) are classic cutaneous findings in neurofibromatosis and are part of the diagnostic criteria for neurofibromatosis-1.

    Lisch nodules (**choice D**) are pigmented hamartomas of the iris and are part of the diagnostic criteria for neurofibromatosis-1.

    A port wine stain (**choice E**) is a vascular nevus found along the distribution of the trigeminal nerve. It is a manifestation of Sturge-Weber syndrome, a neurocutaneous syndrome associated with these port wine stains and seizures.

26. **The correct answer is C.** Maintaining adequate tissue oxygenation is an important component of the emergency management of stroke. Hypoxia leads to anaerobic metabolism and depletion of energy stores, increasing brain insult. Although there is no reason to give supplemental oxygen, the potential need for oxygen should be assessed using pulse oximetry or an arterial blood gas measurement.

    Heparin (**choice A**) and other antithrombotic drugs must be used with caution and after a baseline head CT scan rules out an intracerebral bleed, followed by a repeat CT scan in 48 hours.

    Corticosteroids (**choice B**) as yet are not an indication for the management of cerebral edema and increased intracranial pressure after stroke.

    Optimizing cardiac output is a high priority in the immediate hours after a stroke. Cerebral perfusion may occur if the blood pressure is dropped further and therefore aggressive management with an antihypertensive is not indicated (**choice D**) unless the systolic blood pressure is greater than 220 mm Hg.

    Hypovolemia can exacerbate cerebral hypoperfusion, so there is no need to restrict oral fluid intake (**choice E**).

27. **The correct answer is A.** The courts will accede to his request. This patient is mentally capable and therefore has a right to refuse treatment. The disease is incurable and prolonging his life is not in his best interests. Furthermore, the state does not have a compelling reason to choose life over death. If the patient had dependent minors, then of course, the scales of justice would tilt in favor of life. The raison d'etre comes under the ambit of futility. Futility, in the parlance of medical ethics, implies a unilateral decision on the part of a physician or a patient to withhold or withdraw medical treatment or intervention. Physiologic futility takes into consideration that prolonging treatment or introducing interventions would not in any way alter the ultimate course of the disease, and is determined by the physician. Medical futility affects the quality of life during or after treatment and is determined by the patient or his surrogate. If there is no physiologic futility involved in a given case, the patient should be given the opportunity to decide what he considers is futile treatment. In order to make that decision, it is incumbent on the physician to provide all the information available without being judgmental.

    Referring the matter to an expert panel (**choice B**) is not an option, nor is turning down his request or not admitting the case.

    The clergy (**choice C**) does not sanction death but celebrates life, no matter how dismal that may be.

    Human rights groups (**choice D**) cannot breach the sanctity of an individual's right to refuse treatment. That can only be executed by the state whenever its interests are involved.

    It is unlikely that the court will turn down his request (**choice E**).

28. **The correct answer is C.** The patient has an essential tremor, which is one of the most common movement disorders. This postural tremor may have its onset anywhere between the second and the sixth decades of life. Its prevalence increases with age. It is slowly progressive over a period of years. It may be familial with autosomal dominant penetrance. The frequency of the tremor is typically 5 Hertz. It typically affects the hands and also the head, voice, tongue, and legs. It may be alleviated by alcohol.

    An alcoholic withdrawal tremor (**choice A**) affects only the hands, unlike the multiple sites of involvement of essential tremor.

    A cerebellar tremor (**choice B**) is an intention or goal-directed tremor. It increases in severity as the extremity approaches a target.

    A parkinsonian tremor (**choice D**) typically occurs at rest.

    Psychogenic tremor (**choice E**) includes an abrupt onset, static course, spontaneous remission, and unclassified tremors. They often increase in frequency and amplitude with attention and decrease with distraction.

29. **The correct answer is D.** The patient most likely had a vasovagal syncope that typically presents with prodromal symptoms such as nausea, diaphoresis, pallor, and lightheadedness. These symptoms tend to occur before the loss of consciousness. A quick recovery after an episode of loss of consciousness makes it more likely that this was a syncopal episode rather than a seizure, as seizures are followed by a postictal period of residual confusion. An otherwise healthy individual who had a vasovagal syncope probably does not need any further diagnostic testing; only reassurance is needed.

    In patients experiencing syncopal episodes, head CT scans are unlikely to reveal the diagnosis (**choice A**).

    An echocardiogram (**choice B**) is not indicated in this case as the history and normal study results are most consistent with vasovagal syncope.

    Unless there is any evidence to suspect that this was a seizure, a routine electroencephalogram is also of no benefit (**choice C**).

    Although the abrupt onset of syncope without warning does raise the possibility of cardiac arrhythmias, particularly in patients with known heart disease, 24-hour Holter electrocardiogram monitoring (**choice E**) is rarely diagnostic and would not be indicated in this case.

30. **The correct answer is A.** This is an open-ended question that allows the physician to explore the likely possibility of alcoholism as a cause of her peripheral polyneuropathy. Alcoholism is one of the most common causes of peripheral neuropathy in the outpatient setting.

    Asking about tiredness and fatigue (**choice B**) is vague and may not pertain to any particular diagnosis or cause of the neuropathy. It merely expands on the review of her symptoms. Hypothyroidism and hyperthyroidism may present with fatigue and can cause peripheral polyneuropathy, but if the physician had these in mind a more searching question (e.g., for hyperthyroidism) may be to ask about tremor, weight loss, and increased appetite and heat intolerance.

    Asking about thirst would be appropriate if you suspected diabetes mellitus (**choice C**), another common cause of polyneuropathy, but the patient denies it and her hemoglobin A1c is normal. Diabetes insipidus, which also presents with polydipsia, does not cause peripheral neuropathy.

    Asking about injuries (**choice D**) explores trauma as a common cause of a localized injury to a *single* nerve or mononeuropathy. Pressure or entrapment paralysis usually affects superficial nerves (ulnar, radial, peroneal) at bony prominences or at narrow canals (e.g., carpal tunnel syndrome).

    Medications may cause peripheral neuropathy (e.g., cisplatin, isoniazid, ethambutol, vincristine, metronidazole) but trying to chase what pain medications she takes (**choice E**) for her burning pain will not get you closer to the cause of the peripheral neuropathy when compared with choice A. Neuropathy secondary to outpatient analgesia is extraordinarily rare.

31. **The correct answer is C.** In chronic neuropathy, tricyclic antidepressants such as amitriptyline or anticonvulsants (e.g., carbamazepine, phenytoin), sometimes in conjunction with phenothiazines like fluphenazine, may be required. Treatment of peripheral neuropathies otherwise includes specific treatment of the underlying disease process (e.g., vitamin B_{12} deficiency), along with general supportive measures.

    Amiloride (**choice A**) is a diuretic that can cause hyperkalemia and muscle cramps.

    Amiodarone (**choice B**) is a class III antiarrhythmic that is used for life-threatening ventricular fibrillation. Its side-effects profile is large, affecting the lungs (pulmonary fibrosis), liver (toxic), and heart (heart block or failure). It may potentiate peripheral neuropathy.

Amlodipine (**choice D**) is a calcium-channel blocker that has no efficacy in the treatment of neuropathy. Its side effects include peripheral edema and headache.

Gabapentin (**choice E**) is an anticonvulsant that has recently had successful trials for treatment of neuropathy in diabetic patients.

32. **The correct answer is B.** This question asks for the test with the highest sensitivity, or for identifying all of the patients who are at risk. The highest sensitivity given here is 0.93. For this issue, specificity, positive predictive value, and negative predictive value are not relevant. Specificity seeks to identify the healthy individuals. Positive predictive value gives the chance that a patient with a positive test is truly diseased. Negative predictive value gives the chance that a patient with a negative test is truly disease-free. **Choices A, C, D,** and **E** have a lower sensitivity than choice B and are therefore incorrect.

33. **The correct answer is A.** The patient's history of a short spell, focal neurologic symptoms (facial twitching), unresponsiveness, and a post-ictal state are all consistent with a complex partial seizure. The site of origin is likely from the left side of the brain, causing an aphasia and right-sided twitching. Partial seizures may or may not secondarily generalize.

    Hypoglycemia (**choice B**) can cause seizures, but there is nothing in this patient's history that would point to that diagnosis. In the acute setting, a fingerstick glucose should be checked in all patients with seizures.

    Migraine headaches (**choice C**) can sometimes be associated with focal neurologic symptoms, but this is usually weakness or numbness. Twitching or convulsive activity is more suggestive of a seizure.

    Loss of awareness differentiates a complex partial seizure from a simple partial seizure (**choice D**). Consciousness is retained in a simple partial seizure.

    Transient ischemic attacks (**choice E**) may be confused for seizure activity, especially in elderly patients. However, patients are typically older than 50 and have other risk factors for ischemia (hypertension, diabetes mellitus).

34. **The correct answer is A.** This patient has evidence of a peripheral neuropathy, particularly in the legs. The hands are also affected. He has a history of difficulty running, muscle atrophy and weakness are noted on examination, there are questionable sensory changes in his hands, and the EMG reveals decreased nerve velocity. There also seems to be a history of family members with some sort of diseases that could be neuromuscular (his mother is seeing a neurologist and her sister is in a wheelchair). A sural nerve biopsy and genetic testing will most likely lead to a diagnosis of an inherited progressive peripheral neuropathy such as Charcot-Marie-Tooth disease. There is also a commercially available blood test for Charcot-Marie-Tooth disease that can be done before a biopsy.

    Ordering muscle enzymes such as CPK is not the best answer (**choice B**). It would be helpful in cases of myopathies associated with other diseases such as connective tissue disorders, polymyositis, muscular dystropy, or metabolic diseases; however, there is evidence to support that this is not a primary muscle disease.

    Although it is true that certain types of drug abuse or use may give hyporeflexia and weakness (e.g., alcohol and barbiturates), they would also cause other symptoms, such as ataxia. This vignette supports a diagnosis of a specific type of peripheral neuropathy with a positive family history (**choice C**).

    Lead poisoning in young children classically has symptoms of encephalopathy with behavioral and psychiatric changes (**choice D**). The toxic effects of lead may cause peripheral neuropathy with severe limb weakness and sensory symptoms. This case did not give information about any possible home, occupational, or hobby exposures to lead. Again, the positive family history suggests a different diagnosis. Also, Charcot-Marie-Tooth disease usually is associated with greater neuropathic involvement of the lower extremities compared with the upper ones.

    A Tensilon or edrophonium testing would be conducted if one suspected myasthenia gravis. Myasthenia gravis, however, would not have sensory neurologic deficits. Myasthenia gravis would usually present with hypotonia and ptosis (**choice E**).

35. **The correct answer is E.** This patient has acute angle closure glaucoma. The main tenets of therapy are breaking the attack and lowering the intraocular pressure. This can be accomplished with topical pilocarpine, beta-blocker, and alpha-2-agonists and intravenous or oral acetazolamide. A hyperosmotic agent, such as mannitol, is sometimes necessary.

    Enucleation (or removing the eye) will not likely be required (**choice A**).

    Definitive surgical therapy will likely be required after averting an acute attack. Clearly, offering no treatment (**choice B**) is incorrect. Any patient with simply acute loss of visual acuity even without all of the other findings requires immediate medical attention.

Ophthalmology consultation "first thing in the morning" (**choice C**) is not quick enough, as these patients need immediate attention. An ophthalmology consultation should be sought as soon as possible.

Topical erythromycin (**choice D**) can be used in some cases of acute conjunctivitis; however, those patients should not generally have clouding of the pupil or decreased visual acuity, and certainly not increased intraocular pressure.

36. **The correct answer is E.** Most children with cerebral palsy are term infants and appropriate for their gestational age. Cerebral palsy is a static or nonprogressive neuromuscular disease having many causes that relate to prenatal, perinatal, or postnatal events. This 9-month-old infant has persistence of the Moro and ATNR reflexes that should be absent after 6 months of age.

    APGAR scores that are low at 1 and 5 minutes have been shown to have poor correlation with the development of cerebral palsy (**choice A**).

    Research has not supported that cerebral palsy is caused by a genetic disorder (**choice B**).

    Some parents would like to attribute their child's cerebral palsy to medical negligence or mismanagement during labor and delivery. Although some cases may be caused by perinatal asphyxia, most are not (**choice C**).

    Only a few children who are diagnosed with cerebral palsy have a history of being premature or small for gestational age (**choice D**).

37. **The correct answer is B.** This patient is exhibiting a classic case of amaurosis fugax, which manifests as acute non-painful monocular visual loss. It is caused by an embolus to the central retinal artery. It is often transient, and the embolus usually comes from carotid artery plaque. Alternatively, if the patient has a left atrial thrombus such as in the setting of atrial fibrillation, this too can be a source of emboli. The resolution of symptoms is analogous to a transient ischemic attack in the brain, while if the visual loss is permanent from infarction, it is similar to a stroke. Many patients at high risk for other sources of atherosclerotic disease will undergo carotid artery ultrasound prior to bypass grafting surgery because when the patients are placed on the bypass machine they are at a high risk of stroke. The patient in this scenario falls into this category and should definitely receive an ultrasound prior to coronary artery bypass grafting in the morning (**choice C**). If significant plaque or stenosis is found a carotid endarterectomy will typically be performed prior to or at the time of the bypass surgery.

    Systemic thrombolytics (**choice A**) are used in acute stroke, but their efficacy in central retinal artery occlusion has not been extensively studied. In any case, this patient has had resolution of the symptoms, so thrombolytics are clearly not indicated. She should be on aspirin and heparin already for her unstable angina.

    Carotid angiogram (**choice D**) would certainly be good for evaluating any source of plaque in the carotid arteries, however ultrasound is a much less invasive test, and this does not need to be done emergently.

    MRI of the brain (**choice E**) is a test that can sometimes be used in acute stroke, but it would likely not provide useful information in this case.

38. **The correct answer is D.** This patient's history and examination are consistent with a cervical myelopathy. Myelopathies can be caused by either intrinsic or extrinsic spinal-cord lesions. In this case, a herniated cervical disc causing spinal cord dysfunction is a likely etiology. Examination findings may reveal lower motor neuron signs at the level of the lesion, a sensory level, and upper motor neuron signs below the level of the lesion. The nipple line is approximately at the T4 level, and a sensory deficit to this level would imply a cervical or high thoracic pathology. Therefore, an MRI of the cervical spine would be an appropriate test to evaluate this patient.

    EMG and nerve conduction studies (**choice A**) are useful in differentiating lesions in peripheral nerves, the plexi, and the nerve roots. If other tests are unrevealing, this may be a helpful test; however, it should not be the first test ordered.

    A lumbar puncture (**choice B**) may be indicated, especially if the MRI of the cervical spine shows intrinsic spinal cord pathology, suggestive of demyelinating or inflammatory disease. However, it should not be the first test ordered.

    An MRI of the brain (**choice C**) would not be indicated, as the patient does not likely have a process in his brain as the etiology for his symptoms.

    An MRI of the lumbar spine (**choice E**) would not be indicated. As mentioned, the physical exam findings, especially the increased tone and hyperactive reflexes in the lower extremities, suggest a higher spinal cord localization.

39. **The correct answer is E.** The diagnosis of type I neurofibromatosis requires two or more of the following criteria: (*1*) 6 or more café-au-lait macules of more than 5 mm in greatest diameter in prepubertal individuals and more than 15 mm in diameter in postpubertal individuals; (*2*) 2 or more neurofibromas of any type or one plexiform neurofibroma; (*3*) freckling in the axillary and/or inguinal region; (*4*) optic glioma; (*5*) 2 or more Lisch nodules; (*6*) a distinctive osseous lesion, such as sphenoid dysplasia or thinning of the long bone cortex with or without pseudoarthrosis; and (*7*) a first-degree relative (parent, sibling or offspring) with the disease. Mutation of the *NF1* gene on chromosome 17 causes von Recklinghausen disease. The *NF1* gene is a tumor suppressor gene; it encodes a protein, neurofibromin, which modulates signal transduction through the *ras* GTPase pathway. Patients with NF1 are at increased risk of developing nervous-system neoplasms, including plexiform neurofibromas, optic gliomas, ependymomas, meningiomas, astrocytomas, and pheochromocytomas. Neurofibromas may undergo secondary malignant degeneration and become sarcomas.

Ash leaf macules (**choice A**) are a cutaneous hallmark of tuberous sclerosis. They are present at birth in 85% of patients with this common, inherited, autosomal dominant disease with variable penetrance. Other features include adenoma sebaceum, mental deficiency, epilepsy, periungual fibromas, shagreen plaques, oral papillomatosis, skin fibromas, and café-au-lait macules.

Bamboo hair (trichorrhexis invaginata) (**choice B**) along with an ichthyosiform dermatitis and atopic diathesis are diagnostic of Netherton syndrome, an autosomal recessive disorder. These patients are usually severely ill and many die in their childhood.

Von Hippel-Lindau syndrome is an autosomal dominant disorder consisting of retinal angiomas (**choice C**), cerebellar medullary angioblastic tumors, pancreatic cysts, and renal tumors and cysts. Usually, the skin is not involved, although occasionally angiomas may occur in the occipitocervical region.

Subtle, faint, hypochromic or atrophic Blaschko-linear lesions on the extremities (**choice D**) are seen in the fourth and last stage of incontinentia pigmenti, an X-linked dominant disease that is believed to be lethal in utero in boys. It appears in girls during the first weeks of life and evolves through a vesicular (inflammatory), verrucous, and pigmentary stage. A fourth, hypopigmented and/or atrophic stage, may be seen in some adult women.

40. **The correct answer is D.** Patients with Down syndrome are more likely to develop dementing illness that is markedly similar both clinically and pathologically to Alzheimer disease. A notable clinical feature of this presentation is that patients with Down syndrome who develop dementia do so much earlier in life than most Alzheimer patients.

The patient's normal laboratory values, including chemistries, make a diagnosis of dementia secondary to renal failure (**choice A**) unlikely.

The patient does not demonstrate a presentation consistent with Huntington disease. Separate chromosomes are involved in the pathogenesis of Huntington disease (**choice B**) and Down syndrome.

This patient does not demonstrate a presentation that is consistent with Parkinson dementia (**choice C**), such as tremor, rigidity, bradykinesia.

The patient does not have known risk factors such as hypertension or hyperlipidemia that would make him at any greater risk for developing vascular dementia (**choice E**).

41. **The correct answer is D.** The patient's symptoms and signs are typical of sciatica due to a herniated disc between the third and forth lumbar vertebra. Herniated disc at this level affects the L4 nerve root. In an isolated herniated disc of the lumbar spine, as in this patient, an MRI scan provides the best examination of soft tissues including the intervertebral disc and nerve roots.

A bone scan (**choice A**) is not indicated for an isolated extremity symptom. Bone scan is useful in evaluating an infection or tumor when suspected.

A CT scan (**choice B**) may be helpful in suspected cases of spondylolysis or spondylolisthesis, but is not indicated in this patient.

An electromyogram (**choice C**) may be used in cases of suspected peripheral neuropathy or cervical or lumbar radiculopathies, however an MRI scan is the most appropriate test at this time.

X-rays of the spine (**choice E**) are helpful in diagnosing an acute compression fracture but may not be helpful in the evaluation of a herniated disc.

42. **The correct answer is C.** The clinical triad of ipsilateral ptosis, miosis, and decreased facial sweating (anhydrosis) is called Horner syndrome. It is related to decreased sympathetic innervation caused by involvement of the stellate ganglion. This can sometimes be a complication of Pancoast superior sulcus tumors of the lung, for which this patient has a high risk (he is a chronic smoker). Therefore, a chest x-ray is indicated.

Determining acetylcholine receptor antibody level (**choice A**) would be useful for myasthenia gravis that can also present with ptosis, but it would not help isolate a diagnosis of Horner syndrome.

A fasting glucose level (**choice B**) is useful in ruling out diabetes mellitus but diabetes does not commonly present with Horner syndrome.

Similarly, a [^{131}I] thyroid scan (**choice D**) can be used to evaluate for thyroid disease, but also does not present with Horner syndrome.

At this point an MRI scan of the brain (**choice E**) is not indicated as a first-line diagnostic test compared with a chest x-ray even though Horner syndrome may accompany some intracranial pathology (Wallenberg syndrome).

43. **The correct answer is B.** A multiple sleep latency test (MSLT) is useful to diagnose narcolepsy. Narcolepsy is characterized by the onset of sleep with REM phase and decreased sleep latency.

Electromyogram (**choice A**) is not a part of diagnostic tests for narcolepsy.

Brain CT (**choice C**) is not a standard test to confirm the diagnosis of narcolepsy. Given the history and the symptoms present and the absence of other indications of any medical or neurological disorder it may not be necessary.

Electrocardiogram (**choice D**) is ordered in other sleep disorders such as sleep apnea. In narcolepsy an EKG is not necessary to diagnose the disorder, but may be ordered to rule out other conditions.

HLA testing (**choice E**) is not necessary even though almost all narcoleptics with cataplexy are HLA DR2.

44. **The correct answer is B.** This patient most likely has carpal tunnel syndrome, which is an entrapment of the median nerve as it passes through the carpal tunnel at the wrist. Symptoms often begin with paresthesias and numbness in a median nerve distribution on the hand, which includes the first 3 digits. Later in the course of severe cases, patients will develop weakness and atrophy of the median-innervated muscles of the hand. Symptoms are typically worse at night. Some conditions may predispose patients to develop carpal tunnel syndrome; these include diabetes mellitus, thyroid disease, and pregnancy. Occupations involving repetitive hand-wrist actions are also a risk factor.

A brachial plexopathy (**choice A**) would be expected to produce more physical exam findings consistent with other nerve root and peripheral nerve involvement.

Cervical spondylosis (**choice C**) would more likely present with neck discomfort and atrophy of the intrinsic hand muscles. Reflexes below the lesion would likely be hyperactive.

Diabetic peripheral neuropathy (**choice D**) is a distal, symmetric, peripheral neuropathy, and the main symptoms are numbness and pain in a stocking-glove distribution.

This patient's history, specifically the chronicity of her symptoms, is not suggestive of stroke (**choice E**).

45. **The correct answer is D.** This patient's history and complaints are suggestive of optic neuritis. Optic neuritis is an inflammation of the optic nerve, causing pain and visual loss. It is frequently one of the first symptoms of multiple sclerosis, which is an idiopathic demyelinating disease. Young women are most frequently affected. Multiple sclerosis is defined by demyelinating episodes "separated in time and space." Therefore, it would be helpful to know if the patient has had similar visual losses or any other transient neurologic symptoms in the past.

Asking about family history (**choice A**) may be important, but hereditary causes of optic neuropathy are much less common than multiple sclerosis.

Obtaining a smoking history (**choice B**) would be important in regard to the patient's general health, and if this patient were older, it would be helpful in diagnosing an ischemic optic neuropathy. However, ischemic optic neuropathy has a more acute presentation.

Unless the patient specifically had trauma to her eye or a penetrating trauma that may have affected her optic nerve, head trauma (**choice C**) is not likely to cause subacute, painful visual loss in one eye.

The patient's personal history of wearing glasses (**choice E**) is not likely to help in the diagnosis of a subacute process.

46. **The correct answer is B.** This patient's complaints are suggestive of giant-cell (or temporal) arteritis, an inflammatory condition involving the arteries. It usually occurs in elderly patients, and typical symptoms include headache, jaw claudication, and visual loss. It should be considered in any elderly person who presents with new headaches and visual complaints. Constitutional symptoms, such as low-grade fevers and weight loss, can be seen.

Brain tumors (**choice A**) should be considered when an elderly patient presents with new headaches, but the pain may vary throughout the course of the day and change with position (i.e., bending over). The other symptoms associated with temporal arteritis are usually not seen.

It would be unusual for an elderly patient to present with new-onset migraine headaches (**choice C**). Migraines are usually unilateral and have associated nausea and photophobia.

Pseudotumor cerebri (**choice D**), or idiopathic intracranial hypertension, usually presents in young, obese women. It typically has other features of increased intracranial pressure and when left untreated can result in visual deficits.

Subarachnoid hemorrhage (**choice E**) presents with the acute onset of the worst headache of a patient's life. Other symptoms include photophobia and neck stiffness.

47. **The correct answer is B**. This patient's symptoms are suggestive of carpal tunnel syndrome, or a median neuropathy at the wrist. Both diabetes mellitus and hypothyroidism may be risk factors for this. Typical symptoms are numbness over the thumb and the first two-and-a-half digits of the hand, and there may be weakness in the action of the abductor pollicis brevis. Treatments for carpal tunnel syndrome include pain medications, splinting, and surgery. The first step in confirming the diagnosis of carpal tunnel syndrome is an EMG and nerve conduction studies. This test will help localize the pathology to the median nerve at the wrist and will help to rule out radiculopathy or plexopathy.

A CT scan of the brain (**choice A**) would not be indicated, as the problem is more likely to be peripheral in nature, not secondary to brain pathology.

A lumbar puncture (**choice C**) is used to evaluate a patient for meningitis and may be used in other conditions, such as multiple sclerosis, but it would not help in confirming the diagnosis of carpal tunnel syndrome.

An MRI scan of the brain (**choice D**) would not be indicated, as the problem is more likely to be peripheral in nature, not secondary to brain pathology.

An MRI of the cervical spine (**choice E**) may be indicated, but only if the EMG and nerve conduction studies show a radiculopathy instead of the expected median neuropathy.

48. **The correct answer is A.** This patient has a typical history for migraine headache. She has already failed two classes of pharmacologic prophylaxis (calcium channel blocker and tricyclic antidepressant). A daily beta-blocker such as propranolol is a good choice to try next for headache prophylaxis. Propranolol will not usually be effective at headache onset (**choice E**).

Daily metaxalone (**choice B**) is a good treatment for tension-type headaches.

Oral corticosteroids (**choice C**) may be used to abort status migrainosus.

A narcotic such as oxycodone (**choice D**) is rarely a good choice for migraine treatment. In any case it should never be used for headache prophylaxis and in this case the patient already has a good abortive treatment.

49. **The correct answer is A.** This patient is presenting with classic signs and symptoms of bacterial or viral meningitis. Clinically, he has headache, fever, photophobia, a nonspecific abnormal neurological exam, and leukocytosis with bandemia. The most important diagnostic step for this patient is the analysis and culture of spinal fluid; however, it is not necessary to await results (**choice B**) before initiating treatment. Some clinicians obtain a CT of the head to rule out a posterior fossa mass before a lumbar puncture is performed. A posterior fossa mass is a contraindication to lumbar puncture (LP) because this could lead to brain herniation. Once a mass is ruled out, the LP is essential to look for white blood cells and organisms in the cerebrospinal fluid. This is an emergency and antibiotics should be started immediately. A standard fever workup including chest x-ray, urinalysis, and blood cultures should be obtained secondarily. Even if antibiotics are given several hours before the lumbar puncture, this should not significantly alter the analysis.

An MRI of the brain (**choice C**) is not necessary in this acute setting. The patient may need a CT of the head to rule out signs of increased intracranial pressure before a lumbar puncture is performed. The most important step after the CT is performed is the analysis and culture of the spinal fluid. MRI of the brain would be useful to further characterize any abnormalities detected on the CT.

This patient has no complaints of abdominal pain, and x-ray of the abdomen (**choice D**) is not necessary.

This patient has no signs of heart failure or new cardiac murmurs and the lungs are clear. A chest x-ray (**choice E**) is a standard part of the fever workup, but not strictly necessary at this time.

50. **The correct answer is C.** This patient has clearly sustained a concussion but likely has a cervical spine injury. He has already had insufficient care by the EMS personnel because of a failure to immobilize the cervical spine. Cervical spine injuries are not uncommon in contact sports and the findings on physical exam in this patient should be very concerning. Your job as an emergency medicine physician in this case is to prevent further injury (always immobilize the cervical spine in the trauma patient). Radiographs will likely show this patient's pathology, but if no fractures or dislocations are noted an MRI would be the appropriate next step.

    Admission to the hospital for observation (**choice A**) is not adequate because the cervical spine has not been immobilized or evaluated.

    Informing the patient and his family that the patient has sustained a very mild concussion and that when his family takes him home they should watch him closely for any headaches, nausea, or vomiting (**choice B**) is incorrect management at this time, as he is not going home now because a missed cervical spine injury may result in permanent paralysis.

    Because of the need for immediate immobilization of the cervical spine in all trauma patients, scheduling a CT scan for Monday (**choice D**) is inappropriate management. An emergent CT scan may be considered reasonable by some physicians for severe concussions with residual neurologic findings on exam but not until the patient has had his cervical spine immobilized.

    Depending on which concussion guidelines a physician chooses to follow, this patient should not return to contact sports for 1 week, but should not be discharged from the emergency department (**choice E**). This patient should likely be observed in a hospital setting regardless of the cervical spine problem due to his severe concussion with loss of consciousness and persistent retrograde amnesia.

Obstetrics/Gynecology: **Test One**

1. A 16-year-old girl comes to the office because of irregular vaginal spotting. Her menstrual periods have always been normal and she never had bleeding between periods in the past. She has no other medical problems and takes no medications besides a daily oral contraceptive pill that you prescribed 2 months ago. She has no known drug allergies. Physical examination including pelvic examination is unremarkable. A urinary pregnancy test is negative. At this time you should

   (A) determine serum follicle stimulating hormone level

   (B) determine serum thyroid stimulating hormone level

   (C) perform an endometrial biopsy

   (D) perform pelvic ultrasonography

   (E) reassure her and encourage pill continuation

2. A 58-year-old woman comes to the office because of concerns regarding breast cancer. She has been menopausal for the past 3 years and has been taking estrogen replacement therapy. Her past surgical history is significant for a hysterectomy, which she had at age 43 secondary to pelvic pain and pressure caused by a large fibroid uterus. She has heard that the addition of progesterone can help to prevent "female cancers," and she wants to know more about hormones and breast cancer. In counseling the patient, the most appropriate response is:

   (A) "Hormone replacement therapy is contraindicated in your case."

   (B) "Progesterone does not appear protective against breast cancer."

   (C) "Progesterone should be added to your hormone replacement regimen."

   (D) "You have a high risk of developing breast cancer while on estrogen."

   (E) "You should not have had a hysterectomy."

3. A 22-year-old woman comes to the emergency department because of irregular vaginal bleeding and abdominal pain that started 3 hours ago. The pain is described as generalized and crampy, and initially the patient thought that this was her period. However, the bleeding is much heavier than her normal period, so she came in for evaluation. She reports that her last menstrual period was "over 4 months ago," but says she has always had irregular menstrual periods. She is sexually active and has had three partners in the last 6 months. Her partners use condoms "most of the time," and she is on no hormonal contraception. Her temperature is 37.0 C (98.6 F), blood pressure is 115/65 mm Hg, pulse is 80/min, and respirations are 18/min. Her abdomen is soft, with minimal lower quadrant tenderness. There is no rebound or guarding. Pelvic examination reveals blood in the vaginal vault. The cervical os is closed. There is no cervical motion tenderness, adnexal masses, or tenderness. The size of the uterus on examination is 12 weeks' gestation. On your way out of the room, the nurse informs you that the patient's urine pregnancy test is positive. The most appropriate next step in management is to

   (A) arrange for a dilatation and curettage for the patient's missed abortion

   (B) arrange for immediate surgery for the patient's ectopic pregnancy

   (C) determine the patient's blood type and order an obstetric sonogram

   (D) prescribe ceftriaxone and doxycycline for pelvic inflammatory disease

   (E) prescribe methotrexate for the patient's ectopic pregnancy

4. A 28-year-old white woman comes to the satellite health center because of a persistent vaginal itch and discharge. She first noted the symptoms 2 days ago and they have been worsening since. She also complains of pain with urination. She has no chronic medical problems, but recently had a sinusitis that was treated with amoxicillin. She takes no medications currently and has no allergies to medications. Physical examination reveals well-demarcated erythema of the vulva with edema. Speculum examination demonstrates a thick white discharge. A 10% potassium hydroxide (KOH) microscopy is performed, which reveals pseudohyphae. The most appropriate management at this time is to

(A) perform ampicillin vaginal lavage
(B) perform a vulvar biopsy
(C) treat with oral azithromycin
(D) treat with topical (vaginal) clotrimazole
(E) treat with topical (vaginal) metronidazole

5. A 58-year-old woman comes to the office because of hot flashes. She first noted these hot flashes about 6½ months ago and since then they have been getting progressively worse. Her hot flashes come on at various times throughout the day, but they are especially intense during the night. She had her last menstrual period approximately 6 months ago. Her medical history is significant for a pulmonary embolus at the age of 34 and severe depression. She takes sertraline for depression and has no allergies to medications. She smokes 1 pack of cigarettes per day. Physical examination is unremarkable, including an entirely normal pelvic examination. The most appropriate pharmacotherapy at this time is

(A) clonidine
(B) estrogen and progesterone
(C) estrogen only
(D) raloxifene
(E) tamoxifen

6. A 29-year-old gravida 2, para 1 is on the labor and delivery floor with contractions every 3 minutes for the past hour. She is 29 weeks' gestation and has had an uncomplicated prenatal course. She is a smoker and has been unable to quit during this pregnancy. You cared for her during her first pregnancy, which resulted in a 32-week cesarean section delivery of a female infant. At the time of delivery, you noticed that the patient has a bicornuate uterus. Now, you examine her and find that there is good fetal movement, no leaking of fluid, and no vaginal bleeding. Her temperature is 37.0 C (98.6 F), blood pressure is 110/70 mm Hg, pulse is 80/min, and respirations are 16/min. Fetal heart tones are 140/min with good variability. Uterine contractions are occurring every 3 minutes. A sterile vaginal examination found the cervix dilated to 3 cm. You remember that last week her cervix was closed. Ultrasound confirms a vertex presentation. At this time you should

(A) administer betamethasone, penicillin, and magnesium sulfate
(B) attempt an external version, administer betamethasone, penicillin, and magnesium sulfate
(C) continue to monitor the patient for signs of preterm labor
(D) inform the patient that she will need a repeat cesarean section now
(E) place an intrauterine pressure catheter to better monitor the strength of the contractions

7. A 72-year-old woman comes to the clinic complaining of vulvar itching that has been worsening for the last 3 years. She states that she has been to numerous physicians with this complaint and that they have diagnosed her with a yeast infection and have prescribed antifungal medication. She has had no vaginal bleeding since she underwent menopause at the age of 54. She smokes 1 pack of cigarettes per day. On physical examination, she has a raised, pigmented lesion on the left labia majora. The rest of the examination is otherwise normal. The most appropriate course of action is to

(A) biopsy the lesion
(B) perform a vulvectomy
(C) prescribe an antibiotic
(D) prescribe steroid cream
(E) refer to psychiatry

8. A 25-year-old primigravid woman at 39 weeks' gestation comes to the clinic because she thinks she may have ruptured her membranes. You notice in her chart that she had an outbreak of genital herpes at 34 weeks' gestation. A sterile speculum examination shows a pool of fluid in the vagina that is nitrazine-positive. Examination also demonstrates an ulcerated lesion on the anterior lip of the cervix. On further questioning the woman notes that starting yesterday, she has felt a tingling in her genital area. At this time the most correct statement about her condition is:

(A) The fetus is already infected
(B) The lesion is not infectious
(C) She should be sent home and advised to return when she is contracting
(D) She should be started on oxytocin immediately to expedite delivery
(E) She should have a cesarean delivery as soon as possible

9. A 59-year-old woman comes to the office because of vaginal pain during intercourse and a persistent vaginal itch. Her last menstrual period was at 51 years of age. She takes thyroxine for hypothyroidism. She has no other medical problems and no known drug allergies. A pelvic examination is performed that demonstrates the vaginal mucosa to be pale with no rugae present. The vagina is dry with no discharge present. A potassium hydroxide (KOH) and normal saline wet preparation is negative for pseudohyphae, clue cells, and trichomonads. The most appropriate next step is to

(A) explain that no treatment is available
(B) refer the patient for sexual counseling
(C) treat with clotrimazole vaginal cream
(D) treat with estrogen vaginal cream
(E) treat with metronidazole vaginal cream

10. A 17-year-old white girl comes to the clinic for a prenatal visit. She is at 10 weeks' gestation based on her last menstrual period and a 9 week ultrasound that showed a live intrauterine pregnancy with a fetal heart rate of 156/min, and a 2-cm right ovarian complex cyst. She is concerned because she has been experiencing significant nausea each day for the past few weeks. She has not been vomiting and has been able to eat three times each day. Physical examination is unremarkable including a benign abdominal and pelvic examination. The most appropriate course of action is to

(A) admit to the hospital for intravenous fluids and antiemetics
(B) admit to the hospital for total parenteral nutrition
(C) check a serum thyroid stimulating hormone level
(D) reassure the patient that nausea in early pregnancy is common
(E) recommend laparoscopy with removal of the cyst

11. A 28-year-old woman, gravida 2, para 1, at 39 weeks' gestation, comes to the emergency department because of 3-hour history of abdominal pain. She states that the pain comes approximately every 10 minutes, lasts for about 1 minute, and resolves completely in between. She has missed her last few prenatal appointments. Her obstetrical history is significant for a prior classic cesarean delivery 3 years ago. Examination shows her to be in some distress during the episodes of pain, but comfortable otherwise. Her temperature is 37.0 C (98.6 F). Her abdomen is soft, nontender, and gravid with a 39-week uterus. Her cervix is 2 cm dilated and 50% effaced. The most appropriate course of action is to

(A) advise her to return with increasing contractions
(B) arrange for cesarean delivery as soon as possible
(C) begin a course of betamethasone
(D) obtain a surgical consult to rule out appendicitis
(E) recommend acetaminophen and warm packs

12. A 22-year-old nulligravid woman comes to the emergency department because her partner's condom broke during intercourse earlier in the evening, and she is very clear that she does not wish to become pregnant. The patient has been in a monogamous relationship with her partner for the past 3 years. She has no medical problems. She had an appendectomy 2 years ago for an episode of acute appendicitis. She was on the oral contraceptive pill (OCP) 2 years ago, but currently takes no medications and has no allergies to medications. She has a family history of diabetes. Physical examination, including pelvic examination, is unremarkable. Urine hCG is negative. The most appropriate next step is to

    (A) advise her to get another pregnancy test in 1 week
    (B) offer emergency contraception with an oral contraceptive pill
    (C) recommend placement of an intrauterine device
    (D) treat with intramuscular ceftriaxone
    (E) treat with oral azithromycin

13. A 52-year-old woman comes to the office because of increasing tiredness. For the past several months she has noted difficulty with sleeping. She states that she awakens several times during the night, often covered in sweat. She also notes mood lability throughout the day. These symptoms have come intermittently over the last few months. The symptoms seem to be related to her menses although she has not had a period for 2 months. She has asthma for which she uses an albuterol inhaler. She is status post right ovarian cystectomy for a dermoid cyst. Physical examination, including pelvic examination, is entirely within normal limits. Urine hCG is negative. The most appropriate next step is to

    (A) check serum follicle stimulating hormone (FSH)
    (B) check serum human chorionic gonadotropin (HCG)
    (C) explain that no treatment is available for her symptoms
    (D) prescribe fluoxetine for the patient
    (E) refer the patient for psychotherapy

14. A 34-year-old primigravid woman comes to the hospital at 35 weeks' gestation because of increasing contractions. Her prenatal course was unremarkable except for an elevated maternal serum alpha-fetoprotein test followed by a normal ultrasound. She has no medical problems and has never had surgery. She takes prenatal vitamins and has no known drug allergies. Cervical examination shows her to be 6 cm dilated and 100% effaced with the fetus in a vertex position. The fetal heart rate is in the 140s/min and reactive. She is found to be contracting every 3 minutes. At this time you should

    (A) administer corticosteroids
    (B) perform a cesarean delivery
    (C) prepare for forceps delivery
    (D) start intravenous oxytocin
    (E) start intravenous penicillin

15. A 65-year-old woman comes to the office complaining of a 3-week history of intermittent vaginal bleeding that she says is similar to the way her menses used to be before menopause. She has no other complaints. Her last period was at the age of 53. She has depression for which she takes fluoxetine and no other medical problems. Past surgical history is negative. Physical examination is unremarkable. Pelvic examination reveals some blood in the vaginal vault that appears to be coming out the cervical os. There are no uterine or adnexal masses or tenderness. The most appropriate course of action is to

    (A) fit the patient with a pessary
    (B) perform an endometrial biopsy
    (C) prescribe estrogen replacement therapy
    (D) reassure the patient that the bleeding is normal
    (E) schedule the patient for a hysterectomy

16. A 33-year-old woman at 36 weeks' gestation with her second pregnancy comes to the office because of worsening generalized itching that began about 2 weeks ago. The itching is worse at night and especially marked on the palms and soles. She states that it is driving her crazy and that she cannot sleep at night. She has not noticed any rash. She has had no fever, chills, nausea, vomiting, or abdominal pain. Her pregnancy has been uncomplicated to this point. Past obstetrical history is significant for a normal spontaneous vaginal delivery 3 years ago. She has no medical or surgical history. She takes a prenatal vitamin daily and has no known drug allergies. Physical examination is remarkable only for excoriations on the upper and lower extremities. Her cervix is closed and the fetus is in vertex presentation. The most appropriate next step in management is to

(A) check liver function tests and bile acids
(B) reassure the patient that her symptoms are normal
(C) refer the patient to a dermatologist
(D) refer the patient to a psychiatrist
(E) schedule a cesarean delivery

17. A 42-year-old woman at 27 weeks' gestation comes to the office because of vaginal spotting that she first noticed 12 hours ago. She has no other complaints. Her pregnancy has thus far been uncomplicated. Her temperature is 37.3 C (99.1 F), blood pressure is 110/68 mm Hg, pulse is 82/min, and respirations are 12/min. Her abdomen is soft and nontender with a fundal height of 28 cm. Speculum examination reveals scant blood in the vagina with no evidence of active bleeding or polyps. Laboratory studies show: leukocyte count $11,500/mm^3$, hematocrit 32%, and platelet count $155,000/mm^3$. Her blood type is A and Rh type is negative. The fetal heart rate is in the 130s/min and reactive. A sonogram rules out placenta previa. The most appropriate next step in management is to

(A) administer a dose of intramuscular RhoGAM
(B) give 2 units of fresh frozen plasma (FFP)
(C) prepare the patient for cesarean delivery
(D) reassure and then discharge the patient
(E) start intravenous penicillin

18. A 33-year-old woman with fibromyalgia comes to the clinic for a prenatal visit at 30 weeks gestation. Her pregnancy has thus far been uncomplicated. Her past obstetrical history is significant for a low-transverse cesarean delivery at 39 weeks for a breech fetus. Her past surgical history is significant only for the cesarean delivery. She takes no medications and is allergic to penicillin. Physical examination demonstrates a blood pressure of 100/64 mm Hg, trace protein in the urine, a fundal height of 31 cm, fetal heart rate in the 150s/min, and the fetus in vertex presentation. She is uncertain whether or not she wishes to attempt a vaginal birth after cesarean (VBAC) with this delivery or have an elective repeat cesarean delivery. Among the many issues that you discuss with her, you should counsel her that

(A) repeat cesarean delivery is best for her
(B) she is likely to fail a VBAC attempt
(C) she must attempt VBAC given her history
(D) uterine rupture is a risk of VBAC
(E) VBAC is contraindicated given her history

19. A 57-year-old woman comes to the office because of burning and pain with intercourse and vulvar itching. These symptoms started a few months ago and have been worsening since. She had her last menstrual period at the age of 50 and has had no episodes of postmenopausal bleeding. She has a history of migraine headaches. Surgical history is significant for a cholecystectomy 10 years ago. She takes no medications and is allergic to sulfa drugs. Physical examination demonstrates thin labia majora and virtually absent labia minora. The entire vulva is atrophic and whitish in appearance. This whitish area extends around the perianal region in a butterfly pattern. A potassium-hydroxide and normal saline "wet prep" smear of the discharge is negative. The most appropriate pharmacotherapy for this condition is

(A) clotrimazole
(B) estrogen cream
(C) isoniazid
(D) metronidazole
(E) topical testosterone

20. A 26-year-old woman comes to the office for a 6-week postpartum visit. Her baby is doing well. She is breastfeeding exclusively. Her prenatal course was unremarkable and she had a normal spontaneous vaginal delivery. Her past surgical history is significant for an appendectomy 12 years ago. She takes no medications and has no known drug allergies. Physical examination is unremarkable. The patient states that she has been having intercourse for the past week, but is uncomfortable because of vaginal dryness. In addressing this issue, the most appropriate next step is to

    (A) advise her to stop having sexual intercourse until 10 weeks postpartum
    (B) discuss with her starting hormone replacement therapy
    (C) explain to her that she may have premature ovarian failure
    (D) reassure her that vaginal dryness is common with breastfeeding
    (E) refer the patient and her partner for couples counseling

21. A 29-year-old primigravid woman comes to the clinic for a prenatal visit on her due date. Her pregnancy has thus far been significant for nausea and vomiting in the first trimester, which resolved by the mid-second trimester. She has had no other problems during the pregnancy. She has no medical problems. Her past surgical history is significant for an appendectomy at age 13. She takes prenatal vitamins and has no allergies to medications. The fetus is moving well. She has had no bleeding from the vagina, loss of fluid, or contractions. Her weight is 150 lb. Blood pressure is 110/70 mm Hg. She has no protein or glucose in her urine. The fetal heart rate is 140s/min. Her fundal height is 44 cm. Cervical examination demonstrates that her cervix is long, thick, and closed. Estimated fetal weight by Leopold maneuvers is greater than 10 lb. An ultrasound reveals an estimated fetal weight of 5100 g. The most appropriate next step in management is to

    (A) offer primary cesarean delivery for macrosomia
    (B) offer induction of labor for pending macrosomia
    (C) offer primary cesarean delivery for postterm pregnancy
    (D) offer induction of labor for postterm pregnancy
    (E) perform stat cesarean delivery for fetal distress

22. A 37-year-old woman, gravida 2, para 1, at 38 weeks' gestation, comes to the office for a routine visit. Her pregnancy was complicated by hyperemesis gravidarum in the first trimester, which subsequently resolved. A 36-week perineal culture shows her to be group-B streptococcus positive. Her past obstetrical history is significant for a forceps-assisted vaginal delivery of an 8-pound male. She states that she would like to fly across the country to visit her friends this weekend. The most important factor in your decision not to recommend air travel for this patient is her

    (A) age
    (B) gestational age
    (C) group B streptococcus status
    (D) history of a forceps delivery
    (E) hyperemesis gravidarum

23. A 31-year-old woman comes to the emergency department because of a 36-hour history of abdominal pain and vaginal spotting. She has no significant past medical or surgical history and is unsure of the date of her last menstrual period. She is allergic to erythromycin. Her temperature is 37.0 C (98.6 F), blood pressure is 116/78 mm Hg, pulse is 82/min, and respirations are 14/min. Her abdomen is nontender, soft, and nondistended. Pelvic examination shows a small amount of blood in the vagina, a closed cervical os, no pelvic masses, and left-sided pelvic tenderness. Laboratory studies show a leukocyte count of 5600/mm^3, hematocrit of 39.5%, and a platelet count of 179,000/mm^3. The next step in evaluating her symptoms is to order

    (A) an abdominal/pelvic CT
    (B) an abdominal x-ray
    (C) an electrocardiogram
    (D) serum hCG
    (E) serum thyroid stimulating hormone

24. A 29-year-old white woman at 34 weeks' gestation with her third child comes to the emergency department because of a headache that began yesterday and has steadily worsened. She has no other symptoms. Her pregnancy has been uncomplicated up to this point. Past obstetrical history is significant for two spontaneous vaginal deliveries at term. Past medical history is significant for hypothyroidism for which she takes thyroxine. She has no known drug allergies. Her temperature is 37.2 C (99 F), blood pressure is 140/90 mm Hg, and pulse is 80/min. Physical examination shows abdominal right upper quadrant tenderness and a cervix that is 2 cm dilated and 50% effaced. Laboratory studies show:

Hematocrit	25%
Leukocyte count	13,000/mm^3
Platelet count	81,000/mm^3
Serum ALT	550 U/L
Serum AST	470 U/L
Urinalysis	3+ protein

The most appropriate next step in management is to

(A) initiate an induction of labor
(B) manage the patient expectantly until 37 weeks
(C) perform a liver biopsy
(D) start sumatriptan therapy
(E) treat with phenytoin for seizure prophylaxis

25. A 62-year-old woman with coronary artery disease comes to the office to discuss menopause. She had her last menstrual period 8 years ago. She experienced some hot flashes for several months after her last period, but these no longer bother her. She does note some increasing fatigue over the past few years. She underwent an angioplasty 3 years ago and an appendectomy at the age of 19. She takes a beta-blocker and a baby aspirin every day and has no known drug allergies. Physical examination, including pelvic examination, is unremarkable. She has heard many conflicting things regarding hormone replacement therapy (HRT) and wants to know what benefits it could have for her. You should advise her that:

(A) HRT could increase her likelihood of developing osteoporosis
(B) HRT could increase her likelihood of having a cardiovascular event
(C) HRT will decrease her symptoms of fatigue
(D) HRT will reduce her risk of venous thromboembolism
(E) HRT will reduce the progression of atherosclerosis

26. You are driving to the hospital to evaluate one of your obstetric patients who called and said that she was contracting every 7 minutes. She says that she has no vaginal discharge but has been feeling "lots of fetal movement". You remember that she is a G2P1001 woman at 38 weeks' gestation. She was unsure of her last menstrual period, so a first trimester ultrasound was done to establish her due date. There were no abnormalities seen at the time of the ultrasound. Upon arriving on labor and delivery, you learn that on the way to the hospital the patient's car rear-ended another car at low speed. She was a belted passenger. She has developed moderate vaginal bleeding and more severe contractions that are now occurring "one on top of the other". Her abdomen is tender with a reddened area from her lap belt. Her temperature is 37.0 C (98.6 F), blood pressure is 90/60 mm Hg, pulse is 110/min, and respirations are 22/min. The fetal heart rate is being monitored and the baseline is 180/min. Uterine contractions are occurring every 60 seconds and are lasting 45 seconds. At this time you should

(A) administer betamethasone
(B) give magnesium sulfate for tocolysis
(C) manage the labor expectantly
(D) prepare for a cesarean section while stabilizing the patient
(E) order an ultrasound to rule out placenta previa

27. A 28-year-old primigravid woman who is at 38 weeks' gestation comes to the office for a routine examination. She has had an uncomplicated pregnancy. She had an ultrasound done in the first trimester for an unsure last menstrual period, and no abnormalities were noted. You notice that the patient's weight has increased by 5 pounds in the last week and her blood pressure is 160/100 mm Hg. The patient reports good fetal movement, no contractions, no leaking of fluid, and no vaginal bleeding. She has noticed some increased edema over the last week and has had a severe headache since early in the morning. She denies any visual changes or abdominal pain. The fetal heart tones are found to be 140/min. The nurse then enters the room with the results of the patient's urinalysis. It shows 3+ protein. At this time you should

(A) have the patient admitted to labor and delivery for betamethasone and magnesium sulfate therapy
(B) have the patient admitted to labor and delivery for a cesarean section
(C) have the patient admitted to labor and delivery for magnesium sulfate therapy and induction of labor
(D) send the patient home with instructions for strict bedrest and reevaluate her blood pressure in 24 hours
(E) send the patient home with a prescription for lisinopril for her hypertension

28. A 32-year-old woman comes to the office because she has not had a menstrual period in 7 weeks. A pregnancy test and physical examination confirm a first trimester pregnancy. She has had three pregnancies in the past and all three ended in spontaneous miscarriages in the first trimester. A thorough physical examination, including a pelvic examination, is normal. There is no history of miscarriage or fetal deformities in her family. A prior hysterosalpingogram did not reveal any uterine abnormality. Her serum prolactin level and thyroid function tests are normal. Lupus anticoagulant test is negative. The most appropriate next investigation to evaluate her history of miscarriages is

(A) anticardiolipin antibody
(B) antinuclear antibody
(C) antisperm antibody
(D) glucose tolerance test
(E) histocompatibility locus antigen

29. A 25-year-old college student comes to the student health center because of a lack of menses for the past year. Her menarche started at age 13 and she has always had regular menstrual cycles. She has never been pregnant. For the past year and a half she has been training for the New York marathon, which she successfully completed this year. She was given medroxyprogesterone acetate by another physician a few months ago but did not experience withdrawal bleeding. Physical examination, including pelvic examination, is normal. No galactorrhea is noted. She is 5 ft 2 inches tall and weighs 112 lb. Serum gonadotropin and prolactin levels are within normal limits. Serum follicle stimulating hormone and luteinizing hormone levels are low. The most likely cause of this patient's amenorrhea is

(A) hypothalamic amenorrhea
(B) a pituitary tumor
(C) polycystic ovary disease
(D) premature ovarian failure
(E) prolonged use of intrauterine device

30. A 16-year-old girl is brought to the office because her menstrual periods have not started yet. She does not have any other medical complaints and denies any sexual intercourse. She was born via normal vaginal delivery and has never had any medical problems. Her mother and older sister started their menstrual periods at the age of 13 and their cycles have been regular. Her blood pressure is 110/70 mm Hg. She is 5 ft tall and weighs 120 lb. Physical examination reveals normal breast size and normal pubic and axillary hair. The most likely cause of her amenorrhea is

(A) hypothalamic dysfunction
(B) imperforate hymen
(C) pituitary dysfunction
(D) testicular feminization syndrome
(E) vaginal and uterine agenesis

31. A previously healthy 26-year-old woman comes to the office complaining of 6 months of severe menstrual cramping and pain. She does not have any bleeding between cycles. She had menarche at the age of 14 and since then has had regular menstrual cycles until 6 months ago. Nonsteroidal anti-inflammatory drugs give her only moderate relief. There is no family history of similar symptoms. She has been sexually active and always uses condoms. She says that she has been monogamous and there is no history of sexually transmitted disease either in her or in her partner. Her temperature is 37.0 C (98.6 F). Physical examination, including pelvic examination, is normal. A pelvic ultrasound done in the office is normal except for a small, simple cystic area in the right ovary. The most likely diagnosis is

    (A) endometriosis
    (B) endometritis
    (C) pelvic inflammatory disease
    (D) ruptured ovarian cyst
    (E) uterine fibroids

32. A 30-year-old woman comes to the clinic complaining of "dribbling" of urine. She has had recurrent urinary tract infections over the past 11 months, which were treated with antibiotics. She has been following safe sex practices and denies any history of sexually transmitted diseases but complains of moderate pain during intercourse. Physical examination, including pelvic examination, is normal. The most appropriate next investigation in this patient is

    (A) a CT scan of the abdomen and pelvis
    (B) laparoscopy
    (C) pelvic sonography
    (D) renal sonography
    (E) a voiding cystourethrogram

33. A 42-year-old woman comes to the office complaining of shortness of breath and abdominal distention for the past 2 months. She reports a 5 to 8-lb weight gain in the past 3 months despite a decreased appetite. She underwent an appendectomy at the age of 12 years and a cholecystectomy at the age of 30. Both surgical procedures were uneventful and she had a regular postoperative recovery. Physical examination reveals decreased breath sounds in the right chest, slight abdominal distention, and ascites. Pelvic examination reveals fullness in the right lateral fornix and no tenderness. Complete blood count and metabolic panels are within normal limits. CA-125 level is normal. A chest x-ray shows a right pleural effusion. Ultrasonography of the abdomen shows ascites and an enlarged right ovary with no lesions in the liver. The most appropriate next step in management is

    (A) bilateral salpingo-oophorectomy
    (B) bilateral salpingo-oophorectomy and hysterectomy
    (C) excision of the right ovary
    (D) excision of the right ovary, right tube thoracostomy, and abdominal paracentesis
    (E) ovarian biopsy and right tube thoracostomy

34. A 32-year-old woman comes to the office complaining of a 3-month history of increased bleeding during menstruation and some "spotting" between periods. There is no associated pain or discomfort during menstruation. Menarche was at 14 years of age. Since then she has been having regular menstrual cycles. She denies any bleeding history. A complete blood count reveals microcytic hypochromic anemia. A coagulation profile is normal. Urine hCG is negative. The most likely cause of her excessive menstrual bleeding is

    (A) anovulatory bleeding
    (B) a coagulopathy
    (C) endometrial hyperplasia
    (D) an endometrial polyp
    (E) a threatened abortion

35. A 19-year-old primigravid woman with an unsure last menstrual period comes to the labor and delivery floor because she has been "leaking clear fluid" for the past 12 hours. She thinks that she is "7 months" pregnant but has had no prenatal care. She denies vaginal bleeding, abdominal pain, contractions, or fever. She reports adequate fetal movement. Her temperature is 37.0 C (98.6 F), blood pressure is 110/70 mm Hg, and respirations are 18/min. The fetal heart rate is 150/min with no evidence of uterine contractions. Her abdomen is soft and her fundal height is measured at 28 cm. You perform a sterile speculum examination and see pooling of clear fluid in the vaginal vault with a pH of 7.45. Her cervical os is visually closed. When viewed under the microscope the dried vaginal fluid makes a ferning pattern. The most appropriate intervention at this time is

(A) cesarean section to prevent chorioamnionitis
(B) sterile vaginal examination
(C) treatment with magnesium sulfate
(D) treatment with oxytocin
(E) ultrasound examination of the fetus

36. A 24-year-old primigravid woman at 8 weeks' gestation comes to the office for a prenatal visit. She has had some mild nausea and vomiting, but is able to tolerate food and fluids and has no other complaints. She takes no medications and has no known drug allergies. Physical examination is consistent with an 8-week pregnancy. She is an active woman who has been exercising daily for all of her adult life and loves scuba diving. She has many friends who have told her that she cannot continue these activities during pregnancy. She wants to know your advice on exercise during pregnancy. You should advise her that:

(A) Exercise during pregnancy is prohibited
(B) Exercise during pregnancy may lead to gestational diabetes
(C) Scuba diving is not prohibited during pregnancy
(D) She can do 30 minutes of moderate exercise daily
(E) She should exercise no more than 20 minutes twice weekly

37. A 21-year-old woman with asthma comes to the community-based health center for a follow-up visit. One week ago you saw her for a routine annual examination. At that time, she had no health complaints. Her mother died from a myocardial infarction at the age of 54, and her father died from a myocardial infarction at the age of 48. She has two male sexual partners. Physical examination, including pelvic examination, was normal. Yesterday, the results from the studies performed at the last visit returned as follows: Pap smear normal, gonorrhea negative, and chlamydia positive. The most accurate statement about her condition is:

(A) Asymptomatic disease is not associated with complications
(B) Hospitalization is required for her given her age
(C) No treatment is necessary since she is asymptomatic
(D) She should receive treatment as well as her sexual partners
(E) The result is most likely a false positive and no treatment is needed

38. A 56-year-old woman comes to the office because of disturbed sleep. Over the past 2 months she finds herself waking up at night with a feeling of "flushing and heat" throughout her body. These happen during the day also and typically last for a few minutes. Her last menstrual period was 6 months ago. She has no other symptoms. She has migraine headaches for which she takes sumatriptan and underwent an uneventful cholecystectomy 10 years ago. She has no known drug allergies. She has no family history of cancer or heart disease. Physical examination, including breast and pelvic examination, is normal. Her friends have told her that she is having "hot flashes" and that she should take estrogen, but she has read that estrogen can cause blood clots and cancer. She wants to know your opinion on the matter. Your counseling of this patient should include that:

(A) Hormone replacement therapy may decrease the risk of developing a thrombosis
(B) Hormone replacement therapy may increase the risk of developing breast cancer
(C) Hormone replacement therapy may worsen the hot flashes
(D) The estrogen component of hormone replacement therapy will help to prevent breast cancer
(E) The progestin component of hormone replacement therapy will help to prevent breast cancer

39. A 27-year-old woman who is 5 days postpartum from a primary cesarean delivery, performed because she presented in labor with a breech fetus, comes to the office for staple removal. She states that overall she is doing well but over the past couple of days she has been a little more irritable than usual and more emotionally labile, often crying very easily. She is sleeping and eating normally and has been enjoying having her friends and family over to visit the new baby. She has no thoughts of hurting herself or the baby. Her past medical and surgical histories are unremarkable. Physical examination is unremarkable. You remove the staples and notice that the incision is clean, dry, and intact. This patient is most likely suffering from

(A) mild preeclampsia
(B) postpartum blues
(C) postpartum nonpsychotic depression
(D) postpartum psychotic depression
(E) posttraumatic stress disorder

40. A 31-year-old woman who is at 20 weeks' gestation comes to the office for a prenatal visit. She feels well except for some occasional nausea. Her first pregnancy, 3 years ago, resulted in a low transverse cesarean delivery for a non-reassuring fetal heart tracing during labor. She has no medical problems. She had a diagnostic laparoscopy for pelvic pain at the age of 22. She takes prenatal vitamins and is allergic to sulfa drugs. Her blood pressure is 110/70 mm Hg. Her urine dip is negative. Her fundus is at her umbilicus. The fetal heart rate is 140/min. She asks if vaginal birth after cesarean (VBAC) is an option for her with this pregnancy. The hospital where she will be delivering has 24-hour access to emergency cesarean delivery and anesthesia. The statement that should be emphasized in discussing mode of delivery with her is:

(A) A repeat cesarean delivery is absolutely contraindicated for her
(B) A repeat cesarean delivery is the recommended mode of delivery for her
(C) A vaginal birth must be attempted based on current insurance regulations
(D) VBAC is absolutely contraindicated given her past obstetrical history
(E) VBAC is a reasonable option in her case and the decision is up to her

41. A previously healthy 16-year-old girl comes to the office because of a 1-week history of abdominal pain that began 1 week following her most recent menses, which was normal in character. She describes the pain as "achy", and localizes it to the suprapubic area. She has no dysuria or hematuria but does complain of a foul-smelling, greenish vaginal discharge. Her last office visit was 6 months ago for her routine Pap smear, which she has had since becoming sexually active 1 year ago. She and her partner use condoms "almost always," but she has been resistant to your suggestion to start oral contraceptives because of fears that her parents will find out. As she walks to the examining table, you notice that she has a shuffling gait due to her abdominal discomfort. Her temperature is 38.5 C (101.3 F), blood pressure is 90/60 mm Hg, pulse is 70/min, and respirations are 12/min. Her abdomen is extremely tender in both the suprapubic area and the right upper quadrant. Pelvic examination reveals pus at the cervical os and cervical motion tenderness. There are no adnexal masses. You send cultures of the discharge for *Neisseria gonorrhoeae* and *Chlamydia trachomatis*. Urine hCG is negative. At this time the most correct statement about this patient's condition is:

(A) Antibiotic therapy should result in resolution of her symptoms within 48 hours
(B) Gonococcal perihepatitis ("Fitz-Hugh-Curtis") syndrome is a surgical emergency, requiring prompt drainage
(C) Her risk of subsequent ectopic pregnancy will increase even further if she has recurrent episodes of PID
(D) In the absence of a positive cervical culture, empiric therapy should be discontinued
(E) This episode of PID is likely to have made her infertile, so prescription of a contraceptive method at this time is unnecessary

42. A 38-year-old physical therapist comes to the office because of lower back pain that began after extensive cleaning around her house 2 days ago. The pain is localized around the ischial spines and ischial tuberosity. Your physical examination is consistent with lumbar muscle spasm and you recommend carisoprodol. She returns to clinic a few hours later and hesitantly tells you that she might be pregnant, as her last menstrual period was 8 weeks ago. She looked up carisoprodol in the prescribing reference book and noticed that it is in "risk factor category C" medications for pregnancy. She asks you what this means. In terms of safety during pregnancy, "category C" means that:

(A) Animal studies do not demonstrate a fetal risk but there are no controlled studies in pregnant women.

(B) Animal studies show an adverse effect (other than a decrease in fertility) that was not confirmed in controlled studies in women in the first trimester.

(C) Controlled studies in pregnant women fail to demonstrate a risk to the fetus in the first trimester (and even subsequent trimesters), and the risk of fetal harm is remote.

(D) Studies in animals or humans demonstrate fetal abnormalities and the drug is contraindicated in pregnancy.

(E) There is uncertain safety during pregnancy because animal studies show adverse effects on the fetus (teratogenic), but there are no controlled studies in women; or animal and human studies are not available.

(F) There is positive evidence of human fetal risk but the benefits for use in pregnancy may outweigh the risks.

Items 43-44

43. A 32-year-old woman comes to the emergency department with excessive vaginal bleeding that has required 10 pads/day for the past 8 days. She suffers from depression, systemic lupus erythematosus, and hypothyroidism and is currently taking L-thyroxine and fluoxetine. She has one sexual partner and no previous sexually transmitted diseases. She has one child and is convinced that she is not pregnant. She denies pain and explains that her periods have been irregular over the past 3 months. She is not on the oral contraceptive pill. Her hemoglobin is 7.2 mg/dL and hematocrit is 22.2 mg/dL.

The most likely cause of her abnormal bleeding is

(A) adenocarcinoma of the endometrium

(B) anovulation

(C) coagulation defects

(D) pelvic inflammatory disease

(E) pregnancy

44. On physical examination, she appears pale, her temperature is 37.0 (98.6 F), blood pressure is 95/70 mm Hg, pulse is 86/min, and respirations are 16/min. Her heart sounds are normal, breathing is clear, and abdomen is soft and nontender with no palpable masses. Her reflexes are brisk. A speculum examination demonstrates a normal cervix with bleeding from the cervical os. There is blood in the posterior fornix. A urinary bhCG is negative. Laboratory studies show:

Hemoglobin	7.2 g/dL
Hematocrit	22.2 g/dL
Leukocyte count	8000/mm^3
Platelets	200,000/mm^3
Sodium	141 mEq/L
Potassium	4.0 mEq/L
Bicarbonate	104 mEq/L
Chloride	22 mEq/L
BUN	20 mg/dL
Creatinine	1.2 mg/dL

A pelvic sonogram shows a normal uterus and ovaries. The most appropriate therapy at this time is

(A) conjugated estrogen, 2.5 mg by mouth 4 times a day
(B) estrogen, 25 mg intravenously every 6 hours
(C) ethinyl estradiol/levonorgestrel, 1 tablet daily
(D) ibuprofen, 800 mg by mouth 4 times a day
(E) medroxyprogesterone acetate, 10 mg by mouth daily

45. A 15-year-old girl comes to the office alone because of a 3-day history of vaginal discharge. She is sexually active with a "couple of guys" at school and they use condoms "when someone remembers to bring them." She has been a patient of yours for 10 years and she typically comes to scheduled appointments with her mother. This time she asks you not to even tell her mother that she was here because she does not want her mother to know that she is sexually active. Physical examination shows a frothy green vaginal discharge, deeply erythematous vaginal mucosa, and numerous petechiae on the cervix. A wet mount of the discharge shows motile, flagellated organisms. You counsel her about sexually transmitted diseases and offer HIV testing. After testing her for other common sexually transmitted diseases, the most appropriate next step is to

(A) administer ceftriaxone intramuscularly and prescribe oral doxycycline
(B) call the patient's mother to obtain consent for treatment because she is a minor
(C) contact child protective services for suspected sexual abuse
(D) prescribe oral metronidazole and advise her to tell her sexual partners to be treated
(E) send a culture of the vaginal discharge to establish a definite diagnosis

46. You are called to evaluate a patient in the obstetrics floor because she is exhibiting bizarre behavior. The patient is a 25-year-old white woman who delivered her first child 2 days ago. The patient has no known psychiatric history but since this morning has been making bizarre statements such as, "the baby isn't mine...I don't know whose it is...it belongs to a spirit." The patient's husband states that he has never seen the patient act in this manner before. On mental status examination, the patient is poorly related, disheveled, and continues to assert that her child is not hers. She also appears to be responding to internal stimuli. Vital signs and physical examination are within normal limits. Laboratory studies, including urine toxicology, chemistries, and complete blood count, are normal. The patient and her baby are scheduled to be discharged in the morning. The next appropriate step in management is to

(A) give the patient a 2-week prescription for fluoxetine for "postpartum blues"
(B) have the patient's baby brought into the room to observe mother-child interaction
(C) make an outpatient psychiatry appointment for the patient on discharge
(D) put her on immediate observation and call for a psychiatric consultation with possible transfer to an inpatient psychiatric unit
(E) sedate the patient with diazepam and reassess the patient prior to discharge

47. At the request of a family member, you are called to assess a patient who does not want to accept chemotherapy treatment for breast cancer. The patient is a 55-year-old woman with no known past psychiatric or substance abuse history. She has agreed to mastectomy and radiation therapy for a stage IV breast malignancy, but adamantly states that she does not want chemotherapy because she saw her brother, "suffer horribly," during chemotherapy for lung cancer. On meeting the patient's family prior to evaluation, you are asked to try to convince the patient to undergo chemotherapy. The most appropriate next step is to

(A) agree to convince the patient to undergo chemotherapy
(B) offer the patient psychiatric hospitalization while making this decision
(C) state that an assessment of the patient's capacity to make this decision will be performed
(D) tell the patient that she may only be allowed to leave the hospital if given a psychiatry appointment as an outpatient
(E) temporarily sedate the patient and reassess the patient after she has slept

48. A 16-year-old girl comes to the emergency department in the middle of the night because of progressively severe lower abdominal pain. She vomited once earlier in the evening when she tried to take an extra-strength acetaminophen tablet. She denies other medications. She has had no diarrhea, runny nose, cough, sore throat, or dysuria. She reports her menses have been normal; however, occasionally she gets menstrual cramps. Her last menstrual period was 9 days ago with regular flow. She denies vaginal discharge and states, "no, I do not have a boyfriend and I have never had sexual relations." Physical examination shows a teenage girl in mild discomfort and distress from her abdominal pain. Her temperature is 38.9 C (102.0 F), blood pressure is 128/72 mm Hg, pulse is 112/min, and respirations are 24/min. Her abdomen is flat with tenderness and guarding in the right and left lower quadrants. No masses or hepatomegaly is appreciated, but there is some rebound tenderness that is referred to the lower quadrants. Rectal examination reveals definite tenderness anteriorly. Pelvic examination shows cervical motion tenderness and bilateral adnexal tenderness, particularly in the right adnexal area, and vaginal discharge. Laboratory studies reveal a hematocrit of 39.6%, a leukocyte count of 16,800 mm^3 with 80% segmented neutrophils, 8% neutrophil bands, 10% lymphocytes, and 2% monocytes. Examination of the discharge reveals many leukocytes and bacteria, but no gram-negative intracellular diplococci are seen on Gram stain. A β-hCG is negative. Of the information in this case so far, the most convincing evidence that this girl may have pelvic inflammatory disease is

(A) adnexal tenderness
(B) cervical motion tenderness
(C) a fever over 38.9 C (102.0 F)
(D) no significant prodrome of nausea and vomiting
(E) vaginal discharge

49. A 39-year-old obese woman comes to the office because of new hair growth on her upper lip and chin over the past 6 months. During this time, her menstrual cycles were initially longer with heavy bleeding, however, she had no menses in 10 weeks. She has hypertension and takes hydrochlorothiazide and atenolol. She has a family history of obesity, diabetes, and heart disease but not any menstrual irregularities or cancer. Physical examination shows frontal thinning of her hair and coarse facial hair over her upper lip and chin. Her voice is unchanged, she has a few scattered pustules over her back, which are unchanged from her last visit, and she has abdominal striae. Breast examination shows no masses, and there is no nipple discharge. She has normal ovaries and some clitoromegaly. The testosterone level is elevated. DHEA-S level is within normal limits. The most appropriate next step in management is to

(A) determine free testosterone level
(B) determine luteinizing hormone/follicle stimulating hormone (LH/FSH) ratio
(C) determine prolactin level
(D) order a pelvic ultrasound
(E) provide reassurance

50. A 55-year-old woman comes to the office because of a palpable lump in her right breast. She is otherwise feeling well and denies any pain, breast discharge, fevers, or weight loss. She has no history of prior breast abnormalities and has never had a mammogram. She has no family history of breast cancer, has one child who is 30, and began menopause at age 50. On examination, you confirm a lump in the axillary region of the right breast that is nontender, mobile, and approximately 2 cm in diameter. There is no lymphadenopathy, other masses, or any other abnormalities appreciated on examination. She is sent for a mammogram, which is read as "without abnormalities." An ultrasound also fails to locate any abnormalities. The next best step is

(A) excisional or needle biopsy
(B) reassurance and repeat mammogram in 6 months
(C) reassurance and repeat mammogram in 1 year
(D) reassurance and repeat physical examination in 6 months
(E) reassurance and repeat ultrasound in 6 months
(F) risk stratify by gene testing for BRCA-1 and -2

Obstetrics/Gynecology Test One: **Answers and Explanations**

ANSWER KEY

1. E
2. B
3. C
4. D
5. A
6. A
7. A
8. E
9. D
10. D
11. B
12. B
13. A
14. E
15. B
16. A
17. A
18. D
19. E
20. D
21. A
22. B
23. D
24. A
25. B
26. D
27. C
28. A
29. A
30. E
31. A
32. E
33. C
34. D
35. E
36. D
37. D
38. B
39. B
40. E
41. C
42. E
43. E
44. B
45. D
46. D
47. C
48. B
49. D
50. A

1. **The correct answer is E.** One of the most common reasons for adolescents to stop taking the oral contraceptive pill (OCP) is what is known as breakthrough bleeding. This is irregular spotting and bleeding that occurs during the first months of OCP use. Breakthrough bleeding is often due to missed pills but can also occur in patients who take the pill every day as the body adjusts to the OCP. Adolescents must be reassured that breakthrough bleeding is not harmful to their health, that it is most common in the first months of use, and that it usually resolves with a few months of OCP use. They should also be reminded to take the pill every day at about the same time each day.

   Determining serum follicle stimulating hormone level **(choice A)** would not be necessary in this patient. FSH concentration can be a useful test to determine ovarian reserve (e.g., in cases of infertility or menopause). However, in this healthy 18-year-old with a history of normal periods, it would not be necessary.

   It is often useful to determine serum thyroid stimulating hormone level **(choice B)** in patients with irregular menstrual periods, as thyroid abnormalities can lead to menstrual dysfunction. However, this patient has a history of normal menstrual periods and a much more likely cause for her irregular bleeding (i.e., breakthrough bleeding).

   To perform endometrial biopsy **(choice C)** would be an unnecessary and potentially risky diagnostic approach for this patient. Endometrial biopsy is often used in cases of irregular bleeding. This diagnostic approach, however, is more appropriate for patients at risk for endometrial cancer (e.g., postmenopausal patients). This young woman is at very low risk for endometrial cancer, and endometrial biopsy has the risks of bleeding, infection, and perforation.

   Pelvic ultrasonography **(choice D)** would not be indicated in this patient as there is no evidence of pelvic pathology on the physical exam, and intermittent vaginal spotting is a common complaint among young women starting the OCP.

2. **The correct answer is B.** There is a well-established link between unopposed estrogen (i.e., estrogen not taken with progesterone) and endometrial hyperplasia and cancer. Progestins have been found to help to prevent the development of endometrial cancer in patients who are taking estrogen. This is the "female cancer" to which the patient is likely referring. Breast tissue, however, appears to differ significantly from endometrial tissue in that progesterone does not appear to protect against the development of breast cancer in patients on estrogen replacement therapy. In fact, progesterone appears to increase a woman's risk of developing breast cancer over estrogen alone. Therefore, this patient, who has had a hysterectomy, should not be placed on progesterone.

   To state that "hormone replacement therapy (HRT) is contraindicated in your case" **(choice A)** is incorrect. Hormone replacement therapy is recommended as treatment to relieve vasomotor symptoms (i.e., hot flashes) and genitourinary atrophy, as well as to reduce the risk of osteoporosis and, possibly, cardiovascular disease. There does appear to be some small increased risk of breast cancer among HRT users, but this does not make it contraindicated.

   To state that "progesterone should be added to your hormone replacement regimen" **(choice C)** is incorrect. As noted above, progesterone should be added to estrogen to protect against the development of endometrial cancer. This patient, who is status-post hysterectomy, does not need this protection.

   To state that "you have a high risk of developing breast cancer while on estrogen" **(choice D)** is incorrect. General estimates are that the projected absolute lifetime risk for non-estrogen users is about 10 cases of breast cancer per 100 women. With estrogen use, this increases to 12 cases per 100 women.

   To state that "you should not have had a hysterectomy" **(choice E)** is incorrect. Pelvic pain and pressure with a large fibroid uterus is a reasonable indication for hysterectomy.

3. **The correct answer is C.** This patient's clinical picture is consistent with a threatened abortion. She is pregnant, but has not passed any products of conception and her cervical os is closed. Determination of blood type is important because first trimester miscarriage is an indication for administration of RhoGAM to prevent alloimmunization. A sonogram will help differentiate a threatened abortion from a missed abortion.

   A missed abortion **(choice A)** is defined as retention of the fetal tissue after fetal death has occurred. Fetal death should be confirmed by ultrasound prior to dilatation and curettage. There is no indication that this patient has a missed abortion.

   Ectopic pregnancy should be suspected in any patient with abdominal pain and a positive pregnancy test. It can occasionally be treated surgically **(choice B)** or with methotrexate **(choice E)**. However, this diagnosis should be confirmed with ultrasound prior to either treatment.

Pelvic inflammatory disease (**choice D**) can occasionally present with mild lower abdominal pain and irregular bleeding, and the medications in choice D are appropriate treatment for this infection. However, physical exam usually reveals fever, cervical motion tenderness, or adnexal tenderness. The patient has none of these findings and therefore choice D is incorrect. The patient should, however, be screened for sexually transmitted diseases given her high-risk behaviors. Additionally, doxycycline, typical treatment for pelvic inflammatory disease, should not be used in pregnancy because of adverse affects on fetal bones and teeth in addition to other congenital defects.

4. **The correct answer is D.** This patient has a classic presentation for candidiasis. The usual cause of candidiasis is *Candida albicans.* Most patients with candidiasis will have itching, irritation, or both. The irritation is often associated with dysuria, as the contact of the urine on the irritated mucosa causes significant discomfort. Patients with candidiasis also commonly complain of discharge, which is usually described as thick, white, and cottage cheese-like. Symptoms often begin just prior to the menses and candidiasis is often associated with use of immunosuppressives or steroid therapy, diabetes mellitus, pregnancy, hormone replacement therapy, oral contraceptive agents, and antibiotics. This patient's recent antibiotic use could certainly have contributed to her developing candidiasis. Physical examination demonstrates erythema and edema of the genital area as well as the discharge. Potassium hydroxide (KOH) application to a sample of the discharge leads to lysis of the normal cellular elements; the pseudohyphae and buds of the *Candida* are then revealed. Treatment is with a topical vaginal agent such as clotrimazole or with an oral azole fungal agent.

To perform ampicillin vaginal lavage (**choice A**) would not be correct. This is not a commonly accepted procedure in gynecologic practice. Furthermore, ampicillin is not a treatment for candidiasis. In fact, antibiotic usage can often contribute to the development of candidiasis.

To perform a vulvar biopsy (**choice B**) would not be appropriate. Vulvar biopsy can be used in cases of uncertain diagnosis or when there is concern for malignancy. This patient has a classic presentation for candidiasis and vulvar biopsy would not be needed.

To treat with oral azithromycin (**choice C**) would not be correct. Azithromycin is commonly used in gynecology for the treatment of infections with *Chlamydia trachomatis.* This patient has candidiasis and, therefore, should not be treated with azithromycin.

To treat with topical (vaginal) metronidazole (**choice E**) would not be correct. Topical metronidazole is most often used in gynecologic practice for the treatment of bacterial vaginosis or trichomoniasis. This patient does not have bacterial vaginosis or trichomoniasis and should not, therefore, be treated with topical metronidazole.

5. **The correct answer is A.** This patient has a presentation that is most consistent with perimenopausal hot flashes (or hot flushes as they are sometimes referred to). The exact pathophysiology that underlies the hot flash is unknown. However, studies have shown that women at menopause and men that undergo orchiectomies experience these symptoms. Therefore, it is assumed that it is the withdrawal of normal levels of sex steroids from the circulation that results in the hot flash. These hot feelings are experienced as a "flushing" that can last from several seconds to many minutes. The first-line treatment for most women is with hormone replacement therapy (HRT). HRT has been shown to be effective for the relief of hot flashes. However, estrogen is contraindicated in this patient given her history of pulmonary embolus. The fact that she is a current smoker also places her at greater risk of developing a thrombus if she were to take hormones. Progestins alone have also been shown to relieve hot flashes. However, progestins may worsen depression and cause other mood changes in patients. Therefore, an alternative treatment is needed for her. Clonidine has been used with success by many women for relief from hot flashes. It is a blood pressure medication, but it has been shown to be effective against hot flashes when used in low doses.

As described above, estrogen and progesterone (**choice B**) should not be used in this patient because of her history of a pulmonary embolus (PE). Estrogen has been shown to increase the risk of clot formation in patients. This has been shown in patients on oral contraceptive pills, as well as in patients on hormone replacement therapy. With her history of thrombosis and current smoking, this patient would be at a particularly increased risk.

Estrogen only (**choice C**) would be contraindicated in this patient for two reasons. First, as detailed above, estrogen would increase her risk for thromboembolic disease. Second, her uterus is still in place and unopposed estrogen would place her at greater risk for endometrial hyperplasia and cancer.

Raloxifene (**choice D**) is a selective estrogen modulator (SERM), which is currently recommended for osteoporosis prevention. It can worsen hot flashes and should not be used for this patient.

Tamoxifen (**choice E**) actually brings about hot flashes in many patients. It therefore would not be the treatment of choice in a patient whose chief complaint is hot flashes.

6. **The correct answer is A.** Betamethasone, penicillin, and magnesium sulfate are used in the treatment of preterm labor. This patient has multiple risk factors for preterm labor, including tobacco abuse, history of preterm labor, and uterine anomalies. Preterm labor can be difficult to diagnose, but uterine contractions with cervical dilation of greater than 2 cm, prior to 37 weeks' gestation is indicative of this disorder. The goal of this therapy is to stop contraction (magnesium sulfate) to allow time to promote fetal lung maturity (betamethasone). Preterm labor is also an indication for group B streptococcal prophylaxis and for this the patient should receive penicillin.

   Because of the advanced cervical dilatation, continuing to monitor the patient for signs of preterm labor (**choice C**) is incorrect. Continued monitoring would be appropriate in patients with contractions and no cervical dilatation, but at this time, tocolytic therapy should be instituted.

   External versions (**choice B**) are attempted in breech fetuses to facilitate vaginal delivery. We have not confirmed the position of the fetus, and cessation of contractions, not delivery, is our current goal. An external version is not indicated at this time.

   Because of the patient's history of prior cesarean delivery (**choice D**), she and her physician may choose to deliver by repeat cesarean section if her labor continues. This will depend on the position of the fetus and the patient's wishes. Labor in women with prior history of uterine surgery does increase the risk of uterine rupture, which may be dangerous and even lethal to the mother and her child. However, without evidence to support the diagnosis of uterine rupture, which would necessitate emergency surgical delivery, the best course of action would be to attempt to arrest the labor and promote fetal lung maturity with steroids.

   The patient shows no signs of ruptured membranes. Intrauterine pressure catheters (**choice E**) do allow for more accurate evaluation of uterine contractions, but require ruptured membranes to place. However, rupturing the patient's membranes at this time would increase the risk of infection and promote stronger contractions and is therefore incorrect.

7. **The correct answer is A.** Patients with squamous cell carcinoma of the vulva commonly present with a history of chronic vulvar itching. Other features may include a discharge, pain, or bleeding. The lesions can appear to be raised, ulcerated, or pigmented, although, infrequently there is no lesion at all. This lesion may also be malignant melanoma. Any postmenopausal woman with a chronic vulvar itch should have a biopsy performed to rule out malignancy.

   To perform a vulvectomy (**choice B**) would not be indicated at this point. The patient does not have a known malignancy requiring vulvectomy. But her symptoms are concerning enough, given their chronicity, to merit a biopsy.

   To prescribe an antibiotic (**choice C**) would be inappropriate management. This patient does not have the diagnosis of an infection that would require antibiotic treatment. Moreover, an attempt at treatment with antibiotics (like the numerous attempts with antifungals) could lead to a further delay in having the biopsy performed.

   To prescribe a steroid cream (**choice D**) would also be inappropriate management. Some vulvar lesions in postmenopausal women (e.g., lichen sclerosis) would respond to steroid cream. However, in this patient's situation, it is most important to first establish a diagnosis with a biopsy prior to starting treatment.

   To refer to psychiatry (**choice E**) would not be appropriate. To ascribe this patient's itching to a possible psychiatric process without first trying to establish a diagnosis by biopsying the lesion would be incorrect.

8. **The correct answer is E.** Herpes simplex virus can infect a neonate and cause severe neonatal morbidity and mortality. This infection may occur as a fetus passes through an infected birth canal in which virus is being shed. This patient appears to be having an outbreak of genital herpes, based on her symptoms of tingling in the genital area, as well as the lesion that is present on her cervix. In order to prevent the fetus from becoming infected, she should have a cesarean delivery as soon as possible.

   To state that the fetus is already infected (**choice A**) is incorrect. There is a small chance that transplacental infection has already taken place earlier in the pregnancy or that ascending infection from the birth canal has already taken place. However, while there is a chance of this, it is far from being certain. Cesarean delivery will hopefully prevent the fetus/neonate from becoming infected.

To state that the lesion is not infectious (**choice B**) is not correct. An active herpes lesion has a significant chance of having active, infectious virus in it. Furthermore, the patient may be shedding virus from other areas of the genital tract (i.e., the vagina or the labia) now that she appears to be having an outbreak.

To state that she should be sent home (**choice C**) is not correct. This patient has ruptured her membranes on the basis of her history of a gush of fluid, along with the Nitrazine positive pool of fluid in her vagina. With ruptured membranes and an active herpes outbreak she should undergo cesarean delivery as soon as possible.

To state that she should be started on oxytocin (**choice D**) is incorrect. Vaginal delivery is contraindicated in this patient with an active herpes outbreak and ruptured membranes at term. Oxytocin is used to cause uterine contractions when a vaginal delivery is indicated. Oxytocin would be inappropriate for this patient.

9. **The correct answer is D.** Patients with atrophic vaginitis tend to suffer from vaginal dryness, pruritus, and dyspareunia. Therefore, this patient's signs and symptoms are most consistent with atrophic vaginitis. Atrophic vaginitis affects women that are estrogen deficient. Menopause represents an estrogen-deficient state for most women. Consequently, atrophic vaginitis is most common in this age group. Estrogen is the hormone that helps to keep the vaginal mucosa lubricated and well supported. Without estrogen the mucosa becomes pale and thin with diminished rugae. Treatment with estrogen vaginal cream would represent the most appropriate course of action for this patient. Systemic hormone replacement therapy (with an estrogen-progesterone combination) could also be used, as it would also help to keep the vaginal mucosa moist and well supported.

To explain that no treatment is available (**choice A**) is not correct. Too often, menopausal women are told that their symptoms are simply a normal part of aging and that nothing can be done about them. This is particularly not true for this patient who has atrophic vaginitis and could benefit from estrogen vaginal cream.

To refer the patient for sexual counseling (**choice B**) would be premature. This patient's complaints and physical examination findings point to a diagnosis of atrophic vaginitis. If this is treated correctly, she very well may not have further dyspareunia and would not, therefore, need to be referred for sexual counseling.

To treat with clotrimazole vaginal cream (**choice C**) would not be appropriate. This patient does have pruritus, but she does not have findings on physical examination that would be consistent with *Candida* infections. For example, she does not have the thick, white vaginal discharge or erythema of the vulvovaginal area that are often seen with a Candida infection. Moreover, she has no pseudohyphae on KOH preparation.

To treat with metronidazole vaginal cream (**choice E**) would not be correct. Bacterial vaginosis (BV) or trichomoniasis may be treated with metronidazole. This patient does not have the symptoms (e.g., a vaginal discharge) or examination findings (e.g., malodorous vaginal discharge, or clue cells or trichomonads on wet preparation, or vaginal pH >4.5) that would support the diagnosis of trichomoniasis or BV.

10. **The correct answer is D.** Nausea during pregnancy is a very common complaint. Estimates are that as many as 80% of women experience significant nausea at some point during their pregnancy. The nausea usually takes place in the first and early second trimesters and has often resolved by 16 weeks, although many women continue to suffer from nausea beyond this time. The etiology of the nausea is unclear, although many believe that it is directly related to the high levels of hCG that are found during early pregnancy. This nausea and vomiting can become a significant problem during the pregnancy when it is severe enough to cause dehydration or malnutrition in the patient.

Admitting her to the hospital for intravenous fluids and antiemetics (**choice A**) is not required. While this patient does have nausea, she has had no vomiting and has no evidence of dehydration that would require intravenous fluids to treat.

To admit her to the hospital for total parenteral nutrition (**choice B**) would be incorrect. Again, the patient does have significant nausea but she is eating regularly and there is no evidence that she is suffering from malnutrition. Some patients with severe hyperemesis gravidarum do require parenteral nutrition, but this patient would not require such intervention at this point.

Checking serum thyroid stimulating hormone (TSH) level (**choice C**) is not necessary at this point. Hyperemesis can be caused by hyperthyroidism, but this patient has no other signs or symptoms of this disease. Furthermore, the TSH level can often be depressed in early pregnancy as a result of the hormonal changes of early pregnancy.

Recommending laparoscopy with removal of the cyst (**choice E**) is not correct. A small, complex, unilateral cyst during early pregnancy most likely represents a corpus luteum cyst. The corpus luteum is essential for progesterone production and the overall health of the pregnancy. Laparoscopy with removal of the cyst should, therefore, not be performed.

11. **The correct answer is B.** This patient has had a prior classic cesarean delivery. Patients who have a history of this type of uterine surgery are at a significant risk for uterine rupture during labor (and even before labor). This patient has missed several prenatal appointments and is now at 39 weeks' gestation. Under normal circumstances (i.e., had this patient been attending her weekly prenatal appointments) she would have been scheduled for cesarean delivery around 37 weeks' gestation. Unfortunately, she missed these appointments and is now at increasing risk for uterine rupture as the pregnancy continues. She now appears to be going into labor, with her regular contractions. A patient with a prior classic cesarean delivery should not be allowed to labor, as the risk of uterine rupture during labor increases significantly. A cesarean delivery should be arranged for this patient as soon as possible.

    To advise her to return with increasing contractions (**choice A**) would be incorrect. For most women who are in early labor, it is appropriate for them to present to the labor and delivery ward when their contractions increase in frequency and intensity. However, a patient with a prior classic cesarean should not be allowed to labor at all.

    To begin a course of betamethasone (**choice C**) would not be necessary. Corticosteroids are given to patients between 24 and 34 weeks' gestation who may deliver within the next week. Corticosteroids help to prevent respiratory distress syndrome in the neonate. This patient, at 39 weeks, does not require corticosteroids.

    To obtain a surgical consult to rule out appendicitis (**choice D**) would be unnecessary. This patient has abdominal pain that corresponds to her uterine contractions. In between contractions she is pain free. She also has no temperature and no abdominal tenderness. These findings are consistent with labor and not suggestive of appendicitis.

    To recommend acetaminophen and warm packs (**choice E**) would not be correct. Tylenol and warm packs can be used for some types of abdominal discomfort in pregnancy, but this patient is in labor at 39 weeks with a prior classic cesarean delivery and requires another cesarean delivery as soon as possible.

12. **The correct answer is B.** Emergency contraception refers to therapy given to women who experience an act of unprotected sexual intercourse and do not wish to become pregnant. It has also been referred to as the "morning-after pill." A potential candidate for emergency contraception is any reproductive age woman who has had unprotected intercourse within 72 hours of the time of presentation (independent of the time of the menstrual cycle) and does not desire pregnancy. Several regimens have been used over the years, but most involve the patient taking two to four oral contraceptive pills followed by a repeat dose in 12 hours. Nausea is very common with emergency contraception; therefore, patients should be advised to take an antiemetic agent 1 hour before each dose to prevent nausea and vomiting. There are no currently established contraindications for the use of emergency contraception, except if the patient is currently pregnant. This patient, who has had an episode of unprotected intercourse within the last 72 hours, is a good candidate for emergency contraception and it should be offered to her.

    To advise her to get another pregnancy test in 1 week (**choice A**) would be incorrect. If she were to become pregnant from this episode of unprotected intercourse, her pregnancy test would most likely not become positive for at least 2 weeks. Therefore, a repeat pregnancy test in 1 week would not be useful.

    To recommend placement of an intrauterine device (**choice C**) would not be advisable. Placement of an intrauterine device (IUD) can be used as a form of emergency contraception. However, the intrauterine device is not generally used as the first-line for emergency contraception, particularly for a nulliparous patient. The IUD is considered to be more appropriate for the multiparous patient because there is some concern that a uterine infection in the setting of an IUD can lead to infertility.

    To treat with oral azithromycin (**choice E**) or to treat with intramuscular ceftriaxone (**choice D**) would not be indicated. This patient does not have current evidence of infection with chlamydia or gonorrhea. She states that she has been in a monogamous relationship for the past 3 years. Therefore, she does not require antibiotics for sexually transmitted disease, but should be offered emergency contraception.

13. **The correct answer is A.** Given this patient's symptoms, the most likely diagnoses include perimenopause, premenstrual syndrome (PMS), depression, and anxiety. Her sleep disturbance is most likely caused by hot flashes. Hot flashes are often experienced as a sudden feeling of intense warmth. The skin may become red and the patient can often break out in a sweat. Hot flashes vary in

frequency and intensity. They average about 5 minutes long, although they can last for as long as 10 minutes. The frequency of hot flashes varies from one an hour to one each week. They are believed to be caused by the decrease in estrogen that occurs at the time of a medical or surgical menopause. Insomnia, irritability, depression, and mood lability are all symptoms that are consistent with PMS. When these symptoms are cyclic in nature and occur in the luteal and menstrual phase of the cycle then the diagnosis of PMS can be made. This patient, however, is 52 years old and has been having irregular menstrual cycles that may represent the climacteric (the months around the menopause). The treatment for PMS and perimenopause are very different. In particular, hormone replacement therapy is used to treat hot flashes and not used to treat PMS. Thus, it is important to know if this patient is perimenopausal. A serum FSH should therefore be checked and if it is significantly elevated, the patient can be offered hormone replacement therapy.

Checking serum human chorionic gonadotropin (HCG) **(choice B)** is unnecessary for this patient. This patient has a negative urine hCG, and there is no reason to suspect that this negative urine test is wrong. If there were a reason to suspect pregnancy, for example if this patient had a 14-week sized uterus to go along with her missed menses of 3 months, then a serum HCG check would be reasonable.

To explain that no treatment is available **(choice C)** would be incorrect. If this patient is experiencing hot flashes, then hormone replacement therapy may be used. It has proven to be very effective for the treatment of hot flashes.

To prescribe fluoxetine for the patient **(choice D)** would not be correct at this point. This medication has been used in the treatment of PMS. There is substantial evidence that fluoxetine is effective in the treatment of PMS. However, it is not at all clear that this patient has PMS. In fact, her symptoms may be more consistent with perimenopause.

To refer the patient for psychotherapy **(choice E)** would be premature at this point. This patient may simply be suffering hot flashes, which can seriously disrupt sleep and cause mood changes in a patient. If treatment with hormone replacement therapy were effective, then referral to psychotherapy would not be necessary.

14. **The correct answer is E.** Group B streptococci (GBS) is a gram-positive bacterium that can cause significant morbidity and mortality in newborn infants. Infants can become infected with this bacterium while passing through a birth canal that is colonized with GBS. Therefore, women at risk for having a neonate develop GBS disease should be given intravenous penicillin during labor to help prevent this. According to the centers for disease control (CDC) protocol, at risk women include: Women with a history of having an infant with GBS sepsis, women with GBS in their urine culture, women delivering preterm (<37 weeks), women with ruptured membranes for greater than 18 hours, and women with an intrapartum temperature greater than 100.4 F. If a patient does not have either of the first two risk factors, a vaginal/perineal/anal culture may be taken between 35 to 37 weeks and treatment based on the results of that culture. This patient is presenting in active labor at 35 weeks. She, therefore, has risk factor #3 and should receive penicillin to prevent her neonate from developing GBS disease.

    To administer corticosteroids **(choice A)** would be incorrect. Corticosteroids (betamethasone or dexamethasone) should be given to patients between 24 and 34 weeks' gestation who are at risk of delivering in the next 7 days. This patient is at 35 weeks' gestation and would, therefore, not be a candidate for corticosteroids.

    To perform a cesarean delivery **(choice B)** would not be correct. This patient is progressing well (6 cm dilation) in active labor at 35 weeks' gestation with a fetus that appears to be tolerating the labor well (i.e., has a reactive fetal heart tracing). She should be allowed to continue in labor and hopefully have a vaginal delivery.

    To prepare for forceps delivery **(choice C)** is unnecessary. There is no current indication in this case to use forceps. The fetus appears to be tolerating the labor well. Furthermore, forceps are not used in obstetrics unless the cervix is fully dilated. Preparation for forceps delivery is not needed at this time.

    To start intravenous oxytocin **(choice D)** would also be unnecessary. Oxytocin is commonly used in obstetrics to stimulate contractions to help with a dysfunctional labor or to induce a patient's labor. This woman appears to be in effective labor as she has dilated to 6 cm with 100% effacement. Intravenous oxytocin would, therefore, not be necessary at this time.

15. **The correct answer is B.** Postmenopausal bleeding is abnormal and can be the first symptom found in patients who have endometrial cancer. Other conditions on the differential diagnosis for postmenopausal bleeding include endometrial atrophy, endometrial polyps, infection, trauma, coagulopathy, and medication exposure. Women who present with post-

menopausal bleeding must have an evaluation of their endometrium performed. This evaluation can be done by ultrasound, in which the endometrial stripe is measured. The traditional method for evaluation of postmenopausal bleeding, though, is with endometrial biopsy. An endometrial biopsy may be performed in the office with a thin suction device that is placed through the cervix and into the uterine cavity. Rotation of the device 360 degrees as it is being removed from the uterus allows an adequate sampling of the entire endometrial cavity. The sample is then sent to pathology for evaluation. This 65-year-old patient should have an endometrial biopsy performed to rule out endometrial hyperplasia or cancer. Early identification of these conditions will allow for faster treatment and improved prognosis.

To fit the patient with a pessary (**choice A**) would be incorrect. Pessaries are used in gynecology to treat patients with pelvic organ prolapse. This patient has postmenopausal bleeding and not pelvic organ prolapse. She, therefore, needs an endometrial biopsy and not fitting of a pessary.

To prescribe estrogen replacement therapy (**choice C**) would be contraindicated. This patient has postmenopausal bleeding. This may be a sign of endometrial hyperplasia or cancer. Estrogen would worsen both of these conditions. Furthermore, in postmenopausal women who have not had a hysterectomy, progesterone must be given along with estrogen to prevent the development of endometrial hyperplasia or cancer.

To reassure the patient that the bleeding is normal (**choice D**) is absolutely incorrect. Postmenopausal bleeding is not normal, may represent endometrial cancer, and certainly requires evaluation.

To schedule the patient for a hysterectomy (**choice E**) would not be correct at this point. This patient may be having a single episode of vaginal bleeding and may have no evidence of hyperplasia or cancer on biopsy. If this episode does not recur and there is no evidence of concerning pathology on the biopsy, hysterectomy is not indicated.

16. **The correct answer is A.** Intrahepatic cholestasis (ICP) of pregnancy is a very important condition because there is a significant association between ICP and stillbirth (i.e., fetal death). ICP is a condition that develops in pregnancy, which is characterized by intense pruritus, often worse at night and on the palms and soles. There are often either no findings on physical examination or excoriations from the patient's constant itching. Laboratory testing can often show abnormal liver function tests and elevated bile acids. Other conditions on the differential diagnosis for generalized pruritus in pregnancy include hepatitis and gallbladder disease. This patient, though, has no history or examination findings that would suggest hepatitis or gallbladder disease. Therefore, this patient should have her liver function tests and bile acids checked. It is very important to identify this disease because patients with ICP should undergo fetal testing and early delivery to prevent stillbirth.

To reassure the patient that her symptoms are normal (**choice B**) is absolutely incorrect. Too often, patients with ICP are ignored and told that itching in pregnancy is normal; this can lead to significant morbidity and mortality for the fetus. Patients with generalized pruritus in pregnancy must be taken seriously and an evaluation performed to check for ICP.

To refer the patient to a dermatologist (**choice C**) would not be the most appropriate next step in management. This patient's presentation is classic for intrahepatic cholestasis of pregnancy, and she should have liver function tests and bile acids checked. Referral to a dermatologist may result in a delay in diagnosis.

To refer the patient to a psychiatrist (**choice D**) would not be indicated at this time. Her generalized pruritus may represent hepatic dysfunction and to ascribe it to psychiatric illness at this time would not be correct.

To schedule a cesarean delivery (**choice E**) would not be indicated. This patient has a fetus in vertex position and a prior vaginal delivery. If delivery is indicated for her, she may have a vaginal delivery.

17. **The correct answer is A.** Any pregnant woman with vaginal bleeding must have a blood type checked. This is true because pregnant women who are Rh negative are at risk for developing Rh isoimmunization when they have bleeding during pregnancy. The Rh or Rhesus antigen is found on the red blood cells of most women. However, some women do not have this antigen present and they are called "Rh negative." When an Rh-negative mother becomes exposed to the red blood cells of an Rh-positive fetus, Rh isoimmunization may occur as the mother mounts an immune response to the fetal Rh antigen. This exposure can occur in a variety of situations during pregnancy including vaginal bleeding, trauma, amniocentesis, and delivery. If the mother becomes sensitized, she will make antibodies against the Rh antigen. These antibodies typically do not affect the first Rh-positive fetus (i.e., during the initial pregnancy of the exposure). Yet, in a future pregnancy, if the

fetus is also Rh positive, the mother's antibodies may cross the placenta and "attack" the Rh antigen on the fetal red blood cells causing a hemolytic anemia in the fetus. Therefore RhoGAM, which is anti-D immune globulin and helps to prevent a maternal immune response to the Rh antigen, should be given to any Rh-negative woman who has an episode of bleeding during pregnancy.

To give 2 units of fresh frozen plasma (FFP) (**choice B**) would not be necessary. FFP is used in patients when there is evidence of a clotting disorder and a need for clotting factors to be given. This patient has minimal vaginal bleeding and does not require FFP.

To prepare the patient for cesarean delivery (**choice C**) would not be correct. This patient is having a small amount of vaginal bleeding at 27 weeks' gestation with a fetus with a reactive heart tracing. There is no indication for delivery in this patient.

To reassure and then discharge the patient (**choice D**) would be incorrect. This Rh-negative woman with vaginal bleeding must receive RhoGAM prior to discharge.

To start intravenous penicillin (**choice E**) would not be indicated. There is a normal leukocytosis of pregnancy with white cell counts ranging from 5000 to 12,000/mL. This patient has no evidence of infection and, therefore, penicillin would not be indicated.

18. **The correct answer is D.** Women who have had a prior cesarean delivery are candidates for vaginal birth after cesarean (VBAC) if they meet the following selection criteria:

    1. One or two prior low-transverse cesarean deliveries
    2. Clinically adequate pelvis
    3. No other uterine scars or previous rupture
    4. Physician available to monitor the labor and perform emergency cesarean
    5. Anesthesia and personnel available for emergency cesarean

    This patient, based on her history, meets these criteria. However, it is essential to counsel any patient considering VBAC of the risks and benefits. The major risk is uterine rupture, which is estimated to occur in 0.2 to 1.5% of women with previous low-transverse incisions. Another risk is that patients who fail a trial of labor are at increased risk for infection and morbidity. The benefit is that when VBAC is successful, it is associated with less morbidity than elective repeat cesarean delivery. Patients should be educated regarding the risks and benefits of VBAC and allowed to make their own decisions.

    To counsel her that repeat cesarean delivery is best for her (**choice A**) is incorrect. There are risks and benefits with both VBAC and elective repeat cesarean delivery. It is the physician's duty to fully educate the patient regarding those risks and benefits and to allow the patient to make her decision.

    To tell her that she is likely to fail a VBAC attempt (**choice B**) is not correct. Most published reports estimate that 60 to 80% of trials of labor after previous cesarean result in a successful vaginal delivery. Therefore, she should be counseled that, statistically, she is likely to have a successful attempt.

    To tell her that she must attempt VBAC given her history (**choice C**) is absolutely incorrect. The American College of Obstetricians and Gynecologists (ACOG) has made it clear that global mandates for VBAC (e.g., by insurance companies) are not appropriate.

    To counsel her that VBAC is contraindicated given her history (**choice E**) is incorrect. Contraindications to VBAC include:

    1. Prior classic cesarean or T-shaped incision, or transfundal surgery
    2. Contracted pelvis
    3. Medical or obstetric complication that precludes vaginal delivery
    4. Inability for emergency cesarean to be performed

    This patient does not have these contraindications and is a candidate for VBAC.

19. **The correct answer is E.** This patient's presentation is most consistent with that of patients with lichen sclerosis. Patients with lichen sclerosis typically complain of burning, itching, and dyspareunia. The examination of patients with lichen sclerosis reveals a whitish vulvar area with atrophy of both the labia majora and labia minora. The lesion sometimes includes the perianal area in a "butterfly-like" pattern. Diagnosis is by history, physical examination, and biopsy. There is some association between lesions of this type and cancer, so suspicious lesions should be biopsied. Treatment is with potent topical testosterone.

    Clotrimazole (**choice A**) is an antifungal that is often used in gynecology for the treatment of Candida vulvovaginitis. While this patient does have itching and burning, she has no evidence of yeast infection on examination or on microscopic evaluation of her discharge.

Estrogen cream (**choice B**) is often used to treat atrophic vaginitis. This patient, however, does not have atrophic vaginitis but rather lichen sclerosis. While generalized atrophy is present in both disorders, lichen sclerosis is a white lesion that often extends around the anus. Atrophic vaginitis does not present in this fashion.

Isoniazid (**choice C**) is used to treat tuberculosis. There is no evidence that this patient has tuberculosis.

Metronidazole (**choice D**) is most often used to treat bacterial vaginosis (BV) or trichomoniasis. Bacterial vaginosis can be diagnosed based on symptoms and the presence of clue cells on the "wet prep". Trichomoniasis can also be diagnosed based on symptoms and the presence of trichomonads on the "wet prep". This patient has a negative "wet prep" and history and physical consistent with lichen sclerosis.

20. **The correct answer is D.** When sexual activity should be resumed postpartum depends on the patient's desire and comfort. There is no exact time that can be considered ideal for resuming sexual relations postpartum. Patients who are breast-feeding exclusively have a prolonged period of suppressed estrogen production from the ovary. The result of this decreased estrogen production can be vaginal atrophy and vaginal dryness. During sexual arousal there will, therefore, be decreased vaginal lubrication. The patient should be reassured that this is not abnormal or uncommon and that lubricants can be used to diminish the symptoms.

To advise her to stop having sexual intercourse until 10 weeks postpartum (**choice A**) is incorrect. As noted above, there is no set time postpartum at which patients should resume having sexual intercourse. Intercourse at 6 weeks postpartum is fine if that is the patient's desire.

To discuss with her starting hormone replacement therapy (**choice B**) is not correct. Her vaginal dryness is occurring because of decreased estrogen levels brought about by breast-feeding, but the solution is not to give hormone replacement therapy, which could affect breast-feeding and cross over to the infant.

To explain to her that she may have premature ovarian failure (**choice C**) is incorrect. It is not uncommon for a 26-year-old woman to have vaginal dryness during breast-feeding. This is the most likely explanation for her symptoms. Premature ovarian failure in a 26-year old woman, 6 weeks' postpartum, is very unlikely.

To refer the patient and her partner for couples counseling (**choice E**) would not be correct. This patient has stated that intercourse is uncomfortable because of vaginal dryness. There is a good explanation for her dryness in her case, and a referral to couples counseling is not indicated at this time.

21. **The correct answer is A.** Fetal macrosomia is concerning to patients and obstetricians because fetal macrosomia is associated with increased rates of cesarean delivery as well as increased rates of shoulder dystocia and infant brachial plexus injury. Shoulder dystocia occurs when the fetal head is delivered but the shoulders become lodged against the maternal pelvis. This represents an obstetrical emergency because if delivery is not brought about as soon as possible, fetal asphyxia can result. Also, the efforts to bring about delivery during a shoulder dystocia can lead to injury to the fetus including fractured bones, as well as brachial plexus injury. Unfortunately, shoulder dystocia is very difficult to predict. Even though the risk of shoulder dystocia does increase with increasing birth weight, most cases of shoulder dystocia do not occur in macrosomic infants. The current recommendation from the American College of Obstetricians and Gynecologists is that patients should be offered a cesarean delivery for macrosomia if they are nondiabetic patients with a fetus with an estimated fetal weight greater than 5000 g or diabetic patients with a fetus with an estimated fetal weight greater than 4500 g. This patient, who is nondiabetic and has a fetus with an estimated fetal weight greater than 5000 g by exam and ultrasound, should be offered primary cesarean delivery for macrosomia.

To offer induction of labor for pending macrosomia (**choice B**) is not correct. First, induction of labor for pending macrosomia has not been shown to be an effective approach. Second, this patient appears to have actual macrosomia (and not pending, or developing, macrosomia) given the estimated fetal weight.

To offer primary cesarean delivery for postterm pregnancy (**choice C**) or to offer induction of labor for postterm pregnancy (**choice D**) is incorrect. Postterm pregnancy is most often defined as later than 42 completed weeks of gestation. This patient is at her due date, which is 40 completed weeks of gestation. This patient, though, should be offered cesarean on the basis of her estimated fetal weight, and not based on her gestational age.

To perform stat cesarean delivery for fetal distress (**choice E**) would not be appropriate. There is no evidence of fetal distress requiring stat cesarean delivery for this patient.

22. **The correct answer is B.** Air travel until 36 weeks' gestation is considered to be safe for most pregnant women. There are, however, some exceptions to this rule. Women with a history of pregnancy-induced hypertension, preterm delivery, poorly controlled diabetes, and sickle cell disease or trait may be at significantly increased risk from flying at any time during pregnancy. Also, patients with significant medical problems should exercise caution. In a healthy woman with an uncomplicated pregnancy, air travel up to 36 weeks appears to be safe. After 36 weeks the risks of labor, and some third trimester pregnancy complications, are high enough to make airplane travel not advisable at this point.

Her age (**choice A**) of 37 years does not make flying contraindicated for her. Women older than 35 years of age are considered to be of advanced maternal age and their risks for certain conditions increase (e.g., a fetus with Down syndrome). If she were not 38 weeks' gestation, air travel would be allowed.

Her group B streptococcus status (**choice C**) is important because she will need to receive antibiotics (penicillin or clindamycin or gentamicin) during labor. These antibiotics will be given to prevent group B streptococcal disease of the newborn. This does not factor into prohibition of air travel.

Her history of a forceps delivery (**choice D**) is noncontributory, as far as flying is concerned. Flying would have been acceptable for her prior to 36 weeks.

Her hyperemesis gravidarum (**choice E**) during the early pregnancy does not make flying inadvisable. Nausea and vomiting during early pregnancy is a common complaint. When the nausea and vomiting are so severe that metabolic derangements result, this is termed hyperemesis gravidarum. Normally this condition resolves during the second trimester.

23. **The correct answer is D.** It is an essential principal of emergency medical care that any woman of childbearing age who presents with abdominal pain or vaginal bleeding should have a pregnancy test (urine or serum hCG) sent as one of the very first steps in her evaluation. Ectopic pregnancy is a potentially fatal condition in which a pregnancy develops outside of the uterus. Most often ectopic pregnancies are located in the fallopian tube (the so-called "tubal" pregnancy) but they can also be located on the ovary, in the cervix, and in the peritoneal cavity. Bleeding per vagina and abdominal pain are the two most common presenting complaints for women with an ectopic pregnancy. A woman can have an ectopic pregnancy and appear relaxed and non-acute on examination with stable vital signs and a benign examination. Early diagnosis, however, is absolutely essential in ectopic pregnancy to avoid the significant morbidity and mortality that can result from an ectopic pregnancy that enlarges or ruptures.

Abdominal/pelvic CT (**choice A**) is an effective study for identifying masses in the abdomen and pelvis. It is, however, not the study of choice for diagnosing an ectopic pregnancy. It tends to be used in cases where the differential diagnosis includes appendicitis, abscess, or tumor. For this patient, though, prior to scheduling a diagnostic study, the physician must determine the patient's hCG level.

Abdominal x-ray (**choice B**) is a useful study for identifying many conditions including kidney stones and gallstones, intestinal obstruction or perforation, and some abdominal masses. In this patient, though, the physician would first want to know the result of the pregnancy test (hCG) prior to ordering any diagnostic study. If the pregnancy test is positive in a woman with bleeding and abdominal pain, the correct next study would be pelvic ultrasound and not abdominal x-ray.

Electrocardiogram (EKG) (**choice C**) is a useful test to determine cardiac rate, rhythm, axis, and evidence of ischemia, along with other information. However, in this young, otherwise healthy woman with bleeding and abdominal pain (not chest pain), EKG would not be the most appropriate next step.

Serum thyroid stimulating hormone (**choice E**) is an appropriate test to send as part of an outpatient evaluation on a woman who is having menstrual irregularities because hypo- or hyperthyroidism can cause irregular bleeding. However, the most important and urgent determination to make on a young woman with abdominal pain and irregular bleeding is whether the patient is pregnant or not.

24. **The correct answer is A.** This patient has HELLP syndrome. HELLP is the acronym for the syndrome characterized by hemolysis, elevated liver enzymes, and low platelets. This patient certainly has elevated liver enzymes and a low platelet count. She may also have hemolytic anemia with her hematocrit level of 25%. HELLP is a syndrome that is believed to be closely related to pre-eclampsia and it is often associated with hypertension and proteinuria, which characterizes pre-eclampsia and which this patient demonstrates. However, while some patients with pre-eclampsia may be managed expectantly to try to gain further maturity for the fetus, patients with HELLP syndrome are at an even higher risk for sig-

nificant morbidity and mortality and should be delivered expediently. This patient is a multiparous woman with a favorable cervix at 34 weeks' gestation, and therefore an induction of labor should be initiated. Along with the induction of labor, the patient should be started on magnesium sulfate to prevent a maternal seizure. Delivery of the fetus usually results in rapid maternal improvement over several hours to days.

It is incorrect to manage the patient expectantly until 37 weeks (**choice B**). Expectant management of a woman with HELLP syndrome at 34 weeks' gestation is not appropriate. Expectant management may be undertaken in a woman with mild pre-eclampsia who is stable and with a healthy fetus. This expectant management is done to allow more time for fetal maturation.

To perform a liver biopsy (**choice C**) is incorrect. A liver biopsy is unnecessary to make the diagnosis in this case and would be potentially dangerous for the patient.

To start sumatriptan therapy (**choice D**) is incorrect. This patient's headache is likely related to her HELLP syndrome. Sumatriptan is used for the treatment of migraine headaches and would not be appropriate for this patient.

To treat with phenytoin for seizure prophylaxis (**choice E**) is incorrect. Patients with HELLP syndrome or pre-eclampsia should be treated with magnesium sulfate during the peripartum period to prevent a maternal seizure. Magnesium sulfate has been demonstrated to be superior to phenytoin for the prevention of seizure in patients with pre-eclampsia.

25. **The correct answer is B.** Many observational studies had found lower rates of coronary heart disease in women taking estrogen compared with women not taking estrogen. It was believed that estrogen provided a cardioprotective effect by altering cholesterol levels and the formation of atherosclerotic plaques. However, when a randomized-controlled trial was performed to look at whether hormone replacement therapy was useful as secondary prevention of coronary heart disease (i.e., preventing a worsening of disease in patients with established coronary heart disease), it demonstrated a significant increase in the number of cardiovascular events in women taking hormone replacement therapy in the first years of treatment. One possible explanation for this is that hormone replacement therapy increases a woman's risk for thrombosis. This patient has coronary heart disease. She should, therefore, be advised that HRT could increase her likelihood of having a cardiovascular event.

To state that HRT could increase her likelihood of developing osteoporosis (**choice A**) is incorrect. There is substantial evidence that HRT reduces a woman's risk of developing osteoporosis.

To advise this patient that HRT will decrease her symptoms of fatigue (**choice C**) is incorrect. Fatigue is a symptom that can result from a large number of causes. There is no established evidence that HRT will decrease fatigue.

To state that HRT will reduce her risk of venous thromboembolism (**choice D**) is incorrect. HRT has been shown to increase a woman's risk for venous thromboembolism.

To advise this patient that HRT will reduce the progression of atherosclerosis (**choice E**) is incorrect. HRT has not been demonstrated to reduce the progression of atherosclerosis.

26. **The correct answer is D.** This patient is showing evidence of placental abruption secondary to abdominal trauma. Vaginal bleeding, fetal or maternal distress, and uterine hypertonus are all signs of abruption. Abdominal trauma is a common cause of abruption. Both the patient and the fetus are showing signs of distress from volume loss, and delivery must be accomplished rapidly to prevent fetal death and maternal morbidity from hemorrhage and possible death. The patient should be quickly evaluated for other injuries. IV access should be obtained with determination of blood count and coagulation status. Abruption can commonly cause coagulation abnormalities and even DIC. The patient should also be typed and crossed for blood products. Pregnant women are relatively immune to the usual early signs of volume loss, and the tachycardia, tachypnea, and low blood pressures are all ominous signs of significant blood loss. The amount of vaginal bleeding may or may not correlate with the actual blood loss, so you cannot be reassured by the "moderate" bleeding seen.

Betamethasone is indicated to promote fetal lung maturity in preterm infants. This patient is term, confirmed by a first trimester ultrasound. Therefore, betamethasone (**choice A**) is not indicated.

Magnesium sulfate (**choice B**) can be used in the management of preterm labor, but the contractions this patient is having are not consistent with that diagnosis.

The patient was likely in early labor when you spoke to her on the phone, but the increase in contractions is likely secondary to placental abruption and not active labor. If this patient were close to delivery and hemodynamically stable, expectant management of labor would be reasonable. However, there are signs of maternal and fetal compromise; therefore, delivery should be expedited and expectant management of labor (**choice C**) is inappropriate.

Placental previa (placental tissue covering or near the cervical os) can cause bleeding in the third trimester. However, placenta previa (**choice E**) is more commonly seen in early ultrasounds. The majority will resolve through a process called "placental migration." There is differential growth between the lower uterine segment and the rest of the placenta. This causes the edge of the placenta to gradually move away from the cervical os. If placenta previa was not seen in the patient's first trimester ultrasound it is unlikely to be present at this time.

27. **The correct answer is C.** This patient has met the clinical criteria for pre-eclampsia. Her blood pressure is greater than 140/90 mm Hg and she has edema and proteinuria. She should receive magnesium sulfate therapy for blood pressure control. The goal of magnesium therapy is to prevent eclampsia while the patient is induced. Most cases of pre-eclampsia resolve within 48 hours of delivery, so delivery is the ultimate goal in term patients in whom pre-eclampsia develops.

Betamethasone (**choice A**) is not indicated in patients at term. It is used in patients with preterm labor to promote lung maturity.

Pre-eclampsia is not an indication for cesarean delivery (**choice B**). There are currently no signs of fetal or maternal distress. If these were to develop, then surgical delivery may be indicated, but at this time a trial of induction of vaginal delivery is the best choice.

Bedrest (**choice D**) may be appropriate in patients with mildly elevated blood pressures that do not meet the criteria for pre-eclampsia.

Sending the patient home with a prescription for lisinopril for her hypertension is incorrect in that it does not address the need for prompt delivery and blood pressure control in this patient. Also, lisinopril (**choice E**) is not indicated in pregnant women secondary to potential effects on fetal renal blood flow.

28. **The correct answer is A.** Two antiphospholipid antibodies, lupus anticoagulant and anticardiolipin, are associated with first trimester miscarriage.

Antinuclear antibody (**choice B**) is the antibody usually measured to diagnose systemic lupus erythematosus. Antinuclear antibody is no longer routinely ordered in the workup of recurrent early miscarriages because they have not proven to be responsible for recurrent pregnancy loss.

Antisperm antibodies (**choice C**) have not been proven to be associated with early miscarriages. Antisperm antibodies cross-react with living embryos, resulting in spontaneous miscarriages in mice, but this has not proven to be the case in humans.

No study implicates diabetes mellitus (**choice D**) as a cause of recurrent miscarriage. Therefore, a routine glucose tolerance test is not indicated for patients with recurrent first trimester miscarriages.

Histocompatibility locus antigen (**choice E**) is not associated with early recurrent miscarriages and hence need not be investigated.

29. **The correct answer is A.** The patient's history is highly suggestive of hypothalamic dysfunction as the cause of her secondary amenorrhea. Women who exercise vigorously or experience high levels of emotional stress may develop inadequate hypothalamic function. Low levels of follicle stimulating hormone and luteinizing hormone are diagnostic of hypothalamic amenorrhea.

A pituitary tumor (**choice B**) is highly unlikely because of normal serum prolactin levels.

Polycystic ovary disease (**choice C**) is highly unlikely in this patient, as she did not have withdrawal bleeding after treatment with medroxyprogesterone acetate.

This patient does not have premature ovarian failure (**choice D**) as her serum gonadotropin levels were low normal. In premature ovarian failure, these hormone levels are abnormally high.

There is nothing in this history to suggest that her symptoms are associated with intrauterine devices (**choice E**).

30. **The correct answer is E.** Patients with congenital absence of a vagina usually lack a uterus as well and seek medical advice because of primary amenorrhea at puberty or later. The presence of secondary sex characteristics, pubic and axillary hair, rules out other causes of primary amenorrhea in this patient.

Patients with an imperforate hymen usually complain of cyclical lower abdominal pain that worsens progressively because of uterine and vaginal dysfunction with accumulated obstructed menstrual flow (**choice B**); therefore, imperforate hymen is highly unlikely in this patient.

This patient's secondary sex characteristics developed at a normal age and it is therefore unlikely that she has hypothalamic (**choice A**) or pituitary dysfunction (**choice C**).

Patients with testicular feminization syndrome have scant or absent pubic hair. In this syndrome, testicles produce testosterone and the target cells in the hair follicle are believed to lack androgen receptors; therefore, testicular feminization syndrome (**choice D**) is unlikely in this patient.

31. **The correct answer is A.** Oligomenorrhea, severe menstrual cramping (dysmenorrhea), and increased menstrual flow during the periods are classical symptoms of endometriosis.

Endometritis (**choice B**) is unlikely in this patient without any associated systemic symptoms, such as fever.

Pelvic inflammatory disease (**choice C**) causes moderate-to-severe lower abdominal pain associated with menstrual cramping. Increased menstrual flow is unlikely in pelvic inflammatory disease.

A ruptured ovarian cyst (**choice D**) is usually an acute presentation associated with severe lower abdominal pain. A pelvic ultrasound may show free fluid in the pelvis with a ruptured cyst.

Uterine fibroids (**choice E**) typically cause excessive bleeding associated with normal menstrual cycle. In these patients, oligomenorrhea and dysmenorrhea are unlikely.

32. **The correct answer is E.** The classical triad of dribbling, dyspareunia, and dysuria suggest a urethral diverticulum. These women may have a tender suburethral mass. Frequently they can have history of frequent urinary tract infections. Diagnosis is confirmed by urethroscopy or a voiding cystourethrogram.

CT scan of the abdomen and pelvis (**choice A**) is unnecessary, as intra-abdominal or pelvic tumors typically do not give a classical triad of dyspareunia, dribbling, and dysuria.

Laparoscopy (**choice B**) is not indicated, as no pelvic pathology like endometriosis is suspected.

Pelvic sonography (**choice C**) is not indicated, as no associated pathology with the uterus and the ovary is suspected.

Renal sonography (**choice D**) may not show any evidence of a urethral diverticulum.

33. **The correct answer is C.** Meig syndrome refers to the coexistence of hydrothorax, ascites, and an underlying benign tumor, usually a fibroma. The pathophysiology of ascites and pleural effusion is unclear but they may result from lymphatic obstruction. Excision of the ovarian fibroma is usually accompanied by resolution of the findings. Some ovarian malignancies are also associated with ascites and pleural effusion and are reported as malignant Meig syndrome. Once the ovarian benign pathology is confirmed after excision of the ovary, no further treatment is necessary.

Bilateral salpingo-oophorectomy (**choice A**) is not indicated for an isolated ovarian fibroma.

Bilateral salpingo-oophorectomy and hysterectomy (**choice B**) is indicated in case of malignancy, but not essential in the treatment of an ovarian fibroma.

As ascites and pleural effusion disappear after the excision of ovarian fibroma, further therapy by right tube thoracostomy and abdominal paracentesis (**choice D**) is not essential.

Ovarian biopsy (**choice E**) is not the right option as malignancy can also give rise to similar pleural effusion and ascites, and by doing a biopsy malignancy can spread and should be avoided.

34. **The correct answer is D.** This patient had regularly timed cycles, which suggest normal ovulatory function. Heavy menses with regularly timed cycles (menorrhagia) occur due to organic lesions such as submucous fibroids, endometrial polyps, and adenomyosis.

Anovulation (**choice A**) causes irregular cycles because failure to move into the progesterone dominant luteal phase of the cycle gives them prolonged unopposed estrogen exposure.

A coagulopathy (**choice B**) is usually associated with other episodes of heavy bleeding, in addition to heavy menses.

Endometrial hyperplasia (**choice C**) causes postmenopausal bleeding. Hence, postmenopausal women with the onset of vaginal bleeding require thorough endometrial evaluation, as the bleeding may herald malignant or premalignant pathology.

Pregnancy should be ruled out as the first etiology in sexually reproductive women with abnormal bleeding. A threatened abortion (**choice E**) means that the pregnancy is still viable (beta-HCG is doubling appropriately) and the os is closed.

35. **The correct answer is E.** This patient is showing evidence of preterm rupture of membranes. The clinical findings of pooling of vaginal fluid, elevated pH, and ferning confirm rupture of membranes. The patient is showing no signs of labor, and therefore the rupture is preterm. However, she will need an ultrasound evaluation to establish the gestational age of her fetus to help guide management. The fundal height does suggest that the patient may be close to the 7 months' gestation that she states, but she may have a term infant with severe intrauterine growth restriction or a twin gestation with a much earlier gestational age.

Cesarean section to prevent chorioamnionitis (**choice A**) is never indicated in a preterm gestation. If ultrasound confirmed a term gestation, delivery would be reasonable, but surgical delivery is usually not necessary. There is some evidence that prophylactic antibiotics may help prevent chorioamnionitis. However, delivery should be delayed until signs of chorioamnionitis develop to promote further fetal growth and development.

Sterile vaginal examination (**choice B**) in patients with ruptured membranes should be minimized. There is evidence that the risk of chorioamnionitis increases with the total number of vaginal examinations. Since the os was easily seen on speculum examination, there is no need to do a vaginal examination.

Treatment with magnesium sulfate (**choice C**) to prevent preterm delivery may be indicated in patients with confirmed preterm gestation and contractions. The gestational age has not been confirmed and the patient shows no signs of preterm labor (contractions and cervical dilatation).

Treatment of prolonged rupture of membranes with oxytocin (**choice D**) is indicated in confirmed term gestations and in patients with chorioamnionitis. The gestational age will need to be confirmed and there are currently no signs of chorioamnionitis, which include fever, abdominal tenderness, and fetal and maternal tachycardia.

36. **The correct answer is D.** Currently, the American College of Sports Medicine and the Centers for Disease Control and Prevention recommend the accumulation of 30 minutes or more of moderate exercise a day. This accumulation should occur on most, if not all, days of the week. The American College of Obstetricians and Gynecologists (2002) states that in the absence of either medical or obstetric complications, pregnant women also can adopt this recommendation. Absolute contraindications to aerobic exercise during pregnancy include hemodynamically significant heart disease, restrictive lung disease, incompetent cervix/cerclage, multiple gestation, persistent bleeding, placenta previa, premature labor during the current pregnancy, ruptured membranes, and pre-eclampsia or gestational hypertension. A pregnant woman who has no experience with exercising should not immediately jump into a program of 30 minutes of moderate exercise each day. This patient, however, is in excellent physical condition and has a long history of exercise. She can continue her exercise program.

To advise her that exercise during pregnancy is prohibited (**choice A**) is incorrect. As explained above, pregnant women with no medical or obstetric complications can exercise regularly during pregnancy. She should be cautioned however to stop exercising and contact a physician if during exercise she has vaginal bleeding, dizziness, headache, chest pain, muscle weakness, calf pain or swelling, preterm labor, decreased fetal movement, or a loss of amniotic fluid.

To state that exercise during pregnancy may lead to gestational diabetes (**choice B**) is absolutely incorrect. There is good epidemiological data to suggest that exercise may be beneficial in the primary prevention of gestational diabetes.

To advise her that scuba diving is not prohibited during pregnancy (**choice C**) is incorrect. During scuba diving the fetus is at increased risk of decompression sickness because of the inability of the fetal pulmonary circulation to filter bubble formation.

To state that she should exercise no more than 20 minutes twice weekly (**choice E**) is incorrect. As explained above, current recommendations are for the accumulation of 30 minutes or more of exercise per day on most, if not all, days of the week.

37. **The correct answer is D.** *Chlamydia trachomatis* and *Neisseria gonorrhoeae* are organisms that can cause cervicitis, pelvic inflammatory disease, sepsis, pelvic pain, infertility, and ectopic pregnancy. There is also increasing evidence that these organisms can serve as cofactors, increasing the likelihood of transmission of human immunodeficiency virus (HIV). Infection with these organisms is sometimes characterized by pelvic pain, a malodorous or purulent vaginal discharge, and dysuria. However, in many cases, infection with these organisms is asymptomatic. Estimates are that in some populations the rate of asymptomatic infection may be as high as 15%. Other studies estimate an even higher rate and suggest that the number of asymptomatic sexually transmitted

diseases (STDs) exceeds the number of symptomatic infections. This patient has an asymptomatic infection. That is, she is having no complaints but has a positive chlamydia test. However, even though the infection is asymptomatic, such an infection can still lead to serious sequelae including pelvic inflammatory disease and infertility and can also lead to infection of her sexual partners and further spread of the organism. This patient should therefore be treated (with azithromycin). Also, her two partners must also be identified and treated as well.

To state that asymptomatic disease is not associated with complications (**choice A**) is not correct. As noted above, there is evidence that chlamydia, even when asymptomatic, can cause serious complications including infertility, ectopic pregnancy, and pelvic inflammatory disease.

To state that hospitalization is required for her given her age (**choice B**) is incorrect. In many cases of pelvic inflammatory disease, hospitalization is indicated. This may especially be true in a young woman to ensure that she is fully treated, if you are unsure of appropriate followup. This patient, however, does not have pelvic inflammatory disease. She has an asymptomatic chlamydia infection that requires antibiotics and not hospitalization.

To state that no treatment is necessary since she is asymptomatic (**choice C**) is inappropriate. A patient with chlamydia infection, whether or not she is symptomatic, should be treated, as should her sexual partners.

To state that the result is most likely a false positive and no treatment is needed (**choice E**) is incorrect. While it is true that any screening test will have a false positive rate, a positive chlamydia screen should not be assumed to be a false positive. This patient and her partners should be appropriately treated.

38. **The correct answer is B.** The possible relationship between estrogen replacement therapy (ERT) and hormone replacement therapy (HRT), which contains both an estrogen and progestin component, is somewhat controversial and has been the subject of much study. Thousands of patients have been evaluated as part of several studies to determine the effect, if any, of estrogen and progestin on breast cancer rates. It appears from this data that there may be a modest increase in the rate of developing breast cancer for women using HRT. However, the patient should also be counseled that the decision whether or not to use HRT is a very complex one that involves not only considerations regarding breast cancer but also considerations concerning osteoporosis, heart disease, vaginal dryness, mental functioning, and family history, among other issues. For some patients the "correct" choice is obvious, but for most patients there is no one easy solution, and counseling must involve presenting them with all of the risks, benefits, and alternatives.

To counsel her that HRT may decrease the risk of developing a thrombosis (**choice A**) is incorrect. There is good evidence that estrogen increases the risk of thrombosis and thromboembolic disease. Perhaps the most well known example of this is in women taking the oral contraceptive pill (OCP). While HRT contains a lesser amount of hormone than the OCP, it still does appear to increase thrombosis risk.

To counsel her that HRT may worsen the hot flashes (**choice C**) is not correct. While any given patient may experience variable effects from a medication, HRT is considered a treatment for hot flashes.

To advise her that the estrogen component of HRT will prevent breast cancer (**choice D**) is not correct. As stated above, the effects of HRT on breast cancer are not completely clear. Yet, estrogen is not considered protective.

To advise her that the progestin component of HRT will prevent breast cancer (**choice E**) is also incorrect. Progestins have been found to protect postmenopausal women on ERT from developing endometrial cancer. In breast tissue, however, they have not been shown to have such an effect and may, in fact, increase the risk of breast cancer.

39. **The correct answer is B.** Postpartum blues are estimated to occur in 50% or more of women who have recently given birth. It is a state of heightened emotional reactivity with moments of joy and happiness alternating with sadness, irritability, and tearfulness. These "blues" often start 3 to 5 days after delivery and can last for weeks. A leading hypothesis for the explanation of postpartum blues is the abrupt hormone withdrawal in the days after delivery. It is important to distinguish postpartum blues from postpartum depression, which is characterized by severe sadness or emptiness, withdrawal from family and friends, anhedonia, fatigue, sleep difficulty, loss of appetite, lack of interest in the infant, or thoughts of hurting oneself or the infant. Postpartum depression requires more intensive monitoring and treatment, usually with a selective serotonin reuptake inhibitor (SSRI). All postpartum women should be asked directly about their mood and well being to evaluate for postpartum depression.

Mild pre-eclampsia (**choice A**) is characterized by hypertension (systolic blood pressure >140 mm Hg or diastolic blood pressure >90 mm Hg) with proteinuria (>300 mg in 24 hours). Based on the case presentation, this patient has no evidence for mild pre-eclampsia, which most often resolves with delivery.

Postpartum nonpsychotic depression (**choice C**), which is also called postpartum depression, is characterized by intense sadness and sleep and appetite disturbances, along with other life-altering changes. This patient has a presentation more consistent with postpartum blues than postpartum depression.

Postpartum psychotic depression (**choice D**) is a psychosis characterized by delusions, hallucinations, or both occurring within 3 weeks of birth. This patient does not have these manifestations.

Posttraumatic stress disorder (**choice E**) is characterized by the repeated reliving of an event, avoidance behavior, and other symptoms, such as sleep difficulty, that are also seen in postpartum depression. This patient does not exhibit these symptoms.

40. **The correct answer is E.** In the past, patients who had undergone a cesarean delivery were considered to always need a cesarean for future deliveries. In the late 20th century, however, this approach changed such that patients who had had prior cesarean deliveries were allowed to attempt a VBAC (vaginal birth after cesarean). VBAC has been shown to be sufficiently safe and effective (with success rates around 70%) that it can be offered as an option to women who have had a prior cesarean so long as there are no absolute contraindications. Potential candidates are women who have had one or two prior low transverse cesarean deliveries, a clinically adequate pelvis, and no other uterine scars or previous rupture. Furthermore there should be a physician immediately available throughout active labor capable of monitoring labor and performing an emergency cesarean delivery, and anesthesia available for emergency cesarean delivery. Yet, while VBAC may be *offered* to these patients, such patients should also be apprised of the risks of VBAC. The major risk of VBAC is uterine rupture, which, based on most studies, averages around 1%. Furthermore, there is the risk that the VBAC attempt could fail and that the woman will need a cesarean delivery anyway. Thus, the patient should be counseled that VBAC is an option for her. She should also be counseled, however, that the decision is hers to make.

To state that a repeat cesarean delivery is absolutely contraindicated for her (**choice A**) is incorrect. Absolute contraindications include a prior classic or T-shaped uterine incision or other transfundal uterine surgery, a contracted pelvis, medical or obstetric complication that precludes vaginal delivery, and inability to have an emergency cesarean delivery performed. None of these contraindications are relevant in her case.

To state that a repeat cesarean delivery is the *recommended* mode of delivery for her (**choice B**) is not correct. When it comes to the topic of VBAC, the choice is very much up to the patient, provided there are no contraindications. If, for example, she values the experience of vaginal delivery more than anything else, then she should attempt a VBAC. If the risk of uterine rupture scares her most, then elective repeat cesarean delivery would likely be best.

To counsel her that a vaginal birth must be attempted based on current insurance regulations (**choice C**) is absolutely incorrect. At one time, in certain states, insurance companies attempted to force patients into attempting VBAC. This is no longer the case.

To advise her that VBAC is absolutely contraindicated given her past obstetrical history (**choice D**) is incorrect. As detailed above, she has no absolute contraindications to VBAC.

41. **The correct answer is C.** This patient's clinical symptoms are most consistent with a diagnosis of pelvic inflammatory disease (PID). PID most frequently is the result of infection with sexually transmitted pathogens, including *Neisseria gonorrhoeae* and *Chlamydia trachomatis*. However, other organisms, including vaginal flora, have been implicated in some cases. There is no definitive diagnostic test for PID, but the clinical signs seen in this case, including abdominal pain, vaginal discharge, and fever, are consistent. Treatment for PID is antibiotics directed at the likely pathogens. However, even with prompt treatment there is an increased risk of ectopic pregnancy in women who have had even one episode of PID. This risk increases greatly with each subsequent episode, and has been estimated to be as high as 50% following three episodes of PID.

Institution of antimicrobial therapy is of great importance in minimizing the sequelae of PID, but clinical improvement may lag by days to weeks (**choice A**). Some patients require intravenous antibiotics, while select milder cases may be managed as outpatients.

The right upper quadrant pain in this patient is suggestive of gonococcal perihepatitis (**choice B**), one sequela of ascending infection. This inflammation of the liver capsule can be severe, but permanent hepatic damage is rare. Surgical treatment may be indicated if there is abscess formation, but most cases are managed medically.

Cervical cultures are often useful in helping to confirm the diagnosis of PID, but a substantial proportion of cases may be culture negative. In addition, one or no organisms may be grown from fluid sampled at the os, while there may be a polymicrobial infection in the upper reproductive tract. For this reason, cervical cultures are not used to guide length of treatment for PID (**choice D**).

While infertility is one of the most feared complications of PID, it is certainly not a universal sequela of this clinical syndrome (**choice E**). This patient's history of unprotected sex puts her at risk for unwanted pregnancy as well as sexually transmitted diseases, and discussion of the best method of contraception is appropriate at this time.

42. **The correct answer is E.** Patients will ask this frequently. The definitions of risk factor categories are assigned to all drugs based on the level of risk the drug poses to the fetus and are used by the Food and Drug Administration. They are:

Category A: Controlled studies in pregnant women failing to demonstrate a risk to the fetus in the first trimester (and even subsequent trimesters), and the risk of fetal harm is remote. Animal reproduction studies not demonstrating a fetal risk but there are no controlled studies in pregnant women (**choice C**).

Category B: Either animal reproduction studies have not demonstrated a fetal risk but there are no controlled studies in pregnant women; or animal reproduction studies have shown an adverse effect (other than a decrease in fertility) that was not confirmed in controlled studies in women in the first trimester (**choices A and B**).

Category C: Either the studies in animals revealed adverse effects on the fetus (teratogenic) with no controlled studies in women; or animal and human studies were not available (**choice E**).

Category D: Positive evidence of human fetal risk, but the benefits for use in pregnancy may outweigh the risks (**choice F**).

Category X: Studies in animals or humans have demonstrated fetal abnormalities and the drug is contraindicated in pregnancy (**choice D**).

43. **The correct answer is E.** Pregnancy (along with contraceptive complications) is the most common cause of abnormal bleeding in this age group (i.e., childbearing years from age 16 to early 40s). Even though she tells you that she is not pregnant, a test should be performed to evaluate her for pregnancy.

Adenocarcinoma of the endometrium (**choice A**) is not as common as pregnancy in this age group. It is typically a disease of postmenopausal women with approximately 85% of the patients being over 50 years of age. With longer life expectancy for American women, the disease is becoming increasingly important. Menopause after age 52, nulliparity, obesity, diabetes, previous radiation, and the administration of unopposed estrogen and tamoxifen are the main factors that predispose to this type of cancer.

Anovulation (**choice B**) is a common cause of dysfunctional uterine bleeding in teenagers and women during and after their late 30s. It is also associated with polycystic ovary syndrome and obesity.

Coagulopathies (**choice C**) are rare causes of abnormal vaginal bleeding, although this should be sought in this patient's history (e.g., abnormal bruising), along with thyroid, renal, and hepatic disease, and stress, exercise, and weight changes.

Fever and pelvic pain are typically present with pelvic inflammatory disease (**choice D**). It is not the most common cause of bleeding in this age group.

44. **The correct answer is B.** Patients with hypovolemia or a hemoglobin level below 7 g/dL should be hospitalized for hormonal therapy and iron replacement (ferrous gluconate). Hormonal therapy consists of estrogen intravenously until bleeding stops. If bleeding continues, vasopressin should be administered. A blood transfusion may also be required in severe hemorrhage. Then, an oral contraceptive pill such as conjugated estrogen (**choice A**) should be administered every 6 hours for 7 days, followed by a tapering slowly to one pill once daily. Oral contraceptives are effective in higher than usual doses. At this point, conjugated estrogen can control heavy dysfunctional bleeding. Contraindications include pregnancy and hypertension. In patients over the age of 35 with a similar presentation, before hormonal therapy is given, endometrial sampling should be performed to rule out endometrial carcinoma or hyperplasia.

One tablet of ethinyl estradiol/levonorgestrel daily (**choice C**) will be sub-therapeutic. Oral contraceptives are only effective in menorrhagia at higher than usual doses.

Nonsteroidal anti-inflammatory agents, such as ibuprofen (**choice D**), are useful first choice agents in menorrhagia for outpatient therapy. They are well tolerated and do not have the hormonal effects of oral contraceptives.

Medroxyprogesterone acetate (**choice E**) is less reliable and slower acting.

45. **The correct answer is D.** This patient has *Trichomonas vaginalis*, which is a sexually transmitted disease that often presents with vaginal discharge. The treatment is metronidazole and can be prescribed for this adolescent patient even though she is a minor. Parental consent is not needed in the treatment of sexually transmitted diseases. Sexual partners should be treated to reduce recurrences and reinfection.

If this patient had gonorrhea, it would be appropriate to administer ceftriaxone intramuscularly and prescribe oral doxycycline (**choice A**). The ceftriaxone is to treat the gonorrheal infection and the doxycycline is for the presumptive coinfection with chlamydia, which often occurs. These antimicrobials are not used to treat *Trichomonas*, which the patient in this case has.

Even though this patient is a minor, it is unnecessary to call the patient's mother to obtain consent for treatment (**choice B**). Parental consent is not needed in the treatment of sexually transmitted diseases.

There is no reason to suspect that this adolescent is being sexually abused, so it is inappropriate to contact child protective services for suspected sexual abuse (**choice C**). Many 15-year-olds are sexually active and do not want their parents to know about it.

The vaginal discharge showed motile, flagellated organisms, which is distinctive for a *Trichomonas* infection; therefore, it is unnecessary to send a culture of the vaginal discharge to establish a definite diagnosis (**choice E**). This is usually only done if you have a high index of suspicion and the wet mount is negative. The wet mount is typically positive in 40 to 80% of cases and the culture is positive in 95% of the cases. However, the wet mount is cheaper and quicker so it is the usual first step in trying to establish the diagnosis.

46. **The correct answer is D.** Postpartum psychosis is a true psychiatric emergency, which, if left untreated, can have fatal outcomes for both mother and child. The patient should be placed on observation immediately pending psychiatric evaluation for the protection of mother and child.

The patient is clearly psychotic. Therefore, a prescription for fluoxetine, an antidepressant (**choice A**), as an outpatient is inappropriate.

The psychotic postpartum patient with paranoid ideation regarding her child should absolutely not be in physical contact with her child (**choice B**). This is an extremely dangerous situation and should be avoided at all costs.

The patient cannot be discharged (**choice C**) and will likely require involuntary psychiatric hospitalization. Discharging the patient as planned with psychiatric followup is incorrect.

The patient requires immediate psychiatric attention due to the potential for danger to self and her newborn child. Therefore, sedating the patient and reassessing her later (**choice E**) is incorrect.

47. **The correct answer is C.** The patient is not giving irrational reasons for not wanting to have chemotherapy. The most appropriate step in the management of this patient would be to assess her decision-making capacity, and if she has this capacity, to abide by her wishes.

Patients have an intrinsic right to self-determination of care unless their decision-making capacity is impaired. This patient should not be automatically coerced or goaded into making a decision simply because it is in accordance to what her medical team wants. Therefore, agreeing to convince the patient to undergo chemotherapy (**choice A**) is incorrect.

There is no evidence from the narrative that the patient is an imminent danger to self or others. There is not even any direct evidence that the patient is depressed, and therefore psychiatric hospitalization (**choice B**) is not indicated at this time.

This patient should not be given a discharge contingent on psychiatric followup (**choice D**). Treatment of this sort cannot be mandated in a patient who will likely demonstrate medical decision-making capacity.

Nothing from the narrative indicates that there is an indication to sedate this patient (**choice E**). She was not described as agitated or even anxious. Sedation at this point would likely constitute treatment against the patient's will without an imminent indication.

48. **The correct answer is B.** Pain on cervical motion during a pelvic examination in a case such as this may be the strongest evidence in favor of pelvic inflammatory disease (PID). In this case, the tenderness noted anteriorly on rectal examination also implied a tender cervix. PID is a clinical diagnosis. Major criteria include lower abdominal pain, pain on palpation during abdominal examination, and cervical motion tenderness on pelvic examination. Other supportive evidence for the diagnosis may include: fever, vaginal discharge, elevated white count, elevated sedimentation rate or C-reactive protein, and the feeling of an adnexal mass or fullness on pelvic examination.

Adnexal tenderness (**choice A**) may be suggestive of PID but may also be present in other gynecological diseases, such as ectopic pregnancy or ovarian cyst. Not alone, but together with cervical motion tenderness it would support a diagnosis of PID.

A fever over 38.9 C (102 F) (**choice C**) is more characteristic of PID than acute appendicitis, but high fevers are common in other conditions, such as a perforated appendicitis.

The absence of significant nausea and vomiting (not just vomiting after one dose of medication) (**choice D**) is more compatible with PID than with appendicitis, but sometimes patients with appendicitis have no history of nausea or vomiting.

Although vaginal discharge (**choice E**) may be supportive of PID, cervical mucus smears and Gram stains are not entirely reliable. Vaginal discharge is not a major criterion in the diagnosis of PID. Obviously in this case it will be important to obtain cervical cultures for both gonorrhea and chlamydia.

49. **The correct answer is D.** Hirsutism, or excessive male pattern hair growth, is common and affects approximately 10% of women of reproductive age. Causes include polycystic ovarian syndrome (PCOS), medications, adrenal and testosterone secreting tumors, elevated prolactin levels, hyperprolactinemia, and pregnancy. It may also be idiopathic. Although it is rarely due to a seriously underlying cause, key aspects of the history and physical exam may indicate need for further testing. In this case, fairly rapid onset signs of virilization should lead to concern about adrenal or ovarian neoplasm. The patient has frontal balding and clitoromegaly; other virilizing features include acne and increased muscle mass. A DHEA-S can be used for concern about adrenal tumor, usually with elevated cortisol as well. The concern for an androgen-secreting tumor should lead to an evaluation for ovarian malignancy, in this case an ultrasound.

The free testosterone may be helpful in cases of high or low sex hormone binding globulin, but given the level of elevation of testosterone in this case it is not the most important next step (**choice A**).

PCOS is one of the most common causes of hirsutism. Oligo or amenorrhea is a hallmark of the disease, and symptoms usually begin near puberty and are not of rapid onset. Testosterone levels are often elevated and there can be signs of virilization, but usually not the marked elevation as in this case. The increased LH/FSH ratio (**choice B**) seen in PCOS may or may not be seen secondary to pulsatile gonadotropins and would not be a sensitive test for PCOS even if that were the prime concern.

A prolactin (**choice C**) level should be one of the first laboratory tests sent in evaluations for amenorrhea, but it is a less common cause of hirsutism. In this case the serum testosterone already is worrisome for an ovarian neoplasm as a primary cause of this patient's symptoms, and she would be unlikely to have a coexisting hypothalamic tumor.

In many cases, hirsutism is not worrisome, and simple reassurance can be given (**choice E**). A careful history and physical can determine those who will need laboratory testing and further workup and, as stated above, this patient requires further evaluation.

50. **The correct answer is A.** A breast mass suspicious for malignancy should be biopsied; several techniques exist, including fine needle aspiration, core needle biopsy, and excisional biopsy. The most common causes of a breast mass vary with age. While patients under the age of 40 are most likely to have a benign finding, the incidence of cancer may be less than 1%. Above 50, the incidence rises to approximately 40%. Therefore, a mass in a woman of this age should not be ignored or simply followed.

Reassurance and repeat mammogram in 6 months (**choice B**) or reassurance and repeat mammogram in 1 year (**choice C**) are incorrect. Failure to detect the lesion on mammogram does not preclude further evaluation or mean that repeat mammography will be of benefit. Mammography should be done, however, as part of the evaluation of a breast mass, as the presence of other abnormalities may affect the workup. Similarly, ultrasound can be used to distinguish cystic from solid masses and guide needle aspiration. Its failure to locate the mass again does not obviate the need for biopsy; therefore, a repeat ultrasound in 6 months (**choice E**) is incorrect.

Reassurance and repeat physical examination in 6 months (**choice D**) is incorrect for the reasons stated above, although in a young woman if the initial history and physical exam were consistent with a benign lesion, plans should be made for follow up in the next one or two menstrual cycles.

Further risk stratification (**choice F**) is not useful in assisting in the decision to evaluate this mass. In addition, the patient has no family history to raise any suspicion for the BRCA-1 or -2 mutations. Decisions about genetic testing are complicated and clearly not indicated in this patient.

Obstetrics/Gynecology: **Test Two**

1. A 48-year-old woman receives meperidine intramuscularly for pain management every 4 hours after a hysterectomy. You decide to switch her to oral medication on the fourth day after surgery. The following afternoon she complains of inadequate pain relief and tells you that she wants "the shots" again. The patient has no prior psychiatric history or history of substance abuse. The nurse is concerned that the patient is now drug seeking and developed iatrogenic addiction. In reviewing the case you should explain to the nurse that

    (A) oral meperidine has lower potency than the intramuscular injection form, thus the oral dose should be adjusted

    (B) the patient has developed placebo effect from injection and no dose adjustment is needed

    (C) the patient has developed tolerance to meperidine and the dose must be increased to control the pain

    (D) psychiatry should be consulted because she has histrionic personality traits

    (E) psychiatry should be consulted because she may need detoxification from the opiates

2. A previously healthy 17-year-old girl comes to the clinic with right-sided lower abdominal pain and vaginal bleeding. The pain has been "on and off" for 3 days and she has had scanty white vaginal discharge. She thinks her last menstrual period was about 4 or 5 weeks ago. Her periods are usually regular for 5 days, but a few times a year her period is irregular, either early or late. One year ago she had a chlamydia infection that resolved after therapy. She has had one steady boyfriend for the past 8 months and her periods have been regular. The most important first step in the evaluation of this patient is

    (A) pelvic examination

    (B) a pregnancy test

    (C) a stat CBC

    (D) an ultrasound

    (E) urinalysis and urine culture

3. A 15-year-old girl comes to the emergency department with a 2-week history of vaginal discharge. She is not a great historian, but tells you that the discharge smells "awful and is dirty looking." Her menstrual periods are regular, occurring every month and lasting 5 to 6 days, and her last one was 2 weeks ago. She denies a past history of sexually transmitted diseases. She has one steady boyfriend who usually wears a condom. An abdominal examination is benign and pelvic examination reveals a scanty amount of vaginal discharge. Her uterus is normal, cervix is nontender, and the adnexa are unremarkable. A wet prep of the vaginal discharge reveals several epithelial cells that seem to be studded with bacteria. On the basis of your evaluation at this point you send cultures off for chlamydia and gonorrhea, but feel the best next step is to begin treatment with

    (A) ceftriaxone

    (B) ciprofloxacin

    (C) clotrimazole

    (D) doxycycline

    (E) metronidazole

4. A 27-year-old woman comes to the office complaining that she is "losing all her hair" and will "go bald" if it does not stop. She used to have a full head of hair up to 3 months ago when it started falling out suddenly. Now, she is afraid to wash it and she gathers a handful on her hairbrush every time she brushes it. She has no significant past medical history and takes only sertraline and a multivitamin daily. About a month before her office visit, she had a nasty cold with fever of 38.0 C (100.4 F) and a sore throat for which she took over-the-counter cold medication and it resolved within days. She started working 2 months ago, when her newborn baby was 3 months old. Her job is not particularly stressful, but she is not too happy with her nanny and is thinking about transferring her baby to a day-care facility in the vicinity of her firm. You examine her and note that there is diffuse thinning throughout the entire scalp with no visible changes on the skin. The "pull test" yields 23 hairs in the parietal, temporal, and occipital area combined. Microscopic examination reveals mostly club hairs. The most likely cause of her hair loss is

(A) childbirth that occurred 5 months earlier
(B) a side effect of pseudoephedrine in the cold medication
(C) a side effect of sertraline
(D) a sore throat with fever 4 weeks earlier
(E) stress related to problems with the nanny

5. A 53-year-old woman comes to the emergency department with fever, chills, and left lower quadrant pain that has been worsening over the last 36 hours. Her appetite is markedly decreased. She has not been to a physician in 15 years and admits to smoking 2 packs of cigarettes a day. Her temperature is 38.5 C (101.3 F), blood pressure is 129/90 mm Hg, pulse is 102/min, and respirations are 18/min. She is in moderate distress from abdominal discomfort, and her heart is tachycardic, regular, and no murmurs are present. Lungs are clear. Her abdomen is soft, with voluntary guarding and moderate tenderness over the left lower quadrant and hypoactive bowel sounds. Rectal examination has brown stool that is guaiac positive. Laboratory studies show a hematocrit of 40%, platelets of 300,000 /µL, and a leukocyte count of 15,900/mm^3. She is diagnosed with diverticulitis and treated with metronidazole and ciprofloxacin. Since she has no regular physician, she is scheduled to follow up for a new patient evaluation and monitoring of therapy of her diverticulitis in the clinic in 3 days. During her new-patient evaluation she should be scheduled for

(A) a chest x-ray
(B) a mammogram every year for the first 2 years, then every 5 years
(C) a Pap smear
(D) yearly colonoscopies
(E) yearly electrocardiograms

6. A 19-year-old homeless woman comes to the emergency department complaining of lower abdominal pain for the past 24 hours. She admits to many recent unprotected sexual encounters. Her temperature is 38.3 C (101.0 F). Physical examination shows cervical motion and adnexal tenderness and mucopurulent vaginal discharge. Erythrocyte sedimentation rate is 40 sec and leukocyte count is 17,000/mm^3. She is admitted to the hospital. The most appropriate therapy is

(A) ampicillin IV and gentamicin IM
(B) cefoxitin IV and erythromycin orally
(C) ceftriaxone IM and doxycycline orally
(D) ceftriaxone IM and erythromycin orally
(E) clindamycin IV and gentamicin IV

7. A 35-year-old woman, who had her second baby about a month ago, comes to the clinic with her husband. Both of them have noticed that she is moody, depressed, and tearful for apparently no reason. This did not happen after the birth of her first child. She initially thought that she was tired because of breast-feeding and the difficult pregnancy. However, she reports that she has had little interest in the baby, feels tired, is not motivated to do anything, and has a poor appetite. She feels guilty that she is feeling this way and wants to discuss treatment options. She is adamant about continuing to breast-feed and wants to know if she can still take medication because she feels she cannot continue "like this any more." The most correct statement about the use of antidepressants during lactation is:

(A) Long half-life antidepressants should be prescribed so that fewer pills need to be taken
(B) MAO inhibitors are the first line of treatment of postpartum depression
(C) Nefazodone is safe to use in breast-feeding mothers
(D) An SSRI with a short half-life should be prescribed
(E) The use of antidepressants is safe because most psychotropic medications are not secreted into milk

8. A 16-year-old girl at 40 weeks' gestation comes to the hospital because the "baby is coming out." She had a previous abortion and one normal vaginal delivery. She has gestational diabetes but has been noncompliant with all medical interventions that you advised. The labor is advanced and almost precipitous because you can see the baby's head crowning. One minute later the patient is in severe pain and you note that the baby's head is in the left occipitoanterior position. There are several deep, late decelerations on the fetal heart tracing. Each time the mother pushes with the contraction to deliver the rest of the baby, the head retracts back into the birth canal coinciding with another late deceleration. You are alone in the room with the patient. The most appropriate next step in management is to

(A) apply suprapubic pressure as the mother pushes to deliver the baby
(B) call for assistance
(C) enter the introitus to adduct the baby's shoulder and rotate the baby
(D) enter the introitus to free the baby's posterior arm
(E) enter the introitus to rotate the baby counterclockwise to deliver the posterior shoulder
(F) evaluate for an episiotomy
(G) push the head back into the birth canal and begin an urgent caesarian section
(H) push the mother's legs as far back as possible.
(I) roll mother onto her hands and knees

9. A 23-year-old primigravid woman who is at 17 weeks' gestation comes to the health center for a routine prenatal visit. She feels well but is concerned because she feels no fetal movement. She has had no bleeding per vagina, loss of fluid, or contractions. The pregnancy has been uncomplicated to this point. She has no medical problems. She had an appendectomy at the age of 16 and an ovarian cystectomy at the age of 20. She takes prenatal vitamins and has no known drug allergies. Her blood pressure is 100/60 mm Hg. Her urine dip shows no glucose, protein, or nitrites. She has gained 2 pounds since her first prenatal visit. Her fundal height feels appropriate for 17 weeks. The fetal heart rate is in the 150s/min. In addressing the issue of fetal movement, the most appropriate next step is to

   (A) initiate induction of labor for vaginal delivery
   (B) obtain a biophysical profile (BPP)
   (C) obtain a non-stress test (NST)
   (D) prepare the patient for cesarean delivery
   (E) reassure the patient that this is normal

10. A 29-year-old woman comes to the health center for an annual examination and contraceptive counseling. She has been married for 9 years, is in a monogamous relationship with her husband, and has three healthy children. She thinks she is done with childbearing, but is not 100% sure. She has no medical problems and her only surgical history is two cesarean deliveries. She takes no medications and has no allergies. She smokes a half pack of cigarettes per day. Physical examination, including breast and pelvic examination, is normal. When you are finished examining her, she tells you that she needs an effective contraceptive but that she is afraid of developing cancer. In counseling this patient about contraceptive options, you can advise her that long-term use of the IUD has been most often shown to be associated with decreased rates of

   (A) breast cancer
   (B) cervical cancer
   (C) endometrial cancer
   (D) lung cancer
   (E) ovarian cancer

11. A 23-year-old woman with insulin-dependent diabetes mellitus comes to the health center for an annual examination. She has no complaints. She has regular menstrual cycles with her period coming every 28 days. She takes subcutaneous insulin daily and is somewhat compliant with maintaining her blood glucose levels in the desired range. She exercises about twice a week on a treadmill. Physical examination, including breast and pelvic examination, is unremarkable. She informs you that she and her husband would like to become pregnant in the upcoming year but she is concerned about complications caused by her diabetes. To prevent this patient from having a fetus with congenital anomalies, the most important factor for this patient is

   (A) avoidance of first-trimester insulin
   (B) preconception glucose control
   (C) second-trimester exercise
   (D) third-trimester insulin treatment
   (E) tight glucose control during labor and delivery

12. A 33-year-old woman who is at 24 weeks' gestation comes to the office because of a lesion on her right forearm. She has had "a mole" there ever since she can remember, but that over the past few months she has noticed that it has darkened in color and occasionally bleeds. Her past medical history is significant for hypothyroidism for which she takes thyroxine. She has no past surgical history and no known drug allergies. Past obstetrical history is significant for a normal spontaneous vaginal delivery of an 8-pound male, 3 years ago. Examination of the forearm shows a 7-mm, irregularly pigmented, asymmetric lesion with an ulceration on its left lateral border. The remainder of the physical examination is unremarkable. The most appropriate next step in management is to

   (A) apply topical 5-fluorouracil to the lesion
   (B) counsel the patient to terminate the pregnancy
   (C) counsel the patient to terminate the pregnancy and have permanent sterilization
   (D) reassure the patient that the finding is normal
   (E) recommend an excisional biopsy

13. A 20-year-old pregnant woman with schizophrenia and a history of substance abuse comes to the emergency department. She is at 28 weeks' gestation and claims she is suicidal because she has no place to go. She threatens to kill herself if she is discharged. She is no longer able to stay at her cousin's house because she was caught stealing and selling their things for drugs. When asked about her last use of drugs she begins to scream that she doesn't remember because the "voices" are bothering her. While she is waiting for the psychiatry consult she begins to complain of severe abdominal pain. She then admits that she had been smoking crack with her boyfriend earlier in the day. Given the patient's history and condition, the most appropriate next step in management is to

(A) call security and wait for a psychiatrist to evaluate her for suicidality and delusions
(B) check her vital signs and order immediate external fetal monitoring
(C) get a social worker because she needs to find housing
(D) order basic tests because she is pregnant and let her rest in the emergency department until the crack is eliminated from her system
(E) send her out because she is malingering in order to have a place to stay

14. A 33-year-old woman comes to the office complaining of 8 months of amenorrhea. Prior to this she has had normal menses starting at 15 years old, accompanied by normal sexual development. She denies fatigue, change in libido, hirsutism, or nipple discharge. She is currently sexually active but has been using condoms for pregnancy prevention. Her temperature is 37.0 C (98.6 F), blood pressure is 120/80 mm Hg, pulse is 80/min, and respirations are12/min. Her weight is 55 kg (131 lb) and her height is 65 inches. Physical examination is within normal limits without evidence of hyperandrogenism or acne. Laboratory studies show:

Serum Beta HCG	Negative
Prolactin	8 ng/mL (normal 2-15 ng/mL)
TSH	1.24 μU/mL (normal 0.4-5 μU/mL)
FSH	120 mU/mL (normal 1.4-9.6 mU/mL)

You prescribe progestin 10 mg each day for 7 days and she does not have subsequent withdrawal bleeding. You then prescribe estrogen and progestin and she returns to the office to tell you that she "finally has menstrual bleeding." The most likely cause of this patient's amenorrhea is

(A) Asherman syndrome
(B) gonadal agenesis
(C) hypothalamic dysfunction
(D) polycystic ovary syndrome
(E) premature gonadal failure

15. A 53-year-old woman comes to the office for a periodic health maintenance examination. She had a hysterectomy performed for large fibroids a few years earlier. She now reports that she is experiencing new onset hot flashes, vaginal dryness, and mood swings. She wants to know if she should begin hormone replacement therapy (HRT). She has read "mixed things about HRT on the Internet" and she wants your advice. With the above information, it is appropriate to advise this patient that:

(A) HRT does not increase the risk of breast cancer
(B) HRT would reduce her symptoms while increasing HDL, decreasing LDL, and increasing bone density
(C) She can safely begin full-dose HRT
(D) She should begin HRT with low-dose progestin therapy
(E) Treatment with HRT will have an early cardio-protective effect

16. You are seeing a 25-year-old woman in your office for her first prenatal visit at approximately 8 weeks' gestation. She and her husband are pleased that they are expecting their third child. She has no medical problems and her other pregnancies were uncomplicated. She has no family history of medical problems. She is employed as a nurse. Other than some mild nausea, she has been generally well. Laboratory studies return a few days later and show:

Blood type	A negative
Antibody screen	Negative
Hct	41%
Rubella	Antibody detected
VDRL	Nonreactive
HBsAg	Negative
PAP smear	Within normal limits
Urine culture	>100,000 CFU group B streptococci

At her next visit, you should advise her that:

(A) She shows no evidence of protection against hepatitis B, and you recommend that she start the vaccination series during her pregnancy because she is a health care worker
(B) She will need antibiotics for her urine infection and also when she goes into labor
(C) She will not need RhoGAM during this pregnancy because she shows no evidence of antibody formation from her other pregnancies
(D) These results indicate rubella infection. She should consider elective termination to prevent congenital rubella syndrome
(E) You do not recommend screening for Down syndrome because she is not of advanced maternal age

17. A 24-year-old woman comes to the emergency department complaining of abdominal pain. Her last menstrual period was a month and a half ago. Her vital signs are: blood pressure 80/40 mm Hg and pulse is 110/min supine and 123/min sitting up. Abdominal examination shows rebound tenderness and guarding. Pelvic examination reveals cervical motion tenderness. Hemoglobin is 11.3 mg/dL and urine chorionic gonadotropin is positive. Transvaginal ultrasound shows fluid in the cul-de-sac, a 2.5-cm mass is seen in the right adnexa, and no structures are found within the uterus. The most appropriate next step in management is

(A) laparoscopy
(B) laparotomy
(C) methotrexate
(D) mifepristone (RU-486)
(E) observation

18. A 28-year-old gravida 7, para 7 woman just delivered a 4300-gram infant. She has been bleeding profusely from the vagina since delivery of the placenta, which appears intact. Her temperature is 36.6 C (97.9 F), blood pressure is 140/100 mm Hg, pulse is 100/min, and respirations are 22/min. On physical examination, her uterus appears smooth, enlarged, and soft. The most appropriate initial step in management is to

(A) administer methylergonovine, intravenously
(B) administer oxytocin , intravenously
(C) administer prostaglandin F2 alpha, intramuscularly
(D) perform a uterine massage
(E) prepare her for an immediate hysterectomy

19. A 20-year-old woman comes to the emergency department complaining of lower abdominal pain that started at the end of her last menstrual period, which ended 1 week ago. She normally has menstrual periods every 30 days and they usually last 5 days. She is sexually active and has three children. Her temperature is 39.0 C (102.2 F), blood pressure is 134/76 mm Hg, pulse is 97/min, and respirations are 22/min. She has diffuse abdominal tenderness and pain around her cervix on bimanual examination. Sterile speculum examination reveals thick, mucopurulent discharge in the posterior fornix and in the external os of the cervix. Her inguinal lymph nodes are not palpable. The most likely cause of her condition is

(A) bacterial vaginosis
(B) *Candida albicans*
(C) *Chlamydia trachomatis*
(D) Lymphogranuloma venereum
(E) *Neisseria gonorrhoeae*

20. A 13-year-old girl comes to the clinic requesting oral contraceptive pills (OCP). She has been sexually active for the past 4 months with her first boyfriend. She says they both "hate" condoms and have only used them once. Menarche was at age 10 and she has been having regular periods for the past year. She also tells you that she has very strict parents and they would not approve of her sexual activities. She asks that you do not tell her parents abut this visit. She is holding a pamphlet that describes the risks and benefits of OCPs and tells you that she read all about it in the waiting room and knows that she should also use condoms to prevent sexually transmitted diseases. The most appropriate next step in management is to

(A) prescribe oral contraceptive pills and then inform her parents
(B) prescribe oral contraceptive pills for 1 month and tell her you will giver her 1 month to figure out how she will tell her parents about her sexual activities and re-schedule a return visit in 1 month
(C) prescribe oral contraceptive pills and assure her that you will not inform her parents
(D) refuse to prescribe oral contraceptive pills and tell her you are obligated to inform her parents because of her age
(E) refuse to prescribe oral contraceptive pills and tell her that condoms are not only a good form of contraception, they also protect against sexually transmitted diseases

21. A 22-year-old gravida 3, para 2 at 30 weeks' gestation comes to the office complaining of constant, mild abdominal pain. She says she recently emigrated from a small village in Mexico and while living there she used to work with her hands making colorful pottery. She has no family history of diseases. She has no other complaints other than constipation for 2 months. She also relates that other people in her village have had similar complaints for which the doctor prescribed "a large medicinal drink." Her vital signs are: temperature 37.0 C (98.6 F), blood pressure 115/77 mm Hg, pulse 93/min, and respirations are 18/min. You notice a grayish discoloration of her gums. She has mild, diffuse abdominal tenderness to deep palpation but no rebound or guarding. Her hematocrit is 29%, mean corpuscular volume (MCV) of 79, red cell distribution width (RDW) is normal, and her peripheral smear shows microcytic, hypochromic red blood cells. The study most likely to be helpful in establishing the diagnosis is

(A) serum ferritin
(B) serum folate
(C) serum free erythrocyte protoporphyrin (FEP)
(D) serum electrophoresis
(E) an x-ray of her femur

22. A 37-year-old gravida 4, para 4 woman comes to the office to discuss long-term birth control options. She says she wants to use a birth control method that does not have any side effects and does not interfere with "the mood of foreplay." She has chronic obstructive pulmonary disease (COPD) with reduced functional capacity and had an appendectomy 20 years ago. She has smoked 2 packs per day for the past 14 years, drinks 3 to 4 glasses of wine per day, and denies use of illicit drugs. She has been married for over 13 years. Her family history and physical examination are unremarkable. The best contraceptive method for this patient is

(A) condoms
(B) the intrauterine device (IUD)
(C) medroxyprogesterone acetate injections
(D) oral contraceptive pills
(E) tubal ligation

23. A 20-year-old nulligravid woman calls your office with a question about birth control pills. She says she began taking the pill 2 months ago for the first time in her life. She makes sure she takes a pill every night just before she goes to sleep. Last month she remembers getting her period near the end of the month when she was taking the "white pills." This month she has not had her period and is on her 6th white pill. From your inquiry you find out that she is sexually active and that she claims to be in a monogamous relationship. She had her first period at the age of 12. She gets her periods "like clockwork" every 30 days. Her periods are light and last 4 days. She does not smoke, drink, or use any illicit drugs. The last time she used any medication was 4 months ago when she had a cold. You should tell her to

(A) continue taking the pills as usual
(B) continue taking the pills as usual and use a condom
(C) stop taking the pills and resume after 7 days
(D) stop taking the pills and immediately go to the emergency department
(E) take an additional pill tomorrow

24. A 24-year-old nulliparous woman who is at 39 weeks' gestation is in labor. Her cervix was dilated 4 cm at 5 PM. At 11 PM her cervix was dilated 7 cm and the fetal vertex was at –1 station. It is now 3 AM and her cervix is dilated 7.5 cm and the fetal head is not engaged. Fetal heart rate monitoring shows a normal pattern, and an intrauterine pressure catheter shows adequate but painful contractions occurring every 2 to 3 minutes. Estimated fetal weight by obstetrical ultrasound at 37 weeks' gestation was 7.8 lb. The woman is 5 feet 1 inch tall and weighs 99 lb. Her vital signs are all stable. The most appropriate management at this time is

(A) cesarean section
(B) epidural placement
(C) forceps delivery
(D) meperidine, intravenously
(E) oxytocin, intravenously

25. A 16-year-old nulligravid girl calls your office because she is worried she may be pregnant. She tells you that she had intercourse with her boyfriend on May 17 and used a condom. After the event, she noticed that the condom had a tear on one side. She says she had her first period when she was 12 years old. She gets her periods every 28 days "like clockwork" and her periods always last 5 days. The first day of her last menstrual period was May 1. She took a home pregnancy test today (May 22), which was negative. She is still worried that she may be pregnant because she has heard that home pregnancy tests are unreliable. You should advise her to

(A) bring a urine sample to the office and you will do a urine pregnancy test today
(B) come to the office to evaluate for fetal heart tones by Doppler
(C) come to the office for quantitative beta-hCG levels today
(D) come to the office in 3 or more days to repeat the pregnancy test
(E) go to the radiologist for a transvaginal ultrasound

26. A 21-year-old primigravid woman comes to the clinic for her first prenatal visit. She has no past medical history and no past surgical history. Her last menstrual period was about 7 weeks ago. She does not drink or smoke. She is very athletic and health conscious. In fact she runs 5 km races regularly and is one of the best players on her college tennis team. She asks you about exercise and diet during pregnancy. You advise her to

(A) avoid supine exercises after the first trimester
(B) discontinue exercise after 30 weeks' gestation
(C) increase fat intake
(D) increase protein intake
(E) maintain a heart rate less than 120 beats per minute

27. A 24-year-old primigravid woman who is at 32 weeks' gestation comes to the emergency department because of right upper quadrant pain. She also has nausea and has vomited several times. She has felt irregular uterine contractions since this morning. An obstetrical ultrasound was performed at 20 weeks' gestation by last menstrual period with the following results: Femur length 20 weeks 2 days, abdominal circumference 19 weeks 5 days, biparietal diameter 20 weeks 0 days; adnexa are normal; no fluid in the cul-de-sac. On physical examination of the abdomen, there is diffuse tenderness in all quadrants but mostly in the right mid abdomen. Her temperature is 36.6 C (97.9 F), blood pressure is 99/65 mm Hg, pulse is 98/min, and leukocyte count is 12,400/mm^3 with increased immature forms. Urinalysis reveals 3 white blood cells and 2 red blood cells per high power field. The most likely diagnosis is

(A) acute pancreatitis
(B) appendicitis
(C) pyelonephritis
(D) right renal stone
(E) torsion of right ovarian cyst

28. A 58-year-old postmenopausal woman has been treated with carboplatin and paclitaxel chemotherapy for ovarian cancer for the last 3 years. She is aware of her terminal condition and is not prepared for any heroic measures if her body cannot function on its own. She has not, however, communicated this wish to anyone, nor has she written down her current beliefs. Shortly after initiation of the 12th cycle of chemotherapy, she develops shortness of breath, becomes diaphoretic, hypotensive, and has cardiac arrest. The code team is called to the ICU floor. The head nurse cannot locate an advanced directive. At this time, the best way to ensure that the patient receives the type of care that embodies her current values is a/an

(A) instructional directive
(B) living will
(C) patient self-determination doctrine
(D) proxy directive

29. A 37-year-old gravida 2, para 2 woman comes to the office seeking genetic counseling because she is planning on getting pregnant. She has two teenage sons who attend a special school for the mentally challenged. She describes her sons as having long, narrow faces, large jaws and ears, and enlarged testicles. They both have repetitive speech and are abnormally short-tempered. She says that her sons' facial features were quite normal when they were younger and have become more noticeable with age. The typical pattern of inheritance of this condition is

(A) autosomal dominant
(B) autosomal recessive
(C) a gene mutation
(D) polygenetic and multifactorial
(E) X-linked recessive

30. A 24-year-old pregnant mother of two is seen for the second time in your office for a prenatal care visit. While reviewing results of her first-visit prenatal laboratory studies you discover she is hepatitis B surface antigen positive. She denies current sexual promiscuity, intravenous drug use, or a history of blood transfusions. On physical examination her vital signs are stable, sclera are anicteric, and abdominal examination fails to reveal hepatomegaly. Her hematocrit is within normal range, bilirubin is high normal, and AST and ALT are high normal. She plans to breast-feed as she did with her previous two children. The most appropriate advice regarding breast-feeding with this condition is that it is

(A) allowed and poses no risks
(B) allowed but the infant should receive both the hepatitis B immune globulin (HBIG) and hepatitis B vaccine
(C) allowed if mother has low titers of hepatitis B e antigen (HBeAg)
(D) contraindicated in hepatitis B infection
(E) contraindicated in any hepatitis infection

31. A 27-year-old woman who delivered a viable male infant 1 week ago complains of breast pain and fever. She is breast-feeding her newborn. Her vital signs are: temperature 38.2 C (100.8 F), blood pressure 110/72 mm Hg, pulse 89/min, and respirations 18/min. On examination you discover a localized 2-cm area that is tender in the left breast near the areola. The rest of the examination is unremarkable. Her past medical history and her physical examinations during the pregnancy were unremarkable. The most likely diagnosis is

(A) a breast abscess
(B) breast engorgement
(C) a clogged milk duct
(D) inflammatory breast carcinoma
(E) mastitis

32. An 18-year-old girl is brought to your office by her mother because she has not started menstruating yet. Physical examination reveals Tanner stage II breasts with widely separated nipples and Tanner stage III pubic hair development. The girl is 54 inches tall and weighs 110 pounds. As you review the other characteristics of this condition, you should look for

(A) coarctation of the aorta and a wide space between the first and second toes
(B) coarctation of the aorta and a low-lying hairline
(C) an endocardial cushion defect and epicanthal folds
(D) an endocardial cushion defect and neck webbing
(E) a ventricular septal defect and long, thin extremities

33. A 23-year-old gravida 2, para 1 woman comes to the office at 17 weeks' gestation. After performing a full physical examination and reviewing her prenatal laboratory studies you discuss her plans for this pregnancy. She says she breast-fed her firstborn and would like to do the same with this baby but is not sure if it is possible. She has been angry with herself because 3 months before becoming pregnant she underwent breast augmentation mammoplasty. A trusted friend recently told her that she would not be able to breast-feed her infant successfully with breast implants. You should advise her that:

(A) Breast-feeding after augmentation is generally not recommended
(B) Breast-feeding after augmentation is recommended after biopsy confirms intact acinus-lactiferous units
(C) Breast-feeding after augmentation is recommended and is always successful
(D) Breast-feeding after augmentation is recommended and is usually successful
(E) Successful breast-feeding after augmentation depends on the type of implant

34. A 38-year-old primigravid woman at 39 weeks' gestation comes to the emergency department complaining of a severe headache. Her obstetric history is significant only for A1 gestational diabetes diagnosed at 28 weeks. Her temperature is 37.0 C (98.6 F), blood pressure is 160/90 mm Hg, pulse is 88/min, and respirations are 12/min. Physical examination is normal except for 3+ symmetric deep tendon reflexes. A urine dipstick shows 3+ proteinuria. You order a complete blood count, electrolytes, and liver function tests which all come back within normal limits. The most likely diagnosis is

(A) gestational hypertension
(B) HELLP syndrome
(C) pre-eclampsia
(D) migraine headaches
(E) subarachnoid hemorrhage

35. A 30-year-old woman comes to the office for follow-up after a spontaneous abortion of an anencephalic fetus at 15 weeks' gestation. She has no complaints. Physical examination is normal. She wants to try to conceive again. You recommend waiting for 2 normal menses before trying to conceive and dietary supplementation with

(A) calcium carbonate
(B) ferrous sulfate
(C) folic acid
(D) vitamin A
(E) vitamin C

36. An 18-year-old woman comes to the emergency department complaining of fever, nausea, vomiting, and severe abdominal pain that has worsened over the last 2 days. She has no significant medical history and has had no prior surgeries. She has recently become sexually active and reports having two sexual partners. She does not use barrier contraception consistently. Her vital signs: temperature 38.7 C (101.6 F), blood pressure 130/78 mm Hg, pulse 112/min, respirations 16/min. Her abdominal examination is benign. On sterile speculum examination you visualize a purulent cervical discharge and cervical cultures are taken. A wet prep reveals motile, flagellated organisms. On pelvic examination she has cervical motion tenderness and bilateral adnexal tenderness. No masses are palpable. Urine hCG is negative and a complete blood count is pending. The most appropriate next step is to

(A) admit her to the hospital for intravenous therapy with cefotetan and doxycycline
(B) admit her to the hospital for intravenous therapy with cefotetan, doxycycline, and metronidazole
(C) admit her to the hospital for observation
(D) treat her as an outpatient with intramuscular ceftriaxone and oral doxycycline
(E) treat her as an outpatient with intramuscular ceftriaxone and oral metronidazole

37. A 36-year-old primigravid woman at 38 weeks' gestation is brought to the emergency department by ambulance complaining of abdominal pain and vaginal bleeding after a motor vehicle accident that occurred approximately 1 hour ago. She was a belted passenger sitting in the front seat when the vehicle she was in hit a tree at 40 miles per hour. The patient remembers hitting her abdomen but reports no other injuries. Her temperature is 36.5 C (97.7 F), blood pressure is 90/60 mm Hg, pulse is 118/min, and respirations are 18/min. The fetal heart rate is 120/min with late decelerations and she is contracting every minute on the monitor. Her uterus is tender to palpation. Sterile speculum examination shows a large amount of blood in the vaginal vault and it is difficult to visualize the cervix. An abdominal sonogram reveals a fundal placenta with a retroplacental clot. Her cervix is closed on bimanual exam. You suspect a placental abruption, and an immediate cesarean section is performed. At the end of the procedure you notice that the bleeding is difficult to control. PTT and PT levels are elevated approximately 1.5 times normal. Fibrinogen is 70 mg/dL. Stat complete blood count shows hemoglobin of 6.0 g/dL and platelets of 90,000/mm^3. In addition to packed red blood cells, you should transfuse

(A) cryoprecipitate
(B) Factor VIII
(C) Factor X
(D) fresh frozen plasma
(E) platelets

38. A 35-year-old gravida 3 para 3 woman comes to the office for contraceptive counseling. She desires a very effective form of contraception but does not want permanent sterilization. She is in a monogamous relationship with her husband of 10 years. She had a deep venous thrombosis 3 years ago during one of her pregnancies. A thrombophilia workup at that time showed a Factor V Leiden mutation. The rest of her medical history is unremarkable. She has regular menses and her last menstrual period was 3 weeks ago. On physical examination her uterus is normal in size and no adnexal masses are palpable. The best contraceptive method for this patient is

(A) barrier contraception
(B) copper intrauterine device (IUD)
(C) injectable monthly contraceptive containing 25 mg of medroxyprogesterone acetate and 5 mg of estradiol cypionate
(D) low-dose oral contraceptive pills
(E) periodic abstinence

39. A 25-year-old gravida 2, para 1 woman comes to the emergency department at 30 weeks' gestation complaining of vaginal bleeding that started 3 hours ago. She tells you that she has been soaking through one maxi pad every hour. She explains that she has been on bedrest but is unsure why. You elicit no other significant past medical history. She does not complain of any uterine contractions. Her first child was delivered by cesarean section secondary to fetal distress. Her vital signs are: temperature 37.3 C (99.2 F), blood pressure 90/60 mm Hg, pulse 110/min, and respirations 18/min. You place an intravenous line, send a complete blood count, and type and crossmatch. She does not appear to be contracting on the monitor and the fetal heart rate is 130/min and reactive. The most appropriate next step in management is to

(A) order an MRI of the abdomen and pelvis
(B) perform an abdominal/pelvic ultrasound
(C) perform a bimanual examination
(D) perform colposcopy
(E) prepare her for uterine artery embolization

40. A 49-year-old woman with borderline hypertension comes to the emergency department because of heavy vaginal bleeding and lightheadedness. She has a history of irregular menses for 2 years and is not on any hormonal contraception or hormone replacement therapy. Her past surgical history is significant for a dilatation and curettage 2 years ago. She was diagnosed with endometrial hyperplasia at that time, but never followed up for further treatment. Her vital signs are: temperature 37.0 C (98.6 F), blood pressure 80/40 mm Hg, pulse 144/min, and respirations 20/min. On sterile speculum examination you find that she is bleeding profusely from her cervix. Urine hCG is negative and hemoglobin is 7 g/dL. You start intravenous resuscitation with 0.9 normal saline and type and crossmatch her for 2 units of packed red blood cells. The most appropriate next step in her management is

(A) dilatation and curettage
(B) intravenous estrogen
(C) observation
(D) oral estrogen
(E) oral progesterone

41. An 18-year-old woman comes to the office for her first gynecologic examination. She is sexually active with three partners. Her last menstrual period was 3 weeks ago. She uses condoms for contraception but desires oral contraceptive pills. She has no significant past medical history. Physical examination is unremarkable. You perform a Pap test and gonorrhea and chlamydia DNA probe. You discuss safe sex and although you prescribe oral contraceptive pills, you advise her to continue to use condoms, informing her that condoms do not prevent all sexually transmitted diseases. Three days later her chlamydia test comes back positive. The appropriate pharmacotherapy for this infection is

(A) azithromycin 1 g PO
(B) benzathine penicillin G 2.4 mU intramuscularly
(C) ceftriaxone 125 mg IM
(D) metronidazole 500 mg PO BID for 7 days
(E) valacyclovir 1 g PO BID for 7 days

42. A healthy 19-year-old woman comes to the office for annual gynecologic examination. She has no complaints and is not sexually active. She has had one sexual partner in the past. Her father had a myocardial infarction at age 40 and her maternal grandmother had breast cancer at age 80. The patient weighs 115 lb and is 5 feet tall. Her blood pressure is 90/60 mm Hg, pulse is 60/min, and respirations are 12/min. Her physical examination is significant only for fibrocystic breasts with no distinct mass. In addition to her Pap smear, the most appropriate screening test at this time is

(A) cholesterol testing
(B) fasting glucose
(C) human immunodeficiency virus (HIV) testing
(D) mammography
(E) thyroid stimulating hormone (TSH) testing

43. A 23-year-old woman comes to the emergency department because of vaginal bleeding. Approximately 10 hours ago she noticed some spotting of blood in her underwear and began having mild abdominal cramping. Her last menstrual period finished 8 weeks ago. Her temperature is 37.0 C (98.6 F), blood pressure is 110/80 mm Hg, pulse is 80/min, and respirations are 16/min. Her abdomen is soft with minimal bilateral lower abdominal tenderness. No fetal heart tones can be heard transabdominally. Pelvic examination shows blood at the cervical os and the os is closed. There is no cervical motion tenderness. Laboratory studies show: leukocyte count 6100/mm^3, platelets 310,000/mm^3, hematocrit 45%, BUN 20 mEq/L, and creatinine 0.7 mEq/L. A urine hCG is positive. An ultrasound shows an intrauterine gestational sac, a yolk sac, and fetal pole with heart motion present. A small, crescent-shaped hypoechoic area next to the gestational sac is identified. The most likely cause of the patient's bleeding is

(A) blighted ovum
(B) extrusion of fetal part due to abortion in progress
(C) pelvic inflammatory disease
(D) rupturing ectopic pregnancy
(E) subchorionic hemorrhage

44. A 30-year-old woman comes to the clinic with a 1-week history of an asymptomatic, but "ugly," full body rash. She describes scaly plaques on her trunk as well as on her palms and soles, which she found very odd. When questioned, she admits to being sexually promiscuous and having a small ulcer on her genitals a few months ago. It was painless and healed quickly so she never received medical attention for it. She tells you that besides this she is usually very healthy. She does not drink alcohol or smoke cigarettes. She is allergic to dogs, cats, and penicillin. A biopsy of one of the lesions is performed and returns as secondary syphilis. The most appropriate treatment, if any, for this patient is

(A) no treatment is warranted since secondary syphilis is a self-limited cutaneous dermatoses without internal involvement
(B) no pharmacologic medicine is necessary; one only needs to follow the RPR to ensure it falls to normal once the patient recovers from secondary syphilis
(C) penicillin G, intravenously for 10 days
(D) tetracycline, orally
(E) ultra micronized griseofulvin, orally

45. A 30-year-old pregnant prostitute comes to the emergency department with an "unsightly," mildly pruritic full body rash. She states the rash started in one area and then quickly spread to involve her trunk, arms, legs, palms, and soles. When questioned, she denies ever having a genital ulcer. The best assessment of her non-specific scaly rash is diagnosed as pityriasis rosea (PR). She is sent home with a mild antihistamine for pruritus and told to follow up with her regular physician at the clinic as soon as possible. By her 30-week appointment, which is a few weeks later, the rash is gone. Having heard about her emergency department visit, you order an RPR. This test comes back positive and then an FTA-Abs is ordered which was also positive. She is concerned about the health of her baby. She should be advised that in the immediate neonatal period

(A) babies born to mothers who have had pityriasis rosea during pregnancy will test positive to hepatitis C and have hepatomegaly
(B) her baby will likely have delirium, gummas, and nodular syphilid
(C) her baby will likely have Hutchinson teeth, saber shins, and a saddle nose
(D) her baby will likely have rhagades, snuffles, and neurosyphilis
(E) the baby will likely be fine because babies born to mothers who have had pityriasis rosea during pregnancy do not have any sequelae. Patients with pityriasis rosea (PR) often have a false positive RPR.

46. A 30-year-old woman comes to the office for an annual examination. She has been feeling well over the past year but is concerned regarding her weight. She is 5 feet 2 inches and weighs 200 pounds. She has tried various weight loss programs over the past several years with little success. Her past medical history is unremarkable. Past surgical history is significant for a left ovarian cystectomy 4 years ago. She takes no medications and has no allergies. Physical examination, including breast and pelvic examination, is normal. She is concerned because she plans to become pregnant in the next year. She would like to know what risks her obesity poses for pregnancy. The patient should be counseled that obese patients are at greater risk for

(A) developing hypotension during pregnancy
(B) having a fetus with increased activity syndrome
(C) having a fetus with intrauterine growth restriction
(D) having a fetus with neural tube defects
(E) insufficient weight gain during the pregnancy

47. A 28-year-old woman who is at 12 weeks' gestation comes to the office for an initial prenatal visit. She has some mild nausea and is feeling somewhat fatigued, but otherwise has no complaints. Her obstetrical history is significant for a 28-week intrauterine fetal demise (IUFD). Her past medical history is significant for a false positive rapid plasma reagin (RPR) test and a positive high-level IgG anticardiolipin antibody. She has never had surgery, takes no medications, and is allergic to penicillin. Physical examination reveals a 12-week-sized uterus, but is otherwise unremarkable. Fetal heart tones are heard and are 150s/min. After thorough counseling, this patient should be offered treatment with

    (A) daily oral terbutaline
    (B) daily oral warfarin
    (C) daily subcutaneous heparin
    (D) monthly intramuscular ceftriaxone
    (E) monthly intravenous doxycycline

48. A 25-year-old woman comes to the health center to discuss contraception. She has three healthy children ages 6, 4, and 1. She has tried the oral contraceptive pill and depot medroxyprogesterone acetate, but had to discontinue both secondary to mood changes and menstrual irregularities. She has had pelvic inflammatory disease on two occasions and is not currently in a monogamous relationship. She is certain that she does not wish to have any more children and would like to discuss tubal ligation. Physical examination, including breast and pelvic examination, is normal. In addressing the risks associated with tubal ligation, the patient should be counseled that:

    (A) The risk of failure of the procedure is as high as 5%
    (B) The risk of failure of the procedure is less than 0.1%
    (C) The risk of regret is less than 0.1%
    (D) Tubal ligation increases the risk of ovarian cancer
    (E) Tubal ligation is likely to cause menstrual irregularities.

49. You are involved in a surgical case, wherein a laparotomy is being performed on a 28-year-old woman for removal of a twisted ovarian cyst. The surgeon decides that while she is "in there," she may as well remove the appendix so that the woman will not have to bother with the problem of acute appendicitis in the future. She asks your opinion regarding this. You should suggest that she

    (A) discuss this with the patient's husband before proceeding
    (B) first make sure that the insurance company will pay for the procedure
    (C) not remove it
    (D) remove it but don't tell the patient about it
    (E) remove it so as to avoid unnecessary surgery later on

50. A 29-year-old woman comes to the office for a periodic health maintenance examination. She has no complaints. She has no significant past medical history and takes no medications. She has been in a monogamous relationship for the past 5 years and does not smoke cigarettes or drink alcohol. She has had consistently normal, annual Pap smears for the past 11 years. Physical examination, including pelvic examination, is unremarkable. The results of the Pap smear, which return in 1 week, show no cytologic abnormalities, but there were no endocervical cells present on the smear. The most appropriate next step in management is to

    (A) explain to her that even though the results of the Pap smear are valid, she should come back to the office as soon as possible for you to resample her endocervix
    (B) have her come back to the office as soon as possible to resample her endocervix because the results of the Pap smear are invalid
    (C) recommend increased monitoring and a repeat Pap smear in 6 months
    (D) recommend resampling of her endocervix at her annual exam next year
    (E) schedule her for a colposcopic examination of her cervix

Obstetrics/Gynecology Test Two: **Answers and Explanations**

ANSWER KEY

1. A
2. B
3. E
4. A
5. C
6. E
7. D
8. B
9. E
10. C
11. B
12. E
13. B
14. E
15. B
16. B
17. B
18. D
19. E
20. C
21. C
22. B
23. A
24. A
25. D
26. A
27. B
28. D
29. C
30. B
31. C
32. B
33. D
34. C
35. C
36. B
37. D
38. B
39. B
40. A
41. A
42. A
43. E
44. D
45. D
46. D
47. C
48. A
49. C
50. D

1. **The correct answer is A.** The patient has legitimately poor pain control since oral meperidine has lower potency than injection form. In order to solve this, dose adjustment of the oral form should be made.

   Even though placebo effect can be powerful (**choice B**) one should consider other possible reasons for complaints first.

   Tolerance to meperidine (**choice C**) develops over a longer period of time, not 4 days. The dose should be adjusted because of the reasons mentioned above, not because of the tolerance.

   Histrionic personality traits (**choice D**) can be considered in the absence of any other Axis I disorder. In this case pain with psychological complications may be considered on Axis I. Psychiatry consult will probably not relieve this patient's pain.

   Detoxification form opiates (**choice E**) may be needed if a patient stays on opiates longer and develops dependency. However, receiving opiates over a few days postoperatively may not necessarily warrant the need for detoxification, since gradual tapering of the pain medication can be done by the team and following the decreased needs of the patient.

2. **The correct answer is B.** In any postmenarche female with abdominal pain and vaginal bleeding, pregnancy must be ruled out first—particularly in this case since this young woman may be at high risk for an ectopic pregnancy because of her history of chlamydia and possible late period.

   This teenager will obviously need a pelvic exam (**choice A**), but the most important first step is the pregnancy test. She should have both chlamydia and gonorrhea cultures performed. If she turns out to have pelvic inflammatory disease and had some bleeding from either cervicitis or endometritis, one would expect her to have cervical motion tenderness. Alternatively, a diagnosis of ectopic pregnancy can be very difficult to make. On pelvic exam an ectopic might be suspected when there is unilateral pelvic tenderness or a mass, but no marked cervical tenderness.

   It may be important to get a CBC (**choice C**), but this is not the first step in evaluating this patient. Although it may be important to establish how anemic the patient is, a CBC will not be so helpful in differentiating between diagnoses such as pelvic inflammatory disease and appendicitis.

   An ultrasound may be helpful in sorting out pregnancy-related illness from pelvic inflammatory disease and appendicitis, but it is not the first step (**choice D**).

   A urinalysis and urine culture would not be very helpful in the work up of this case (**choice E**). Pregnancy needs to be ruled out first and pelvic assessment needs to take place. There is no good history given by this patient to suggest that there is cystitis or another urinary problem.

3. **The correct answer is E.** Metronidazole tablets or intravaginal gel should be the therapy of choice to treat this case of bacterial vaginosis. An alternative therapy would also be clindamycin intravaginal cream. The tip-off that this is a case of bacterial vaginosis is the finding of "clue cells." Clue cells are epithelial cells that have many bacteria adhering to the outside cell surface. They almost look speckled around the edges. Bacterial vaginosis also is characterized by discharge that is of gray-white color, a pH greater than 4.5, and there is a characteristic fishy odor after the addition of 10% KOH (the so-called whiff test).

   Ceftriaxone is used to treat uncomplicated gonorrhea and also is part of the combination therapy for pelvic inflammatory disease (**choice A**).

   Ciprofloxacin is an acceptable treatment for uncomplicated gonorrhea (**choice B**).

   Clotrimazole is commonly used for vulvovaginal candidiasis (**choice C**).

   Doxycycline is a treatment of choice for chlamydia trachomatis infection (**choice D**).

4. **The correct answer is A.** This patient has typical postpartum telogen effluvium. Telogen effluvium is early and excessive loss of normal club hairs from resting follicles in the scalp. This excessive hair loss results from traumatization of the normal hair follicles by a stimulus, such as parturition, surgery, fever, drugs, or traction. The stimulus hastens the anagen phase to prematurely turn into catagen, and then telogen phase. Alternatively, follicles may remain in prolonged anagen rather than normally cycling into telogen. This occurs in pregnancy. With delivery, these follicles are released into telogen, and increased shedding occurs some months later. The usual time interval for this delayed telogen is 2 to 6 months. Whatever the cause, the patient sees the hair loss as "lots of hairs coming out at the roots." Loss is diffuse and clinically visible thinning occurs when more than 50% of the hairs are lost. The telogen count is estimated by the "pull test": grasping

approximately 40 to 50 hairs between the thumb and forefinger firmly and close to the scalp, a slow pull is performed. A count greater than four to six club hairs is abnormal, although it may be influenced by recent hair washing, brushing, and the stage in which the telogen effluvium currently is (resolving or entering a chronic phase). A normal scalp has approximately 100,000 hairs; of these, 100 to 150 are lost daily. In telogen effluvium, the patient loses between 150 and 400 or greater. Postpartum telogen effluvium begins 2 to 6 months after delivery. The hair loss may continue for over 6 months, but should eventually resolve and the normal, or almost normal, hair growth is eventually regained. Drug-induced telogen effluvium has been described with amphetamines, aminosalicylic acid, bromocriptine, captopril, coumarin, carbamazepine, cimetidine, danazol, enalapril, etretinate, lithium carbonate, levodopa, metoprolol, propranolol, pyridostigmine, and trimethadione. Other causes of dramatic hair loss have been kwashiorkor or a starvation diet, secondary to protein deprivation. Hypothyroidism and renal dialysis with secondary hypervitaminosis A are other possible causes. There is no specific therapy for telogen effluvium; in most cases it will stop spontaneously within several months and normal hair growth will ensue.

Neither pseudoephedrine (**choice B**) nor sertraline (**choice C**) have been known to cause telogen effluvium. Drug-induced telogen effluvium has been described with amphetamines, aminosalicylic acid, bromocriptine, captopril, coumarin, carbamazepine, cimetidine, danazol, enalapril, etretinate, lithium carbonate, levodopa, metoprolol, propranolol, pyridostigmine, and trimethadione.

Hyperpyrexia has been known to induce telogen effluvium, but a fever of 38.0 C (100.4 F) accompanied by a sore throat (**choice D**) does not qualify as a sufficiently powerful stimulus, and the time frame is inappropriate, too, since she had already had hair loss for 2 months when the intercurrent illness happened.

This patient's telogen effluvium had already started when she went back to her job and started leaving her baby with a nanny. The patient's account of the problems with the nanny, i.e., " she is thinking about transferring her baby to a day-care facility" (**choice E**) does not imply a major stress-inducing event. Stress, as encountered during a major surgical event, may cause telogen effluvium.

5. **The correct answer is C.** Current recommendations vary, but in general, Pap testing to screen for cervical cancer should be performed every 1 to 3 years at the physician's discretion. Screening may be discontinued at age 65 if past studies have been consistently normal.

   Chest x-rays (**choice A**) are not used for screening in standard health maintenance.

   A mammogram (**choice B**) should be ordered for her, but recommendations are for yearly mammograms to appropriately screen for breast cancer. Some people recommend every 2 years.

   Standard screening recommendations for colon cancer are fecal occult blood testing with flexible sigmoidoscopy every 3 years. Some people do use colonoscopy (**choice D**) when screening, but yearly examinations are not standard.

   Yearly electrocardiograms (**choice E**) are not recommended screening tests.

6. **The correct answer is E.** The preferred therapy for inpatient PID is cefoxitin 2 gm IV every 6 hours and doxycycline IV every 12 hours. An alternative regimen may include clindamycin 900 mg IV every 8 hours and gentamicin 2 mg/kg loading dose followed by 1.5 mg/kg every 8 hours.

   Ampicillin and gentamicin are used frequently to treat neonatal sepsis, not PID (**choice A**).

   Cefoxitin and parenteral doxycycline are a first-line combination therapy and erythromycin can be used if doxycycline cannot be used. However, parenteral therapy would be preferred (**choice B**).

   Ceftriaxone IM and oral doxycycline can be used for outpatient therapy for PID, but are not used for inpatient therapy (**choice C**).

   Similarly, ceftriaxone and oral erythromycin are not used for inpatient therapy of PID (**choice D**).

7. **The correct answer is D.** All SSRIs are excreted in breast milk. Because their concentration peaks several hours after the dose, an SSRI that has no active metabolites and has a shorter half-life would be desirable. This would allow a shorter nursing interval and the milk would be free of the medication.

   Long half-life antidepressants (**choice A**) are not desirable because of the long period the mother would need to refrain from nursing in order to avoid excretion in milk.

   MAO inhibitors (**choice B**) are not used as the first-line treatment because of dietary restrictions and potential for hypertensive crisis.

   Nefazodone (**choice C**) effects on breast-feeding are not known.

The use of antidepressants (**choice E**) is generally *not* safe because most psychotropics are excreted in breast milk.

8. **The correct answer is B.** This is a shoulder dystocia (impingement of baby's anterior shoulder on mom's symphysis pubis) probably due to gestational diabetes causing macrosomia. Once recognized as a shoulder dystocia the first priority is to call for help (**choice B**). This would be to help push mother's legs back as far as possible (**choice H**) as part of McRoberts maneuver. Next, quickly evaluate mother for an episiotomy (**choice F**) to increase the passage size. Then apply suprapubic pressure each time mother pushes with a contraction (**choice A**). If this fails to deliver the anterior shoulder then enter the introitus to either adduct the baby's shoulder and rotate the baby (**choice C**), or turn the baby counterclockwise (**choice E**). These maneuvers are to deliver the posterior shoulder first. If this fails then sweep the baby's posterior arm across its chest and deliver the posterior arm first (**choice D**), rotating baby into an oblique position to deliver the anterior shoulder. If this fails then roll mother onto her hands and knees and try delivering the posterior shoulder this way (**choice I**). If unsuccessful then push the head back into the birth canal for an urgent caesarian section (**choice G**).

9. **The correct answer is E.** Most women are able to perceive fetal movement at some time between 16 to 20 weeks (menstrual age). First-time mothers often perceive this movement later than multiparous patients. The first movements that are felt are usually small fluttering movements felt in the abdomen. The day that these movements are first recognized by the pregnant woman is designated as the day of quickening. Over time these movements increase in intensity. This patient is at 17 weeks' gestation with her first pregnancy and, therefore, it is not surprising that she has not felt fetal movement yet. She should be reassured that the absence of fetal movement at this gestational age is normal and that she should begin to appreciate more fetal movements over the next few weeks.

   To initiate induction of labor for vaginal delivery (**choice A**) would be incorrect. A fetus at 17 weeks' gestation is previable. That is, it cannot survive once it is delivered. Moreover, there is no indication for induction, as lack of fetal movement at 17 weeks is normal.

   To obtain a biophysical profile (BPP) (**choice B**) is not correct. The biophysical profile is a method of antepartum fetal testing that uses ultrasound to look for fetal breathing movements, fetal body movements, fetal tone, and the amniotic fluid volume. These four parameters are combined with a non-stress test. The BPP is a useful method to monitor a viable fetus when there is an indication to monitor. This patient, at 17 weeks' gestation, does not require a BPP.

   To obtain a non-stress test (NST) (**choice C**) would be incorrect. The non-stress test is a method of antepartum fetal testing in which the fetal heart rate is measured. If the heart rate accelerates 15 beats per minute for 15 seconds and does this twice in 20 minutes, the test is considered normal. The NST is also a useful method to monitor a viable fetus (especially later in the third trimester) when there is an indication to monitor.

   To prepare the patient for cesarean delivery (**choice D**) is incorrect. Delivery at this gestational age would result in a nonviable neonate. Again, the absence of fetal movement at 17 weeks' gestation is not abnormal.

10. **The correct answer is C.** In the United States, endometrial cancer is the most common gynecological malignancy. A number of case-control studies have demonstrated a protective effect of the IUD against the development of endometrial cancer. It is difficult to evaluate a cause-effect relationship from case-control studies, but there are at least six case-control studies from the 1990s that all point in the same direction; that is, that the IUD is associated with decreased rates of endometrial cancer. The exact mechanism for this association is unknown. Endometrial cancer is believed to most often result from the effect of hormones on the endometrial lining. For example, when postmenopausal women are exposed to unopposed estrogen (i.e., without a progestin) they have a significantly increased risk of developing endometrial hyperplasia and endometrial cancer. One theory for the protective effect of the IUD is that it changes the intrauterine environment to interfere with the response of the endometrium to hormones or that the IUD alters the amount or nature of the hormones produced. Another theory is that the sterile inflammatory reaction, which is produced by the IUD, works against atypical endometrial histology that could possibly lead to endometrial cancer. Whatever the reason, this patient should be counseled that there is an association between IUD use and decreased rates of endometrial cancer.

    There is no established relationship between the IUD and breast cancer (**choice A**). There is much controversy surrounding contraception and breast cancer, but this centers on hormonal contraception (i.e., the oral contraceptive pill) and not the IUD.

    The relationship between IUD use and cervical cancer (**choice B**) is incompletely established. A few studies have shown what appears to be a possible protective effect, but none were statistically significant.

There is no established relationship between the IUD and lung cancer (**choice D**). This patient would be best advised to quit smoking to reduce her chances of developing lung cancer.

There is substantial evidence that oral contraceptive pill use provides significant protection for women against ovarian cancer (**choice E**). This protection has not been demonstrated with the IUD.

11. **The correct answer is B.** It is well established that infants of diabetic mothers have an increased risk of having congenital anomalies. Estimates are that the risk for diabetic mothers is approximately doubled as compared with the "background" level of risk in infants whose mothers do not have diabetes. There is good evidence that this risk relates directly to glycosylated hemoglobin values during the first trimester. First trimester glycosylated hemoglobin values, in turn, are directly related to the level of glucose control that the patient has preconceptionally. Thus, a diabetic patient can significantly decrease her chances of having offspring with congenital anomalies by having good control of her blood glucose levels prior to, and at the time of, conception. Studies have shown that women with diabetes who receive preconceptional counseling regarding the importance of good glucose control prior to conception are more likely to have lower glycohemoglobin values. Unfortunately, many diabetic women do not receive intensive counseling regarding diabetes and congenital anomalies until they present for their first prenatal visit, at which time it is often too late to gain the optimal level of glucose control for organogenesis. Fortunately, this patient has presented preconceptionally, and provides an excellent opportunity for counseling and intervention regarding improved glucose control to prevent congenital anomalies.

Avoidance of first-trimester insulin (**choice A**) is not the most important factor to prevent having a fetus with congenital anomalies. Insulin does not cross the placenta and is not linked to birth defects. Insulin requirements may change during the first trimester, but it should not be avoided.

Second-trimester exercise (**choice C**) or, for that matter exercise through most of pregnancy, is fine for most women. However, second-trimester exercise will not alter the development of congenital anomalies in offspring of diabetic mothers.

Third-trimester insulin treatment (**choice D**) can be especially important in some diabetic women to avoid the development of a macrosomic fetus. Third-trimester insulin will not, however, do anything to affect the development of congenital anomalies.

Tight glucose control during labor and delivery (**choice E**) is important in diabetic women to avoid the development of neonatal hypoglycemia. Glucose control during labor and delivery will not affect the likelihood of congenital anomalies.

12. **The correct answer is E.** Cancer during pregnancy is an uncommon occurrence because most malignancies occur in older women. However, malignant melanoma is one malignancy that can present in younger age groups. The changes in nevi that are associated with melanoma are described by the ABCD signs: asymmetry, irregular borders, color changes, and diameter greater than 5 mm. This young woman has a lesion that demonstrates some of these changes; therefore, she should undergo an excisional biopsy to determine the exact nature of the lesion. It is important to emphasize that pregnancy provides an excellent opportunity for providers to perform a full evaluation of the skin in women who otherwise may not seek medical care. When a concerning lesion is noticed it should be appropriately evaluated and the patient should not receive substandard care because of her pregnancy.

To apply topical 5-fluorouracil to the lesion (**choice A**) is incorrect because this is a topical chemotherapeutic agent used to treat non-melanotic skin cancers and actinic keratoses. This patient, however, has a nevus which is concerning for melanoma and, therefore, the lesion must be biopsied.

To counsel the patient to terminate the pregnancy (**choice B**) would be incorrect. First, without a biopsy, it cannot be certain what the nature of the lesion is. Second, in spite of the widely held myth, pregnancy does not confer a worse prognosis on the disease, even if this is melanoma.

To counsel the patient to terminate the pregnancy and have permanent sterilization (**choice C**) would also be incorrect. Again, at this point, it is not clear what type of lesion this is. Furthermore, even if this were melanoma, exact recommendations regarding future pregnancies would depend upon the stage of the disease.

To reassure the patient that the finding is normal (**choice D**) is incorrect. An asymmetric nevus of 7 mm with irregular pigmentation and ulceration is not a normal finding and must be evaluated further. It is important not to delay diagnosis during pregnancy due to the false notion that all changes in nevi are due to the pregnancy itself.

13. **The correct answer is B.** The patient admits to smoking crack cocaine. This could cause placental abruption, which may be fatal. Vitals signs monitoring and external fetal monitoring while she is transferred to ob-gyn care should be done immediately.

Calling security and waiting for a psychiatrist (**choice A**) may be appropriate only in the absence of described symptoms of abdominal pain provided that the patient is actively endangering herself or somebody else. Psychiatry consult should be called for the assessment of suicidality and further disposition only after she has been medically stabilized in the ER. If not, psychiatry consult should be called upon admission to the unit and patient placed on 1:1 until further evaluation.

A social worker (**choice C**) can be consulted for assistance concerning housing only after medical and psychiatric issues are resolved.

Ordering basic tests (**choice D**) and letting the patient stay while crack is metabolized and excreted is a poor choice of management in this case since patient has severe symptoms and deserves full evaluation.

Malingering (**choice E**) is sometimes seen in homeless psychiatric patients with substance abuse problems.

However, all other conditions should be ruled out first. In this case there is little evidence for malingering even though there is clearly an interest to stay in the hospital.

14. **The correct answer is E.** This patient has premature gonadal failure. The workup of secondary amenorrhea begins with a pregnancy test. If the pregnancy test is negative, evaluation for thyroid disease and prolactinoma is required. If both of these tests are normal, a progesterone challenge can be performed which involves giving the woman 5 to 7 days of oral progestin or 10 days of IM progestin and then observing for withdrawal bleeding. Absence of withdrawal bleeding suggests a defect in endogenous estrogen production. Treatment with alternating estrogen then progestin should be attempted. Subsequent bleeding should suggest either hypothalamic dysfunction or premature ovarian failure. Determination of FSH should be performed. High FSH levels are consistent with premature ovarian failure. Premature ovarian failure is easily distinguished from hypothalamic etiologies of amenorrhea by FSH level. Hypothalamic etiologies (**choice C**) would have a normal or low FSH level.

Asherman syndrome (**choice A**) is the only uterine cause of secondary amenorrhea. It is an acquired scarring of the uterine lining. It occurs in women after postpartum hemorrhage or endometrial infection. The diagnosis should be suspected in women who don't have withdrawal bleeding after a course of estrogen and progestin. It can be confirmed by ultrasound.

Gonadal agenesis (**choice B**) is a cause of primary amenorrhea. This patient cannot have this diagnosis because prior to 8 months ago she was having normal menses.

Polycystic ovarian syndrome (**choice D**) should be suspected in women with signs of hyperandrogenism such as acne, hirsutism, obesity, or striae. The definition of PCOS is vague but most people agree that both menstrual irregularity and virilization (physically or biochemically) must be present. Our patient is not virilized, and therefore doesn't meet criteria for PCOS.

15. **The correct answer is B.** HRT remains a controversial topic in medicine. Studies have shown that HRT can increase HDL levels, decrease LDL levels, and increase bone density initially at rates of 1 to 2% each year. HRT is also effective at decreasing symptoms of menopause such as vaginal dryness and hot flashes.

The debate about increased risks of breast cancer with HRT are at the forefront of most women's minds while deciding if HRT is right for them. The latest data suggests that HRT might slightly increase the risk of breast cancer but the increase is not statistically significant. Therefore, it is not appropriate to tell patient that they have no increased risk for breast cancer (**choice A**), since at the very best we are not sure. Patients need to be given this information and allowed to decide what is best for them.

We cannot tell this patient that it is safe to begin HRT (**choice C**) until we have more information. Contraindications include history of estrogen-dependent cancers. Relative contraindications include patients with hypercoagulable states. Patients are at increase risk for gallbladder disease if on HRT. Patients are also at risk for endometrial cancer if they have a uterus.

Unopposed estrogen treatment increases the risk of endometrial cancer. Therefore, patients on HRT need to have progesterone added to decrease this risk. This patient does not need combined therapy (**choice D**) because she has had a hysterectomy in the past.

Treatment with HRT has been shown to decrease cardiovascular mortality with long-term use but there is a small but significant increase in coronary events, which occur during the first two years of therapy with estrogen (**choice E**).

16. **The correct answer is B.** Patients with evidence of Group B Strep infection need prophylaxis against transmission to the fetus at the time of delivery. Usually, this is screened for during the third trimester with vaginal and rectal cultures, but GBS urinary infection any time during pregnancy is also an indication for prophylaxis during labor.

HBsAg is a marker of hepatitis infection and is not a measure of protection from past immunization and **choice A** is incorrect.

All Rh-negative women should be given RhoGAM for every pregnancy and **choice C** is incorrect. This antibody screen is evidence that isoimmunization has not occurred in past pregnancies, but does not predict it in this pregnancy.

Without any clinical evidence of recent rubella infection, this patient's results are evidence of protection against rubella from immunization or remote infection and **choice D** is incorrect. Congenital rubella syndrome may result in deafness and cardiac anomalies, and elective termination should be offered to patients that you suspect have rubella infection during their pregnancy.

All women regardless of age should be offered screening for Down syndrome and **choice E** is incorrect. The patient's individual risk is low given her age, but testing should still be offered.

17. **The correct answer is B.** This patient has an ectopic pregnancy in the right fallopian tube as seen on ultrasound. Since her vital signs are unstable (low BP and high pulse), there is fluid in the cul-de-sac, and her abdominal exam shows rebound tenderness, you suspect a ruptured ectopic. The best management is a laparotomy with linear salpingostomy if ectopic is found in the ampullary region of the tube, or a segmental resection if the ectopic is found in the isthmus of the tube.

Laparoscopy (**choice A**) is not indicated at this time because laparoscopy is absolutely contraindicated in a hemodynamically unstable patient. If the patient had been stable, even in the presence of intraabdominal hemorrhage (by ultrasound), she would be a candidate for laparoscopy.

Medical treatment in the form of methotrexate (**choice C**) is useful for an ectopic pregnancy if all of the following are satisfied: stable vital signs, low quantitative beta hCG levels (usually less than 10,000 mU/mL), adnexal mass <3.5 cm, absence of fetal cardiac activity, and no active medical problems especially of liver, kidney, or lung. Methotrexate is usually administered at a dose of 50 mg per square meter of body surface area. It is contraindicated in this unstable patient.

Mifepristone (**choice D**) is incorrect. There are only anecdotal reports of ectopic being treated with RU-486. There have been no published studies in the literature.

Observation (**choice E**) of a hemodynamically unstable patient is not only inappropriate but also worthy of litigation.

18. **The correct answer is D.** This patient has two risk factors for uterine atony. She is a grand multiparous and she just delivered a large newborn. Since the placenta is intact, you can rule out bleeding from a retained succenturiate lobe. The first and quickest step in managing her postpartum hemorrhage (PPH) is to vigorously massage the uterus.

Not only is methylergonovine (**choice A**) not the first step in treating PPH, it is contraindicated in this patient because she is hypertensive (140/90). This drug could produce hypertensive encephalopathy in this patient. Methylergonovine would be the next step in management if uterine massage and oxytocin fail to control her PPH *and* she is not hypertensive.

Oxytocin (**choice B**) is not the initial step. It is, however, the second step in management of PPH. There are many oxytocin receptors in the myometrium near term. Oxytocin causes contraction of the smooth muscle fibers, which squeeze the bleeding vessels that run within the myometrium, thus halting PPH.

PG-F2 alpha (**choice C**) would be the next step if uterine massage and oxytocin fail. PG-F2 alpha causes vasoconstriction of spiral arterioles in the myometrium of the uterus, thus preventing further loss of blood.

Hysterectomy (**choice E**) is the last resort in management of PPH. If all medical therapies have failed and ligation of uterine or hypogastric artery has not been attempted or has failed, then you proceed to do a hysterectomy.

19. **The correct answer is E.** This patient has acute pelvic inflammatory disease (PID). *Neisseria gonorrhoeae* (NG) is more symptomatic than chlamydia in that there is greater pain, higher temperature, and thicker discharge associated with NG. Also, infections that start near the end of the last period are more common to be NG because the sloughing tissue during a period is a growth medium for NG.

Bacterial vaginosis (BV) **(choice A)** usually produces thin, grayish vaginal discharge that is often mildly pruritic and malodorous. It is rarely associated with fever. The discharge found in BV has a pH >4.5, clue cells on wet mount (with leukocytes), and positive whiff test with 10% KOH.

Candida albicans (CA) **(choice B)** usually presents as thick, adherent, "cottage cheese-like" discharge. It is associated with pruritus and no fever. Microscopically you can see pseudohyphae with budding yeast.

Although chlamydia **(choice C)** also causes acute PID, it is typically associated with milder symptoms than NG. Chlamydial PID often presents with diffuse, low-grade abdominal pain, low-grade fever (e.g., 100.8 F), slight cervical motion tenderness, and thin, if any, cervical discharge.

Lymphogranuloma venereum (LGV) **(choice D)** produces a painless papular lesion on the perineum or around the vaginal introitus. It is also associated with enlarged inguinal lymph nodes, which can eventually ulcerate through the skin or form a fistula. LGV is rarely found in the United States.

20. **The correct answer is C.** This question deals with physician-patient confidentiality in the adolescent patient. The physician is obligated to maintain confidentiality. Only under certain conditions, such as a life-threatening emergency, would the physician breach this confidentiality. Most states allow a minor to obtain certain medical services without the need of parental consent. These include contraceptive services, interventions dealing with mental health, STD, and alcohol and drug abuse management. You should remind the patient that her parents might find out about her visit to the doctor from insurance or laboratory billing practices; however, this is out of your control.

It is inappropriate to prescribe oral contraceptive pills and then inform her parents **(choice A)**. Deceiving an adolescent is not only unethical, it breaks patient-physician trust. Adolescents are already a group who are the least likely to visit a doctor. Deception will only aggravate this reality.

It is inappropriate to prescribe oral contraceptive pills for 1 month and tell her you will give her 1 month to figure out how she will tell her parents about her sexual activities and re-schedule a return visit in 1 month **(choice B)**. This answer choice avoids the problem at hand. The patient may not return in a month out of fear that the physician will inform or force her to inform her parents. Alternatively, the patient may return in a month but still be adamant about not wanting her parents involved.

It is inappropriate to refuse to prescribe oral contraceptive pills and tell her you are obligated to inform her parents because of her age **(choice D)**. Adolescents do not need parental consent for certain interventions (see above). This includes obtaining counseling for and receiving OCP.

It is inappropriate to refuse to prescribe oral contraceptive pills and tell her that condoms are not only a good form of contraception, they also protect against STDs **(choice E)**. The patient stated that both she and her boyfriend do not like using condoms. It is appropriate to educate her about condoms, but if she insists on using OCPs you should prescribe them for her. Don't forget that the U.S. has the highest adolescent pregnancy rate in the developed world.

21. **The correct answer is C.** In lead-poisoning anemia, serum lead levels would be diagnostic, but this is not one of the options listed. FEP is a heme precursor. It is significantly elevated in lead-induced anemia, but only mildly elevated in iron deficiency anemia. Certain decorated pottery (especially those made in Mexico), wall paint used on houses built in the mid-1900s, battery fluid, lead bullets, film processing solutions, and make-up used by Indian women called *sura* have been known to contain high levels of lead.

Decreased ferritin (measure of stored of iron) **(choice A)** would be helpful in iron deficiency anemia, which is more microcytic (MCV <80; MCV is a measure of the average size of red blood cells on a peripheral smear) and has a significantly elevated RDW (RDW is a measure of the spectrum of red blood cell sizes found on a peripheral smear).

Anemia caused by folate deficiency **(choice B)** is a macrocytic anemia (MCV >100). It is accompanied by a low reticulocyte count, may have hypersegmented neutrophils evident on peripheral smear, and demonstrates an elevated LDH level.

Serum electrophoresis **(choice D)** is not indicated. It is useful if you suspect sickle cell, sickle C, or any of the thalassemias.

An x-ray of the femur **(choice E)** or long bones in lead-induced anemia may reveal a "lead line," especially in the femur or tibia. However, this only occurs at higher levels of toxicity and thus is not the most sensitive test for lead exposure. It is not the most appropriate study at this time.

22. **The correct answer is B.** The intrauterine device is a good contraceptive method for a monogamous, multiparous patient seeking long-term contraception. Although it may cause a bit of cramping immediately after placement, it is technically easy to place and doesn't have many side effects as long as the patient doesn't have dysmenorrhea and there are no contraindications to its placement such as history of pelvic inflammatory disease, history of ectopic pregnancy, or undiagnosed vaginal bleeding. Having multiple sexual partners is a contraindication to the placement of an IUD. The copper-containing IUD is effective for 10 years and the new progesterone-containing IUD used in Europe is good for 5 years.

    Condoms (**choice A**) are not the best option since of all the contraceptive methods, it is the only one that requires placement just before coitus and thus may interfere with "the mood of foreplay."

    Medroxyprogesterone acetate injection (**choice C**) is incorrect because it has the most side effects of the choices listed. Patients on medroxyprogesterone acetate may experience irregular vaginal bleeding (usually spotting), weight gain, or breast tenderness; are prone to osteoporosis; and may be more prone to major depression if they have a psychiatric history.

    Oral contraceptives (**choice D**) are incorrect because combined oral contraceptives are contraindicated in patients older than 35 years of age who are smokers due to increased risk of thromboembolic events.

    Tubal ligation (**choice E**) is not the best method listed because a bilateral tubal ligation is a minor surgical procedure. It is best for a patient with COPD with decreased pulmonary functions to stay away from the operating room if other options are available.

23. **The correct answer is A.** Occasionally, following correct use of a full cycle of pills, withdrawal bleeding may fail to occur. This is called "silent menses." Pregnancy is very unlikely. She should be advised to finish her inert (white) pills as usual. If, however, a second consecutive period is missed (the next month) she should see her doctor because she may be pregnant.

    Continue taking the pills as usual and use a condom (**choice B**) is incorrect. Since she has been taking her pills correctly every day, you can assume that she is unlikely to have an unintended pregnancy. The theoretical failure rate of oral contraception is 0.1% (i.e., 0.1% of women experience an unintended pregnancy within the first year if they use the pill perfectly). The actual failure rate is 5%, mainly due to inconsistencies of taking the pill every day and taking other drugs simultaneously, which may diminish the effectiveness of the pill (i.e., certain antibiotics and over-the-counter medications). She should consider using a condom if she forgot to take her pill for 2 to 3 consecutive days during a cycle.

    Stop taking the pills and resume after 7 days (**choice C**) is incorrect. There is no reason to stop her pill since she is currently one inert pill away from starting a new cycle. The inert pill was designed to keep women on track in terms of when to stop taking the pill (in order to have a period) and when to start a next cycle of pills.

    Stop taking the pills and immediately go to the emergency room (**choice D**) is incorrect. Although she did not have a period this month, statistically it is more likely that she had a "silent menses" and not a pregnancy given the fact that she took her pill every single day at the same time and has not used any medications while she has been on the pill. Reasons for "immediate" medical attention while on the pill include, but are not limited to: a painful swollen calf (sign of thrombophlebitis), hemoptysis (sign of pulmonary embolus), and sudden blindness (sign of thrombosis of retinal artery). Had the answer choice said "go see your doctor to rule out a pregnancy," this answer choice would have been more tempting.

    Take an additional pill tomorrow (**choice E**) is incorrect. She is on the inactive pill. There is no need to take an additional pill. Only someone taking the active pills and who forgot to take one pill should take an additional pill immediately when she remembers or the next day.

24. **The correct answer is A.** This patient has arrest of descent and secondary arrest of dilatation with adequate uterine contractions. This small-framed woman is carrying a large fetus (since the fetus was 7.8 lb. at 37 weeks, it must be much larger now at 39 weeks) and has cephalopelvic disproportion (CPD). The fact that the head is not engaged supports this diagnosis. CPD is an indication for cesarean section.

    Epidural placement (**choice B**) is not correct. An epidural is usually placed early in active phase of labor (usually 4 to 5 cm of dilation). Placement of an epidural may help only a small amount in alleviating her pain, but may slow her labor progression.

    Meperidine (**choice D**) is incorrect. This patient has arrested in the active phase of labor. Contractions can be painful during the active phase of labor despite pain medication via IV or epidural. Meperidine would not help.

    Forceps delivery (**choice C**) is absolutely contraindicated when the fetal head is not engaged, at –1 station (high forceps), and the cervix is not dilated. Due to the medico-legal climate in the United States, forceps deliveries are dwindling and only the most experienced obstetricians will do forceps delivery if vertex is +2 station or higher (i.e., low and outlet forceps delivery). The use of mid and high forceps delivery has a high rate of morbidity for the fetus.

This patient has CPD and is already having adequate contractions. There is no reason to augment uterine contractions with oxytocin (**choice E**).

25. **The correct answer is D.** The patient is correct in assuming that home pregnancy tests are unreliable because the tests can be falsely normal 25% of the time. Since this patient has a 28-day cycle and since the luteal phase of the menstrual cycle is always constant (14 days), ovulation must have occurred on day 14. Sperm can survive up to 48 hours and therefore the earliest she could have conceived would be about May 17. The earliest that hCG can be detected in maternal serum or urine is 8 to 9 days after ovulation. Hence the earliest detection of pregnancy would be May 23 to 24.

    Today is too early to detect hCG by a urine pregnancy test (**choice A**) or quantitative hCG (**choice C**), which is more sensitive than a standard urine test. Additionally, since this is not a clinical emergency, a costly test such as the quantitative hCG is unwarranted.

    The earliest a Doppler can detect fetal heart activity (**choice B**) is late first trimester to early second trimester.

    The earliest that fetal heart activity can be seen on transvaginal ultrasound (**choice E**) is approximately 5 weeks of gestation. This corresponds to about 1500 mU/mL.

26. **The correct answer is A.** After the first trimester, exercise in the supine position can compress the vena cava, which can decrease venous return to the heart and thus decrease cardiac output and uterine perfusion.

    In the absence of antepartum complications and medical problems, exercise can be safely continued throughout all of pregnancy and the postpartum period. She does not have to discontinue exercise after 30 weeks' gestation (**choice B**).

    There is no need to increase fat (**choice C**) or protein intake (**choice D**) because of exercise during pregnancy. Normal metabolic changes during pregnancy will require an additional 300 kilocalories a day for the needs of pregnancy and a greater amount of kcal will be required in a pregnant person who exercises. In particular, carbohydrate needs will be greater, not protein.

    There is no data in the obstetrical literature to support limitation of exercise intensity or lower target heart rates (**choice E**) during pregnancy.

27. **The correct answer is B.** Acute appendicitis is the most common extrauterine complication of pregnancy requiring surgery. It is associated with preterm labor and spontaneous abortion. Appendicitis is frequently misdiagnosed during pregnancy because there are no diagnostic signs, symptoms, lab values, or radiographic images. Many times, other diagnoses have to be ruled out. Also interesting is that sometimes the appendix is displaced laterally and upward during pregnancy, producing right mid to upper quadrant pain.

    Acute pancreatitis (**choice A**) in pregnancy is rare. Nausea and vomiting do occur along with abdominal pain but the pain is in the mid-abdomen and it radiates to the back and last several hours. Elevated liver function tests, lipase, and especially elevated amylase levels would have been given in the question to help with the diagnosis of pancreatitis.

    Because pyuria is often seen in pregnant women with appendicitis, these women are often misdiagnosed as having pyelonephritis (**choice C**). The patient described may have pyelonephritis, but in the absence of fever or chills and costovertebral angle tenderness, this diagnosis is hard to make.

    Renal stone pain (**choice D**) is excruciating pain that frequently cause patients to writhe in pain. It is usually more often found in men and is almost always associated with hematuria. This patient only has 2 RBC/hpf, which can be found in a normal person or someone with appendicitis.

    This patient had no adnexal masses detected on obstetrical ultrasound. Since no ovarian cyst (**choice E**) was detected at 20 weeks' gestation, it is unlikely that she has had torsion of an ovarian cyst at 32 weeks' gestation.

28. **The correct answer is D.** An advance directive is the formal mechanism by which a patient may express her values regarding her future health status. It may take the form of a proxy directive or an instructional directive. A proxy directive or "durable power of attorney for health care" is when the patient designates a surrogate to make medical decisions on her behalf when the patient is no longer competent to express her choices. Since a patient's goals of care are very likely to change with time and differing clinical circumstances, appointment of a proxy who knows the patient's interests and accepts the role of surrogate decision maker is the best way of ensuring that the patient's wishes will be carried out.

An instructional directive (**choice A**) is a valid form of advanced directive that focuses on the types of life-sustaining treatment that a person would or would not choose in various clinical circumstances (for example, CPR yes or no, ventilator yes or no, tube feedings yes or no, etc.). An instructional directive is not, however, the best way to reflect the patient's most current beliefs and values.

A living will (**choice B**) is an example of an instructional directive. See explanation above.

The Patient Self-Determination Act (PSDA) was passed in December 1991. It requires all Medicaid and Medicare participating health care institutions to inform all adult patients of their rights "to make decisions concerning medical care, including the right to accept or refuse medical or surgical treatment and the right to formulate an advance directive." The inherent value of individual autonomy is encompassed by PSDA (**choice C**).

29. **The correct answer is C.** Fragile X syndrome has been described as "X-linked dominant with reduced penetrance in females." Its mechanism of inheritance was elucidated via the DNA-based molecular analysis techniques of Southern blot and PCR. The best way to account for the pattern of inheritance is by looking at the Fragile X mental retardation-1 gene (FMR-1) on the long arm of the X chromosome, which contains within it a three-base CGG repeat. Transmission of the disease (>200 CGG repeats) depends on two factors: sex of the parent and the number of CGG repeats. When a female carries a "premutation" (50-200 CGG repeats) and the premutation has a length that exceeds 90, there is a high likelihood that the repeats will expand to over 200 in the offspring and thus result in the birth of an affected child. Males transmit the premutation gene to their children, but expansion to a full mutation does not occur in the offspring.

In an autosomal dominant disease (**choice A**) such as Huntington, inheritance of the abnormal chromosome from either parent is enough to result in disease. The chance that the offspring will have the disease is 50%. Most autosomal dominant diseases have varying severity of disease manifestation in the offspring and some can present with symptoms for the first time after the age of 30, as in the case of Huntington disease.

In an autosomal recessive disease (**choice B**) such as sickle cell, an offspring must inherit two copies of a defective chromosome to render the disease. Hence, the chance that the offspring will have the disease is 25%.

Neural tube defects and cleft lip with or without cleft palate are both examples of PMF inheritance (**choice D**). The disease comes about as result of the interactions of many genes with the environment (e.g., folic acid deprivation contributing to neural tube defect). The chance that the next offspring will be affected is 1 to 3%.

Although at first glance at this question, it appears that the inheritance pattern is X-linked recessive (**choice E**) since both sons of the phenotypically normal carrier mother have the disease, it is not true with Fragile X syndrome. Examples of X-linked recessive diseases are hemophilia, Duchenne muscular dystrophy, and glucose-6-phosphate dehydrogenase (G6PD) deficiency.

30. **The correct answer is B.** None of the hepatitis infections preclude breast-feeding. With appropriate immunoprophylaxis, breast-feeding is allowed and poses no additional risk for the transmission of hepatitis B virus. There are, however, certain infections which preclude breast-feeding and even contact with the infant. These include active tuberculosis (no contact allowed), active varicella zoster (no contact allowed), active herpes zoster, and active herpes simplex. Breast-feeding is, however, allowed with cytomegalovirus infection because both the virus and maternal antibody are present in breast milk.

Although breast-feeding is allowed in hepatitis B infection, it does pose a theoretical risk (**choice A**). This is why both HBIG and hepatitis B vaccine should be administered to the infant as soon as possible after birth.

Although high titers of HBeAg (**choice C**) reflect the high infectivity potential of the mother who has hepatitis B, it is not currently used in management decisions regarding breast-feeding.

Breast-feeding is not contraindicated (**choice D**) with maternal hepatitis B infection.

None of the hepatitis infections preclude breast-feeding (**choice E**). Maternal HCV is not considered a contraindication to breast feeding nor is acute hepatitis A infection as long as the infant receives immune serum globulin and vaccine against hepatitis A.

31. **The correct answer is C.** The most likely diagnosis is a clogged milk duct. This diagnosis is not only based on physical findings, but is also derived through exclusion of other diagnoses. A clogged milk duct presents in a breast-feeding mother within the first 1 to 2 weeks postpartum as a localized, tender mass in one breast that is not erythematous and usually not firm. It can be accompanied by a fever, as in this patient.

An abscess (**choice A**) is a palpable, hardened mass that is fluctuant and follows an untreated or an incompletely treated mastitis. It can be suspected in a patient being treated for mastitis especially if there is failure to defervesce within 48 to 72 hours of antibiotic therapy. It should be treated with incision and drainage followed by prolonged antibiotic therapy. It is the only circumstance during which breast milk should be discarded for the first 24 hours after surgery.

Breast engorgement (**choice B**) presents very similarly to clogged milk duct except that there is generalized involvement of both breasts instead of a localized tender area. Breast engorgement occurs most commonly in the first 2 weeks postpartum.

Inflammatory breast carcinoma (**choice D**) can be similar in presentation to breast engorgement. The major feature that differentiates it from inflammatory breast cancer is the knowledge of previous negative breast examination results during pregnancy. Inflammatory breast cancer can present as unilateral erythema, heat, and induration that is more diffuse and recurrent. It is a lethal disease process.

Mastitis (**choice E**) generally occurs between the first and fifth weeks postpartum, but may be seen any time throughout the first year. Mastitis is manifested by a sore, reddened area on one breast and often is accompanied by chills, fever, and malaise. A segment of the breast becomes hard and erythematous. The fever can be high and mother feels ill.

32. **The correct answer is B.** The features described in this patient are those of Turner syndrome (XO). In addition to the aforementioned characteristics, children with Turner syndrome have streak gonads (nonfunctional or soon to be nonfunctional ovaries) and may present with swelling of the hands and feet in the newborn period as a result of congenital lymphedema of the extremities. Coarctation of the aorta occurs in 15% of Turner children and most have a low-lying hairline.

    Coarctation of the aorta can be present in 15% of patients with Turner syndrome. However, a wide space between the first and second toes (**choice A**) is seen in Down syndrome.

    Endocardial cushion defects of the heart occur in greater than 30% of Down syndrome babies. Other features that may be present in Down syndrome children include: Brushfield spots of the iris, small ears, redundant skin of neck (nuchal fold in prenatal ultrasound), upslanting palpebral fissures, epicanthal fold (**choice C**), and short hands.

    An endocardial cushion defect (**choice D**) of the heart is present in Down syndrome. Webbing of the neck is unique to Turner phenotype.

    Ventricular septal defect of the heart is present in many chromosomally abnormal children as well as many genetically normal children with congenital heart defects. Long, thin extremities (**choice E**) are features of Marfan disease. Children with Marfan disease are tall by stature and tend to have complications of the aorta (aortic aneurysm, aortic root dilation, aortic regurgitation) and have ectopic lentis (subluxation of the ocular lens).

33. **The correct answer is D.** The American College of Obstetrics and Gynecology (ACOG) recommends breast-feeding in all circumstances except when the mother *1*) takes street drugs or abuses alcohol, *2*) has infant with galactosemia, *3*) is infected with HIV, *4*) has active untreated tuberculosis, *5*) is taking certain antineoplastic, thyrotoxic, and immunosuppressive medications, and *6*) is undergoing treatment for breast cancer. Many women may breast-feed after reduction mammoplasty or augmentation mammoplasty with implants, and most women can breast-feed after breast biopsies.

    Augmentation mammoplasty with implants is not a contraindication to breast-feeding (**choice A**).

    Even after undergoing surgery, there is never a need to biopsy the breast in order to confirm lactation (**choice B**).

    Breast-feeding is not always successful (**choice C**) after breast surgery (reduction, augmentation, or other). Lactation is not possible for women who have had breast surgery inadvertently involving the complete severing of the lactiferous ducts. Some, but not all, women successfully breast-feed after surgery.

    Breast-feeding is recommended even in patients with silicone breast implants. It is not dependent on the type of implant (**choice E**). A study done in Toronto, Canada, comparing silicone levels in blood and milk of 15 silicone-implanted women versus mean silicone levels in cow's milk or infant formula showed no significant differences. In fact, silicone levels were higher in cow's milk and even infant formula than in breast milk of mothers with silicone implants.

34. **The correct answer is C.** Pre-eclampsia is characterized by hypertension (BP >140/90) during pregnancy *with* proteinuria. This patient presents with a headache. Other symptoms of pre-eclampsia include visual changes, epigastric pain, and pathologic edema (i.e., hands and face). The cause of pre-eclampsia is

unknown; however, vasospasm leads to elevated blood pressure and end organ damage. This patient has multiple risk factors for developing pre-eclampsia, including nulliparity, advanced maternal age, and gestational diabetes. Other risk factors are a history of chronic hypertension, chronic renal disease, antiphospholipid antibody syndrome, and twin gestation. The treatment of pre-eclampsia is delivery. Intravenous magnesium sulfate is used to prevent eclampsia.

Gestational hypertension (**choice A**) is defined as hypertension first developing after midpregnancy *without* proteinuria. Many of these patients will subsequently develop pre-eclampsia so the final diagnosis is made postpartum.

HELLP syndrome (**choice B**) is a variant of pre-eclampsia characterized by hemolysis, elevated liver enzymes, and low platelets. Approximately 10% of severe pre-eclamptics will develop HELLP syndrome. This patient has no evidence of HELLP by laboratory evaluation.

Migraine headaches (**choice D**) can appear for the first time during pregnancy in 15% of cases. In this patient, however, the elevated BP and proteinuria support the diagnosis of pre-eclampsia.

Subarachnoid hemorrhage (**choice E**) is bleeding into the subarachnoid space. The most common causes of subarachnoid hemorrhage in pregnancy are rupture of a cerebral aneurysm or arteriovenous malformation. This is an unlikely diagnosis in this patient; however, if the patient had neurologic findings on exam or an altered level of consciousness SAH should be ruled out with at CT scan of the head.

35. **The correct answer is C.** Folic acid is recommended for all women of childbearing age to prevent neural tube defects which include anencephaly, spina bifida, and encephalocele. The recommended dose is 0.4 mg per day starting 1 month prior to conception. Risks for first occurrences are slightly increased in couples with a close relative with a neural tube defect, in patients with insulin-dependent diabetes mellitus, and in women taking valproic acid or carbamazepine for seizure disorders. This patient has no risks for having a child with a neural tube defect, which is the case in 95% of neural tube defects. In those women with a previous infant affected the risk of recurrence is 2 to 3% and the recommendation of folic acid is 4 mg per day starting 1 month prior to pregnancy and continuing for the first 3 months of pregnancy.

Calcium carbonate (**choice A**), ferrous sulfate (**choice B**), vitamin A (**choice D**), and vitamin C (**choice E**) have not been shown to be effective in the prevention of neural tube defects. Also, vitamin A in high doses (10,000-50,000 IU) can be teratogenic and is not recommended in pregnancy.

36. **The correct answer is B.** This patient has pelvic inflammatory disease (PID) and should be admitted to the hospital for intravenous therapy with cefotetan, doxycycline, and metronidazole. To make this diagnosis there must be a history of lower abdominal pain, cervical motion tenderness, and bilateral adnexal tenderness plus one of the following additional criteria: temperature, abnormal cervical or vaginal discharge, elevated sedimentation rate, elevated C reactive protein, or lab diagnosis of gonorrhea or chlamydia. PID can be managed with outpatient antibiotics in some cases; however, inpatient management is indicated in the following cases:

- If the patient is noncompliant with outpatient therapy
- If outpatient therapy has failed
- If nausea or vomiting preclude administering oral antibiotics
- If the diagnosis is uncertain
- If the patient is pregnant
- If the patient is immunodeficient
- If the infection is severe (i.e., peritoneal signs, suspected tubo-ovarian abscess, shock)

The most appropriate antibiotic regimen to treat this patient's PID is cefotetan and doxycycline. Since PID is often polymicrobial in nature cefotetan 2 g IV q 12 and doxycycline 100 mg IV q 12 allow broad-spectrum antibiotic coverage in addition to covering gonorrhea and chlamydia. Alternative antibiotics as recommended by the CDC are clindamycin 900 mg IV q 8 hr with gentamicin 2 mg/kg followed by 1.5 mg/kg q 8 h. Metronidazole is added to this regimen to treat the trichomonas infection. Any patient with one sexually transmitted disease is at risk for others, therefore this patient should also be tested for syphilis, HIV, and hepatitis B and C. If she has not been vaccinated for hepatitis B, then it should be offered. Before the patient is discharged from the hospital she should be counseled on the prevention of sexually transmitted diseases and her partners should be informed that they need treatment.

Admit her to the hospital for intravenous therapy with cefotetan and doxycycline (**choice A**) is the appropriate management for PID but the patient also has a trichomonas infection, which is treated with metronidazole.

Admission for observation (**choice C**) alone would be inappropriate management because antibiotics as above are necessary to treat the infection.

Treat her as an outpatient with intramuscular ceftriaxone and oral doxycycline (**choice D**) is inappropriate in this patient because she cannot tolerate oral antibiotics because of her nausea and vomiting; therefore, inpatient treatment is necessary. Also, there is no coverage for trichomonas in this regimen.

Treat her as an outpatient with intramuscular ceftriaxone and oral metronidazole (**choice E**) is inappropriate as above. Plus, chlamydia in not adequately treated in this regimen.

37. **The correct answer is D.** The patient has disseminated intravascular coagulation (DIC). This is a complication of her placental abruption. Placental abruption is premature separation of the placenta from its implantation site. Thromboplastin release is thought to be the cause of DIC related to placental abruption. In this case, the placental abruption is a result of external maternal trauma. Other risk factors for placental abruption are multiparity, increasing age, pre-eclampsia, premature rupture of membranes, sudden uterine decompression, cigarette smoking, thrombophilias, cocaine, and uterine leiomyomas. In managing DIC it is important to replace blood losses to increase the oxygen carrying capacity. Each unit of packed red blood cells will increase the hemoglobin by 1 g/dL (or hematocrit by 1-3%). The coagulation abnormality is best corrected with fresh frozen plasma (FFP), which contains all of the coagulation factors including fibrinogen. It usually comes in a volume of 200 to 250 cc per unit. Each unit increases fibrinogen by 25 mg/dL. The usual starting dose is 2 units.

Cryoprecipitate (**choice A**) is incorrect. Although cryoprecipitate can be used to restore clotting factors, a bleeding patient such as the patient above needs volume replacement as well. Cryoprecipitate is similar to FFP but concentrated into a volume of 10 to 15 cc. It specifically contains Factor VIII, Von Willebrand factor, Factor XIII, fibrinogen, and fibronectin.

Factor VIII (**choice B**) and Factor X (**choice C**) are incorrect because they are single coagulation factors that by themselves will not correct this patient's DIC.

Platelets (**choice E**) is incorrect because the patient's platelet count is 90,000. Although she is thrombocytopenic, her platelets should still be functioning normally and this is not the cause of her bleeding. Platelet transfusions are usually not started until the platelets drop below 50,000 in a bleeding patient. One unit of platelets contains approximately 5.5×10^{10} platelets and will increase the platelet count by 5 to 10,000. The usual starting dose is 6 to 10 units.

38. **The correct answer is B.** The copper IUD is the best option for this patient. The failure rate is less than 1%. The copper IUD is effective for up to 10 years. It is safe to use and can be easily inserted in the office. The main risks are of infection related to insertion and of expulsion. The contraceptive effects of the IUD are easily reversible by removing the IUD.

Barrier contraception (**choice A**) is incorrect because barrier contraceptives have a high failure rate. Examples of barrier contraception are condoms, the diaphragm, and the cervical cap. The in-use failure rates are 12% for condoms, 18% for the diaphragm, and up to 36% for cervical cap in multiparous women.

Injectable monthly contraceptive containing 25 mg of medroxyprogesterone acetate and 5 mg of estradiol cypionate (**choice C**) and low-dose oral contraceptive pills (**choice D**) are incorrect because they both contain estrogen. Estrogen in any form is an absolute contraindication in this patient because of her history of deep venous thrombosis and Factor V Leiden mutation.

Periodic abstinence (**choice E**) is incorrect because it has an extremely high failure rate. Periodic abstinence is avoiding intercourse during the fertile phase of the menstrual cycle. The failure rate, however, is 40%.

39. **The correct answer is B.** The two most common causes of antepartum hemorrhage are placental abruption and placenta previa. Placental abruption is premature separation of the placenta from its implantation site. It usually presents as bleeding associated with uterine tenderness and contractions. Placenta previa is when the placenta implants over or very near the internal os of the cervix. It usually presents as *painless* vaginal bleeding without contractions. Both can cause significant bleeding and maternal and fetal morbidity or mortality. It is extremely important to rule out placenta previa before performing an internal exam. If the placenta is exposed, an internal exam may worsen the bleeding to the point that delivery may be necessary immediately. The best diagnostic tool for ruling out placenta previa is ultrasound. Abdominal ultrasound is 95% accurate for diagnosing placenta previa. If the ultrasound shows that the placenta is not over or near the cervix an internal exam can then be performed. Although abdominal ultrasound is accurate in diagnosing placenta previa, it only diagnoses approximately 15% of abruptions.

A magnetic resonance imaging (MRI) (**choice A**) is incorrect. It is accurate in diagnosing placenta previa; however, ultrasound is less expensive and more readily available. Most emergency rooms have access to a portable ultrasound unit. A patient who is bleeding heavily should be monitored continuously and not sent out of the emergency department for an MRI.

A bimanual examination (**choice C**) should not be performed if placenta previa is suspected.

Colposcopy (**choice D**) is an instrument used to magnify the cervix in the evaluation of cervical dysplasia or carcinoma. This is an unlikely reason for this patient's bleeding.

Uterine artery embolization (**choice E**) is a technique performed by interventional radiologists. Embolization of the uterine artery decreases blood flow to the uterus. This technique is contraindicated during pregnancy. It may be used for cases of postpartum hemorrhage.

40. **The correct answer is A.** Dilatation and curettage (D&C) is the most appropriate management in this patient. She is bleeding and unstable. The D&C is the quickest way to stop the bleeding and it also gives you the opportunity to collect a specimen for pathologic evaluation. This woman has a history of endometrial hyperplasia, which can be a precursor for endometrial cancer.

    Although IV estrogen (**choice B**) can stop the bleeding in a patient with dysfunctional uterine bleeding, it does not work rapidly enough to stop the acute bleeding that this patient is experiencing. Both oral (**choice D**) and intravenous estrogen cause the endometrial lining to thicken and stop the bleeding. This is appropriate therapy in a stable patient where there is no suspicion for endometrial carcinoma or other pathology.

    Observation (**choice C**) is incorrect because the patient is unstable and observation will not stop her bleeding.

    Progesterone (**choice E**) is not used to stop acute bleeding.

41. **The correct answer is A.** Of the choices above, the most effective treatment for chlamydia is azithromycin 1 g PO. Alternative regimens are doxycycline 100 mg PO BID for 7 days, erythromycin 500 mg PO QID for 7 days, and ofloxacin 300 mg PO BID for 7 days.

    Benzathine penicillin G (**choice B**) at this dose is the treatment for primary syphilis.

    Ceftriaxone (**choice C**) at this dose is the treatment for gonorrhea.

    Metronidazole (**choice D**) at this dose is effective against trichomonas and bacterial vaginosis (which is generally not thought to be sexually transmitted).

    Valacyclovir (**choice E**) at this dose is treatment for primary herpes simplex infection.

42. **The correct answer is A.** Cholesterol testing is important in this patient because her father has a history of premature coronary artery disease. In low-risk groups, cholesterol testing should be performed every 5 years beginning at age 45. In patients who are high risk, cholesterol should be checked prior to age 45. Patients at high risk are those with familial lipid disorders, family history of premature coronary heart disease, or personal history of coronary heart disease. In addition to cholesterol testing, lipid profile assessment is recommended because she has a first-degree relative with premature coronary heart disease.

    Fasting glucose (**choice B**) is incorrect. The patient, by history and physical exam, has no risk factors for developing diabetes. Screening for diabetes generally starts at age 45 and is checked every 3 years thereafter for low-risk patients.

    HIV testing (**choice C**) is not necessary in this low-risk patient.

    Mammography (**choice D**) is incorrect. The recommendations by the American College of Obstetrics and Gynecology and United States Preventive Services Task Force are mammography starting at age 40. If there is a strong family history of breast cancer (first-degree relative or multiple other relatives who have a history of premenopausal breast or breast and ovarian cancer) mammography is started earlier. The fact that this patient has fibrocystic breasts does not increase her risk for developing breast cancer.

    Thyroid stimulating hormone (TSH) (**choice E**) is incorrect. Thyroid screening is recommended in patients with a family history of thyroid disease or autoimmune disease.

43. **The correct answer is E.** The most life-threatening thing to rule out in a woman early in pregnancy who has abdominal pain and bleeding is an ectopic pregnancy. In this case, an intrauterine gestational sac is identified, making ectopic pregnancy (**choice D**) exceedingly unlikely (approximately 1:30,000, or 1:4000 if the patient is on fertility drugs). The ultrasound findings of rupturing ectopic pregnancy are free pelvic fluid, an adnexal mass, and no intrauterine gestational sac. This patient does have an intrauterine gestational sac, which

contains a yolk sac and a fetal pole, thus confirming an intrauterine pregnancy. The fetal pole also has heart motion confirming that it is alive. Subchorionic hemorrhage is present (crescent-shaped hypoechoic area next to the gestational sac). The subchorionic space is in direct communication with the endometrial canal allowing blood to exit the cervical os. Thus, patients with subchorionic hemorrhage often present with vaginal bleeding. Many patients with this type of hemorrhage will have a spontaneous abortion, but many will also have completely normal pregnancies. The fact that a living embryo is present makes extrusion of fetal parts from an abortion in progress (**choice B**) incorrect.

A blighted ovum (**choice A**) is also termed a missed abortion. This is when an empty gestational sac is seen by ultrasound and fetal demise has already occurred at some point. Again, a living fetus is seen in this case, negating this diagnosis.

Pelvic inflammatory disease (**choice C**) presents with lower abdominal pain, cervical motion tenderness, and signs of infection such as fever and elevated WBC count, none of which are present here.

44. **The correct answer is D.** Secondary syphilis indeed must be treated in an effort to prevent tertiary syphilis, which occurs in approximately 16% of untreated patients. In a penicillin-allergic patient, tetracycline, doxycycline, or erythromycin can be used. They are given orally in secondary syphilis.

No treatment is warranted since secondary syphilis is a self-limited cutaneous dermatosis without internal involvement (**choice A**) is wrong in that secondary syphilis manifests primarily as cutaneous eruptions (condyloma lata, alopecia, mucosal ulcerations, depigmented spots) but a patient can also have hepatitis, meningitis, deafness, optic neuritis, fever, and lymphadenopathy.

It is important to follow the RPR to be sure it is falling back to normal in a patient being treated for syphilis but **choice B** is wrong for two reasons. For one, the VDRL serologic test is a better test to follow in patients being treated for syphilis; and secondly, these patients need pharmacologic treatment. If the VDRL titer is not decreasing, these patients need to be retreated. Secondary syphilis can develop into latent syphilis where 60 to 70% of all patients will remain for the rest of their lives or it can progress to tertiary syphilis. Either way, these patients are highly infectious.

If there is an effective alternative treatment to penicillin, a penicillin-allergic patient should not receive penicillin (**choice C**). If equally effective and safe alternatives to penicillin (or any other medications) do not exist, investigate exactly what the allergy is and consider using the medication if warranted. It is possible to desensitize a patient for penicillin allergy when appropriate. However, there are multiple, equally effective alternatives to penicillin for treating secondary syphilis.

Griseofulvin, whether ultramicronized or not, is an antifungal medicine and will not kill the spirochete *T. pallidum* that causes syphilis (**choice E**).

45. **The correct answer is D.** This patient indeed has secondary syphilis. The clinical clues are the palm and sole extension of the rash, the resemblance to PR, and the fact that she is at high risk as a prostitute to this and any sexually transmitted diseases. The fact that she denies a preceding ulcer is common. The ulcer of primary syphilis is asymptomatic and is often missed in women who may not see it on their cervix or on their vaginal wall. The ulcer heals without a problem and patients go untreated. In this case, the unborn child is undoubtedly infected, as the spirochete can cross the placenta after the fourth month and this patient was 6-months pregnant when she showed signs of secondary syphilis. The typical signs of early congenital syphilis are snuffles, rhagades, and neurosyphilis, which may or may not be symptomatic. The babies can have positive CSF serologies, meningitis, hydrocephalus, optic atrophy, and iritis.

This patient does not have pityriasis rosea (PR) (**choice A**). PR is most likely due to a virus, but the specifics of this unknown virus are yet to be determined. PR has not been shown to be related to hepatitis C virus. Babies born to mothers who have had PR during pregnancy have absolutely no sequelae or stigmata.

Delirium, gummas, and nodular syphilid (**choice B**) are seen in tertiary syphilis.

Hutchinson teeth, saber shins, and saddle nose (**choice C**) are commonly found in late congential syphilis, which is seen at the age of 2 years and above.

There are many reasons for false positive RPRs (**choice E**) but PR is not one of them. One of the reasons the RPR test is ordered first is that it is a screening test for syphilis. If this is positive, the FTA-Abs test is checked which is much more specific for syphilis and can confirm the diagnosis. Although PR and secondary syphilis can look quite similar clinically, the positive FTA-Abs test clinches the diagnosis of syphilis.

46. **The correct answer is D.** Obesity is a major problem in the United States and throughout the world and its prevalence is rising. Many women of childbearing age are obese, which makes obesity one of the more common factors complicating pregnancy. Numerous studies have been done to determine whether and how obesity increases maternal and fetal morbidity and mortality. There is now substantial evidence that maternal obesity is a risk factor for the development of gestational diabetes and hypertensive disorders of pregnancy. Maternal obesity also appears to place the patient at greater risk for needing a cesarean delivery and of having anesthetic and postoperative complications. Maternal obesity also places the fetus at increased risk of having a neural tube defect. The reason for this is unknown. Fetuses of obese mothers also appear to be at increased risk of macrosomia and stillbirth. For all of these reasons, this patient would be well advised to begin a diet and exercise program to lose weight prior to becoming pregnant.

    Obese patients do not appear to be at risk of developing hypotension during pregnancy (**choice A**). As noted above, obesity during pregnancy places a woman at increased risk for developing hypertension during pregnancy.

    Obese patients do not appear to be at risk of having a fetus with increased activity syndrome (**choice B**). This is not an established fetal syndrome in obstetrics. In fact, obese women are often less able to appreciate fetal movement and, as noted above, obese women appear to be at increased risk of stillbirth.

    Obese patients are at increased risk of having a fetus with macrosomia and not of having a fetus with intrauterine growth restriction (**choice C**).

    Obese patients do not appear to be at increased risk for insufficient weight gain during the pregnancy (**choice E**). Optimal weight gain for obese patients has not been established by definitive studies.

47. **The correct answer is C.** This patient meets the clinical and laboratory criteria for antiphospholipid syndrome. According to the recent (1999) international consensus statement on criteria for the antiphospholipid syndrome, a patient is considered to have antiphospholipid syndrome if he/she has one clinical criterion and one laboratory criterion. The clinical criteria are an episode of thrombosis, a fetal death after 10 weeks, a premature birth before 34 weeks, or three or more spontaneous abortions before 10 weeks' gestation. The laboratory criteria are anticardiolipin IgG or IgM antibodies or lupus anticoagulant antibodies. This patient meets the criteria for antiphospholipid syndrome on the basis of her IUFD at 28 weeks and her positive IgG anticardiolipin antibody. Most experts now view antiphospholipid syndrome as a treatable cause of recurrent pregnancy loss. The recommended treatment is daily subcutaneous heparin or low molecular weight heparin.

    This patient should not be offered treatment with daily oral terbutaline (**choice A**). Oral terbutaline is sometimes used in patients with a history of preterm labor or with recurrent preterm contractions. However, it has never been proven to be effective in a randomized controlled trial and is not recommended treatment.

    This patient should not be offered treatment with daily oral warfarin (**choice B**). Warfarin is contraindicated during pregnancy, as it is a known cause of birth defects.

    This patient should not be offered treatment with monthly intramuscular ceftriaxone (**choice D**). Ceftriaxone is used to treat gonorrhea. This patient does not have gonorrhea and has no indication for ceftriaxone.

    This patient should not be offered treatment with monthly intravenous doxycycline (**choice E**). Doxycycline is contraindicated during pregnancy as it can cause permanent discoloration of the teeth of the offspring.

48. **The correct answer is A.** Tubal sterilization is considered to be a safe and effective method of contraception for many women. It can be performed during a cesarean delivery, immediately postpartum (usually through a small umbilical skin incision), or at any other time (usually by laparoscopy). As with most surgeries, the risks of the procedure are bleeding, infection, and damage to internal organs. However, tubal ligation also has the risks of regret and failure of the procedure. Estimates are that between 5 and 20% of women who have a tubal ligation will later regret having done so. Risk factors for poststerilization regret include young age, recent pregnancy, and black race. Failure of the procedure with a resultant pregnancy is also a significant risk of tubal ligation. Estimates for the rate of failure vary depending on the study, the age of the woman, the method chosen, and other factors. However, some studies have found the rate of failure for some methods (especially bipolar coagulation in a young woman) to be as high as 5%. This patient should be counseled regarding all of the risks, as well as benefits, of the procedure and allowed to make her own decision.

    To counsel her that the risk of failure of the procedure is less than 0.1% (**choice B**) would be incorrect. As noted above, most estimates of the failure of interval laparoscopic tubal ligation are considerably higher than this.

To counsel her that the risk of regret is less than 0.1% (**choice C**) is also incorrect. As stated above, the risk of regret after tubal ligation is considerably higher than this. This is especially true for this patient given her age.

To counsel this patient that tubal ligation increases the risk of ovarian cancer (**choice D**) is incorrect. There is substantial evidence that tubal ligation decreases a woman's lifetime risk of developing ovarian cancer.

To counsel this patient that tubal ligation is likely to cause menstrual irregularities (**choice E**) would not be correct. There has been much discussion and many anecdotal reports over the years regarding a "post-tubal ligation syndrome" characterized by menstrual irregularities. However, in well-conducted studies, there appears to be no increased risk of menstrual irregularities after tubal ligation.

49. **The correct answer is C.** It would be inappropriate to remove the appendix without having obtained consent to do so, as charges of battery could be brought against the physician. It is mandatory for a physician to ensure that a patient capable of making such a judgment—or, when indicated, his/her duly appointed surrogate—is informed about the nature of his/her medical condition, the objectives of the proposed treatment, treatment alternatives, and possible outcomes and risks involved. These issues should be spoken in a language that the patient can understand clearly and fully in order to make a decision. The physician should not modulate this information to suit his/her own personal therapeutic preferences, nor should clinical judgment be clouded by fiscal considerations or financial incentives, as these will raise a conflict of interest.

    The husband (**choice A**) has no legal right to make a decision.

    The question of payment by the insurance company (**choice B**) should not be an issue. The primary duty of any physician is to tend to the sick, and monetary or other reward is and should be a secondary concern. The same principle applies if the patient happens to be uninsured or underinsured, or in cases in which an institution limits expenditure.

    Removing the appendix without first obtaining consent (**choices D and E**) would be construed as battery.

50. **The correct answer is D.** The presence of endocervical cells on a Pap test is regarded as evidence of adequate sampling of the transformation zone during cytologic screening of the cervix. When these cells are absent, it indicates that this area may not have been sampled. This is considered a satisfactory but limited smear. In patients with no known risk factors (i.e., prior abnormal Pap, multiple sexual partners, smoking) the American College of Obstetricians and Gynecologists recommends that the physician may defer to repeating the Pap test in 12 months.

    It is inappropriate to tell the patient that she needs increased monitoring (**choice C**) because these results do not indicate any abnormality; it is simply a sampling error.

    If this were a high-risk patient (i.e., prior abnormal Pap, multiple sexual partners, smoking) a resampling of the endocervix (**choice A**) only would be the appropriate next step. However, since she is not at a high risk, you can wait for 1 year.

    It is inappropriate to tell her that the results of this test are not valid (**choice B**) because they are valid, just not complete.

    A colposcopic examination of the cervix (**choice E**) would be appropriate if this patient had abnormal cells on her smear, indicating a precancerous lesion.

Obstetrics/Gynecology: **Test Three**

1. A 34-year-old Indian woman comes to the clinic at 32 weeks' gestation for a scheduled prenatal visit. She has no complaints and she tells you that she is due to go on vacation to visit her mother soon. She had an elective abortion 2 years ago and her mother has type 2 diabetes mellitus. Her only current medication is a daily multivitamin. Her temperature is 37.0 C (98.6 F), blood pressure is 130/80 mm Hg, pulse is 72/min, and respirations are 16/min. Fundal height is 34 cm and the fetal heart rate (Doppler) is approximately 140/min. A sonogram done at 12 weeks' gestation was consistent with dates. Her updated prenatal tests are as follows: HIV negative, syphilis serology nonreactive, Rubella titer immune, HepB surface antigen negative, Gonorrhea and Chlamydia screen negative, and 1-hour glucose tolerance test serum glucose of 203 mg/dL. The most appropriate next step in management is to

    (A) begin treatment with long-acting NPH and regular insulin
    (B) obtain a sonogram to obtain an estimated fetal weight and abdominal circumference
    (C) reassure the patient that the prenatal course is going well before she leaves your clinic to go on vacation
    (D) recommend a 3-hour glucose tolerance test before she goes on vacation
    (E) start a diet consisting mainly of complex carbohydrates, low in saturated fats and soluble fiber

2. A 24-year-old female computer consultant comes to the emergency department complaining of a burning feeling when she urinates, along with increased frequency and urgency. She is at 17 weeks' gestation and gets routine prenatal care with a private physician. This is her first pregnancy and she reports that it has been uncomplicated thus far. She has no other medical problems, has never had surgery, takes prenatal vitamins and iron, and does not smoke cigarettes or drink alcohol. A urine dipstick supports your suspicion of a urinary tract infection and on examination you find that she is febrile and has severe right costovertebral angle tenderness. You send urine for culture and admit her for therapy with intravenous antibiotics. Once the patient defervesces, the most appropriate next step in management to prevent morbidity is to

    (A) obtain a formal renal consult
    (B) order a cystoscopy
    (C) order a renal ultrasound
    (D) prescribe suppression therapy for the remainder of her pregnancy
    (E) urge her to increase fluid consumption and to empty her bladder frequently, and return again with the first sign of any infection

3. A 67-year-old woman comes to the office for a routine checkup. She is in good health, exercises three times a week, and experienced menopause 15 years ago. She takes calcium and iron, does not smoke cigarettes, and drinks a glass of wine nearly every night with dinner. Physical examination is unremarkable, except for a small area of white skin discoloration on her left labia majora. When you question her about it, she states that she never noticed it. You suspect that it is lichen sclerosis. The most appropriate next step in management is to

   (A) do a local office biopsy of the area
   (B) give her estrogen cream to apply to the area before bedtime and have her return in 2 weeks
   (C) inform her that this is a normal finding on post-menopausal women and continue with other health maintenance issues
   (D) prescribe boric acid vaginal suppositories and have her return in 2 weeks
   (E) tell her to apply hydrocortisone cream twice a day and have her return in 2 weeks

4. A 23-year-old graduate student comes to the clinic complaining of vague, cramping pain in the lower left quadrant. She is nulliparous and is not currently sexually active. Her last menstrual period was 2 weeks prior to this visit. Her gynecological history is negative except for an abnormal Pap smear 3 years ago for which she had a benign colposcopic examination. She has mild exercise-induced asthma that she uses an inhaler for, has never had surgery, and takes no other medications. She denies alcohol, tobacco, or drug use. Pelvic examination is benign other than a slight fullness in the left adnexa. You decide to perform a bedside transvaginal ultrasound which confirms a left ovarian simple cyst that measures 4 × 5 cm. The most appropriate next step in management is to

   (A) draw and send a serum CA-125
   (B) repeat the pelvic examination and ultrasound in 6 weeks
   (C) schedule the patient for a diagnostic laparoscopy and possible cystectomy
   (D) send the patient for a CT scan of the abdomen and pelvis
   (E) start the patient on oral contraceptives and follow up in 3 months

5. A 27-year-old woman comes with her husband to the clinic because they have been trying to conceive for 18 months without success. She states that she has even used basal body temperature kits to determine the best times to have intercourse. Her gynecologic history is significant only for an elective abortion 7 years ago. She has no other significant medical, surgical, or social history. Her physical examination, including pelvic examination, is unremarkable. The most appropriate next step in management is to

   (A) arrange an appointment for her husband so that you can discuss semen analysis
   (B) draw serum prolactin
   (C) draw serum thyroid stimulating hormone
   (D) evaluate her uterus with a hysteroscope
   (E) perform a diagnostic laparoscopy and chromotubation

6. A 30-year-old woman comes to the clinic complaining of mild sinusitis. She is at 18 weeks' gestation with her second child, and receives routine prenatal care at your facility. Her first child was delivered at full term with an uncomplicated vaginal delivery. Her medical, surgical, and social history is entirely negative. She is currently taking prenatal vitamins and iron. The pregnancy has been uncomplicated thus far. You perform a physical examination and diagnose sinusitis, which you treat appropriately. Before you leave the room, the patient asks if you can tell her the results of her triple screen test that was drawn 2 weeks prior. You notice that the test came back abnormal, with an increased alpha-fetoprotein component. She is concerned about what will happen next. You inform her that the most appropriate next step is to

   (A) enroll her in a high-risk obstetrical clinic
   (B) perform an amniocentesis for karyotype
   (C) perform an amniocentesis for amniotic fluid alpha-fetoprotein
   (D) perform a level II anatomy scan
   (E) repeat the blood test

7. A 22-year-old primigravid woman who is at 30 weeks' gestation comes to the office for a prenatal visit. She tells you that the baby is moving well and she has had no bleeding per vagina, no loss of fluid, and no contractions. Her pregnancy has been uncomplicated thus far. She has no medical or surgical history, takes no medications, and has no known drug allergies. Her blood pressure is 110/60 mm Hg. She has no protein on her urine dip. Her fundal height is 26 cm. The fetal heart rate is 140/min. Given the fact that her fundal height is less than her dates, she is sent for an ultrasound that shows a fetus in the 8th percentile. The most appropriate next step in management is to

   (A) have the patient follow up in 4 weeks
   (B) initiate an induction of labor
   (C) obtain Doppler of the umbilical artery
   (D) perform immediate cesarean delivery
   (E) start magnesium sulfate therapy

8. A 29-year-old primigravid woman with phenylketonuria who is 5½ weeks pregnant comes to the office for an initial prenatal visit. She is dated based on an ultrasound performed earlier in the day. She complains of moderate nausea with a few episodes of vomiting, but she is able to tolerate liquids and some solids. Her past surgical history is significant for a left ovarian cystectomy 3 years ago. She takes no medications and is allergic to penicillin. Physical examination, including breast and pelvic examination, is unremarkable. In counseling this patient about interventions to prevent her fetus from developing mental retardation and microcephaly, she should be told

   (A) that no intervention is necessary
   (B) that the father of the baby must be tested for phenylketonuria
   (C) to follow a special diet
   (D) to have an ultrasound each trimester
   (E) to have a weekly nonstress test

9. A 67-year-old woman comes to the health center for an annual examination. She has been in excellent health during the past year. She exercises daily by walking for 30 minutes. She has no medical problems. She had an appendectomy at the age of 29, and no other surgeries. Her last menstrual period was at the age of 49. She takes no medications and has no known drug allergies. She works as a librarian and lives with her husband of 47 years. She does not smoke, drink, or use illegal drugs. Physical examination, including a breast and pelvic examination, is unremarkable. She wants to know if there are any screening tests that she should have done. In addressing this issue, you should

   (A) order a serum CA-125 level for ovarian cancer screening
   (B) order bone mineral density testing for osteoporosis screening
   (C) order urine N-telopeptide for osteoporosis screening
   (D) perform an endometrial biopsy for endometrial cancer screening
   (E) schedule an ultrasound for ovarian cancer screening

10. A 33-year-old primigravid woman comes to the emergency department complaining of left leg swelling for the last 2 days, progressively worsening to the point that she now cannot ambulate comfortably. She is at 16 weeks' gestation, and has had an uneventful course until now. She has no other past medical history or significant family history, and is taking only prenatal vitamins. She denies a history of trauma or recent travel. Her temperature is 37.0 C (98.6 F), blood pressure is 100/60 mm Hg, pulse is 88/min, and respirations are 14/min. Complete blood count and serum electrolytes are within normal limits. A left lower extremity Doppler ultrasound confirms the presence of a deep vein thrombosis, and the patient is started on unfractionated heparin and admitted to the medical service. The most appropriate long-term therapy before discharging the patient is

   (A) daily low-dose aspirin therapy during her pregnancy
   (B) inferior vena cava (IVC) filter placement without further anticoagulation
   (C) low molecular weight heparin for at least the duration of her pregnancy
   (D) subcutaneous heparin 5000 units BID for at least the duration of her pregnancy
   (E) warfarin therapy daily until the INR is 2 to 3 times control, then discontinuation of heparin and continuation of warfarin for at least the duration of her pregnancy

11. A 55-year-old woman comes to the office for follow-up. She has a history of diabetes mellitus, controlled with metformin and glyburide, and has no complaints at this time. She has a family history of breast cancer, and her most recent mammogram 1 month ago revealed a 1-cm opacity with irregular margins. She has since had the mass excised by a breast surgeon and pathology showed it to be infiltrating ductal carcinoma, estrogen- and progesterone-receptor positive. Margins or resection were clear of tumor invasion, and subsequent axillary lymph node dissection did not reveal evidence of spread to the lymph nodes. Aside from referral for evaluation for chemotherapy and radiation, the most appropriate long-term management of this patient is to

(A) recommend no further therapy
(B) recommend screening of this patient's family for the breast cancer gene
(C) refer her to a surgeon for bilateral radical mastectomy
(D) start tamoxifen therapy for 5 years
(E) start tamoxifen therapy for life

12. A 27-year-old pregnant woman in her first trimester comes to the office because of burning on urination. She had noticed that she has been urinating more frequently and there is an odor associated with her urination. She has mild suprapubic discomfort but there are no associated fevers or chills. You start her on clindamycin for her symptoms and send urine for culture and sensitivity. Forty-eight hours later she returns for the results of her culture that shows 40,000 colony-forming units of *E. coli* sensitive to all antibiotics. The most appropriate next step in management is to

(A) begin chloramphenicol
(B) begin tetracycline
(C) change her antibiotic to a fluoroquinolone
(D) continue with clindamycin
(E) defer antibiotics because the colony count is not large enough

13. A 24-year-old nulligravid woman comes to the office for a routine prenatal visit. She is at 9 weeks' gestation and denies any medical problems. Her family history is significant for a few distant relatives with renal failure. She lives with her husband and works in a meat factory as a supervisor. She denies smoking, alcohol intake, or any drug use. She tries to exercise moderately every day and keeps a healthy diet with a moderate amount of fish. The most appropriate advice regarding eating fish during pregnancy is:

(A) All fish should be avoided while pregnant
(B) Raw fish can be eaten as long as she consumes it in less than five meals per week
(C) She should avoid eating cooked shark, swordfish, and other predatory fish
(D) She can eat cooked fish as long as she consumes it in less than five meals per week
(E) There are no restrictions on eating fish

14. A 27-year-old nulligravid falls off her horse and lands on her back while playing polo. She is taken to the hospital where she is found to have partial, severe transection of her spinal cord above level T-10. Years later she gets married and becomes pregnant with her first child. The complication of spinal cord injury that poses the greatest threat to her and her developing fetus is

(A) anemia
(B) autonomic dysreflexia
(C) painless labor
(D) pressure sores
(E) urinary tract infections

15. A 36-year-old gravida 2, para 1 woman at 25 weeks' gestation comes to the office because of "another urinary tract infection." She has had five symptomatic, culture-proven urinary tract infections during this pregnancy and a urologic evaluation did not show any anatomic abnormalities. You decide to put her on daily low-dose nitrofurantoin. You also recommend that she drink 16 ounces of cranberry juice every day. She does not understand why cranberry juice would be helpful in preventing a bacterial infection. While responding to her inquiry, you should explain that

(A) cranberry extract acidifies urine and prevents growth of bacteria
(B) cranberry extract has a diuretic effect that reduces urine stasis
(C) cranberry extract is inherently bacteriostatic
(D) cranberry extract prevents bacteria from adhering to the urinary epithelium
(E) there is no scientific evidence for your recommendation

16. A 20-year-old primigravid woman at 13 weeks' gestation is a passenger in a motor vehicle accident. She is taken by ambulance to your hospital where she is found to be alert and oriented to herself, to time, and to place. She has stable vital signs, two lacerations on her forehead, a few contusions of her right shoulder and left arm, some abdominal and back pain, but no vaginal bleeding and no uterine contractions. To fully evaluate her, you know that you must order diagnostic imaging. The imaging modality with the highest level of radiation exposure and its suitability during pregnancy is

(A) barium enema, not contraindicated during pregnancy
(B) chest x-ray, not contraindicated during pregnancy
(C) CT scan of the abdomen, contraindicated during pregnancy
(D) CT scan of the head, not contraindicated during pregnancy
(E) small bowel series, contraindicated during pregnancy

17. A 20-year-old college student is found unconscious in a fraternity living room. When she awakens, she says she was having an alcoholic beverage with a guy she had just met at a party and then she does not remember much else after a few sips of her drink. She feels achy all over and thinks that she has been sexually violated. Her best friend brings her to the emergency department where she is suspected of being date-raped. The most accurate statement regarding sexual assault is:

(A) Emergency contraception must be used within 48 hours to be effective.
(B) Informed consent need not be obtained before physical examination.
(C) Injuries to the vulva and rectum are commonly found in all age groups.
(D) It is a good idea to include a police officer or a social worker while obtaining a history.
(E) *Trichomonas* infections are the most likely acquired sexually transmissible infection after sexual assault.

18. A 30-year-old gravida 3 woman is undergoing counseling before surgery for a 30-cm abdominopelvic mass. She is reluctant to receive a blood transfusion because of a fear of contracting acquired immunodeficiency syndrome (AIDS). In explaining the risks and benefits of blood transfusions you should tell her that she is at greatest risk for contracting

(A) hepatitis B virus
(B) hepatitis C virus
(C) hepatitis D virus
(D) human immunodeficiency virus
(E) human T-cell lymphotrophic virus

19. A 63-year-old woman with ovarian cancer comes to the emergency department because of 48 hours of nausea and vomiting and the inability to take oral intake. She has voided once today. She denies diarrhea, constipation, or abdominal pain. Two days ago she received intravenous chemotherapy with Taxol and cisplatin. On physical examination she is pale and lethargic, but alert and oriented to self, time, and place. Vitals signs are: temperature 36.5 C (97.7 F), blood pressure 90/50 mm Hg while sitting (baseline blood pressure 110/80 mm Hg), and pulse 124/min. Abdominal examination reveals normoactive bowel sounds. The most appropriate next step in management is to

(A) administer ondansetron
(B) admit her to the hospital for observation
(C) insert a nasogastric tube
(D) order abdominal flat and upright radiographs
(E) start intravenous hydration

20. A 22-year-old woman who is at 18 weeks' gestation comes to the office for a routine prenatal visit. Her pregnancy has been progressing well and she is in a mutually monogamous relationship. Physical examination is normal. Before she leaves the office, she asks you about continuing sexual activity during pregnancy. The most appropriate advice for this patient is that she should

(A) avoid the female-supine positions after 28 weeks
(B) have no coital activity after 34 weeks
(C) have no oral-genital contact after 20 weeks
(D) not alter her sexual practices as there are no restrictions
(E) use condoms

21. A 76-year-old woman requires abdominal surgery for a large complex adnexal mass suspicious for ovarian cancer. She has not been under the care of a physician since age 50 years. Her past medical history is significant for smoking 60 packs of cigarettes per year. She has a productive cough and dyspnea. In addition to a complete history, physical examination, and chest x-ray, initial preoperative evaluation of this patient should include

(A) an arterial blood gas
(B) no additional testing
(C) a PPD and anergy panel
(D) screening spirometry
(E) sputum culture and sensitivity

22. A 20-year-old woman has multiple episodes of vaginal candidiasis. She has used over-the-counter and prescription medications which have only provided temporary relief of symptoms. She now comes to the clinic with thrush-like patches in her vagina and oral pharynx. A wet smear with KOH demonstrates pseudohyphae. The most important diagnostic test at this time is

(A) an HIV test
(B) protein electrophoresis
(C) a 3-hour glucose tolerance test
(D) a type-specific fungal culture
(E) VDRL serology

23. A 26-year-old woman has a 3-month history of painful intercourse. She was sexually active before the onset of this pain and never had any associated symptoms. She denies any gynecologic problems. She has seen other physicians for this problem and has been treated with fluconazole and metronidazole without success. On physical examination there are painful red spots, 2 to 3 mm in size, on the inner aspect of the labia majora. The spots are extremely tender to touch with cotton swab. The remainder of the physical examination is normal. Initial treatment should include

(A) a fentanyl patch
(B) an interferon injection
(C) intensive psychotherapy
(D) tricyclic antidepressants
(E) a vulvar vestibulectomy

24. A 58-year-old woman is worried about ovarian cancer because her third cousin recently died from it. She says she began her menstrual periods at age 11, her periods used to be 30 days in length, and she used to bleed for 3 to 4 days. She thinks she stopped having periods entirely at age 55. She has one child and no past medical or surgical history. She used birth control pills for more than 15 years. She is an ex-smoker of 1 pack per day for 10 years. The factor in this patient's history that most significantly changes her risk of ovarian cancer is

(A) age at first menses
(B) age at menopause
(C) oral contraception use
(D) parity
(E) smoking

25. A 22-year-old woman comes to the office complaining of a 25-pound weight loss despite not attempting to lose weight. She has a history of sexual promiscuity. Her thyroid function tests are normal. Her HIV test is positive. The information about the ELISA test for HIV that would be the most useful for this patient is

(A) negative predictive value
(B) positive predictive value
(C) sensitivity
(D) specificity

26. A 31-year-old woman comes to the office because of irregular bleeding. Over the past 2 months she has several days of spotting followed by a "bleeding-free" interval, followed by more spotting. She has always had normal periods, every 28 days, since she was 16 years old. She has no medical problems. Her past surgical history includes a breast reduction 4 years ago. She started depot medroxyprogesterone acetate (DMPA) 8 weeks ago for contraception. She has no known drug allergies. Physical examination is within normal limits. Pelvic examination demonstrates normal genitalia. There is a scant amount of blood in the vaginal vault. There are no uterine or adnexal masses or tenderness. Urine hCG is negative. The most likely cause of this patient's irregular bleeding, according to the information available, is

(A) depot medroxyprogesterone acetate
(B) endometrial cancer
(C) endometrial hyperplasia
(D) pregnancy
(E) spontaneous abortion

27. You are starting a busy day in your outpatient office when your nurse hands you a message. One of your patients, a 28-year-old nulligravid woman, is concerned that she is pregnant and would like to speak to you this morning. She is in a monogamous relationship with her husband of 2 years and does not wish to become pregnant. You remember that at her last physical examination you discussed various contraception options. The patient and her husband both felt comfortable using condoms. She had tried hormonal contraception in the past, but experienced mild weight gain and she wished to avoid this. While talking to the patient, you find that her last menstrual period was approximately 2 weeks ago. She has monthly periods and has had no irregular vaginal bleeding. She is having no vaginal discharge or abdominal pain, and has used condoms without difficulty every time she and her husband have had intercourse. She is concerned that she may be pregnant because last evening, approximately 14 hours ago, while having intercourse "the condom broke." She and her husband are still not interested in becoming parents and she asks if there is anything she can do now. You advise her that:

(A) Because it has been longer than 12 hours, elective termination is her only option and you can provide her with a list of physicians that will perform the procedure
(B) It is unlikely that she became pregnant given the timing of her last menstrual period and therefore she should be reassured
(C) She should start an oral contraceptive agent like 35 micrograms ethinyl estradiol/0.3 milligrams norgestrel now; she should take one pill daily and this will prevent pregnancy from occurring
(D) She should take 100 micrograms of ethinyl estradiol and 0.5 milligrams of levonorgestrel now and repeat the dose in 12 hours; this will decrease the chance of her becoming pregnant
(E) She should wait until she has missed her period and if this happens she would be a candidate for emergency contraception with 2 doses of 0.75 milligrams of levonorgestrel taken 12 hours apart

28. A 28-year-old primigravid woman who is at 36 weeks' gestation is admitted to the labor and delivery floor because of fever and abdominal tenderness. She began "leaking clear fluid" from her vagina 2 days ago. She reports normal fetal movement and no vaginal bleeding. She has had an uncomplicated pregnancy and had a first-trimester ultrasound that confirmed her due date. Her temperature is 38.0 C (100.4 F), blood pressure is 110/65 mm Hg, pulse is 90/min, and respirations are 16/min. The fetal heart rate is 160/min with good variability and contractions every 10 minutes. Her abdomen is diffusely tender. Sterile speculum examination reveals turbid fluid pooling in the vagina with an elevated pH and a ferning pattern when examined on a slide. Her cervical os is visually closed. Ultrasound evaluation confirms a cephalic presentation. The most appropriate action at this time is to

(A) administer antibiotics
(B) administer antibiotics and oxytocin
(C) administer betamethasone
(D) administer magnesium sulfate
(E) prepare her for a cesarean section

29. A 22-year-old gravida 1, para 1 woman comes to the emergency department because of a 20-day history of heavy bleeding, passing clots for the past 2 days, and weakness. Her menstrual periods are irregularly irregular, with her last one occurring 3 weeks before this bleeding episode. Vital signs are: blood pressure 95/65 mm Hg, pulse 104/min, and respirations 20/min. Her hemoglobin is 9.0 mg/dL. A urine hCG is negative. The most appropriate next step in management is to

(A) advise her to take nonsteroidal anti-inflammatory drugs
(B) advise her to begin taking an oral contraceptive agent
(C) begin therapy with conjugated estrogen
(D) begin therapy with progestin
(E) perform a dilatation and curettage

30. A 53-year-old woman comes to the office for a periodic health maintenance examination. She has no complaints at this time, but tells you that her best friend was recently diagnosed with breast cancer. Your patient is now concerned about her risk for developing this disease. You recall a recent journal article that you read on this topic. To determine the risk factors associated with breast cancer in women over 50 years of age, a study was conducted comparing the past histories of 100 women between the ages of 50 and 60 who had been diagnosed with breast cancer with 200 women who were cancer-free. Eleven percent of the sample refused to answer one or more of the questions asked. Some of the results of the study are presented below:

Factor	Risk	95% Confidence Interval
Positive parental history	2.34	(1.54-3.25)
Positive family history	1.47	(0.71-1.95)
Cigarette smoking	2.81	(1.54-3.25)
Over 5 drinks per week	3.43	(0.88-5.85)
Urban living	1.14	(1.04-1.29)
Pregnancy before age 20	0.64	(0.41-0.86)

Based only upon the results of this specific study, the strongest factor suggesting increased risk for breast cancer in women between the ages of 50 and 60 is most likely

(A) cigarette smoking
(B) family history
(C) more than 5 drinks per week
(D) parental history
(E) pregnancy before age 20
(F) urban living

31. A 20-year-old primigravid woman at 17 weeks' gestation comes to the office because of a small growth on her vulva. She is sexually active with one partner. She denies any history of sexually transmitted diseases. On physical examination you discover a 3 to 4 mm, warty growth on the posterior fourchette. Her vagina and cervix are normal. Application of acetic acid and colposcopic examination reveal several areas of thin, acetowhite epithelium with well-demarcated borders. The most appropriate therapy at this time is

(A) an interferon injection
(B) laser ablation
(C) podophyllin application
(D) trichloroacetic acid application
(E) wide local excision

32. A 20-year-old nulligravid woman comes to the office for a follow-up appointment. She had come to the office 2 weeks ago for abdominal pain, and you ordered an MRI, which failed to demonstrate a cause for her pain. However, the MRI showed that she has a bicornuate uterus. The patient is interested in becoming pregnant soon and is concerned when you tell her about the MRI finding. Appropriate management is to

(A) perform cervical cerclage at 12 weeks' gestation
(B) perform cervical cerclage at 15 weeks' gestation
(C) recommend that she attempt pregnancy without therapy
(D) refer her for hysteroscopic excision of uterine septum
(E) refer her for a uterine reunification procedure

33. A 52-year-old is concerned about her risk of ovarian and breast cancer. She has 2 children that were born vaginally after uneventful pregnancies. Menarche was at age 15, and she entered menopause at age 50. Her mother was diagnosed with breast cancer at age 62 and paternal grandmother was diagnosed with breast cancer at age 70. Her mother's two sisters are both without cancer. At this time, the appropriate management is to

(A) advise her to have a bilateral salpingo-oophorectomy
(B) advise her to have genetic testing
(C) measure CA-125 levels
(D) order periodic transvaginal ultrasounds
(E) recommend routine gynecologic care

34. A 29-year-old nulligravid woman with a 1-year history of dysmenorrhea, dyspareunia, and pelvic pain (despite therapy with oral contraceptive pills [OCP]) seeks your advice. Two years ago, she had laparoscopic surgery for appendicitis, at which time the surgeon noted "chocolate-colored" cystic masses around her uterus and in the cul-de-sac. She wants to avoid further surgery at this time and wishes to become pregnant within the next year. At this time, the most appropriate therapy for her pain is

(A) danazol
(B) depot-medroxyprogesterone acetate
(C) gonadotropin-releasing hormone analogue
(D) mifepristone
(E) OCP

35. A 61-year-old postmenopausal woman comes to the clinic for routine health care. She has no medical problems and is not taking any medications. She has smoked half a pack of cigarettes per day for 40 years. Physical examination is unremarkable. In addition to a Pap smear, fecal occult blood test, and mammography, you should recommend an annual

(A) chest x-ray
(B) cholesterol measurement
(C) influenza vaccine
(D) sigmoidoscopy
(E) urinalysis

36. A 30-year-old gravida 3, para 3 woman comes to the office to discuss contraception options. She has heard "mixed things" about oral contraceptive pills and wants to know your opinion. She is specifically concerned about the risks of cancer associated with its use. You explain that some cancers are actually reduced in women who have taken oral contraceptive pills and that the largest reduction of cancer-related deaths are associated with the

(A) breast
(B) cervix
(C) colon
(D) endometrium
(E) ovary

37. A 25-year-old woman who recently donated blood is notified that her serologic test for syphilis is positive. She had an unexplained, second-trimester fetal loss two years ago and a documented iliofemoral thrombosis, found last year, with no precipitating cause and for which she received heparin. She has no known history of sexually transmitted diseases. Her fluorescent treponemal antibody absorption test (FTA-ABS) is negative. The most likely diagnosis is

(A) antiphospholipid syndrome
(B) antithrombin III deficiency
(C) polymyalgia rheumatica
(D) protein C deficiency
(E) systemic lupus erythematosus

38. A 26-year-old gravida 4, para 3 woman at 38 weeks' gestation has rectal bleeding, perineal pain, and severe anal pruritus. On physical examination, there are 2 to 4-cm, dark purple, and tender masses surrounding the anus. There is no evidence of thrombosis on palpation. The most effective single therapy for her current condition is

(A) hemorrhoid suppositories
(B) hemorrhoid cream
(C) increased dietary fiber
(D) injection of phenol
(E) sitz baths

39. A 21-year-old college student comes to the clinic with a second episode of painful, frequent urination in the past 2 months. She is sexually active with one partner. Her temperature is 36.6 C (97.8 F), blood pressure is 120/85 mm Hg, and pulse is 80/min. Physical examination is unremarkable. Midstream clean catch urine shows 3000/mm^3 WBC and 4 to 5% RBC per high-powered field. Urine dipstick is negative for leukocyte esterase. Urine culture shows <1000 *E. coli*/mL. The most likely diagnosis is

(A) infectious cystitis
(B) interstitial cystitis
(C) traumatic cystitis
(D) urethral syndrome
(E) vulvar vestibulitis

40. A 24-year-old woman at 29 weeks' gestation comes to the office with a 6-hour history of severe, nonradiating, burning epigastric pain. She has also had a mild headache for the past 2 days and one episode of vomiting. She has no visual symptoms. Her prenatal course has been unremarkable, and she has no significant past medical history. On physical examination, she appears pale, diaphoretic, and in mild distress. Her blood pressure is 126/82 mm Hg and pulse is 82/min. Physical examination is unremarkable. She has trace proteinuria and 1+ pitting pedal edema. The most likely diagnosis is

(A) acute cholecystitis
(B) a bleeding peptic ulcer
(C) gastroesophageal reflux
(D) myocardial infarction
(E) pre-eclampsia

41. You have been treating a 26-year-old woman with anticardiolipin antibodies with low-dose aspirin for the past 6 months. When she presented to you initially she had a 1-year history of focal, painful, purpuric lesions of the lower extremities that would ulcerate frequently and slowly heal to leave small, white, stellate scars mainly around the ankles. The skin of the lower two-thirds of her lower legs had a diffuse, purple, reticulated pattern with foci of telangiectasis and brown, hemosiderin-induced pigmentation. A biopsy of the lesions showed segmental hyalinizing vasculopathy of the small blood vessels. On direct immunofluorescence, fibrin, C3, and IgM were detected in vessel walls. At this office visit her husband and the patient tell you that they have decided to try to have a baby again, and remind you that she had 2 miscarriages in the past 3 years. Her skin disease has been under good control lately and they feel that this next anticipated pregnancy might be successful. They are not sure whether aspirin is safe in pregnancy and inquire if there is any other treatment option to prevent recurrence of her skin disease if she discontinues it. The treatment modality that would be the most appropriate in view of the anticipated conception is

(A) continue aspirin
(B) minidose heparin
(C) nifedipine
(D) no treatment is necessary at this time
(E) warfarin

42. An 11-year-old girl is brought to the health center by her mother because of heavy periods. The daughter had her first menses a few months ago. Since that time she has had heavy periods that seem to be growing heavier with each cycle. She is not currently bleeding. She has migraine headaches and no other medical problems. She has never had surgery. She takes acetaminophen for her headaches and she has no known drug allergies. She has no family history of bleeding disorder or other medical problem. She lives at home with her parents and 10 year-old brother. Her physical examination is unremarkable. Pelvic examination reveals normal external female genitalia, a normal vaginal vault, and normal cervix. She has no uterine or adnexal masses or tenderness. Evaluation of her medical record shows that a recent complete blood count was performed that showed:

Leukocyte count 8900/mm^3

Hematocrit 24%

Platelets 210,000/mm^3

The most appropriate next step in the management course is to

(A) order blood tests including ristocetin cofactor assay of vWF function
(B) perform a hysteroscopy and dilatation and curettage in the operating room
(C) reassure the patient that this bleeding is normal and will decrease with time
(D) recommend a hysterectomy as soon as possible
(E) start the patient on the oral contraceptive pill

43. A 34-year-old primigravid woman who is at 12 weeks' gestation comes to the office for a prenatal visit. She feels somewhat fatigued but is otherwise doing well. She has had no bleeding or discharge from the vagina and no complaints. Her pregnancy has been uncomplicated thus far. She has exercise-induced asthma for which she occasionally needs to use an inhaler. Otherwise, she has no medical problems. She has never had surgery and no known drug allergies. Her blood pressure is 100/68 mm Hg. She has no protein or glucose on her urine dip. The fetal heart rate is in the 150s/min. You review with her the laboratory studies from her initial prenatal visit and note that the Pap smear was normal but demonstrated some findings suggestive of bacterial vaginosis. She is currently asymptomatic. The most appropriate management at this time is to

(A) examine the patient if she becomes symptomatic later in pregnancy
(B) treat the patient with intravaginal clindamycin
(C) treat the patient with oral metronidazole
(D) wait until the second trimester and treat with intravaginal clindamycin
(E) wait until the second trimester and treat with oral metronidazole

44. A 36-year-old woman who is at 38 weeks' gestation comes to the hospital complaining of contractions. Her prenatal course was significant for well-controlled chronic hypertension. Her past obstetrical history is significant for a full-term vaginal delivery 3 years ago; that child developed sepsis due to *Streptococcus agalactiae* during the newborn period. Her past medical history is significant for chronic hypertension, which she has had for 2 years. She took no medications during the pregnancy and is allergic to sulfa drugs. Her temperature is 37.0 C (98.6 F), pulse is 90/min, respirations are 12/minute, and her blood pressure is 110/60 mm Hg. Cervical examination shows that she is 5 centimeters dilated, 90% effaced, and at +1 station. The fetal heart rate is in the 130s/min and reactive and the patient is contracting every 3 minutes. The most appropriate next step in management is to admit her to labor and delivery and to

(A) give intrapartum clindamycin
(B) give intrapartum erythromycin
(C) give intrapartum magnesium sulfate
(D) give intrapartum oxytocin
(E) give intrapartum penicillin

45. A 31-year-old primigravid white woman who is at 15 weeks' gestation comes to the office for a prenatal visit. She had some significant fatigue and nausea earlier in the pregnancy, but that these are now improving. Her past medical history is significant for cystic fibrosis. She has never had surgery. She takes oral pancreatic enzyme replacement and she has no known drug allergies. Her blood pressure is 100/60 mm Hg. She has no protein or glucose in her urine. The fetal heart rate is in the 150s/min and her uterine size is appropriate for her dates. The patient and her husband, who is also white, are very concerned about their child having cystic fibrosis. They should be advised that:

(A) Cystic fibrosis is no longer a reason for pregnancy termination.
(B) It is too late in the pregnancy for testing to be performed.
(C) Testing can be performed on the father of the baby.
(D) The fetus cannot have cystic fibrosis.
(E) The fetus likely has cystic fibrosis.

46. A 23-year-old woman who is at 30 weeks' gestation with her third child comes to the office for a prenatal visit. Her pregnancy has been uncomplicated thus far, including unremarkable prenatal labs (e.g., negative HIV and syphilis testing). Her obstetric history is notable for 2 term vaginal deliveries following uncomplicated pregnancies. She has no medical problems. She had a tonsillectomy as a child and an appendectomy as an 18-year-old. She takes no medications and has no known drug allergies. Her family history is unremarkable. The baby is moving well. She has no contractions, bleeding per vagina, or loss of fluid. Her blood pressure is 108/72 mm Hg and she has no protein or glucose on her urine dip. Her fundal height is 31 cm. The fetal heart rate is in the 150s/min. A complete blood count that was sent 2 weeks ago shows:

Leukocyte count	9900/mm^3
Hematocrit	36%
Platelets	84,000/mm^3

The most likely diagnosis is

(A) gestational thrombocytopenia
(B) HIV infection
(C) immune thrombocytopenia purpura (ITP)
(D) pre-eclampsia
(E) pseudothrombocytopenia

47. A 33-year-old woman comes to the health center for an annual examination. She has no complaints at this time. She has sickle-cell anemia with occasional pain crises and a recent history of chlamydia. She has never had surgery, takes no medications, and is allergic to penicillin. She lives with her mother and 2 children. She is sexually active with one partner and intermittently uses condoms for contraception. She does not smoke, drink alcohol, or use illegal drugs. Physical examination, including breast and pelvic examination, is unremarkable. She is concerned because she is sexually active, but does not wish to become pregnant. Some of her friends use the intrauterine device (IUD), others use depot medroxyprogesterone acetate (DMPA), and she wants to know what you would recommend. In discussing contraceptive options with this patient, the most appropriate advice is:

(A) Abstinence is the only appropriate method of birth control
(B) DMPA has been shown to reduce the incidence of pain crises
(C) DMPA is contraindicated in patients with sickle-cell disease
(D) The IUD would be recommended in her case
(E) There is no appropriate contraceptive option for patients with sickle-cell anemia

48. An 18-year-old previously healthy girl comes to the clinic because of fevers and abdominal pain for the past week. She is also complaining of pain on urination. Her last menstrual period was 2 weeks ago and she states that it was more painful than usual. She describes the pain as intermittent, located in the lower abdomen, and nonradiating. She has been sexually active since she was 15 years old, and currently has 2 partners. She is "on the pill" and uses condoms "almost every time." Her temperature is 39.5 C (103.1 F). Examination shows lower abdominal, adnexal, and cervical motion tenderness and a mucopurulent cervical discharge. Urinalysis is unremarkable. At this time the most correct statement about her condition is:

(A) An intrauterine device would be an appropriate form of contraception after this episode
(B) Her risk of infertility will increase if she has repeated episodes of this condition
(C) It is unlikely that her inconsistent condom use contributed to this condition
(D) There is a less than 1% chance of long-term sequelae
(E) There is little association between her condition and sexually transmitted diseases, such as HIV

49. A 19-year-old woman is admitted to the hospital for an asthma exacerbation. On day 2 of her admission she complains to her night nurse of intense pain and pruritus in her genital region and upper thighs. The nurse reports this finding to you, as she knows that the patient will probably be discharged the next day since her asthma is already under control. The patient was given acetaminophen overnight for the pain but its effects have long since worn off. The rash consists of scattered vesicles on the labia minor and majora and on the inner thighs bilaterally. Some are grouped, others are single. Many vesicles are excoriated from being scratched. The mouth and eyes are not involved and there is no other body rash present. The patient adamantly states that she has "never had anything like this before." She does admit to having sexual intercourse for the very first time with her new boyfriend last week. You scrape the base of one of the vesicles with a swab and send it to the lab for a viral culture. You perform a Tzanck smear on another lesion, which you take to the lab yourself to read. The Tzanck smear is positive. The most appropriate management at this time is to

(A) prescribe intravenous acyclovir and keep her in the hospital for a few more days despite her improving asthma exacerbation; she should also be advised to use a barrier method during sexual intercourse but only when she is having an identical outbreak

(B) prescribe oral acyclovir and advise her to use condoms when engaging in sexual intercourse whenever she has an identical herpes simplex outbreak

(C) prescribe oral acyclovir and advise her to use condoms whenever she has sexual intercourse since there is asymptomatic shedding of the herpes virus

(D) prescribe topical penciclovir as there is no need to treat with oral antivirals in this self-limited disease and advise her against having intercourse while these lesions are present, but she can "go about her business" once these lesions are crusted over

(E) send the patient home when she is cleared with her primary team since it is best to await the results of the viral culture (only 1-2 days); herpes simplex type 1 and type 2 are managed differently and this will allow the patient to be treated appropriately; she should be advised to refrain from sexual intercourse during this outbreak only

50. A previously continent 82-year-old woman with diabetes mellitus and hypertension is admitted to the hospital after a left hemispheric stroke resulting in receptive and expressive aphasia and mild weakness of the right upper and lower extremities. After admission she is noted to be incontinent of urine. The incontinence is unrelated to coughing. Her post void residual volume (PRV) is 70 ml. The most appropriate initial management for this patient's urinary incontinence is to

(A) establish a better communication system with her caregivers

(B) insert an indwelling catheter

(C) insert a vaginal pessary

(D) perform clean intermittent catheterization every 8 hours

(E) recommend pelvic floor exercises

Obstetrics/Gynecology Test Three: Answers and Explanations

ANSWER KEY

1. D
2. D
3. A
4. B
5. A
6. D
7. C
8. C
9. B
10. C
11. D
12. D
13. C
14. B
15. D
16. A
17. E
18. B
19. E
20. D
21. D
22. A
23. D
24. C
25. B
26. A
27. D
28. B
29. C
30. A
31. D
32. C
33. E
34. C
35. C
36. E
37. A
38. E
39. D
40. C
41. B
42. A
43. A
44. E
45. C
46. A
47. B
48. B
49. C
50. A

1. **The correct answer is D.** In view of the high serum glucose on the 1-hour glucose test the next most appropriate step would be to get a 3-hour glucose tolerance test to rule out the possibility of gestational diabetes. If this is positive, the patient should then be transferred to the obstetrics clinic as a high-risk pregnancy with gestational diabetes. The management course would then include a discussion with the patient about managing the gestational diabetes through dietary intervention or starting pharmacotherapy with long-acting NPH and regular insulin (**choice A**).

   At this stage, antepartum fetal surveillance in high-risk insulin-dependent diabetes mellitus would include a sonogram (**choice B**) at 4 to 6-week intervals (to rule out macrosomia with an elective caesarian section at full term discussed as an option with the patient), a non-stress test every 2 weeks, contraction stress tests and biophysical profiles if the non-stress test is nonreactive, a lung profile at 37 to 38 weeks, and daily maternal assessment of fetal activity.

   Reassuring this patient that the prenatal course is going well (**choice C**) before the 3-hour glucose test would be inappropriate.

   Start a diet consisting mainly of complex carbohydrates, low in saturated fats and soluble fiber (**choice E**) is incorrect because the recommended dietary management of diabetes in pregnancy generally consists of complex carbohydrates (not simple sugars), soluble fiber, low in fat while reduced in saturated fats.

2. **The correct answer is D.** This patient has pyelonephritis: fever, costovertebral angle tenderness, and signs and symptoms of a urinary tract infection. Occurring in approximately 1 to 2% of all pregnancies, pyelonephritis is an important source of maternal morbidity and is the most common non-obstetric cause of hospitalization during pregnancy. Acute pyelonephritis should be treated on an inpatient basis as soon as the presumptive diagnosis is made. After an episode of acute pyelonephritis, antibiotic suppression should be initiated and continued for the remainder of the pregnancy.

   Since pyelonephritis in pregnancy is not an uncommon, straightforward diagnosis in pregnancy, a formal renal consult (**choice A**) should not be necessary.

   This patient is presenting with a straightforward case of pyelonephritis in pregnancy. There is no reason to suspect a primary bladder lesion or dysfunction at this time, and thus, a cystoscopy (**choice B**) is not warranted.

   A renal ultrasound (**choice C**) is also not indicated, as there is no reason to suspect kidney abnormalities from this one episode of pyelonephritis.

   Pyelonephritis has serious consequences in pregnant women, and should not be dismissed lightly. Advising her to increase fluid consumption, to empty her bladder frequently, and return again with the first sign of any infection (**choice E**) are precautions that should be told to patients, but antibiotic suppression must also be given.

3. **The correct answer is A.** Any woman presenting with a lesion on her vulva must have the lesion biopsied before any treatment begins. An easy office punch biopsy can be done for a definitive tissue diagnosis. The most important thing to rule out is vulvar cancer, which accounts for 5% of all gynecologic malignancies. Average age of diagnosis of squamous cell carcinomas (90% of vulvar cancers) is 65. The most frequent symptom is vulvar itching, but some women present with bleeding, discharge, or dysuria. On physical exam, a vulvar cancer is usually raised and may appear fleshy, ulcerated, leukoplakia, or wartlike. Diagnosis is based solely on biopsy.

   Treatment with estrogen cream (**choice B**) or boric acid (**choice D**) is inappropriate because a biopsy should be performed to rule out a malignancy before any treatment is given.

   Vulvar changes are not normal for any age group (**choice C**), and any lesion must be biopsied.

   Only after an office biopsy is performed can treatment be given. If your suspicion is correct and biopsy confirms lichen sclerosis, then the best treatment is a topical corticosteroid (**choice E**).

4. **The correct answer is B.** The most likely diagnosis for this patient is a physiologic cyst that will likely regress over the next 1 or 2 menstrual cycles. Cysts that are less than 10 cm and have a benign pattern on ultrasound are most likely benign in the premenopausal woman. If the cyst persists over a full cycle, it may represent a benign neoplasia. Repeat exam in 6 weeks will allow for probable regression of the simple cyst.

   CA-125 (**choice A**) is often elevated in women with epithelial ovarian cancer. However, it is a poor screening test for young women as it can often be elevated with benign disease such as endometriosis, fibroids, or even pregnancy. If the patient had a persistent pelvic tumor, a CA-125 may be warranted for determining baseline value prior to definitive therapy.

Subjecting the patient to surgery with a diagnostic laparoscopy and possible cystectomy (**choice C**) at this point is unnecessary, as the visualized cyst is most likely a physiologic cyst that will regress within one or two menstrual cycles. If the cyst grows, persists, or changes its appearance surgery may be an appropriate next step. However, the patient still needs to be reexamined before this decision can be made.

CT scan of the abdomen and pelvis (**choice D**) would not add anything to the management of this case, and would expose the patient to unnecessary radiation. In addition, a pelvic ultrasound is the gold-standard diagnostic tool for the pelvis.

The use of oral contraceptives (**choice E**) would not increase the likelihood of regression of this cyst. In addition, it would be desirable to follow up with this patient before 3 months. Although you want to give the cyst time to change, you don't want to leave too much of an interim period between exams.

5. **The correct answer is A.** The organization of an infertility evaluation requires consideration of each of the factors of reproduction: male, ovulatory, pelvic, and cervical. This patient has achieved a pregnancy in the past, confirming that she has the ability to ovulate and conceive. In addition, if this patient achieves menstruation and a change in basal body temperature every month, she is most likely currently having ovulatory cycles. The most cost-effective and highest yield next step would be an evaluation of male factor. Male factor is responsible for approximately 35% of infertility cases. Sperm analysis includes parameters for motility, ejaculate volume, concentration, and morphology.

   Ovulatory factor is responsible for approximately 20% of cases of infertility. Measuring prolactin (**choice B**) for galactorrhea or TSH (**choice C**) for hyper- or hypothyroidism, along with hirsutism, severe weight loss, obesity, and severe psychological stress should be taken into consideration in infertility patients. However, with a normal review of systems and physical exam, as well as probable ovulatory function as described above, evaluation of male factor is the most appropriate next step for this patient.

   The pelvic organs indeed need to be evaluated as part of a thorough infertility evaluation. However, hysteroscopy (**choice D**) is an invasive procedure that is most often preceded by other methods of structural evaluation. For example, a hysterosalpingogram is a less invasive primary study that allows for visualization of the uterus and tubes. Hysteroscopy does not evaluate tubal patency unless coupled with laparoscopic chromotubation. Again, laparoscopy (**choice E**) is an invasive procedure that is not warranted at this point in this patient's infertility evaluation.

6. **The correct answer is D.** Maternal serum screening is a non-invasive method of obtaining information about fetal development that can be used early in pregnancy. Maternal serum alpha-fetoprotein is elevated in certain fetal malformations, and a lower value is associated with some chromosomal abnormalities. A normal result from this screening test does not insure that the fetus will not have a birth defect, and conversely, a positive result does not mean that the fetus is necessarily affected. A positive result does, however, warrant further evaluation. The most appropriate next step in evaluation is a targeted ultrasound examination. This should include accurate dating (and adjustment of the maternal serum screen appropriately), as well as checking for multiple gestation, fetal demise, and abnormal structural markers. Ultrasound is non-invasive and can often be diagnostic of several fetal abnormalities.

   This patient needs further evaluation of her abnormal screening test. A positive result does not necessarily mean an affected fetus. Once a diagnosis is confirmed, enrollment in a high-risk clinic (**choice A**) may be appropriate.

   Once a suspicion of abnormality is confirmed by ultrasound, the patient may wish to undergo more invasive testing in the form of an amniocentesis. Or, even if no abnormality is found on ultrasound, a patient may elect further invasive testing in the form of an amniocentesis to finalize a negative result. A low maternal alpha-fetoprotein may indicate chromosomal abnormalities, while a high result will indicate fetal abnormalities more often distinct from chromosomal abnormalities, such as neural tube defects. Amniotic fluid alpha-fetoprotein (**choice C**) is a good indicator of a fetal abnormality, with a high value indicating abnormality. Although a karyotype (**choice B**) is more often performed for low results, it would be appropriate to draw a karyotype at the same time as an amniotic fluid alpha-fetoprotein. However, although it may eventually be performed in this patient's case, an invasive amniocentesis is still not the next step in her care.

   There is no indication to repeat the blood test (**choice E**) in this patient at 18 weeks' gestation. It will only delay diagnosis and therefore may limit her choices once a diagnosis is made. If dating is found to be incorrect on the original sample, the lab may adjust it. A new sample need not be taken.

7. **The correct answer is C.** The most commonly used definition of intrauterine growth restriction (IUGR) is a birth weight of less than the 10th percentile. A fetus that is found to be below the 10th percentile during a pregnancy should be a cause of concern because small fetuses have an increased perinatal morbidity and mortality when compared with larger fetuses. Possible causes of IUGR include chromosomal abnormalities, congenital malformations, multiple gestation, infection, placental abnormalities, malnutrition, maternal vascular or renal disease, maternal thrombophilic disorder, drugs, and hypoxia. A preterm fetus that is found to have growth restriction should have an evaluation to determine its status. Numerous randomized trials have shown that checking the Doppler velocimetry of the fetal umbilical artery is a modality that can reduce perinatal death and unnecessary induction of labor. Absent or reversed end-diastolic flow in the umbilical artery of the fetus suggests poor fetal condition and should prompt further action, including delivery. If the flow is normal, the fetus may be followed until later in gestation with frequent testing.

   To have the patient followup in 4 weeks **(choice A)** would be incorrect. A fetus that is found to be below the 10th percentile during pregnancy may be in poor condition and need to be delivered or at least have intensive fetal testing. Followup in 4 weeks would not be appropriate.

   To initiate an induction of labor **(choice B)** would not be correct. While some fetuses that are below the 10th percentile will be in poor condition, others will simply be "constitutionally small"; for example, if the parents are of small stature. To induce labor in a woman at 30 weeks for a constitutionally small fetus would be incorrect. Rather, the fetus should be tested to determine if its small size represents poor condition.

   To perform immediate cesarean delivery **(choice D)** would also be incorrect. Again, it is not clear if this small fetus is in an inhospitable intrauterine environment or simply of small stature. To deliver this fetus so early (30 weeks) solely on the basis of the estimated fetal weight would be incorrect.

   To start magnesium sulfate therapy **(choice E)** would not be correct. Magnesium sulfate is used in obstetrics to prevent seizures in patients with pre-eclampsia or eclampsia (to prevent further seizures) and to stop preterm labor. It would not be indicated in this patient.

8. **The correct answer is C.** Phenylketonuria (PKU) is an autosomal recessive metabolic disorder of phenylalanine metabolism. Patients with this disorder have a deficiency of the enzyme phenylalanine hydroxylase that can lead to elevated blood phenylalanine levels and severe mental retardation. Early dietary therapy can markedly reduce the likelihood of development of mental retardation in affected individuals. Sadly, many women with this disorder stop following the special diet as they get older. If this diet is not followed, the fetus of an affected mother will be exposed to elevated phenylalanine levels and is highly likely to develop mental retardation and/or microcephaly. In fact, estimates are that when women with PKU do not follow their diet before and during pregnancy, infants born to them have a 93% risk for mental retardation and a 72% risk for microcephaly. It is therefore imperative that this patient follow a special diet during the pregnancy.

   To state that no intervention is necessary **(choice A)** is incorrect. As noted above, when no intervention takes place (i.e., when a special PKU diet is not followed) the risk of mental retardation and microcephaly in the offspring is immense.

   To state that the father of the baby must be tested for PKU **(choice B)** is incorrect. While it may be helpful to know what the father's status is to determine if the offspring has a risk of developing the disease, whatever the father's status, the patient must follow a special diet to prevent microcephaly and mental retardation in her fetus.

   To tell the patient to have an ultrasound each trimester **(choice D)** is not an effective strategy to prevent her fetus from developing mental retardation or microcephaly. Ultrasound is useful to diagnose conditions, but it is dietary intervention that is needed for this patient to prevent disability for her offspring.

   To tell the patient to have a weekly non-stress test **(choice E)** is also not an effective strategy to prevent the development of mental retardation or microcephaly. Non-stress testing is a fetal testing modality that can be used to determine the reactivity of the fetal heart rate. It would not prevent mental retardation or microcephaly in this case.

9. **The correct answer is B.** Osteoporosis is a major problem in the United States, accounting for a significant amount of morbidity and mortality. Treatments are available, but identification of patients with osteoporosis can be difficult because it often occurs without obvious symptoms. Therefore, screening is necessary. The most effective method of screening for osteoporosis is

with bone mineral density testing. Current recommendations by the National Osteoporosis Foundation (1998) and the American College of Obstetricians and Gynecologists (2002) are that bone mineral density testing should be recommended to all women aged 65 or over, women younger than 65 with risk factors, and all postmenopausal women with fractures. This 67-year-old patient should, therefore, have bone mineral density testing. Several techniques are available with dual-energy x-ray absorptiometry (DEXA) being considered the "gold standard."

To order a serum CA-125 level for ovarian cancer screening (**choice A**) would not be correct. Using CA-125 levels to screen for ovarian cancer is not currently a recommended standard of care.

To order urine N-telopeptide for osteoporosis screening (**choice C**) would be incorrect. Urine N-telopeptide is one of the biomarkers of bone turnover. These biomarkers have large individual variability, only modest correlation with bone density, and are not currently recommended for use in screening for osteoporosis.

To perform an endometrial biopsy for endometrial cancer screening (**choice D**) would not be correct. Screening for endometrial cancer is not currently recommended. Furthermore, endometrial biopsy is an invasive test with potential infectious and bleeding complications and not an ideal screening test.

To schedule an ultrasound for ovarian cancer screening (**choice E**) would be incorrect. Routine ultrasound for ovarian cancer screening is not currently a recommended standard of care.

10. **The correct answer is C.** Low molecular weight heparin is the drug of choice in this situation. It is convenient and does not require inpatient intravenous infusion, and there is no need for regular blood work to monitor partial thromboplastin time (PTT).

This patient needs full anticoagulation, and aspirin (**choice A**) is simply not enough for her. It has been shown to reduce the risk of recurrent myocardial infarction, and probably stroke, but has no role in this setting.

IVC filter placement (**choice B**) is indicated for a patient who "failed" anticoagulation therapy (e.g., had a DVT while on therapy for heparin or warfarin) or for whom anticoagulation is contraindicated (e.g., GI bleeding or high risk for intracranial hemorrhage).

Subcutaneous heparin 5000 units BID (**choice D**) is incorrect. This is a prophylactic dose and this patient has a DVT and needs full anticoagulation.

Warfarin (**choice E**) is teratogenic, contraindicated in pregnancy, and would prompt a lawsuit!

11. **The correct answer is D.** This patient has stage I breast cancer, as the tumor size is 1 cm and she has no evidence of metastatic disease from the information given. Tamoxifen therapy for 5 years will decrease her risk of developing a subsequent breast cancer by approximately 50%. Patients such as this are at significantly higher risk than the general population for developing another, contralateral, breast malignancy.

No further therapy (**choice A**) is incorrect as she is at increased risk of a new contralateral breast cancer and should take chemoprevention for 5 years.

The decision to test for the BRCA1 and BRCA2 genes (**choice B**) is complicated, subjective, and generally you wouldn't be expected to know any more about this for Step 3 other than referring a patient to a genetic counselor at the patient's discretion. Generally you might only recommend testing a patient who requested it and had more than one first-degree relative diagnosed with breast cancer at a young age. Less than 10% of patients with breast cancer are thought to be positive for the gene.

Lumpectomy with axillary node dissection is as effective in preventing tumor recurrence as radical mastectomy, and a bilateral mastectomy (**choice C**) has no role here. It may play a role if the patient is at very high risk (e.g., strong family history, early menarche, nulliparous, etc.) and desires this treatment, but it is inappropriate in this woman with early-stage disease who may have been cured.

Although tamoxifen is appropriate in this setting, lifelong treatment (**choice E**) unnecessarily increases this patient's odds of developing endometrial cancer, as tamoxifen is estrogenic in certain tissues (e.g., bone, endometrium) while being antiestrogenic in others (i.e., breast). Five years is the current recommended duration of treatment after primary therapy for breast cancer.

12. **The correct answer is D.** Pregnant women are at a high risk for developing pyelonephritis and recurrent bacteriuria. All pregnant women should be screened for urinary tract infections. Because of the increased risk for complications, all pregnant women, symptomatic or asymptomatic, should be treated. She should continue

taking the clindamycin. For this reason, deferring antibiotics because the colony count is not large enough (**choice E**) is incorrect.

Chloramphenicol may accumulate to toxic levels because the fetus lacks the ability to metabolize or excrete the drug. This causes "the gray syndrome" associated with cardiovascular collapse (**choice A**).

Choosing the appropriate antibiotic during pregnancy is crucial. Tetracyclines may cause acute maternal liver decompensation and fetal malformations. Also, the chelating action of tetracycline causes hypoplasia and staining of teeth (**choice B**).

The fluoroquinolones are contraindicated during pregnancy because of the potential adverse effects on cartilage formation (**choice C**).

13. **The correct answer is C.** The U.S. Environmental Protection Agency (EPA) advises women who may become pregnant, nursing mothers, and young children to limit freshwater fish caught by family and friends to one meal per week (i.e., less than 6 ounces for adults and less than 2 ounces for children), to limit ocean fish caught by family and friends, and to avoid eating shark, swordfish, king mackerel, and tile fish. Pregnant women can safely eat an average of 12 ounces per week of fish purchased in stores or restaurants, canned fish, smaller ocean fish, and farm-raised fish.

    Advising her that all fish should be avoided while pregnant (**choice A**) and that there are no restrictions on eating fish (**choice E**) is therefore incorrect.

    Raw fish (**choice B**) and all *raw* meats should be avoided or kept to a minimum during pregnancy because of potential parasitic infections.

    Even *cooked* fish (**choice D**) should be kept to a minimum (see above) because of the organic mercury content. The most important source of methyl-mercury poisoning in the United States is consumption of contaminated fish. In the developing brain, organic mercury (methyl- and ethyl-mercury) is toxic to the cerebral and cerebellar cortex, causing focal necrosis of neurons and destruction of glial cells. Organic mercury is also a teratogen. It interferes with neuronal migration and the organization of brain nuclei and layering of the cortical neurons. In the Minamata Bay (Japan) disaster and the Iraq epidemic, mothers exposed to large amounts of mercury gave birth to infants with psychomotor retardation, blindness, deafness, and seizures.

14. **The correct answer is B.** Although all of the above are prevalent in a patient with spinal cord injury (SCI), autonomic dysreflexia (AD) poses the greatest threat. AD is manifested by hypertension that is associated with headache, bradycardia, cardiac arrhythmia, sweating, flushing, tingling, nasal congestion, and occasional respiratory distress. Uteroplacental vasoconstriction may result in fetal hypoxemia. If severe, it can cause hypertensive encephalopathy, stroke, and even death. AD can be triggered by any stimulus, even distension of the vagina, bladder, bowel, or even simple manipulation such as changing a urinary catheter. It only occurs in incompletely transected spinal cord injuries as a result of loss of hypothalamic control over sympathetic spinal reflexes that occur in viable cord segment distal to the level of injury.

    Although anemia (**choice A**) occurs in 63% of women with SCI, it is not a cause of serious morbidity during pregnancy.

    Transection of the spinal cord above a low thoracic level will make labor pain so reduced in intensity and quality as to make the patient unaware of uterine contractions (**choice C**). The only way these patients know they are in labor is from concurrent sympathetic nervous system symptoms of labor such as abdominal or leg spasms and shortness of breath. This does not cause the greatest threat to her and her developing fetus, however.

    Although decubitus ulcers (**choice D**) are a cause of morbidity, they are not initially life-threatening. Patients should be made aware of the importance of appropriate padding, frequency of position changes, elevation of legs, and range-of-motion exercises.

    Eighty percent of SCI patients have urinary tract infections (**choice E**). Suppressive antibiotic therapy and treatment for concomitant yeast vaginitis may be appropriate in selected patients.

15. **The correct answer is D.** *Vaccinium macrocarpon* is the scientific name for the American cranberry plant, which is a small evergreen shrub. A study done at Harvard reported the results of the first large-scale, placebo-controlled trial that demonstrated the ability of cranberry juice to prevent UTIs. Another study published in *J.A.M.A.* also revealed that participants who drank cranberry juice were more than 50% less likely to show evidence of asymptomatic urinary tract infections. Recent research suggests that cranberry prohibits *Escherichia coli* from adhering to the inner lining of the urinary tract. The study published in the New England Journal of Medicine in 1998 reported that compounds

called proanthocyanidins prevent bacteria from adhering to the wall of the urinary tract. Therefore it is incorrect that there is no scientific evidence for your recommendation (**choice E**).

At one time it was believed that cranberry juice could acidify urine (**choice A**), thereby inhibiting the growth of bacteria and preventing urinary tract infections. This is not, however, our current understanding.

There is no scientific data to suggest that cranberry extract produces diuresis (**choice B**) and that the diuresis is responsible for decreasing UTIs.

There is no evidence that cranberry extract is by itself bacteriostatic (**choice C**).

16. **The correct answer is A.** In evaluating a trauma patient, important life-saving information can be derived from diagnostic imaging. None of the listed imaging modalities is contraindicated during pregnancy. Even nuclear medicine modalities such as ventilation perfusion scans, bone, and renal scans are allowed. The only modality absolutely contraindicated during pregnancy is the use of radioactive isotopes of iodine (specifically [^{131}I]), because they can adversely affect the fetal thyroid gland. Barium enema exposes the fetus to approximately 2 to 4 rad (note: 1 Gy = 100 rad). Although it is one of the highest radiation-producing sources, its use is allowed during pregnancy because the threshold for adverse effect is in the range of 20 to 40 rad and is the most harmful to the developing nervous system between 8 to 15 weeks of gestation.

    A chest x-ray (**choice B**) with two views only exposes the fetus to 0.02 to 0.07 mrad.

    Although a CT scan of the abdomen (**choice C**) can expose a fetus to 3.5 rad, it is not contraindicated during pregnancy.

    A CT scan of the head (**choice D**) exposes the fetus to less than 1 rad.

    A small bowel series (**choice E**) exposes the fetus to 2 to 4 rad but its use is allowed during pregnancy.

17. **The correct answer is E.** There are few studies available to predict the actual risk for acquiring a sexually transmissible infection during sexual assault, but trichomonas infection may be the most likely to be acquired. The risk for acquiring other infections is lower: HIV (<1%), gonorrhea (6-12%), and syphilis (3%).

    Emergency contraception (which consists of 4 oral contraceptive pills with high-dose estrogen given 12 hours apart) used to be recommended up to 72 hours, not 48 hours (**choice A**) after sexual assault, but now some researchers suggest that it can be effective for up to 120 hours.

    Informed consent must be obtained before the examination of a sexual assault victim is begun and specimens are collected (**choice B**). In addition to fulfilling legal requirements, this informed consent process also helps the victim participate in regaining control of her body and her life.

    Injuries may be present around the vulva and rectum because of manipulation of these areas with the hand or penis. Such lesions are more common in children who have not had sexual intercourse before and in older women, and are not commonly found in all age groups (**choice C**).

    A chaperone or a victim advocate, not a police officer (**choice D**) should be present during the history-taking and physical examination to reassure the victim and provide support.

18. **The correct answer is B.** When explaining the risks of blood transfusion, immunologic risk of fever, chills, and urticaria are the most common, occurring in 1 out of 50 to 100 transfusions. Hemolytic transfusion reaction occurs in 1 out of 6000 transfusions because of ABO incompatibility, usually attributable to clerical error. Fatal transfusion reactions occur in 1 out of 100,000 transfusions. The most common infectious risk (accounting for 80-90% of transfusion infections) is hepatitis C. Currently available anti-hepatitis C tests fail to detect up to 10% of HCV-infected blood. Therefore, 1 in every 3300 units of transfused blood may contain hepatitis C virus.

    HBV (**choice A**) accounts for 10% of infections caused by blood transfusion. One out of every 50,000 to 200,000 units of transfused blood will contain HBV.

    Few infections acquired from blood transfusion are caused by HDV (**choice C**). This virus requires simultaneous or prior infection with HBV to be able to infect.

    HIV (**choice D**) accounts for <1% of transfusion-associated infections. One in every 200,000 to 1,000,000 units of blood transfused will contain HIV.

    HTLV (**choice E**) accounts for fewer blood transfusion-related infections than all of the above.

19. **The correct answer is E.** Cisplatin is associated with nausea and vomiting. Gastrointestinal symptoms begin 1 to 6 hours after starting IV infusion and subside within 24 hours. Nausea and vomiting may persist days after infusion. Intravenous hydration before and after chemotherapy will mitigate these symptoms. When prolonged nausea and vomiting are associated with orthostatic changes, intravenous hydration is needed.

    5HT3 receptor antagonists, such as ondansetron (**choice A**), are effective when taken before cisplatin administration to alleviate anticipatory nausea and vomiting. They are, however, ineffective at controlling delayed onset emesis 3 to 5 days after chemotherapy. Metoclopramide is effective for delayed onset emesis.

    It is inappropriate to simply admit her to the hospital for observation (**choice B**) when a patient has intractable nausea, vomiting, orthostatic vital signs, has only voided once during the day, and requires intravenous hydration.

    A nasogastric tube (**choice C**) is not necessary in this case. Intravenous hydration is.

    Absence of gastrointestinal bleeding, obstruction, or pancreatitis makes abdominal flat and upright radiographs (**choice D**) unnecessary. After hydration, serum chemistry, amylase, and lipase may be used to rule out electrolyte imbalance and pancreatitis.

20. **The correct answer is D.** No alteration in sexual practice is advised during pregnancy except if the patient has placenta previa, premature rupture of membranes, or a history of early premature labor.

    Although positions used for intercourse often change based on comfort, there is no evidence that special practices are necessary (**choice A**).

    Although frequency of intercourse may decrease as pregnancy progresses (**choice B**), most of this is because of discomfort, change in interest, and increase in noncoital activity such as holding and caressing.

    Although reports of air embolism from blowing into the vagina have been reported in the literature, oral-genital activities (**choice C**) pose no special risk for mother and fetus.

    Condoms (**choice E**) are not necessary because she is in a mutually monogamous relationship and because she is already pregnant.

21. **The correct answer is D.** Cigarette smoking accounts for 80 to 90% of chronic obstructive pulmonary disease (COPD). Symptoms include productive or nonproductive cough and dyspnea. Preoperative assessment should include a chest x-ray to rule out lung cancer, and pulmonary function testing to assess degree of impairment or obstruction. The diagnosis of COPD is made when FEV_1/FVC is <70%. The patient should stop smoking at least 2 to 3 days before surgery but preferably 8 weeks before.

    Screening preoperative ABG (**choice A**) in a patient with COPD is of value only for a patient undergoing coronary artery bypass graft (CABG) or lung resection.

    No additional testing (**choice B**) is incorrect as this patient should undergo pulmonary function testing.

    PPD and anergy panel (**choice C**) is unnecessary in a patient without risk factors who is about to undergo surgery.

    Sputum culture and sensitivity (**choice E**) is reserved for a patient with productive cough who fails to respond to standard pharmacologic therapy.

22. **The correct answer is A.** Women are the fastest growing population with AIDS in the United States. Certain types of infections or uncommon sites or failure to clear infections despite appropriate therapy should alert to the possibility of HIV. For example, Candida esophagitis and ulcerative HSV occur in AIDS. Recurrent vaginal candidiasis occurs even when CD4 lymphocyte counts are high.

    Protein electrophoresis (**choice B**) is not diagnostically useful in this patient.

    Recurrent infections may prompt a screening test for diabetes mellitus (**choice C**). However, the nature of this infection and the presence of thrush-like patches in her oral pharynx are highly suspect for AIDS.

    Recurrent fungal infection with treatment should prompt fungal typing (**choice D**). This is not the most appropriate diagnostic test, however, as this patient might be infected with HIV and should be diagnosed as soon as possible.

    A significant increase in syphilis has been reported in some areas with high prevalence for seropositivity for HIV. Evaluation for syphilis (**choice E**) is reasonable but it is important to test for HIV first.

23. **The correct answer is D.** Chronic vulvar pain or vulvar vestibulitis consists of severe pain to light touch. It has a high incidence with coexistent fungal vaginitis and it may be sensitive to topical fungal creams. Low-dose amitriptyline and imipramine has been shown to be effective.

Pain should not be treated initially with a narcotic such as fentanyl (**choice A**) until an etiology is found.

Human papillomavirus (HPV) can cause vestibulitis. Therapy with interferon alpha (**choice B**) has an 18% response rate.

Psychologic etiology of vulvar vestibulitis has been proposed. Psychologic problems arising from marital conflict, history of sexual abuse, or somatization has been suggested.

Use of intensive psychotherapy (**choice C**) is not the initial treatment.

Surgery (**choice E**) should be reserved for a patient who has failed conservative therapies.

24. **The correct answer is C.** Women who have used oral contraceptive pills have lower risk for invasive epithelial ovarian cancer than nonusers.

There is no consistent data about early age of menarche (**choice A**) or age at menopause (**choice B**) being risk factors for ovarian cancer.

Although higher parity (**choice D**) and longer duration of breast-feeding have been associated with protection against ovarian cancer, this patient has only given birth once and parity therefore does not affect her risk for ovarian cancer as much as OCPs.

Smoking (**choice E**) has not been as significantly linked to the development of ovarian cancer as it is to cervical cancer.

25. **The correct answer is B.** PPV shows the likelihood that a positive test result (HIV positive test) actually indicates presence of disease. Because her HIV test is positive, this information is most useful for this patient.

Negative predictive value (**choice A**) is the likelihood that a negative test indicates the lack of disease.

Sensitivity (**choice C**) is the proportion of patients with disease who have a positive test. It is a measure of how good a test is at detecting disease in the population.

Specificity (**choice D**) is the proportion of patients without disease who have a negative test; in other words, how good the test is at detecting the nondiseased population.

26. **The correct answer is A.** Irregular bleeding occurs in almost all women using depot medroxyprogesterone acetate (DMPA). In the first months of use, this irregular bleeding and spotting can last up to a week at a time or longer. Typically, with continued use, the irregular bleeding lessens significantly. Fifty percent of women on DMPA for a year will have complete amenorrhea. These rates increase further in users who continue beyond 1 year. Irregular bleeding is an important side effect of DMPA because it is the main cause of discontinuation of this method. The irregular bleeding can be treated with estrogen. Unfortunately, however, the menstrual irregularities recur when the estrogen is stopped. The best way of addressing this common side effect is with patient education: patients must be informed before starting the method that irregular bleeding is likely and that it is very unlikely to represent pregnancy, cancer, or other gynecologic illness. Those patients for whom regular menses are important are better served by another method of contraception.

Endometrial cancer (**choice B**) or endometrial hyperplasia (**choice C**) is not the most likely cause for this patient's irregular bleeding. Endometrial cancer and endometrial hyperplasia are more common in older women and in women with menstrual irregularities (e.g., oligo-ovulation). This woman is a 31-year-old woman with a long history of regular menstrual cycles who has just started DMPA. Therefore, her irregular bleeding is most likely secondary to this method of contraception. Endometrial biopsy, dilatation and curettage, or hysteroscopy would not be indicated for this patient. If, however, the irregular bleeding persists over time or increases, or amenorrhea does not begin to develop in this patient on DMPA, then further evaluation may be warranted.

Pregnancy (**choice D**) is unlikely to be causing this patient's irregular bleeding because her urine pregnancy test is negative. However, it is essential that this pregnancy test be sent because DMPA is not 100% effective as a birth-control method. Any woman of reproductive age with irregular vaginal bleeding should have a urine or serum hCG sent to rule out pregnancy.

Spontaneous abortion (**choice E**) can cause irregular bleeding in reproductive-age patients. This patient, however, has a negative pregnancy test and a far more likely cause for her irregular menses (i.e., DMPA use).

27. **The correct answer is D.** This medication regimen is one of the FDA-approved emergency contraception options for women. Criteria for its use include unprotected intercourse less than 72 hours ago. These medications should not be used in patients in whom you suspect pregnancy. Since this patient has used contraception regularly and has had normal menses, pregnancy is unlikely. This regimen in addition to 2 doses of 0.75 mg levonorgestrel 12 hours apart are dedicated products available for emergency contraception. Both of these methods will prevent approximately 75% of unwanted pregnancies. There are combinations of the usual oral contraceptive pills that can also be used. Additionally, there is some evidence that the insertion of a copper IUD within 120 hours of unprotected intercourse is successful in preventing unwanted pregnancy. Mifepristone (RU-486) was recently approved by the FDA for pregnancy termination. It has been used in other countries for emergency contraception; this is not currently a FDA-approved indication.

    Telling her that because it has been longer than 12 hours, elective termination is her only option and you can provide her with a list of physicians that will perform the procedure (**choice A**) is incorrect because emergency contraception can decrease the incidence of unwanted pregnancies. The earlier these medications are used, the more effective they are. However, taking these medications within 14 hours is still very likely to prevent an unwanted pregnancy.

    Telling her that it is unlikely that she became pregnant given the timing of her last menstrual period and therefore she should be reassured (**choice B**) is incorrect. Women are most likely to become pregnant in the middle of their cycles. This is when ovulation occurs. This patient has regular menstrual cycles with a last menstrual period of 2 weeks ago and is at high risk of becoming pregnant from unprotected intercourse.

    Telling her that she should start an oral contraceptive agent like 35 micrograms ethinyl estradiol/0.3 milligrams norgestrel now; she should take one pill daily and this will prevent pregnancy from occurring (**choice C**) is incorrect because these doses are found in typical oral contraceptive pills. These pills can be used in combination to achieve the doses necessary to reduce the risk of unwanted pregnancy. However, taking them as regular oral contraceptives will not help prevent pregnancy.

    Telling her that she should wait until she has missed her period and if this happens she would be a candidate for emergency contraception with 2 doses of 0.75 milligrams of levonorgestrel taken 12 hours apart (**choice E**) is incorrect. This is an accepted medical regimen for emergency contraception, but should be given immediately, not at the time of a missed period. At that time implantation will have occurred, and this method of emergency contraception will not prevent pregnancy at this stage.

28. **The correct answer is B.** This patient is showing signs of chorioamnionitis (fever, abdominal tenderness, fetal tachycardia). This is likely secondary to prolonged ruptured membranes. The goal in this situation is to treat the infection with antibiotics and to accomplish delivery as soon as possible for both maternal and fetal well-being. Although the patient is contracting, her cervix is still closed and she therefore is not in labor. Induction with oxytocin is indicated.

    Administering antibiotics alone (**choice A**) is not adequate therapy for chorioamnionitis. The source of infection needs to be removed (i.e., delivered) for maternal reasons. It is also advantageous to the fetus to be removed from the "hostile" environment of infection.

    Betamethasone (**choice C**) is not indicated in patients with greater than 34 weeks' gestation. The benefit of steroids is greatest in patients at less than 32 weeks, but some benefit may be seen up to 34 weeks. This patient is at 36 weeks and therefore should not receive steroids.

    The presence of chorioamnionitis is a contraindication for tocolysis with magnesium sulfate (**choice D**).

    Chorioamnionitis alone is not an indication for cesarean section (**choice E**). If fetal or maternal distress occurred and delivery was remote, it may be necessary. However, at this time the mild maternal and fetal tachycardia are likely related to fever and possibly mild fluid deficit secondary to increased insensible losses. These conditions should be corrected with antipyretics, antibiotics, and fluids. Even if they did not correct, they do not currently meet criteria for distress and a trial for vaginal delivery is indicated.

29. **The correct answer is C.** A young woman who presents with a 3-week history of bleeding needs something immediately to control the bleeding because her vital signs are becoming unstable. It is safe to assume that she is not ovulating because her periods are normally "irregularly irregular." Thus, she is most likely experiencing estrogen breakthrough bleeding associated with long periods of unopposed estrogen. The quickest way to stop her bleeding is with high doses of conjugated estrogen, which will provide growth of endometrial tissue. A progestin should be added after the bleeding is under control to provide protection against the carcinogenic effect of unopposed estrogen on the endometrium.

NSAIDs (**choice A**) can help lessen menstrual blood loss in women who ovulate and thus is the first line of therapy. NSAID would be appropriate in a premenopausal woman who is experiencing menorrhagia (excessive bleeding during periods), and who has regular, predictable cycles.

An oral contraceptive (**choice B**) is not as effective in controlling this patient's severe dysfunctional uterine bleeding (DUB) as estrogen alone.

Progestin therapy (**choice D**) may be appropriate for someone who has endometrial hyperplasia secondary to unopposed estrogen.

Dilatation and curettage (**choice E**) is appropriate in someone whom you suspect may have endometrial hyperplasia or carcinoma, such as a perimenopausal woman with irregular bleeding or someone with polycystic ovarian disease.

30. **The correct answer is A.** The correct answer is the one with the highest risk ratio that is statistically significant. Statistical significance can be determined by examining the confidence intervals associated with each risk estimate. If the number 1.0 occurs within the confidence interval, then the interval indicates nonsignificance. If 1.0 is excluded from the interval, then this indicates statistical significance. Although more than 5 drinks per week (**choice C**) has the highest risk ratio (3.43) the confidence interval indicates nonsignificance. This leaves cigarette smoking, with a risk of 2.81 and a confidence interval that excludes 1.0 as the strongest risk factor.

    The risk associated with a positive family history (**choice B**) and parental history (**choice D**) is nonsignificant because the confidence intervals include 1.0.

    Pregnancy before age 20 (**choice E**) is associated with lower risk.

    Although the risk associated with urban living (**choice F**) is statistically significant at 1.14, it is not as strong a factor as cigarette smoking, which in this study has a risk of 2.81.

31. **The correct answer is D.** Cost-effective management of typical HPV-related condylomata is bichloracetic or trichloroacetic acid application.

    Interferon (**choice A**) and laser ablation (**choice B**) are appropriate in patients with resistant or persistent disease *after* biopsy has confirmed condyloma.

    Podophyllin (**choice C**) is contraindicated in pregnancy.

    Wide local excision (**choice E**) and other surgery are reserved for patients with extensive, widespread disease.

32. **The correct answer is C.** Uterine anomalies are found in <0.5% of the general population. Although there is an increased rate of pregnancy loss with müllerian anomalies, many people end up having a normal reproductive outcome.

    Cervical cerclage (**choices A and B**) has been known to improve reproductive outcome in patients with bicornuate uteri who have had previous reproductive losses. However, cerclage has not been evaluated for prophylactic placement in an initial pregnancy.

    Hysteroscopic excision of uterine septum (**choice D**), whether hysteroscopic or abdominal, is not applicable to the treatment of bicornuate uterus. This management procedure is more fitting for septate uteri.

    Surgical correction (**choice E**) is justified in patients with documented histories of poor reproductive outcome. Interestingly, outcomes improve in subsequent pregnancies, even without treatment.

33. **The correct answer is E.** This patient's history is consistent with sporadic, not familial, breast cancer. Routine gynecologic care is the best management.

    The National Institutes of Health (NIH) recommends prophylactic bilateral salpingo-oophorectomy (**choice A**) for women with 2 or more first-degree relatives with ovarian cancer after completion of childbearing and after the age of 35.

    A patient with a history of familial or hereditary breast-ovarian cancer syndrome may benefit from genetic testing (**choice B**) for BRCA-1 (chromosome 17) and BRCA-2 (chromosome 13). Women carrying the BRCA-1 mutation have an increased risk for both breast and ovarian cancer.

    Management of a patient with suspected hereditary breast or ovarian cancer syndrome may include periodic measurement of CA-125 levels (**choice C**) and transvaginal ultrasonography (**choice D**). This is not a recommended screening technique for people with history of sporadic breast cancer in their family.

34. **The correct answer is C.** A gonadotropin-releasing hormone (GnRH) analogue suppresses pituitary gonadotropin secretion and creates a pseudomenopausal state. It is effective for pain relief for endometriosis for a duration of 6 months. It is not recommended beyond 6

months due to the risk of osteoporosis. It is the most appropriate choice for this patient because she doesn't want surgery.

Danazol (**choice A**) is an androgen-derived ethisterone that reduces pituitary secretion, reduces ovarian steroidogenesis, displaces estrogen from its receptors, and inhibits synthesis of sex hormone-binding globulins. It is not typically the most appropriate initial therapy because of its androgenic side effects (weight gain, breast atrophy, hot flushes, and deepening voice).

High-dose progestins such as depot-medroxyprogesterone acetate (**choice B**) suppress the pituitary gland and decrease production of estrogen by the ovary. They are associated with weight gain, headache, and irregular bleeding. They are not appropriate for this patient who desires pregnancy.

RU-486 (mifepristone) (**choice D**) is an antiprogestin and an antiglucocorticoid, but data on its efficacy for endometriosis are lacking.

This patient has already been on oral contraceptive pills (**choice E**) without any improvement of symptoms.

35. **The correct answer is C.** Influenza vaccination is recommended annually for individuals older than 55, residents of chronic care facilities, and persons with cardiopulmonary or metabolic diseases.

There is no effective screening test for lung cancer today. A chest x-ray (**choice A**) is not recommended, even for smokers.

Cholesterol screening (**choice B**) is recommended every 5 years (not annually) in asymptomatic patients.

Sigmoidoscopy (**choice D**) is recommended every 3 to 5 years (not annually) after age 50.

Annual urinalysis (**choice E**) as a screen for cancer of the bladder and kidney (or for any other reason) in an asymptomatic patient is not recommended.

36. **The correct answer is E.** The incidence of ovarian cancer decreases by 40 to 50% in oral contraceptive pill (OCP) users. Although cancer of the ovary is less common than endometrial cancer, the stage of ovarian cancer at the time of diagnosis is more advanced. As a result, ovarian cancer accounts for more deaths than any other gynecologic cancer. Therefore, protection against ovarian cancer afforded by OCP accounts for the greatest reduction of gynecologic cancer deaths.

The relationship between OCP and breast cancer (**choice A**) has been studied extensively; however, it is still controversial.

OCP has been reported to increase risk of cervical cancer (**choice B**).

There is no evidence yet that OCP has an effect on the incidence of colon (**choice C**), gallbladder, or kidney cancer.

Use of OCP has been reported to decrease the incidence of endometrial cancer (**choice D**) by 50%, but not the number of cancer-related deaths.

37. **The correct answer is A.** Three of the following criteria must be met for the diagnosis of antiphospholipid syndrome: a false-positive test for syphilis (RPR-positive but FTA-negative), the presence of lupus anticoagulant or anticardiolipin antibody (IgG or IgM), arterial or venous thrombosis, connective tissue disease, thrombocytopenia, or unexplained pregnancy loss in first trimester.

Antithrombin III deficiency (**choice B**) and protein C deficiency (**choice D**) are associated with thrombotic events but not with a false-positive test for syphilis.

Polymyalgia rheumatica (**choice C**) is not a disease of younger, reproductive-age women. It is also not seen in pregnancy.

Systemic lupus erythematosus (**choice E**) is not typically associated with thrombotic events or second-trimester loss, but a false-positive test for syphilis may be present.

38. **The correct answer is E.** Sitz baths and other forms of moist heat help treat hemorrhoids by reducing swelling and inflammation. Analgesic creams are helpful for the pain.

Over-the-counter hemorrhoid suppositories (**choice A**) and cream (**choice B**) typically contain hydrocortisone, which is only somewhat helpful in decreasing the swelling. These products work best to relieve itching.

Lifestyle modifications such as increasing dietary fiber (**choice C**), increasing fluid intake, and exercising help prevent constipation, which can both cause and aggravate hemorrhoids.

There is no scientific evidence showing any benefit to intrahemorrhoidal injections with phenol (**choice D**).

39. **The correct answer is D.** Symptoms of dysuria and frequency with a negative leukocyte esterase, low bacteriuria, and pyuria (WBC) are consistent with urethral syndrome.

Infectious or lower urinary tract infection (**choice A**) requires a growth of >100,000 coliform/mL on a midstream urine culture.

Interstitial cystitis (**choice B**) involves transmural inflammation of the bladder wall and petechiae of bladder mucosa of unknown etiology. It is associated with urgency, frequency, dysuria, and a normal microscopic examination of urine.

Traumatic cystitis (**choice C**) typically occurs in an estrogen-deficient woman after engaging in intercourse or following diaphragm use or catheterization of the bladder. It is characterized by recurrent symptoms of hematuria/microhematuria without pyuria.

Vulvar vestibulitis (**choice E**) is characterized by severe pain to light touch of vestibule. Urinalysis is normal.

40. **The correct answer is C.** This patient most likely has gastroesophageal reflux disease (GERD), which is common during pregnancy, occurring in about 70% of pregnant women, especially in the third trimester. It is more prevalent in pregnancy because of decreased lower esophageal sphincter tone due to progesterone secreted by the placenta. Also, gastric acid secretion is increased during pregnancy, progesterone decreases esophageal motility, the growing uterus creates increased abdominothoracic pressure, and levels of the hormone motilin are decreased.

Acute cholecystitis (**choice A**) is the number-two, nonobstetric cause for surgery during pregnancy; appendicitis is number one. The pain begins in the right upper quadrant or epigastric region. Fevers and chills may be present, and Murphy sign is evident on palpation. These patients are also intolerant to fatty foods.

A new occurrence of peptic ulcer (**choice B**) during pregnancy is rare. Even if a patient has an active peptic ulcer before pregnancy, it typically improves during pregnancy due to estrogen-mediated effects on the gastric mucosa and placental production of histaminase, which decreases the effect of gastric acid on the mucosa.

Pain in the central chest or epigastrium that radiates to the ipsilateral arm may be caused by a myocardial infarction (**choice D**). It is associated with dizziness, nausea/vomiting, weakness, sweating, and anxiety. It is rare during pregnancy.

Liver involvement in pre-eclampsia (**choice E**) only occurs in 1% of cases. It typically presents with epigastric or low substernal pain. Also, this patient does not have an elevated blood pressure, which is necessary for this diagnosis.

41. **The correct answer is B.** This patient has livedo vasculitis associated with anticardiolipin antibody syndrome, a cause of her secondary hypercoagulable state that already resulted in 2 miscarriages in addition to her skin disease. Clinically, the vasculopathy is characterized by early, focal, painful, purpuric lesions of the lower extremities that frequently ulcerate and slowly heal with stellate, white scars (called atrophie blanche). It may also cause livedo reticularis (violaceous reticulated discoloration of the skin), telangiectasis, and hemosiderin-induced hyperpigmentation. Livedo vasculitis may be idiopathic or secondary to associated systemic diseases, most commonly the anticardiolipin antibody syndrome, protein C deficiency, hepatitis C, and fibrinolytic abnormalities. Histopathologic evaluation shows a segmental hyalinizing vasculopathy of the small blood vessels in the dermis, and direct immunofluorescence usually reveals fibrin, C3, and IgM in the blood vessel walls. Low-dose aspirin (325 mg or 162 mg once or twice daily) and dipyridamole have been effective, as well as nifedipine 10 mg PO tid and pentoxiphylline 400 mg PO tid. In patients who have had multiple miscarriages as part of the syndrome, anticoagulation with mini-dose heparin throughout the pregnancy is the recommended treatment of choice. The usual dose is anywhere from 5000 units every 3 days to 5000 units twice a day and should be tailored to the individual patient.

It would not be prudent to continue the use of aspirin (**choice A**) in pregnancy because of the associated high risk of bleeding complications, especially during childbirth.

Nifedipine (**choice C**) is Pregnancy Category C (uncertain safety: animal studies show an adverse effect; no human studies have been performed). It therefore would not be the treatment of choice in someone trying to conceive.

There is a high risk of recurrence after discontinuation of treatment as long as the underlying cause of the hypercoagulable state is present. In a patient with anticardiolipin antibodies and a history of 2 miscarriages it would not be prudent to discontinue all treatment (**choice D**) in anticipation of conception.

Warfarin (**choice E**) is Pregnancy Category X (highly unsafe: risk of use outweighs any possible benefit). Obviously, use of warfarin is highly contraindicated in pregnancy. In addition to that, warfarin is not used in the treatment of the anticardiolipin antibody syndrome.

42. **The correct answer is A.** This patient has severe menorrhagia, given her history and hematocrit level. Many things, including malignancies, fibroids, polyps, medications, an altered hormonal environment, and coagulopathy, can cause menorrhagia. In an adolescent with such severe menorrhagia at menarche, particular attention should be paid to evaluation for coagulation disorders. As many as one-third of all adolescents presenting with menorrhagia at menarche have been found to have von Willebrand disease. Von Willebrand disease is a hereditary bleeding disorder caused by a deficiency of von Willebrand factor. Von Willebrand factor is essential for platelet adhesion and aggregation, which is necessary for normal blood clotting. Perhaps the best single screening test for von Willebrand disease is the ristocetin cofactor assay of von Willebrand factor (vWF) function. If the patient is found to have von Willebrand disease, treatment options include the oral contraceptive pill, desmopressin acetate, antifibrinolytic agents, and concentrates of vWF. Consultation with a hematologist is recommended for a patient with severe disease.

    To perform a hysteroscopy and dilatation and curettage in the operating room (**choice B**) is not the most appropriate course of action. Dilatation and curettage with hysteroscopy can be beneficial in the evaluation of some patients with menorrhagia. In an adolescent with severe bleeding at menarche, however, an evaluation for a coagulation disorder would be a more appropriate next step.

    To reassure the patient that this bleeding is normal and will decrease with time (**choice C**) is incorrect. This patient has severe menorrhagia and a very low hematocrit. Such bleeding is not normal and an evaluation (and not just reassurance) is needed.

    To recommend a hysterectomy as soon as possible (**choice D**) is not an appropriate course of action. Hysterectomy would render this 11-year-old infertile. A proper evaluation and attempt at more conservative strategies would be recommended.

    To start the patient on the oral contraceptive pill (**choice E**) would not be appropriate until the patient is screened for von Willebrand disease because oral contraceptives can mask the diagnosis.

43. **The correct answer is A.** Bacterial vaginosis is the term given to describe the condition in which there is an alteration in the normal vaginal flora. It can be found in up to 25% of patients in general obstetrical clinics. This patient may possibly have bacterial vaginosis based on her Pap smear findings. Because bacterial vaginosis has been associated with preterm birth, several studies have been done to determine if screening and treatment of bacterial vaginosis in pregnant women would reduce the incidence of preterm delivery. Based on these studies, treatment of women with bacterial vaginosis and no history of preterm birth does not appear to reduce the rates of preterm delivery. However, in the subgroup of women with a prior preterm birth, treatment of asymptomatic bacterial vaginosis may reduce rates of preterm birth. This patient is asymptomatic and has no history of a prior preterm birth. Therefore, she does not require treatment at the present time. If she becomes symptomatic later in pregnancy, she can be examined and treated if bacterial vaginosis is found.

    To treat the patient with intravaginal clindamycin (**choice B**) would not be necessary at this time as she is asymptomatic. If she were having symptoms of bacterial vaginosis (e.g., a foul-smelling vaginal discharge) treatment with intravaginal clindamycin would be appropriate.

    To treat the patient with oral metronidazole (**choice C**) would not be appropriate. First, she is asymptomatic and doesn't require treatment. Second, if treatment were necessary, metronidazole should be avoided in the first trimester.

    To wait until the second trimester and treat with intravaginal clindamycin (**choice D**) would not be appropriate. Again, there is no need for treatment of this patient unless she has symptoms.

    To wait until the second trimester and treat with oral metronidazole (**choice E**) would not be correct. This patient does not require treatment unless she becomes symptomatic. If she is symptomatic in the second trimester, metronidazole is considered acceptable for second-trimester use.

44. **The correct answer is E.** Group B streptococci (GBS) or *Streptococcus agalactiae* is an important cause of significant morbidity and mortality. As many as 30% of pregnant women are colonized with GBS in the vagina or rectum. Vertical transmission can result in infection of a neonate with the organism, which can lead to sepsis, neurologic sequelae, or death. To prevent such morbidity and mortality from GBS, the Centers for Disease Control (CDC) recommends two prevention strategies.

In one strategy, patients with a previous infant with invasive GBS disease, with GBS bacteriuria during the pregnancy, or in preterm labor (<37 wks) are treated with intrapartum penicillin. All other patients are screened with a rectal and vaginal swab between 35 and 37 weeks and only treated with penicillin if positive. In the second strategy, patients are treated if they have had a previous infant with GBS disease, GBS bacteriuria during the pregnancy, preterm labor, ruptured membranes greater than 18 hours, or temperature greater than 100.4 F. There is no screening with rectal and vaginal swab in the second strategy. Regardless of the strategy used, this patient has had a previous infant with GBS sepsis and, therefore, requires treatment.

To give intrapartum clindamycin (**choice A**) or to give intrapartum erythromycin (**choice B**) would be incorrect. Penicillin is the drug of choice for GBS prophylaxis, with ampicillin being an acceptable alternative. However, penicillin is preferred since it has a narrower spectrum. Clindamycin and erythromycin can be used when the patient is allergic to penicillin. This patient is allergic only to sulfa drugs. Therefore, penicillin should be used.

To give intrapartum magnesium sulfate (**choice C**) would not be appropriate. Magnesium sulfate is used in obstetrics to prevent seizures in patients with pre-eclampsia or eclampsia (to prevent further seizures) and to stop preterm labor. This patient does not have evidence of pre-eclampsia and, at 38 weeks, is not in preterm labor.

To give intrapartum oxytocin (**choice D**) is not correct. Oxytocin is used when there is a need to cause contractions. This patient is having regular contractions every 3 minutes and does not require oxytocin.

45. **The correct answer is C.** Cystic fibrosis is an inherited disorder, which is genetically transmitted in an autosomal recessive pattern. It affects the pancreas, sweat glands, and mucous glands in the respiratory, digestive and reproductive tracts. In the United States, approximately 4% of the Caucasian population is heterozygous carriers of the cystic fibrosis gene with the disease occurring in 1 in 3000 live Caucasian births. This patient has cystic fibrosis. If her husband is a carrier of a cystic fibrosis gene mutation, the child will have a 50% chance of having the disease. If her husband carries no mutation, the child will be a carrier but not have the disease. DNA testing can be performed on the father of the baby to determine his status. It is important, however, to counsel the patient that even if the DNA testing does not identify a cystic fibrosis mutation in the father of the baby, there is still the possibility that he carries an unidentified cystic fibrosis mutation and that the child could still have cystic fibrosis.

To advise the patient that cystic fibrosis is no longer a reason for pregnancy termination (**choice A**) is incorrect. This patient understands very well what it is like to have this disease. The decision regarding termination is not for the physician to make.

To advise the patient that it is too late in the pregnancy for testing to be performed (**choice B**) is incorrect. This patient is in the early second trimester. Testing may be performed at this time.

To advise that the fetus cannot have cystic fibrosis (**choice D**) is incorrect. As stated above, cystic fibrosis is an autosomal recessive disorder. If this patient's husband is a carrier of a cystic fibrosis gene mutation, there is a 50% chance that the child will have cystic fibrosis.

To state that the fetus likely has cystic fibrosis (**choice E**) is also incorrect. If the father is a carrier, the risk is 50% that the fetus has cystic fibrosis. If the father does not carry any mutation, the fetus will not have cystic fibrosis.

46. **The correct answer is A.** Thrombocytopenia is a common occurrence during pregnancy with as many as 8% of all pregnant women being affected. The differential diagnosis for thrombocytopenia in pregnancy includes gestational thrombocytopenia, pseudothrombocytopenia, HIV infection, systemic lupus erythematosus, immune thrombocytopenia purpura, pregnancy-induced hypertension, HELLP syndrome, drug-induced thrombocytopenia, thrombotic thrombocytopenia purpura, hemolytic uremic syndrome, disseminated intravascular coagulation, antiphospholipid syndrome, and the congenital thrombocytopenias. Gestational thrombocytopenia is far and away the most common cause of thrombocytopenia in pregnancy. It is characterized by a mild decrease in platelet count, which usually is above 70,000/mm^3, no history of bleeding difficulties, no history of thrombocytopenia outside of pregnancy, and a return of the platelet count to normal 2 to 12 weeks after delivery. Gestational thrombocytopenia poses no risk to the mother or the fetus and requires no therapy. This patient, with her mild thrombocytopenia and unremarkable history (including no hemorrhage with 2 surgeries) most likely has gestational thrombocytopenia.

This patient is unlikely to have HIV infection (**choice B**) given her negative HIV test. While it is possible that her HIV test was a false negative or that she has been infected since the test was obtained, this is not the most likely scenario and the most likely diagnosis is gestational thrombocytopenia.

Immune thrombocytopenia purpura (**choice C**) is characterized by immunologically mediated platelet destruction by IgG antiplatelet antibodies. It is a diagnosis of exclusion. However, most women with ITP have a history of bruising or bleeding which precedes the pregnancy.

Pre-eclampsia (**choice D**) is characterized by blood pressure above 140 mm Hg systolic or 90 mm Hg diastolic with proteinuria (<300 mg/day). This patient has normal blood pressure and no proteinuria.

Pseudothrombocytopenia (**choice E**) occurs when patients have platelet clumping such that the platelet counter doesn't correctly identify all of the patient's platelets. Evaluation of a peripheral smear will rule this out.

47. **The correct answer is B.** In women with sickle-cell anemia, contraception is a very important topic because of the pregnancy complications, chronic debility, and often shortened life expectancy that accompanies sickle-cell anemia. Therefore, it is essential to raise this topic with women who have sickle-cell anemia and to work out an effective approach to contraception. This patient does not wish to become pregnant, but is sexually active and only intermittently using condoms. Therefore, a better solution must be sought. Estrogen-progesterone oral contraceptives have been inadequately studied in women with sickle hemoglobinopathies. There is concern that the estrogen component may increase the risk of vaso-occlusive episodes and venous thrombosis. Studies have shown that DMPA reduces the incidence of pain crises. Also, DMPA does not contain an estrogen component, so it may be particularly appropriate for patients with sickle-cell disease.

To advise this patient that abstinence is the only appropriate method of birth control (**choice A**) is incorrect. Patients with sickle-cell anemia can use barrier methods (e.g., condoms), can have permanent sterilization, and use DMPA. Abstinence is not the only appropriate method for these patients.

To advise her that DMPA is contraindicated in patients with sickle-cell disease (**choice C**) is incorrect. Some investigators feel that the safety issue is unclear with DMPA and sickle-cell disease, but DMPA is widely used in women with sickle-cell disease and is not contraindicated.

To state that the IUD would be recommended in her case (**choice D**) is incorrect. First, her recent history of chlamydia would represent a contraindication to the IUD. Second, many experts feel that the IUD should be contraindicated in women with sickle-cell disease because of an increased risk of infection.

To advise her that there is no appropriate contraceptive option for patients with sickle-cell anemia (**choice E**) is incorrect. As described above, the patients have several options, including DMPA, sterilization, and barrier methods.

48. **The correct answer is B.** This patient most likely has pelvic inflammatory disease (PID) and her risk of infertility will increase if she has repeated episodes. One episode of PID is associated with a 13 to 21% risk of infertility, two episodes are associated with a 35% risk, and three or more episodes are associated with a 55 to 75% risk of infertility.

An intrauterine device is not a better form of contraception after an episode of PID (**choice A**). IUD use increases the risk of PID and must be removed immediately if the diagnosis of PID is made. It can facilitate the direct spread of bacteria.

Inconsistent condom use (**choice C**) also increases the risk of PID. Barrier protection, such as condoms, when used correctly, provides protection from the spread of the bacteria associated with pelvic inflammatory disease.

About 25% of women with PID will have some long-term sequelae of the infection, making **choice D** incorrect. These long-term sequelae include infertility, dyspareunia, and chronic pelvic pain.

Other sexually transmitted diseases, such as HIV, syphilis, trichomoniasis, herpes, and genital warts, can occur concomitantly with PID. Behaviors that increase the risk of PID are often the same behaviors that increase the risk of these other STDs, making their association not uncommon. Therefore, **choice E** is incorrect.

49. **The correct answer is C.** This patient is presumably having the first outbreak of genital herpes. Genital herpes is caused by *either* herpes simplex virus type 1 or 2 and is best treated with oral acyclovir for 7 to 10 days for the first episode and for 5 days for recurrent episodes. Brand names such as Valtrex and Famvir can also be used. The newest studies show that the majority of new infections are caused by exposure to asymptomatic shedders. This means that the infected patient does not show clinical lesions but is nonetheless spreading the virus through contact. Thus, anyone with a history of genital herpes is best advised to use condoms every time they engage in sexual intercourse and not solely during outbreaks (**choice B**).

Intravenous (IV) acyclovir is rarely used but can be given, when appropriate, to intubated patients unable to take oral medication with outbreaks of herpes simplex, herpes zoster, or eczema herpeticum (herpes lesions in eczematous skin of the face, usually seen in inpatients). It can also be used for herpes meningitis when foscarnet is not appropriate. IV acyclovir is not indicated for herpes simplex outbreaks **(choice A)**. Although it is true that the first outbreak of a herpes simplex infection is the worst in terms of numbers of lesions and symptoms such as pain and pruritus, IV medication is not required.

Topical penciclovir (Denavir) and topical acyclovir (Zovirax) are ineffective antivirals and should not be prescribed for genital herpes treatment **(choice D)**. They can be used when the first symptoms are noticed for herpes labialis (cold sores) in an attempt to shorten the outbreak, but studies show they leave a lot to be desired. Once infected with the herpes simplex virus future outbreaks are expected due to the fact that the virus remains latent in the dorsal root ganglion and can be reactivated at any time. One must protect oneself and others against transmission. Although the above patient's lesions will heal and crust over, she still needs to be advised to use condoms with *any* oral–genital contact with another person.

Herpes simplex infections are caused by either herpes simplex virus (HSV) type 1 or type 2. Type 1 has historically caused infection "above the belt" and type 2 has historically caused the lesions "below the belt." However, oral-genital contact can likely create HSV-1 genital lesions and HSV-2 oral lesions. Both types produce identical patterns of infections and are treated identically **(choice E)**. The Tzanck smear identifies characteristic multinucleated giant cells which are keratinocytes infected with the virus. The viral culture confirms the diagnosis of a herpes simplex virus and defines the type. The newest studies show that the majority of new infections are caused by exposure to asymptomatic shedders. This means that the infected patient does not show clinical lesions but is nonetheless spreading the virus through contact. Thus, anyone with a history of genital herpes is best advised to use condoms every time they engage in sexual intercourse and not only during outbreaks.

50. **The correct answer is A.** This patient is suffering from functional incontinence. Functional incontinence is defined as incontinence with a functional cause (i.e., impaired mobility or willingness to reach a toilet). This patient's incontinence started after her stroke and aphasia, is unrelated to coughing, and her PVR is normal. Her inability to communicate with the caregivers prevents her from accessing the toilet, thus making her incontinent of urine.

Bladder outlet obstruction can cause overflow incontinence. Overflow incontinence is more common in men and is characterized by elevated post voiding residual. It is unlikely that this patient has overflow incontinence considering that her incontinence started after she had a stroke and her PVR is normal (less than 100 ml), so an indwelling catheter **(choice B)** or intermittent catheterizations **(choice D)** are not indicated.

Stress incontinence is due to impaired urethral closure and is more common in women. It occurs with increased intra-abdominal pressure (coughing or laughing). It is related to hormone deficiency and multiple childbirths. First-line therapy is usually pelvic floor exercises **(choice E)**. If this treatment fails, a vaginal pessary **(choice C)** can be used.

Pediatrics: **Test One**

1. A 4-year-old boy is brought to the emergency department by his parents who report that he has not been acting normal since yesterday. They say that he has felt hot and has been pulling at his right ear. He has had a runny nose and nasal congestion for 1 week. The child has had 1 previous ear infection 6 months ago. He has no other medical history and no drug allergies. The child is crying and inconsolable. On examination, the patient's temperature is 40.0 C (104.0 F) and he has a rapid, thready heartbeat. Otoscopic examination reveals the presence of a red, immobile, bulging tympanic membrane on the right side. On the left side, the tympanic membrane is dull and immobile, but not acutely inflamed. The physical examination is otherwise unremarkable. The most appropriate next step in management is to

   (A) admit the patient for intravenous antibiotics and close observation
   (B) perform a tympanocentesis for culture and prescribe culture-directed antibiotics
   (C) prescribe amoxicillin for 10 days and have the patient follow up in the clinic
   (D) prescribe ciprofloxacin ear drops in the right ear for 2 weeks and have the patient follow up in the clinic
   (E) reassure the parents and recommend over-the-counter pain medications

2. A 17 year old boy comes to the office for a routine physical examination. He moved to the United States from South Africa 3 years ago and has been in good health. His vital signs and physical examination are within normal limits. A purified protein derivative (PPD) test for tuberculosis shows 20 mm of induration. He denies fever, cough, night sweats, weight loss, or exposure to individuals with known tuberculosis. A chest x-ray shows no evidence of cavitation or of hilar adenopathy. The most appropriate next step in the management is to

   (A) begin 4-drug antituberculosis therapy with isoniazid (INH), rifampin, ethambutol, and pyrazinamide pending the result of daily sputum cultures
   (B) begin treatment with INH alone for 9 months
   (C) monitor antituberculosis antibody titers to assess the stage of disease
   (D) order a repeat PPD in 1 month
   (E) repeat the chest x-ray every 6 weeks to monitor for progression of disease

3. A 14-year-old girl is brought to the emergency department from school. She reports that she was walking outside between classes when she began to feel an "asthma attack" coming on. She had forgotten her albuterol metered-dose inhaler at home and collapsed on the way to the nurse's office. Her temperature is 37.0 C (98.6 F), pulse is 110/min, respirations are 35/min, blood pressure 102/58 mm Hg, and oxygen saturation is 93% on room air. She has moderate air entry bilaterally with diffuse wheezes, a prolonged expiratory phase, and suprasternal and subcostal retractions. She receives 3 treatments with aerosolized albuterol and 1 dose of oral prednisone. She responds to this treatment and now has a pulse of 100/min, respirations of 16/min, and oxygen saturation of 100% on room air. She feels well and is ready to go home. On further history, you learn that this is her third trip to the hospital in the past 3 months (all winter months), that she has nightly cough, and generally uses her albuterol MDI as needed, roughly 3 to 4 times per day. Upon discharge, she should be advised to

(A) continue inhaled albuterol as needed and encouraged to use a spacer device
(B) continue oral prednisone for 4 more days with albuterol as needed, then resume the regimen of inhaled albuterol as needed
(C) take daily oral prednisone until the winter season is over
(D) take oral prednisone for 4 days and inhaled albuterol as needed and to begin therapy with inhaled fluticasone daily as needed
(E) take oral prednisone for 4 days and inhaled albuterol as needed and to begin therapy with inhaled fluticasone daily regardless of symptoms

4. A 9-year-old boy is brought to your office by a social worker. He has just been taken into a nearby refugee camp after fleeing from a war-torn, underdeveloped third-world country. The social worker tells you that he does not see well at nighttime and has been found several times wandering lost after dark. She also points out that his skin is very dry and "bumpy" and asks if you can prescribe something to relieve the dryness. You find the boy to be very quiet and withdrawn. His vital signs are within normal limits, but he is below the fifth percentile for weight. He is 142 cm (4 ft 7 in) tall and weighs 23 kg (51 lb). When you examine his skin you find that his shoulders and extremities are covered with perifollicular keratotic papules. Each papule has a horny keratotic plug in the center that projects as a horny spine. On the face, there are many comedolike lesions. The entire skin is very dry and with fine scale. On ophthalmologic examination you determine there is xerophthalmia, xerosis of the cornea, and nyctalopia. After sending the appropriate serum analysis, the most appropriate treatment for this patient is

(A) vitamin A
(B) vitamin B_2
(C) vitamin B_6
(D) vitamin D
(E) vitamin K

5. A previously healthy 4-year-old boy is brought to the emergency department by his mother for evaluation. She is concerned about his "noisy breathing." She reports that he has had a sore throat over the past 24 hours that has worsened progressively, as well as a fever. In addition, he has refused anything to eat or drink during the past 12 hours. Vital signs are: temperature 38.8 C (101.8 F), blood pressure 115/70 mm Hg, pulse 121/min, and respirations 32/min. His oxygen saturation on room air is 100%. The child appears to be in moderate respiratory distress with inspiratory stridor and is drooling. Physical examination reveals positive and equal breath sounds bilaterally with superimposed upper airway sounds and evidence of retractions with respiratory effort. The most appropriate next step in management is to

(A) begin treatment with intravenous antibiotics
(B) have an intravenous line placed and send blood for complete blood count with differential
(C) make arrangements for direct laryngoscopy and intubation in the operating room
(D) obtain a lateral soft tissue radiograph of the neck
(E) order supplemental oxygen and nebulized albuterol and admit the child for observation

6. An 11-year-old girl is brought to the emergency department after being hit in the nose with a softball. There was no loss of consciousness per her mother, who was present during the accident. Following the injury, she had some bleeding from the nose bilaterally which subsided spontaneously on the way to the hospital. On physical examination, the child is awake, alert, and in no apparent distress. Her vital signs are stable. The pupils are equal and reactive to light and extraocular movements are intact. There is no periorbital tenderness or edema. Examination of the oral cavity is within normal limits. There is no tenderness or mobility of the palate and the mandible is without tenderness or obvious step-off. Her neck is without tenderness, including the cervical spine, and has full range of motion. There is significant bruising and edema over the nasal dorsum. While the nasal dorsum is tender, it appears to be midline and without obvious depression or mobility. Dried blood can be seen around the nares bilaterally. The most important next step is to

(A) administer intravenous sedation and perform manual reduction of a suspected nasal fracture
(B) carefully examine the anterior nasal cavity
(C) obtain a CT scan of the face with axial and coronal views
(D) rule out a fracture with radiographs of the nasal bones
(E) treat with an oral antibiotic and follow up in 1 week

7. A newborn girl is intubated by the neonatal intensive care unit team due to respiratory distress shortly after birth. She was the product of a term delivery and had an uncomplicated prenatal course. Her respiratory status has stabilized now that her airway has been secured. No masses or other anomalies were seen at the time of endotracheal tube placement. Physical examination reveals a coloboma of the right eye and an abnormally formed and low-set right pinna. The external nose and face appear normal, although a 6 French suction catheter cannot be passed transnasally into the oropharynx on either side. Examination of the oral cavity reveals no evidence of cleft palate or mass lesion. The neck examination is also normal, without evidence of a palpable mass. The most appropriate next diagnostic step is

(A) an axial CT scan of the head
(B) flexible bronchoscopy
(C) a karyotype
(D) an MRI of the head
(E) a plain lateral radiograph of the skull

8. A 5-year-old boy is brought to the office by his parents after a parent-teacher conference at his school. The parents tell you that their son suffers from chronic constipation and encopresis and this has become a problem at school, where he gets teased by other children. His development has otherwise been normal and he has always been a healthy child except for the problems mentioned. In further discussion, you learn that the family adopted a baby girl a few months ago. The parents are uncertain if this new addition to the family has caused the worsening or if the problems were there all along but they were not paying enough attention to him. The most appropriate initial step in management is to

(A) evacuate the impacted stool
(B) recommend sitting on the toilet for 30 minutes daily after each meal
(C) refer him to child psychiatrist for play therapy in order to resolve the sibling rivalry
(D) set up a behavioral program with negative reinforcers for incontinence
(E) set up a star reward system for days when he does not soil his pants

9. A 15-month-old girl is brought to the clinic by her mother who is very concerned about the pigeon-toelike appearance of the child's feet. She also says that the child falls a lot when walking; however, there is no history of significant trauma or lower extremity pain. The mother tells you that none of her 3 other children had this problem. The pregnancy and delivery were noncomplicated. Immunizations are up to date and developmental milestones are age appropriate. The patient started walking at age 11 months. Height and weight are stable at the 30th percentile. Physical examination reveals a well-nourished, well-developed, happy, and playful 15-month-old toddler. Gait is independent with a predominance of hip and knee flexion, a foot progression angle of –5 degrees, and intermittent heel strike. Passive range of motion is full at the hips, knees, ankles, and feet. The feet are supple and free of local tenderness. Forefoot inspection reveals a straight lateral foot border. In the prone position the thigh foot angle is –10 degrees, and hip internal and external rotations are 50 and 40 degrees, respectively. At this time the most correct statement about her condition is:

(A) Denis Browne ("bars and boots") footwear is indicated; start with just the shoes at night, then several days later add the connecting bar; several days after that add an external rotation component to the shoe-bar axis; continue nighttime application for 6 months with monthly office checks; adjust the external rotation as needed.
(B) The mother should be reassured about the relatively benign nature of in-toeing; however, just to be sure, recommend orthopedic surgery consultation; offer to follow the patient on a regular basis after orthopedic evaluation.
(C) The mother should be reassured about the relatively benign nature of in-toeing; inform her that the majority of patients improve by 6 years of age; however, if she prefers, a prescription can be made for physical therapy; the therapist could gently stretch the lower extremity muscles.
(D) The mother should be reassured that this is a normal child; no intervention indicated; educate and reassure the mother about the benign nature of in-toeing; offer to follow the patient on a regular basis.
(E) X-rays of the pelvis and feet are indicated to rule out developmental hip dysplasia and tarsal coalition; if the x-rays are negative, proceed with orthopedic consultation.

10. A 16-year-old girl is brought to the office for a routine health maintenance examination. She has no complaints. You ask her mother to leave the room so you can complete the routine history and physical examination that you do with every adolescent patient. The most appropriate screening and anticipatory guidance that should be done during this and all adolescent well visits is

(A) chlamydia and gonorrhea cultures
(B) a dietary history
(C) a drug screen
(D) a head circumference
(E) a urinalysis

11. A 2-year-old boy is brought to the emergency department late at night after his parents found him coughing in their living room. They tell you that they left him playing on the ground for "only a moment." He was coughing quite a bit but his lips never turned blue. He continued coughing for approximately 30 minutes but stopped on the way to the hospital. Now, the boy is sitting in the chair and looks comfortable. Vital signs are: temperature 37.1 C (98.7 F), blood pressure 108/60 mm Hg, pulse 120/min, respirations 18/min, and oxygen saturation 93% on room air. His lungs sound clear, although his breath sounds seem to be louder on the left side. His parents are very tired and would like to take the patient home. The most appropriate next step in management is to

(A) admit the patient to the hospital for observation as a precaution
(B) give the patient something to eat, and if he swallows it without difficulty that will most likely rule out any serious abnormality
(C) obtain a chest x-ray and if that is normal, reassure the parents that anything that made the patient cough has most likely cleared
(D) obtain a chest x-ray, but regardless of its findings consult the otolaryngology team because of your high suspicion of an airway foreign body
(E) reassure his parents that because he seems comfortable in the emergency department and never developed cyanosis that he should be clear to go home with them

12. A 3-year-old boy is brought to the emergency department with a temperature of 39.4 C (103.0 F) and decreased food intake for the past 2 days. His mother tells you that he has been refusing to walk since this morning. He is generally healthy except for a hospitalization at 3 months of age for bronchiolitis. His mother has sickle-cell trait and his father's history is unknown. His leukocyte count is 17,000 mm^3, hemoglobin is 7.9 mg/dL, hematocrit is 30%, platelet count is 255,000 mm^3, and mean corpuscular volume is 70 μm^3. Urinalysis and electrolytes are normal. X-rays of his legs reveal no significant abnormalities. Blood cultures are pending. He is admitted to the hospital for further management. The organism that is most likely causing his infection is

(A) *Pasteurella multocida*
(B) salmonella species
(C) *Staphylococcus aureus*
(D) *Streptococcus pneumonia*
(E) *Streptococcus pyogenes*

13. An 18-year-old female college student who is home for Thanksgiving break comes to the office complaining of fatigue. She denies other symptoms except for mild chest pain and occasional nausea. She does not think she has had any fever, night sweats, or sore throat. She has lost 3 to 4 pounds. Mainly she sleeps 12 hours a night and is too tired to go out on the weekends with her friends. She denies having had sexual intercourse and does not have a boyfriend. Her menstrual periods are sometimes irregular and her last menstrual period was mid-October. Her roommate is not ill, but many of the girls in her dorm have infectious mononucleosis. Physical examination is unremarkable except for mildly enlarged red tonsils with no exudate. The most appropriate next step in management is to

(A) obtain a complete blood count
(B) obtain a Monospot test
(C) obtain a urine hCG
(D) obtain a throat culture
(E) reevaluate the patient in 4 weeks during Christmas break

14. A healthy 13-year-old girl comes to the office for her annual well checkup. She takes no medications, has no allergies, and her immunizations are up to date. While you are conducting her examination she mentions that she has been having "on and off vaginal discharge" for the past 6 months. Her menarche was 4 months ago. She has had only 3 periods, the first two were 3 to 4 days, then she missed a period, and her last menstrual period (LMP) was for 3 days, which finished 1 week ago. There were no cramps with her last menses. She denies any abdominal pain, dysuria, or other complaints. Physical examination reveals that she is sexual maturity rating (SMR) 3 and there is definite white mucoid discharge noted between her labia minora. There is no obvious redness. You test the mucus and note it has a pH of 4-4.5. The wet prep reveals several epithelial cells, and lots of rod-shaped bacteria. The most appropriate next step in management is to

(A) obtain chlamydia and gonorrhea cultures
(B) perform a pelvic examination
(C) reassure her that everything looks normal
(D) treat her with clotrimazole
(E) treat her with metronidazole

15. A 15-year-old goes on a family vacation mountain climbing, whitewater rafting, fishing, swimming, and camping in Colorado. Ten to 14 days after their trip the adolescent becomes sick with abdominal pains and cramping, flatus, and foul-smelling diarrhea. She denies any fever, headache, vomiting, cough, or runny nose. Physical examination reveals that she is well hydrated with normal physical findings. Her mom is quite concerned because school starts next week and she cannot go for more than an hour without running to the bathroom. The mother fears it must be something she ate. In order to get to the "bottom of things" and correct the problem the next best step would be to order

(A) abdominal films
(B) a testing of stool specimen for ova and parasite
(C) a CBC to check for eosinophilia
(D) ELISA (enzyme-linked immunosorbent assay) testing of the stool
(E) a stool culture

16. A 15-year-old boy comes to the office because of dull, achy knee pains for several months. The pains seem worse when he runs and jumps. Physical examination reveals localized soft tissue swelling with warmth and tenderness bilaterally below the patellae. On physical examination the boy is Tanner stage III. The most appropriate management at this time is to

(A) order a CBC and ESR
(B) order a CBC, ESR, and ANA
(C) recommend NSAIDs alone
(D) recommend symptomatic therapy with the use of ice, knee pads, and NSAIDs
(E) send him for x-ray of both knees

17. A 3-month-old infant male has been crying for 12 hours nonstop and his first-time mother instinctively "knows" this is not colic. He has been eating well and his last bottle was 3 hours ago. He drank it furiously but then forcefully vomited a lot of his formula. Now he will not settle down with anything to drink. You determine that the baby is mildly dehydrated. He has a dry diaper and he is mottled but crying with some tears. You check and discover that the ears, nose, and throat are normal. However, as you pull back his diaper you note a large, firm, tender inguinal mass. The most appropriate management at this time is to

(A) obtain an immediate surgery consult
(B) order a stat CBC, BUN, and electrolytes
(C) order a stat CBC and type and cross blood for imminent surgery
(D) order a technetium scan
(E) transilluminate the testes

18. A 14-year-old adolescent is brought to the office for a routine examination. There are no complaints at this time. The adolescent plays tennis and does well in school. In evaluating for scoliosis in this patient, the information that would indicate that the scoliosis may not be idiopathic, but instead is secondary to another underlying disease is

(A) a Cobb angle of 15 degrees
(B) a complaint of back pain that has been present on and off for 3 months
(C) female gender
(D) a rib hump with rotation of the thorax
(E) 3 to 4 café-au-lait spots are noted

19. Late one afternoon a mother brings her 17-year-old son to the office for an acute sick visit after he got into a fist-fight with another boy at school. Your patient swung at the other boy's arm and the other boy struck a return blow with his fist, hitting the boy directly in the eye. The boy is not thrilled to be in your office and he is feeling humiliated by the whole ordeal. The mother is not panicky but wants to be sure that her son is all right. On physical examination there are no injuries noted. There does not seem to be any significant bruising on or around either eye, except for very slight discoloration above the upper eyebrow of the eye that was hit. The conjunctiva are minimally injected without hemorrhages. Both pupils are equal and reactive to light and there is no blood noted in the anterior chambers of either eye. The most appropriate next step in management is to

(A) give them head trauma instructions for the next 8 to 12 hours
(B) recommend ice packs to prevent swelling
(C) recommend rest and observation at home overnight
(D) refer him to an ophthalmologist
(E) provide reassurance but schedule a follow-up visit in 1 week to discuss anger management

20. An 8-year-old boy is brought to the clinic because of a lump in his neck. His past medical history is unremarkable and no one noticed any lump there before. On examination there is a midline, mobile, small cystic swelling that appears to be inflamed. It is slightly tender with some redness and there is a small amount of pus coming from its center. The boy adds an interesting bit of history. As he was inspecting "the lump" in the mirror he noticed that if he stuck his tongue out, it moved. The most appropriate next step in management is to

(A) order a neck ultrasound
(B) order a radioactive iodine uptake
(C) order a T_4 and TSH
(D) refer him to a surgeon
(E) start him on antibiotics

21. A 12-year-old girl comes to the office for a routine examination. As a primary care provider, you know that you should be providing anticipatory guidance regarding healthy lifestyle habits during well-child and adolescent visits. As you promote healthy eating and emphasize the importance of bone health to adolescent patients, you advise that they should be taking a certain amount of calcium each day. Considering this, you should advise this patient that her daily calcium intake should be

(A) 400 mg
(B) 500 mg
(C) 800 mg
(D) 1000 mg
(E) more than 1000 mg

22. A 6-year-old Caucasian girl is brought to the emergency department with a 2-day history of gum bleeding and bruises on her extremities. Her mother tells you that she has had no major medical illnesses and is generally a very healthy and happy child. However, she did have a mild upper respiratory infection 2 weeks prior to this presentation. Her temperature is 37.0 C (98.6 F). On physical examination, you note multiple ecchymoses and diffuse petechiae. There is no lymphadenopathy or hepatosplenomegaly. The most appropriate next diagnostic step is to

(A) determine bleeding time
(B) determine partial thromboplastin time
(C) determine prothrombin time
(D) order a complete blood count
(E) order hemoglobin electrophoresis

23. An 800-gram, 26-week premature infant is delivered to a 23-year-old woman. You are called to the delivery room because the child has developed respiratory difficulties. You supervise an intubation. After initial stabilization, 24 hours later, you are called to the neonatal intensive care unit because the child has developed hypotension, bradycardia, and cyanosis. On physical examination, the child is still intubated and is noted to have a bulging anterior fontanelle. The most appropriate diagnostic test at this time is

(A) a complete blood count with platelets
(B) an echocardiogram
(C) an electroencephalogram
(D) serum prothrombin time
(E) an ultrasound of the head

24. A 2-hour-old, 32-week premature male baby develops progressive grunting, flaring, and cyanosis. The child is also noted to be retracting. A chest x-ray demonstrates poor aeration with a ground-glass appearance. The child is subsequently intubated on standard ventilatory settings. Because of this decline in respiratory status and prematurity, a rule-out sepsis evaluation is performed and antibiotic therapy is initiated. After 2 hours, the child remains on FiO_2 of 50 to 60%. The most appropriate management at this time is to administer

(A) endotracheal surfactant
(B) intramuscular vitamin K
(C) intravenous sodium bicarbonate
(D) intravenous steroids
(E) oral indomethacin

25. A 5-week-old infant is brought to the emergency department by his parents because of vomiting. The patient was born full term by normal spontaneous vaginal delivery at 8 pounds without any complications. He had been doing well until about 1 week ago when he began to have a few episodes of nonforceful, nonbloody, nonbilious emesis a few times a day after feeds. The parents brought the child to the pediatrician, who felt that it was "some reflux" and sent them home with hints on reflux precautions. The baby weighed 9 pounds at that visit. The vomiting continued and over the last 2 days the emesis has progressed to occurring after every feed; it is still nonbilious and nonbloody but has now begun to appear forceful in nature. When asked, the parents report that he appears hungry after each episode of emesis. His vital signs and physical examination are unremarkable, with no signs of dehydration. He has guaiac-negative stool. He weighs 9 pounds 4 ounces. The most appropriate next step in your workup of this infant is to

(A) draw electrolytes
(B) get an abdominal ultrasound
(C) obtain an abdominal x-ray
(D) order an upper GI with small bowel follow-through
(E) reassure the parents that it is reflux and send them home with followup

26. A 1-year-old boy is brought to the emergency department because of increased effort to breathe, hoarseness, and a worsening cough. His mother reports there was a preceding history of diarrhea, tactile fever, and mild cough. The patient has been able to tolerate some solids for dinner, but little else during the day. There have been no sick contacts and no daycare, and there are no pets in the home. His temperature is 38.3 C (101.0 F), pulse is 150/minute, and respirations are 39/min. There is some rhinorrhea, but otherwise his ear, nose, and throat examination is normal. He has some intercostal retractions of the chest and stridor on inspiration and expiration. There is no wheezing present. The most appropriate management at this time is to

(A) admit him for therapy with aerosolized budesonide, racemic epinephrine, and intravenous dexamethasone
(B) admit him for therapy with nebulized albuterol
(C) admit him for therapy with intravenous ceftriaxone
(D) observe him in the emergency department while giving humidified inspired air and then send him home
(E) obtain an immediate otolaryngology consultation for visualization of the epiglottis

27. A 5-week-old male infant is brought to the urgent care clinic by his mother because of "dry diapers for over 15 hours." She took her son to his primary care physician yesterday because of 2 weeks of worsening symptoms including a prominent cough, nasal congestion, and wheezing. He was started on albuterol nebulizers every 4 hours and she was given reassurance that the child had a viral infection and that it would get better. But now she is particularly concerned with his lack of urination. You should advise the mother that the most effective form of oral rehydration is

(A) boiled and then cooled water
(B) milk feedings either as bottle or breast-feeding
(C) oral solution of glucose-electrolyte mixture
(D) oral solution of glucose with water
(E) orange juice

28. A 4-week old girl is brought to the emergency department because of irritability and "difficulty breathing." She has not had any fevers, vomiting, or diarrhea, but is not tolerating breast-feeding or bottle feeding well. She is alert. Her temperature is 36.5 C (97.8 F), pulse is 119/min, and respirations are 40/min. Her mucous membranes are moist and skin has good turgor. She has mild conjunctivitis. There are no lymph nodes noted and her tympanic membranes appear normal. There are rales noted diffusely on auscultation. Her hemoglobin is 12.6 mg/dL, hematocrit is 37.1%, platelet count is 204,000/mm^3, and eosinophil count is 6%. Blood and urine cultures are pending. A chest x-ray shows interstitial infiltrates and hyperinflation. The most likely organism responsible for this infant's condition is

(A) *Chlamydia trachomatis*
(B) human parvovirus
(C) parainfluenza virus
(D) respiratory syncytial virus
(E) staphylococcal species

29. A 5-year-old boy is brought to the clinic by his parents because of "penile pain." The pain is mainly at the tip of the penis and has been going on for the past 24 hours. He has not had any recent fever, burning sensations, or crying during urination. His urine color has been normal. The only thing she recalls is that the child likes playing in the water during bath time and can sometimes sit in the water for over 45 minutes. Two days ago he was playing in the bath for about 1 hour before she took him out. His temperature is 36.1 C (97.0 F). Unfortunately, the child will not let you or the nurse examine him. However, he has good rapport with his parents and while he is sitting on his mother's lap you are able to observe the patient. The penis is of normal size for his age, and is uncircumcised with no obvious deformity, discharge, or trauma. You ask the mother to pull the foreskin back and there is no pain elicited. The glans appears uninflamed and clean. The meatus appears normal too. The testes are palpable, according to mother, and are pain free. There are no other visible abnormalities. A urinalysis is negative for protein, leukocyte esterase, and nitrites. A complete blood count is normal. The most likely cause of the penile pain is

(A) child sexual abuse
(B) irritation to the glans from prolonged stays in the bath
(C) phimosis
(D) urinary tract infection
(E) urolithiasis

30. A 2-year-old girl is admitted to the hospital for mild dehydration following diarrhea, fever, and abdominal pain that began 24 hours ago. There is no significant past medical or surgical history, or family history of disease, nor a history of foreign travel or ingestion of uncooked meat. The child appears fussy and mildly dehydrated. Her temperature is 36.1 C (97.0 F), blood pressure is 105/62 mm Hg, pulse is 84/min, and respirations are 16/min. Her abdomen is soft, non-tender, and without organomegaly or masses. The bowel sounds are normal. Rectal examination reveals green, loosely formed stool mixed with mucus and blood. Laboratory studies show:

Hemoglobin	12.2 g/dL
Hematocrit	36%
Platelets	150,000/mm^3
Leukocyte count	15,000/mm^3 with a neutrophil count of 66% with 6% band cells
Sodium	132 mEq/L
Potassium	3.7 mEq/L
Chloride	100 mmol/L
Bicarbonate	20 mEq/L
BUN	12 mg/dL
Creatinine	0.6 mg/dL
Serum glucose	102 mg/dL

A peripheral blood smear, urinalysis, chest x-ray, and abdominal x-rays are normal. Over the next 24 hours, the child becomes pale and dehydrated. The blood cultures are negative and stool cultures are negative for *Salmonella*, *Shigella*, *Yersinia*, *Campylobacter*, and rotavirus. Over the next 36 hours the child continues to have fever and bloody stools. Her blood pressure remains normal despite worsening dehydration. On day 3 of her hospital stay her laboratory studies show:

Hemoglobin	5.0 g/dL
Hematocrit	15%
Leukocytes	15,000/mm^3
Platelets	28,000/mm^3
Sodium	125 mEq/L
Potassium	5.0 mEq/L
Chloride	100 mmol/L
Bicarbonate	16 mEq/L
BUN	34 mg/dL
Creatinine	2.5 mg/dL
Glucose	100 mg/dL

A urinalysis demonstrates moderate levels of protein and blood with no casts. A peripheral blood smear shows fragmented red blood cells. At this stage, the most likely diagnosis is

(A) Berger disease
(B) hemolytic uremic syndrome
(C) Henoch-Schönlein syndrome
(D) Hirschprung disease
(E) Goodpasture disease

31. A few weeks after a viral illness, a 7-year-old girl develops multiple fine red lesions over her entire torso, arms, and legs, but otherwise seems to feel fine. As you inspect the distribution of these pinpoint lesions you see that they are especially noticeable around her waistline area and at points of pressure. The most appropriate next step in management is to

(A) order a CBC and platelet count
(B) order a CBC, UA, BUN, and creatinine
(C) order a Monospot test
(D) order no tests; the rash is diagnostic
(E) send her for an echocardiogram

32. A 3-year-old girl is brought to the office by her mother because of recurrent episodes of pneumonia. The prior night, she was brought to the emergency department because she had a temperature of 40.0 C (104 F) and was coughing. An x-ray was read as "positive" by the emergency department doctor, and the patient was sent home on oral amoxicillin. The mother says the child is feeling better since last night and is now afebrile, but the family is concerned about the repeated lung infections. Over the past 2 years, the girl has been hospitalized 3 times with fever, tachypnea, and changes on chest x-ray consistent with pneumonia. Other than this issue, her only other medical problems have been a prolonged hospitalization at birth because of a failure to pass meconium and, her mother adds, being "too skinny." In the office, her temperature is 37.0 C (98.6 F), blood pressure is 105/50 mm Hg, pulse is 100/min, and respirations are 30/min. She is 37 cm tall (50th percentile) and weighs 12 kg (10th percentile). Physical examination shows a well-appearing child with faint crackles throughout both lung fields. The most appropriate next step in management is to

(A) determine erythrocyte sedimentation rate
(B) do a follow-up chest x-ray in 2 to 3 days
(C) check peak expiratory flow rate
(D) measure sweat chloride concentration
(E) send her for a rectal biopsy

33. A 14½-year-old girl comes to the office because of irregular menses. Her menarche was 1 year ago and she had 2 or 3 periods that lasted for 4 or 5 days, but then for the past 9 months she has had only a "little spotting." Birth history and early development were unremarkable. Past medical history reveals that she has no chronic illnesses and has been healthy over the past year. However, the mother is very concerned that she has lost 10 pounds over the past few months. She tells you that her daughter is somewhat shy and this year has only two close friends. At this point in the history-taking, the girl says, "Yeah, I have two best friends, but I am definitely not a 'nerd'." She has a very high grade point average and participates in sports. She is very active on the school track team and is also a member of the Spanish club. As the girl is changing into her gown you notice her recorded vital signs in her chart: temperature 36.7 C (98 F), blood pressure 90/60 mm Hg, pulse 48/min, and respirations 18/min. On the growth chart you plot her height at 50th percentile and weight 3rd percentile. As you proceed to examine the girl alone, the review of system questions that will most likely lead you to the likely diagnosis is

(A) headaches, polyuria, visual difficulties, vomiting
(B) heat intolerance, fidgetiness, overactivity, sweatiness, tremor, weakness
(C) cough, fever, night sweats, malaise, rash
(D) constipation, cold intolerance, inactivity, poor academic performance
(E) constipation, cold intolerance, dry skin, hair loss, overactivity

34. A 2½-year old girl was playing with her dad, squealing with delight as he grabbed onto her hands and swung her above his head, around and around in a circle, until she suddenly started to scream in pain. He set her back down feet first on the ground as she shrieked loudly with pain. She continued to cry and sob with tears, refusing to let anyone touch her hand and arm. As her dad rushed her to the hospital he was feeling very guilty. Upon arrival at the emergency department the girl is still in tears, holding her forearm close to her body, extended at the elbow with her forearm in pronation. As the dad retells the story he adds that he may have heard a "snap" just before she started to scream. Upon examination, you note that her arm appears to be particularly painful at the elbow. No bruising or other injuries are apparent. An x-ray of the arm and elbow are obtained and are negative. At this point the next best step is to

(A) call child protective services
(B) order an oblique film of the elbow and x-rays of shoulder
(C) perform mild manipulation of the arm
(D) place the arm in a short arm cast and have her follow up in 1 week
(E) refer to the orthopedist on call

35. A 16-year-old girl has been having heavier than normal menses for the past 2 years. Her periods last 6 to 7 days and she reports using 4 to 5 pads each day. Laboratory studies confirm that she has iron deficiency anemia. If you want to be sure that she is compliant with the treatment and that the iron pills are working as they should, the test that would show the earliest response to therapy is

(A) complete blood count
(B) ferritin
(C) platelet count
(D) reticulocyte count
(E) serum iron

36. A baby girl is born in the hospital and during the first hours of life it is noted that on her physical examination she has edema of both feet. Her cardiovascular examination seems normal except for decreased femoral pulses. The most appropriate next step in management is to

(A) administer digoxin
(B) administer furosemide
(C) observe her in the newborn nursery
(D) obtain a karyotype
(E) supply her with oxygen

37. A 15-year-old boy comes to the office for a routine physical examination. He has no complaints at this time. His review of systems is negative, he takes no medications, and his immunizations are up to date. He reluctantly admits that last year he tried drugs and alcohol but denies current use. His maintained a B average last year, but this year he has slipped to a C+ average. He has dated a few girls, but now has a steady girlfriend for the past 3 months. He admits to being sexually active, but always uses a condom. As you are completing his examination you perform a genital examination. His genital assessment is Tanner stage IV. As you take note of his pubic hair you see that he has several whitish-gray specks scattered throughout his pubic hair area that do not brush off the hair. He claims that he did not see those before, but has been itching a lot lately. You explain that he has an infection that he probably got from his girlfriend. The best treatment for his condition is

(A) clotrimazole
(B) fluconazole
(C) griseofulvin
(D) lindane
(E) permethrin crème rinse

38. An adolescent girl comes to the clinic because of a "rash" on her face consisting of 4 to 5 orange-pink patches with well-demarcated, non-raised borders. On examination you also note flaky eyebrows that she says also are sometimes a problem because they are itchy. A Wood lamp examination and KOH wet prep are negative. The most appropriate therapy for this facial rash is

(A) calcipotriene ointment
(B) low-potency topical corticosteroids
(C) mupirocin ointment
(D) permethrin crème rinse
(E) topical trichloroacetic acid (TCA)

39. A 13-year-old boy is brought to the office for an initial visit. His father works for the foreign service and the family has recently moved back to the U.S. He needs a physical examination before entering high school. He has no complaints but his mother is very worried about his growth. His past medical history is unremarkable. The mother chooses to sit out in the waiting room while you examine and talk to her son. The findings on physical examination or tests that would lead you to evaluate this patient for an endocrine disorder are

(A) his bone age is 12 years 6 months and SMR is 1
(B) his bone age is 14 years 1 month and SMR is 2
(C) if he is very short and very overweight for his age
(D) if he is very tall and overweight for his age
(E) if he is very tall for his age and sexual maturity rating is 3

40. A mother brings her 13-year-old son to your office for a sick visit. She reports that he has been sick for 3 weeks and feels that something must be very wrong. He seemed to have a cold with runny nose for more than a week and then for the following 10 days he began coughing very badly at night. He wakes up everyone in the house. He coughs and coughs so badly that he becomes "beet red" in the face and frequently vomits at the end of the long coughing spells. After coughing he is sweaty all over, but does not seem to have any fever with this illness. The over-the-counter medications do not help. She also tried his sister's asthma medicine to break the coughing spells, but this did not help either. His mother reports that her son's past medical history is unremarkable, but she is unsure about his immunizations, because they recently moved to the U.S. from overseas. His temperature is 37.0 C (98.6 F) and respirations 20/min. Physical examination is unremarkable. The chest is clear to auscultation and there is no lymphadenopathy or hepatosplenomegaly. He looks well, but sounds so sick from what the mother says that you order a complete blood count that shows a leukocyte count of $20{,}000/mm^3$ with 78% lymphocytes. The best therapeutic choice for this patient's condition is

(A) ampicillin
(B) ciprofloxacin
(C) erythromycin
(D) penicillin and corticosteroids
(E) sulfonamide

41. You are writing up the results section of an epidemiologic cohort study in which various variables about a given disease were studied among a sample population of children. Your study population included 183 children less than 21 years of age. Followup was over 20 years. There were 5 children ages 0 to 4, 12 children ages 5 to 9, 70 children ages 10 to 14, and 96 children ages 15 to 19. The best measure of central tendency to describe the age of the population would be the

(A) arithmetic spot
(B) mean
(C) mean of the largest age group (age 15 to 19)
(D) median
(E) mode

42. A mother brings her 10-year-old son to the office because of a facial rash. He is feeling "fine" but this rash is "concerning." She thinks he must be overheated and sweating a lot, or that maybe he has some early form of acne. Vital signs are normal and he is afebrile. Physical examination is unremarkable except for an erythematous rash, mostly on his cheeks. The mother states that the rash started a few days ago as bright red bumps and now upon your examination these bumps are coalesced together to give very red cheeks. The rest of his body is pretty much rash-free except for some lacelike-looking pink areas on his arms. The mother says that she noted the arm rash yesterday and it seems to be most noticeable after he showers. There is no lymphadenopathy or hepatosplenomegaly. After considering possible diagnoses you should advise the mother that:

(A) Her son has a mild virus, but he does not have to stay home from school.
(B) Her has a mild virus, but he should stay home from school until the rash disappears.
(C) This is mild acne on his cheeks and that it should be left alone for now.
(D) This is mild acne on his cheeks and he should use over-the-counter benzoyl peroxide.
(E) Topical antibiotics should be useful in clearing the mild acne on his cheeks.

43. You happen to glance at the appointment book on your way into the office and notice that your entire afternoon is scheduled with adolescents. You remember from your training that the age of onset for puberty, duration between the sexual maturation ratings (SMRs) or Tanner stages, and physical growth are highly variable. In order to provide adequate health care to these adolescents, you must appreciate the normal variations in pubertal development. Of the following teenage cases, the one that would most likely lead you to look for underlying disease is a/an

(A) 11-year-old female with SMR 1 breasts, SMR 1 pubic hair, and history of abdominal pain
(B) 12-year-old male with early SMR 2 genitalia, SMR 1 pubic hair, no axillary hair
(C) 12-year-old male with SMR 3 genitalia, gynecomastia, tall stature, and weight is >95%
(D) 14-year-old female with SMR 4 breasts, SMR 4 pubic hair, dysmenorrhea
(E) 15-year-old female with SMR 2 breasts, SMR 4 pubic hair, irregular menses

44. You are taking care of a young infant who has been on total parenteral nutrition for a long time. While reviewing her chart you notice that a complete blood count shows neutropenia and hypochromic anemia. Iron therapy is initiated for several weeks and there is no change in the anemia. At this time the best test to order to establish a diagnosis is

(A) ceruloplasmin level or copper level
(B) ferritin level
(C) lead level
(D) selenium level
(E) zinc level

45. A 12-year-old boy is brought to the emergency department because something is "terribly wrong." The boy has been sick for a few days with fever, chills, headache, and a mild stomachache, and only now he is complaining that his "privates" hurt. On examination, the boy is in no obvious distress. His temperature is 37.9 C (100.2 F), blood pressure is 105/75 mm Hg, pulse is 78/min, and respirations are 20/min. He has slightly enlarged tonsils, shoddy anterior cervical nodes, and mild swelling over the parotid gland. He also has marked tenderness bilaterally on the neck area just beneath the mandibles. His chest is clear and there is no hepatosplenomegaly, but he does complain of slight abdominal pain with palpation. On genital examination his left scrotum is swollen and there is tenderness over the entire surface of the testis. Of the following, the best diagnostic test for this patient is

(A) CMV serology
(B) EBV serology
(C) HIV testing
(D) mumps serology
(E) serum amylase

46. You are supervising a third-year medical student who jumps right in to see the first patient of the day, who is a 12-year-old boy complaining of chest pain. The student presents the case to you and states that when the boy took off his shirt for examination there was evident gynecomastia. His lungs, however, were clear to auscultation. The young boy denied that he had any past disease and he reports that he takes no medications, does not smoke marijuana or do drugs, and insists that he hates girls and has never had sex. The boy's mother could not be found in the waiting room, so the student was unable to obtain her side of the story. His blood pressure is 120/82 mm Hg, pulse is 88/min, and respirations are 18/min. The conscientious medical student also plotted the boy's height and weight, noting that the boy is greater than 95% in height and 80% in weight. As a supervising physician, you emphasize to the student that the best next step in evaluation of this patient will be

(A) bone age
(B) genital examination
(C) serum testosterone
(D) to find out from the mother whether there is a family history of gynecomastia
(E) urine screen for drugs

47. A 4-month-old baby is brought to the office for a well-child visit. The mother is a 19-year-old girl who just moved here with the baby from Peru and lives with her grandmother. While obtaining the history you discover that the baby was born at home and this is the baby's first visit to a doctor. The mother tells you that the baby likes to sleep a lot, does not eat very well, and stools about once every 5 to 7 days; she also thinks that her tongue is "too big for her mouth." Her vital signs are stable in your office. Physical examination shows macroglossia, large anterior and posterior fontanelles, a reducible umbilical hernia, and dry skin. The most likely diagnosis is

(A) Beckwith-Wiedemann syndrome
(B) congenital hypothyroidism
(C) galactosemia
(D) maple syrup urine disease
(E) urea cycle defect

48. An 18-month-old girl is brought to the office for a well-baby visit. Physical examination is unremarkable, although the child is at the 40th percentile in terms of both height and weight. In reviewing the child's medical history, you notice that the patient has not had any of the recommended childhood immunizations. When questioned, the mother states that she does not believe in immunizations and does not want her child to receive injections. You explain the risks and benefits of vaccinations and she still "absolutely refuses" to vaccinate her child. Faced with this response, the most appropriate next step is to

(A) agree to forgo the immunizations and schedule the child for the next well-child visit
(B) assure the mother that the immunizations are harmless and tell her about the details of the diseases prevented by the immunizations
(C) begin the immunization series in the interests of the child's health
(D) explain to the mother that immunizations are required by law
(E) inform the local public health department
(F) tell the mother that you cannot continue to be her daughter's physician if she will not allow the immunizations

49. A 6-year-old girl is brought to the office by her mother, who is worried that she is not reading at a level appropriate for her age. The patient's reading grades on her report card are always low, and she repeatedly asks that her mother read items for her and she does not like to read books on her own accord. Physical examination is normal and on mental status examination, she seems to be a well-related and happy-appearing child with no observable verbal language deficiencies. The most appropriate next step in establishing a diagnosis of a reading disorder is to

(A) order an electroencephalogram
(B) order neuroimaging studies
(C) send her for a Minnesota Multiphasic Personality Inventory
(D) send her for projective psychological testing
(E) send her for standardized testing of reading achievement and intelligence quotient

50. A 17-year-old boy comes to the office concerned about a rash he has had for the past 2 weeks. He feels fine, but admits that he has been a bit fatigued lately. Physical examination reveals numerous macules on his trunk and upper thighs. The rash is bilateral and symmetric. You also note some scaly lesions present on his palms and soles. The most appropriate next diagnostic study is a

(A) complete blood count
(B) KOH wet prep of scrapings from a macule
(C) rapid strep test and throat culture
(D) RPR
(E) Wood lamp exam

Pediatrics Test One: Answers and Explanations

ANSWER KEY

1. C
2. B
3. E
4. A
5. C
6. B
7. A
8. A
9. D
10. B
11. D
12. C
13. C
14. C
15. D
16. D
17. A
18. B
19. D
20. E
21. E
22. D
23. E
24. A
25. B
26. A
27. C
28. A
29. B
30. B
31. A
32. D
33. E
34. C
35. D
36. D
37. E
38. B
39. C
40. C
41. D
42. A
43. E
44. A
45. D
46. B
47. B
48. A
49. E
50. D

1. **The correct answer is C.** This patient has the classic presentation of uncomplicated otitis media (febrile with a red, bulging tympanic membrane). The proper first-line treatment for otitis media is amoxicillin in non-penicillin allergic patients. Because the patient has serous otitis media in the other ear (dull, immobile tympanic membrane), he needs to follow up with a primary physician to document resolution of both the acute and serous otitis media.

   Admission for IV antibiotics (**choice A**) is not indicated, as the vast majority of cases of acute otitis media resolve with oral antibiotic therapy.

   If the patient returns with recurrent symptoms after completing the course of amoxicillin, a broader-spectrum drug such as amoxicillin-clavulanic acid should be used. If this therapy is unsuccessful, culture-directed antibiotic therapy should be contemplated. Tympanocentesis can be performed in the office or emergency department to obtain material for culture. It is not necessary to perform tympanocentesis for uncomplicated otitis media. Therefore, performing a tympanocentesis for culture and prescribing culture-directed antibiotics (**choice B**) is incorrect.

   Topical antibiotic therapy with ear drops is the treatment of choice for otitis externa (swimmer's ear). There is no role for antibiotic ear drops in acute otitis media with an intact tympanic membrane (**choice D**).

   Although complications of otitis media are rare, facial nerve paralysis, meningitis, and brain abscesses can result from untreated acute otitis media. Therefore, reassurance and over-the-counter pain medications (**choice E**) is incorrect, as acute otitis should be treated with appropriate antibiotics.

2. **The correct answer is B.** This patient has latent tuberculosis infection (LTBI), demonstrated with a highly reactive PPD and a negative chest x-ray. If he had had a cavitary lesion or other pulmonary pathology on chest x-ray, he would have fallen into the category of active tuberculosis disease and required treatment with multiple drugs. Therapy for LTBI is isoniazid as a single drug for a 9-month course. This is curative in most cases.

   In situations in which a patient has active tuberculosis and a high probability of harboring a drug-resistant strain (exposure either to countries or populations with a high prevalence of drug-resistant TB) treatment is recommended with four anti-TB medications pending the results of susceptibility testing. This patient has LTBI, as noted above, and thus multiple drug therapy (**choice A**) is not indicated.

   Anti-tuberculosis antibody testing (**choice C**) is not clinically available and does not help in guiding therapy. Diagnosis of tuberculosis is based on the PPD test and imaging studies, as noted above.

   Once a patient's PPD test is reactive, it is unlikely to revert to a negative state even with proper therapy. The PPD measures a delayed-type hypersensitivity response to tuberculosis antigens, which is positive for life following exposure to tuberculosis. Thus, serial measurements after a positive PPD (**choice D**) are not useful.

   Screening radiographs are an important tool for monitoring the progression of disease in PPD-positive patients after treatment for LTBI. These are used because, as noted above, the PPD will be positive regardless of proper treatment and is not useful for indicating reactivation of disease. However, 6 weeks (**choice E**) would be too frequent an interval for monitoring in an asymptomatic person. Six to 12 months is a more reasonable interval.

3. **The correct answer is E.** This patient has moderate-persistent reactive airway disease, as demonstrated by daily symptoms and use of inhaled beta-agonist medication (albuterol). Thus, she needs to begin maintenance therapy with an inhaled steroid in addition to continuing her as-needed albuterol. Inhaled steroids decrease airway inflammation and improve symptoms in patients with persistent asthma symptoms.

   The use of albuterol alone (**choice A**) is not sufficient therapy for this patient, as demonstrated by her frequent emergency department visits over the past winter. There is no reason to think that she will spontaneously improve on the same regimen that she has been using, and daily therapy is thus indicated.

   Continuation of the oral corticosteroid treatment that was started in the emergency department (**choice B**) will allow for suppression of inflammation over the subsequent several days and for recovery from this acute event. However, as stated above, resumption of a regimen of beta-agonist therapy alone in this patient who has continually failed such therapy is insufficient.

   Long-term use of oral corticosteroids (**choice C**), while potentially effective for reduction of airway inflammation, is associated with adrenal suppression and an unacceptably high rate of side effects. For that reason, inhaled corticosteroids are preferred agents.

   Following the completion of a short course of oral steroids, initiation of an inhaled steroid preparation such as fluticasone is an acceptable therapeutic alternative in this child. However, it is important to note that inhaled steroids are most effective when administered daily, regardless of symptoms, rather than on an as-needed basis (**choice D**).

4. **The correct answer is A.** This child has the classic clinical picture of vitamin A deficiency. Vitamin A is a fat-soluble vitamin found as retinyl-esters in milk, fish oil, liver, and eggs, and as carotenoids in plants. Vitamin A deficiency is common in children in the developing world. In developed countries it is most commonly associated with disease of fat malabsorption, such as Crohn disease, celiac disease, cystic fibrosis, and cholestatic liver disease. Vitamin A is required for normal keratinization of the skin. When deficient, a skin eruption develops that consists of keratotic papules of varying size over the shoulders and extremities. Individual lesions are firm papules containing a central intrafollicular keratotic plug that projects as a horny spine and leaves a pitted depression when removed. It may spread to involve most of the body surface except palms and soles (where there are no pilosebaceous follicles). On the face it resembles acne because of large comedones that develop. The whole skin displays dryness and fine scaling. Eye findings are prominent and often pathognomonic. They include night blindness (nyctalopia), an inability to see bright light, xerophthalmia, xerosis corneae, and keratomalacia. Vitamin A deficiency is a major cause of blindness in children in the developing world. The diagnosis is usually based on typical eye findings, but may be aided by determination of the serum level of vitamin A. The treatment is 100,000 IU/day for 2 days, and an additional 200,000 IU before discharge, after which an appropriate diet should be started.

Vitamin B_2 (**choice B**) deficiency manifests with the oral-ocular-genital syndrome. Angular cheilitis and cheilosis are prominent. The tongue is atrophic and magenta-colored. A seborrheic dermatitislike eruption affects the face. Confluent dermatitis of the scrotum or vulva is present and extends onto the thighs. Photophobia and blepharitis angularis also occur. All the signs respond dramatically to 5 mg of riboflavin (vitamin B_2) daily.

Vitamin B_6 (**choice C**) deficiency occurs in patients with uremia, cirrhosis, and with some medications. The skin changes include a seborrheic dermatitis-like eruption, atrophic glossitis with ulceration, angular cheilitis, conjunctivitis, and intertrigo. The patients may be somnolent, be confused, and display signs of neuropathy.

Vitamin D (**choice D**) deficiency has no skin manifestations except for alopecia.

Vitamin K (**choice E**) deficiency occurs in patients with malabsorption syndromes or liver disease, or as a side effect of certain medications (coumarin, salicylates, cholestyramine). The result is a decrease in the vitamin K-dependent clotting factors II, VII, IX, and X. Purpura, hemorrhage, and ecchymosis occur in the skin. Treatment is with 5 to 10 mg/day of IM vitamin K. In acute, life-threatening situations, fresh frozen plasma provides the deficient clotting factors until their synthesis can be resumed.

5. **The correct answer is C.** This child presents with the classic signs and symptoms of acute epiglottitis. The basic differential diagnosis includes croup (or laryngotracheobronchitis) and bacterial tracheitis. Croup occurs most commonly in children less than 2 years of age and is characterized by a barking cough with inspiratory or biphasic stridor. The stridor is thought to be related to edema of the subglottic region, but only the most severe cases result in acute airway obstruction. Croup is associated with RSV or parainfluenza virus. Bacterial tracheitis can occur at any age and affects the trachea primarily. It is often due to a bacterial superinfection following a severe episode of viral croup and is associated with the organism *Staphylococcus aureus*. Epiglottitis is an infection of the supraglottis and epiglottis that can result in life-threatening airway obstruction. It is most commonly seen in children 3 to 5 years old and is characterized by respiratory distress, inspiratory stridor, and inability to tolerate secretions. It is most commonly associated with *Haemophilus influenzae* and, as expected, has become less common with routine use of the *Haemophilus influenzae* B vaccine. Suspected epiglottitis is an airway emergency and the diagnosis is made clinically. It is generally felt that causing any crying, straining, or further distress of the child may lead to further compromise of the airway and, therefore, the most appropriate initial step is for direct laryngoscopy and securing of the airway in the operating room, either with endotracheal intubation or tracheotomy if necessary. This is the most controlled and ideal setting, if possible. In the OR, an anesthesiologist can administer inhalational anesthesia while maintaining respiratory effort, to allow examination and securing of the airway, as well as subsequent placement of an IV and blood work as necessary.

Placing an IV initially (**choice A**) or obtaining blood work (**choice B**) may lead to crying and further airway congestion and obstruction.

A lateral soft tissue x-ray of the neck (**choice D**) may reveal thickening of the epiglottis or supraglottic soft tissues, but will delay the appropriate management of an impending airway emergency.

Supplemental oxygen is reasonable, although nebulized albuterol will delay appropriate management and is not likely to be helpful. Admitting the child for observation (**choice E**) rather than immediate evaluation and protection of the airway is an incorrect choice.

6. **The correct answer is B.** In any case of trauma to the nose, the anterior nasal cavity and nasal septum should be carefully examined for evidence of a septal hematoma. This can be done with a nasal speculum or an otoscope with a large speculum attached. A septal hematoma will appear as a pale or slightly erythematous midline mass in the anterior nasal cavity and represents a collection of blood between the septal cartilage and mucosal layer. The treatment is drainage with a small incision in a dependent location within the nose under local anesthesia and placement of light nasal packing to prevent reaccumulation of blood. Oral antibiotics that cover *Staphylococcus aureus* are indicated while any nasal packing remains in place. A septal hematoma that is missed and not drained is at significant risk of infection. This can lead to destruction of the septal cartilage with subsequent loss of nasal dorsal support and a saddle nose deformity.

   Reduction of a suspected nasal fracture (**choice A**) is not indicated as there is no evidence on exam of an obvious displaced nasal fracture. The nasal dorsum, although tender, does not appear deviated or mobile. It is possible that several days later, when a majority of the swelling has resolved, a subtle deformity of the dorsum may be appreciated. If this is the case, the child can be scheduled for a closed reduction of nasal fracture in the operating room. This is best performed within 7 to 10 days of the injury, before any significant bony healing has taken place. It is also possible that the child has a non-displaced nasal bone fracture with no deformity of the nasal dorsum. Generally, this would not require any surgical intervention.

   A CT scan of the facial bones (**choice C**) may be reasonable given the mechanism of injury, but a careful physical examination can rule out most other possible facial fractures or injuries.

   Radiographs of the nasal bones (**choice D**) are not felt to be helpful by most otolaryngologists. In general, the diagnosis of a nasal fracture is made on physical exam. Even if a nondisplaced or partial fracture was identified on x-ray, it would likely not require any intervention.

   Treatment with an antibiotic and followup in 1 week (**choice E**) is not a reasonable option. If a septal hematoma were to be missed on initial exam, it would likely be infected by 1 week and the patient would be at risk for the complications described above.

7. **The correct answer is A.** The presentation and physical findings in this newborn indicate a possible choanal atresia. Choanal atresia is a complete obstruction of the nasal cavity resulting from a persistence of the oronasal membrane beyond the 6th week of gestation. Choanal atresia can be membranous (10%) or bony (90%) and is bilateral in approximately one-third of cases. Because the atresia is oriented in the coronal plane, it is best diagnosed with an axial CT scan. Choanal atresia is seen in approximately 1/8000 live births and occurs in females about twice as often as in males. In unilateral cases, the right side is more commonly affected than the left. Choanal atresia is associated with other congenital anomalies in 50% of unilateral cases and 60% of bilateral cases. The most common congenital syndrome associated with choanal atresia is the CHARGE syndrome (coloboma, heart anomalies, choanal atresia, retarded growth, genital hypoplasia, and ear abnormalities). Because newborns are obligate nasal breathers, bilateral choanal atresia can present at birth with episodes of apnea and cyanosis. Unilateral atresia often presents later in childhood with unilateral rhinorrhea and nasal obstruction.

   As this newborn's airway distress was resolved with endotracheal intubation, a flexible bronchoscopy (**choice B**) via the endotracheal tube to evaluate the distal trachea and bronchi would not be expected to yield the diagnosis.

   A karyotype (**choice C**) may be reasonable for this child, although there is no typical chromosomal abnormality associated with choanal atresia or CHARGE syndrome.

   An MRI of the head (**choice D**) might help to make the diagnosis, but CT is preferred because of its superior imaging of bony detail. MRI is often used for better visualization of soft tissues, but takes significantly longer (likely requiring a general anesthetic in this case) and is not necessary for the diagnosis.

   A plain lateral radiograph of the skull (**choice E**) would not be helpful in the diagnosis of choanal atresia. In evaluation of the sinuses, this film is classically used for visualization of the sphenoid sinus.

8. **The correct answer is A.** The first and most appropriate intervention should be to evacuate the impacted stool that is causing the problems. After that, medical and psychological causes should be looked into, starting with medical causes first.

   Prescribing sitting on a toilet after each meal (**choice B**) is usually done if there is a concern that the child is getting distracted and suppressing the bowel movements in order to pursue other more interesting or important things. It may be helpful in younger children that need toilet training, but it would most likely not be helpful in this case.

   Play therapy (**choice C**) is appropriate in treating children of this age in order to work on some conflicts related to family. It can involve different methods. In this case, however, referral to a child psychiatrist should be done if there is a suspicion of other underlying issues going on, once the medical causes are ruled out.

   Negative reinforcers (**choice D**) are used in treatment of severe behavioral problems. They are usually not used for treating constipation.

   Star award system (**choice E**) is a helpful behavioral method used mostly for treatment of enuresis and encopresis. It is mostly useful in younger children and mentally retarded patients, when other medical causes are ruled out. In this case one should first proceed with evacuation of stool and medical workup since encopresis alone is less frequently seen, especially in this age group.

9. **The correct answer is D.** Ten percent of children ages 2 to 5 years have in-toeing. Forty percent recover spontaneously. Rarely does in-toeing which persists into adulthood cause any problems such as arthritis. Management is education and reassurance to the family members. Inquire about other family members. It is very helpful in reassuring the mother when a family elder has asymptomatic in-toeing. A thorough history and physical examination will rule out underlying problems such as cerebral palsy, neuromuscular disorders, or other problems which would necessitate orthopedic consultation. The history of falls is quite common in early walkers. Toddlers are top heavy (center of gravity higher than adults), and they do not lift their toes when walking. Other factors, including poor balance, lead to frequent falls. The mother's statement that her other children did not have this problem is questionable. The origin of in-toeing is essentially from one of three locations: the thigh, leg, or foot. Metatarsus varus is more common in newborns. Increased internal femoral torsion is more common in the school-age child. For toddlers, in-toeing is usually from internal torsion. A combination of these three is possible. The physical exam is relatively simple, telling, and straightforward. The patient is examined as a whole and then in parts. Start with the gait, looking for symmetry, foot angle progression, and ability to lift the toes off the ground at the start of swing phase. Heel strike, an adult gait quality, begins approximately 6 months after the start of walking. Normal foot angle progression is 5 to 7 degrees. A negative angle indicates in-toeing, but not the source of in-toeing (thigh, shin, foot). In the prone position flex the knees up and check the lateral foot border. If the border is straight then metatarsus varus is not present. Next, keep the knee flexed and look down over the bottom of the foot in line with the leg. Imagine straight lines through the anatomic axis of the foot and thigh. This is the thigh-foot angle. Normal in this age group is 20 to 30 degrees. Less than –30 degrees is increased internal tibial torsion. Finally, check femoral torsion by testing internal and external rotation of the hips while in the prone position. For this age group, normal internal rotation is 15 to 60 degrees and external rotation is 45 to 90 degrees. Keep in mind that normal range of motion changes with age. The patient in this question has a completely normal exam.

   Denis Browne splints (**choice A**) are a treatment option but not for a normal patient.

   Orthopedic consultation (**choice B**) is not indicated. Follow the patient. If things progress or the patient develops pain, then consider specialty consultation.

   Physical therapy (**choice C**) has not been shown to be an effective treatment modality for in-toeing. Furthermore, it is not an option for a normal patient.

   Hip dysplasia and tarsal coalition (**choice E**) have different presentations. Newborns, firstborn, and breech babies with a hip "clunk" equals DDH. Tarsal coalitions typically become painful during early adolescence. A foot x-ray in a 15-month-old will show immature bone. Some bones (the navicular, for example) are not radiographic until 2 to 3 years of age.

10. **The correct answer is B.** An adolescent well visit should include an assessment of nutrition. Health providers should ask about diet, physical activity, and the number and balance of meals and snacks. They should assess whether there is adequate intake of calcium and iron. Attention should be placed on cholesterol intake and what is the teenager's body image.

    Cultures for chlamydia and gonorrhea (**choice A**) should be obtained only after a provider determines that an adolescent patient has engaged in intercourse, has symptoms of sexually transmitted disease, or reports that his or her partner has a sexually transmitted infection.

There are many ethical issues with regard to drug screening. The American Academy of Pediatrics does not always recommend voluntary or involuntary testing. They also do not recommend that adolescents should be tested when a parent wants it. Drug screening should be performed according to the individual case at hand (**choice C**).

Head circumferences should be carefully measured during well-child visits until age 2 years. They no longer need to be routinely measured if there has been steady normal growth (**choice D**). If neurologic problems develop or other growth concerns arise, then measurements should be obtained.

A urinalysis including a urine dipstick for glucose and protein and microscopic evaluation is recommended either during the first well visit of an adolescent or during late puberty, but it is not as important as a dietary assessment that should take place during all adolescent well visits. A urinalysis is not the best answer (**choice E**).

11. **The correct answer is D.** Airway foreign bodies are a life-threatening emergency. Children, particularly at the age of 2, due to their curiosity and tendency to place items in the mouth, are at high risk of aspirating both food and non-food items. These objects can lodge anywhere in the respiratory tract and result in airway obstruction as well as infections (pneumonia or lung abscess) over several days or weeks. The assessment of patients for airway foreign bodies is based on the triad of history, physical exam, and radiographic findings. Of these, history is the most sensitive factor. History includes either a witness who saw the patient placing something in the mouth or simply a history of prolonged coughing or choking. Physical exam findings include asymmetric breath sounds (less air movement on the affected side), wheezes, or potentially loud upper airway sounds for tracheal or mainstem bronchus foreign bodies. Finally, radiographic findings can detect radiopaque foreign bodies as well as lung hyperinflation on the affected side due to air trapping, with potential shift of the mediastinum that is most often seen only on an end-expiration x-ray (when the air trapping of the affected side is most pronounced relative to the unaffected side). The treatment for airway foreign bodies is removal through rigid bronchoscopy performed under general anesthesia. Ideally, this is performed as soon as it is safe for the patient to undergo a procedure. Airway edema can progress to complete airway obstruction if not treated expeditiously. Because the risks of untreated airway foreign bodies are so serious, the index of suspicion should be high and consultation should be performed early, with preparation of the patient for a possible procedure under general anesthesia.

Admitting the patient to the hospital for observation as a precaution (**choice A**) is incorrect because patients with a suspected airway foreign body should be evaluated by an otolaryngologist in the emergency department.

Giving the patient something to eat, and if he swallows it without difficulty that will most likely rule out any serious abnormality (**choice B**), is not correct because this is an airway foreign body that often does not produce an associated difficulty with oral intake. In addition, any patient who may undergo general anesthesia in the near future should be on NPO status with IV fluids.

To obtain a chest x-ray and if that is normal, reassure the parents that anything that made the patient cough has most likely cleared (**choice C**), is incorrect. The patient's history is convincing for foreign body aspiration. The cough reflex that is produced by an airway foreign body has the ability to fatigue over time, even if the object remains in place. Therefore, the fact that the patient has stopped coughing does not necessarily suggest that the foreign body has cleared.

Reassuring his parents that because he seems comfortable in the emergency department and never developed cyanosis that he should be clear to go home with them (**choice E**) is not correct because history is the most sensitive factor in assessment of patients for airway foreign bodies and since the history suggests aspiration, he requires further evaluation.

12. **The correct answer is C.** In light of this child's high white count and fever, he most certainly needed further workup. Both his mother's medical history and his hemoglobin indicate that the child is likely to have sickle-cell anemia, despite the fact that we do not know the father's history. The fact that the child is refusing to walk is most concerning, and both septic joint and osteomyelitis must be considered. In patients with sickle-cell anemia, the most common cause of osteomyelitis or septic joint is the same as in all other patients. This is *Staphylococcus aureus.*

Pasteurella multocida (**choice A**) is incorrect because it is not a likely source of osteomyelitis in this setting. It is a common bacteria found in the mouths of dogs and cats.

Salmonella species (**choice B**) is the most common gram-negative organism known to grow in sickle-cell patients with suspected septic joint or osteomyelitis.

Patients should therefore receive appropriate antibiotic coverage. This choice, however, is incorrect because overall *Staphylococcus aureus* is still more common.

Streptococcus pneumonia (**choice D**) is the most common cause of bacterial infections in children ages 3 months to 3 years and should most definitely be covered with antibiotic treatment. However, it is not the most common cause of this infection.

Lastly, *Streptococcus pyogenes* (**choice E**) is a very rare cause of septic arthritis or osteomyelitis.

13. **The correct answer is C.** This patient has a few symptoms to suggest pregnancy. She has history of fatigue and nausea. Her nausea may well explain the few pounds of weight loss. Some women early in pregnancy lose rather than gain weight. The chest pains this patient is experiencing may really represent breast tenderness. Noteworthy in this case is that the patient's last menstrual period was mid-October and it is now the end of November. Even though she denies sexual activity, she may be reluctant to talk about it and the physician must do a pregnancy test.

A complete blood count (**choice A**) might be indicated if the patient appears to have an infectious disease or anemia, but it would not be the first step in this assessment.

Although fatigue is a major complaint with infectious mononucleosis, the absence of physical findings such as cervical lymphadenopathy, exudative tonsillitis, or hepatosplenomegaly would not lead the physician to obtain a Monospot test (**choice B**).

A throat culture or rapid strep test (**choice D**) is not indicated at this time. She denies any fever and other illness symptoms to suggest significant pharyngitis or possible streptococcal disease. Her physical examination does not reveal impressive findings.

If this patient had a negative hCG and was not pregnant, then followup in 4 weeks (**choice E**) would be appropriate. However, she should be advised to seek medical help before then if her symptoms worsen or she develops a fever.

14. **The correct answer is C.** This discharge is consistent with physiological leukorrhea. It is a normal discharge that appears in young premenarchal girls usually 3 to 6 months prior to menarche. It is characterized by white, mucoid, nonmalodorous discharge that has a pH less than 4.5. This girl had her menarche about 2 months after she claims to have noted the discharge. She otherwise seems well without other symptoms or history that would require a pelvic examination. The rodlike bacteria are most likely lactobacilli. These bacteria are found in normal vaginal flora.

At this time there is no indication to culture for sexually transmitted diseases (**choice A**).

In the absence of a history of sexual contact and other genitourinary complaints in this young adolescent female, no pelvic is indicated (**choice B**).

There is not a heavy, white, cottage cheese-like discharge or vulvovaginitis that suggests this girl needs therapy for monilial vaginitis (**choice D**). If this girl had diabetes, was on oral contraceptives, or recently had taken antibiotics, one might be tempted to prescribe therapy for candida.

Metronidazole might be used if the girl has trichomoniasis (**choice E**). No flagellated, motile forms were seen on the wet prep. Clinical features that would suggest trichomoniasis include a frothy, greenish-gray discharge and a high pH of the mucus.

15. **The correct answer is D.** ELISA is the test of choice for *Giardia lamblia*, which is one of the most common causes of diarrhea after exposure to mountain lake and river waters. In fact, persons embarking on whitewater rafting adventures in the mountain rivers and streams are advised to close their mouths if they fall into the river because of *Giardia*.

Radiologic studies will not usually be very helpful in cases of *Giardia* (**choice A**). However, if studies are performed there might be subtle findings such as apparent increased mucosal fold thickness of the small intestine, and this could be suggestive for *Giardia*.

A single stool examination for trophozoites or cysts is helpful, and frequently three different stool examinations are necessary to find *Giardia*, but the use of the ELISA test for the *Giardia* antigen is the better diagnostic test (**choice B**).

Eosinophilia is not a very helpful screening tool for parasitic disease (**choice C**).

Stool cultures for bacterial organisms would not detect *Giardia* (**choice E**).

16. **The correct answer is D.** This patient most likely has Osgood-Schlatter disease. It is frequently encountered during early to mid-adolescence with painful enlargement of the tibial tubercle. It may affect one knee or frequently both knees. Treatment consists of decreasing the swelling with ice, protecting the knee from repeated trauma with the use of special pads, and NSAIDs or acetaminophen for pain relief.

    A CBC and sedimentation rate would not be helpful in screening for disease. These are nonspecific and may even be normal in a variety of diseases (**choice A**).

    A CBC, ESR, and ANA might be appropriate tests to order if one suspects rheumatologic disease (**choice B**). However, in this case there is no history of joint stiffness, no other joint involvement besides the knees, the swellings are below the knees, and extra-articular complaints such as fever, rash, and eye symptoms are absent.

    NSAIDs alone might help alleviate the pain and swelling, but would not be the best answer (**choice C**).

    It is always important to think of malignancy or bone cancer in the differential diagnosis of knee or hip pain. However, if a patient presents with the classic features of Osgood-Schlatter disease, especially when both knees are affected, x-rays are not usually indicated (**choice E**).

17. **The correct answer is A.** This patient most likely has an incarcerated inguinal hernia. The immediate step in this case is to obtain a surgical consult right away. The surgeon needs to determine whether or not it is an incarcerated hernia. Keep in mind that sometimes inguinal lymphadenopathy may mimic an incarcerated hernia. Both may present with tender irreducible groin masses in infants who are crying and irritable. Sometimes bowel gas can be palpated in the groin bulge of the hernia. If it is incarcerated and the surgeon is unable to reduce it then surgery is needed right away.

    CBC, electrolytes, and BUN may be indicated while you are waiting for the surgeon if the infant is significantly dehydrated and listless, but this is not the first-choice answer in this infant who is crying tears (**choice B**). It is best not to upset the infant anymore until the surgeon consults and tries to manually reduce the incarcerated hernia.

    In this case wait for the surgeon before ordering a CBC and type and cross (**choice C**).

    A technetium scan is definitely not indicated here (**choice D**). A technetium scan would be ordered when one wants to determine or demonstrate blood flow to the testes, as in cases of possible testicular torsion.

    Transillumination of the testis might be used to better identify scrotal masses (**choice E**), but would not be very helpful in this case, which is most consistent with an incarcerated inguinal hernia.

18. **The correct answer is B.** Spinal curves that are rapidly progressive and painful require further workup for underlying disease, especially if there are neurologic abnormalities such as asymmetric reflexes. In most cases of idiopathic scoliosis there is not a lot of associated pain.

    The amount or degrees of curvature does not necessarily indicate whether or not the scoliosis is idiopathic or primary or whether it is secondary to other disease (**choice A**). The most common form of scoliosis during adolescent years is idiopathic scoliosis. It may be mild or reach a moderate or severe degree of spine curvature. For managing, decisions as to when a referral to orthopedic surgery is indicated often depend on the physical maturation of the teen (e.g., sexual maturity rating) and the rate of curve progression.

    Female gender is not an indicator that there is other underlying disease (**choice C**). Most idiopathic scoliosis during adolescence occurs among females. If a male teen presents with scoliosis one might want to look more closely for possible secondary disease.

    A rib hump indicates that there is not only linear spinal curvature, but a significant degree of spinal rotation as well. In and of itself, it is not an indicator of other pathological disease (**choice D**).

    Three or four café-au-lait spots are not enough to point to a diagnosis of neurofibromatosis, one possible secondary disease that may be an etiology for scoliosis (**choice E**). One of the criteria for neurofibromatosis-1 in adolescence is the presence of six or more café-au-lait spots that are greater than 15 mm in diameter.

19. **The correct answer is D.** Blunt trauma to the eye should be taken very seriously. It may be associated with anterior chamber bleeding or hyphema, lens subluxation, and importantly, as in this case, retinal tears, edema, or detachment. An additional part of the eye exam (not mentioned in this case) is visual acuity. In cases with severe hits to the eye an immediate referral to the ophthalmologist is important.

    The injury was described to the eye, but this patient should obviously be evaluated for other head injury. No other injuries were noted in this case, so this is the wrong answer (**choice A**).

An ice pack over the area may help to decrease the swelling, but one needs to rule out an internal eye injury right away (**choice B**).

Rest and observation is not the next best step (**choice C**).

It would seem to be an excellent plan to see this young man in followup regarding his anger and how he handles bad situations. However, this is not the initial best step in acute management (**choice E**).

20. **The correct answer is E.** This is an infected thyroglossal duct cyst and the infection needs to be treated first. An appropriate choice of medications would be a broad-spectrum antibiotic to cover streptococcus or staphylococcus bacteria, such as cephalexin.

A neck ultrasound might be useful in some cases to confirm the presence of a normal location for the thyroid or in instances where the thyroid gland seems irregular; however, it is not an important next step in the management of this case (**choice A**).

A radioactive iodine uptake study is not necessary (**choice B**).

A T_3, T_4, and TSH may be ordered when the history or physical findings are suggestive of hypo- or hyperthyroidism (**choice C**).

The infections should be treated before a surgical consult or other evaluations are carried out (**choice D**). Obviously, the surgeon must be certain that it is a thyroglossal duct cyst before removing it. In very rare cases it may be confused with an ectopic thyroid.

21. **The correct answer is E.** Currently, the recommended calcium intake for adolescents is definitely more than 1000 mg. The most recent American Academy of Pediatric guidelines recommend 1300 mg a day for children aged 9 to 18 years. Children with malabsorption, growth hormone deficiency, cerebral palsy, chronic renal disease, and certain other conditions have an increased risk for osteoporosis and need higher daily intakes of calcium.

The recommended vitamin D intake a day is 400 IU, however 400 mg a day of calcium is the wrong amount of calcium needed each day (**choice A**).

A calcium intake of 500 mg a day would be an appropriate choice of calcium intake for a 5-year-old child (**choice B**).

A calcium intake of 800 mg a day would be an appropriate choice of calcium intake for an 8-year-old child (**choice C**).

A calcium intake of 1000 mg a day would not be a sufficiently high calcium intake for an adolescent (**choice D**).

22. **The correct answer is D.** With signs and symptoms such as mucosal bleeding, petechiae, and ecchymoses, a complete blood count will provide useful information such as the platelet and hemoglobin counts.

Bleeding time (**choice A**) is used to screen for small vessel integrity, von Willebrand, and platelet function. This may be useful but not as an initial test.

A partial thromboplastin time (**choice B**) and a prothrombin time (**choice C**) may be useful but not initially. These studies will evaluate whether or not there is a coagulopathy due to deficiency or abnormality of clotting factors (for example, secondary to liver disease). However, the scenario states that there is no hepatomegaly. Also, the patient is experiencing mucosal bleeding versus coagulation-type bleeding. Coagulation factor bleeding, as in the case of hemophiliacs, occurs in deep tissues and joints.

Hemoglobin electrophoresis (**choice E**) would not reveal anything about platelet count or other cell lines. With the symptoms presented, a CBC is most appropriate.

23. **The correct answer is E.** Based on the signs and symptoms, the most likely diagnosis is an intraventricular hemorrhage, hence the tense fontanelle. Intraventricular hemorrhages are associated with extreme prematurity and problems with maintaining blood pressure. The germinal matrices nearest the ventricles are highly vascular are susceptible to spontaneous hemorrhage.

A complete blood count (**choice A**) would be helpful in knowing how low the hematocrit is and whether the child needs to be transfused but it does not provide a diagnosis.

The bradycardia and hypotension are likely due to low perfusion pressure secondary to blood loss in the brain. An echocardiogram (**choice B**) would not reveal the cause of hypotension. An echo would be useful in a primary cardiac problem such as arrhythmias.

An electroencephalogram (**choice C**) is useful for delineating seizure foci and baseline background brain wave activity. In this clinical setting, it would not aid in diagnosis of intraventricular bleed.

A serum prothrombin is useful (**choice D**) if a primary coagulopathy is suspected. In this case, the cause of the bleed is prematurity.

24. **The correct answer is A.** With the advent of surfactant, mortality and pneumothoraces have decreased among infants with hyaline membrane disease, which is the most likely diagnosis in this 32-weeks' gestation baby. Babies who require over 30 to 40% FiO_2 should receive 2 doses 8 to 12 hours apart. With treatment with surfactant, ventilator settings and FiO_2 are significantly decreased

    Vitamin K (**choice B**) is routinely given to newborns to prevent hemorrhagic disease of the newborn, which is caused by a deficiency of the vitamin K clotting factors (2, 7, 9, 10). It occurs in 0.25 to 1.7% of newborns and can lead to intraventricular hemorrhage and ecchymoses. There are not signs and symptoms of this in the vignette.

    Sodium bicarbonate (**choice C**) is used during resuscitation for acidosis that has not responded to oxygen, ventilation, and volume. Though this may be a useful adjunct to endotracheal surfactant, especially if the infant has *documented* metabolic acidosis, the vignette does not offer that information (i.e., a blood gas).

    In the premature infant, intravenous steroids (**choice D**) are given to mothers prior to delivery to aid in lung maturity. Infants whose mothers have received steroids more than 24 hours prior to delivery have less respiratory distress and decreased mortality. There is no role for postnatal steroids.

    Intravenous indomethacin (**choice E**) is used to close a clinically significant patent ductus arteriosus. It is administered every 12 to 24 hours for three doses. A major side effect is transient oliguria as well as transient decreases in intestinal and cerebral blood flow. There is no role for this medication in treatment of respiratory distress syndrome.

25. **The correct answer is B.** This history is typical of pyloric stenosis. Pyloric stenosis is hypertrophy of the pyloric sphincter causing a gastric outlet obstruction. Firstborn males are more commonly affected. Generally, the emesis begins with occasional non-bilious emesis that then progresses to projectile, forceful emesis after almost every feed. The emesis doesn't contain bile because the obstruction is before the ampulla of Vater. On physical exam you should feel for an epigastric olive-shaped mass, but it can be difficult to palpate so an abdominal ultrasound must be done.

    If this child had appeared dehydrated or malnourished then it would be more appropriate to obtain electrolytes to check for the hypokalemic metabolic alkalosis that can come along with a long-standing process. Here, the progressive, forceful emesis was only present for a few days and the baby still appears to be well hydrated and not malnourished, therefore electrolytes would be unnecessary at this point so electrolytes (**choice A**) is incorrect.

    With a typical story for pyloric stenosis, an abdominal x-ray is not needed. If there were a history of bilious vomiting then an x-ray would be necessary to rule out volvulus and malrotation. Since that history is not present in this case, abdominal x-ray (**choice C**) is incorrect.

    A barium study can reveal a narrow pylorus in pyloric stenosis and one may see a "string sign" or a pyloric beak. Although this study can aid in the diagnosis of pyloric stenosis, it is not the first line in imaging studies and therefore an upper GI with small bowel follow-through (**choice D**) is incorrect in this case.

    Reassure the parents that it is reflux and send them home with followup (**choice E**) is incorrect because reflux is generally not a forceful event. Reflux is generally described as non-forceful emesis that was present in the beginning of this case. But being that the nature of the emesis changed, this case is not typical for reflux and therefore choice E is not the correct answer.

26. **The correct answer is A.** The child has the typical features of viral laryngotracheobronchitis (croup) usually secondary to the parainfluenza virus. The cough, respiratory stridor, and distress result from edema of the subepiglottic portion of the upper airway, thus aerosolized epinephrine is indicated along with intramuscular dexamethasone and budesonide.

    Albuterol (**choice B**) is not indicated due to the absence of wheezing. It may also cause further tachycardia.

    Antibiotics (**choice C**) do not have a role in the treatment of viral croup.

    Humidification of inspired air can sometimes be beneficial, but the illness can be complicated by critical upper airway obstruction and the child has stridor with intercostal retractions. The child should not be sent home (**choice D**) until improvement is demonstrated.

    Attempted visualization of the epiglottis (**choice E**) will increase the child's anxiety and worsen the symptoms. The likelihood of it being an epiglottitis is rare.

27. **The correct answer is C.** The child should be given a glucose-electrolyte mixture, which is based on active transport of sodium ions linked with glucose molecules and subsequent diffusion of water from the gut. Flow of sodium into and out of the bowel lumen is primarily responsible for fluid regulation in the gut. With the

addition of glucose to the solution, sodium will be reabsorbed by active coupled transport and dehydration will be prevented. The glucose concentration should be about 5% and the sodium (and potassium) content should be 2 to 3 mEq of each ion per 100 cc of water.

Boiling and then cooling water (**choice A**) might sterilize the water appropriately but will not effectively allow reabsorption to occur since it lacks glucose and sodium to enable active couple transport at the enterocytic level.

Milk feedings would be a less effective form of oral rehydration compared with the glucose electrolyte mixture for the same reason (**choice B**).

Glucose and water (**choice D**) lacks sodium and would not effectively allow for reabsorption of water from the gut. In fact, the introduction of a hyperglycemic solution without adequate sodium may result in diffusion of water *into* the bowel lumen and worsening dehydration. It is for this reason that orange juice (**choice E**) would also not work and might even exacerbate the dehydration.

28. **The correct answer is A.** Chlamydial pneumonia is seen in infants 3 to 16 weeks of age. They are usually sick for several weeks. The infant is nontoxic on exam, afebrile, usually tachypneic, and has a prominent cough. Conjunctivitis is seen in about 50% of cases. The chest film demonstrates diffuse interstitial patches.

Human parvovirus (**choice B**) or parvovirus B19 causes erythema infectiosum typically presenting in an older age group as a low-grade fever, a facial rash with a slapped-cheek appearance, and a lacy, reticularlike, maculopapular rash on the trunks and extremities. Gastrointestinal upset, coryza, and myalgia are associated symptoms.

Parainfluenza virus (**choice C**) presents as upper respiratory infections of several days' duration with a hoarse, croupy cough and inspiratory stridor. The child is restless with retractions evident in severe infections. It usually resolves in 48 to 72 hours and if this progresses longer can manifest as laryngeal obstruction. Steeple sign is seen on a lateral x-ray of the neck with glottic and subglottic narrowing.

Respiratory syncytial virus (**choice D**) begins with pharyngitis and rhinorrhea followed by 1 to 3 days of cough and wheezing. Diffuse rhonchi, fine rales, and wheezing can be auscultated. The chest film is normal. Chlamydial infections may be differentiated from RSV by conjunctivitis and a subacute onset.

Staphylococcal pneumonia (**choice E**) has a sudden onset. The child appears toxic and febrile with an expiratory wheeze at onset, stimulating bronchiolitis. There may also be signs of abdominal distress, tachypnea, dyspnea, and localized or diffuse bronchopneumonia. There is prominent leukocytosis.

29. **The correct answer is B.** Irritation to the glans is the most likely cause of his pain. This is actually common and often occurs after prolonged stays in the bath. This can sometimes cause vulvovaginal irritation in girls.

There is no indication for child or sexual abuse in this history (**choice A**). First of all, the child is brought in quickly after the initial complaint of penile pain. The history has no inconsistencies, the child demonstrates good rapport with his parents, and there are no other members in the household. There is no obvious damage or trauma to the penis on exam, which can sometimes be seen after aggressive handling of the genitalia.

Phimosis (**choice C**) is pain and swelling of the glans. In phimosis, the foreskin effectively "strangulates" the glans and is a cause of severe pain. If not corrected manually then the patient would require operative resection of the foreskin to save the glans. (Always remember to pull back the foreskin after retraction, particularly with adult patients who have had a urethral catheter inserted.)

Urinary tract infections in boys are rare (**choice D**). If confirmed, they point to further workup to rule out urological pathology, including a renal sonogram to rule out hydronephrosis and a voiding cystourethrogram to rule out urinary reflux disease at the pelvic-ureteric junction/valve. The latter is done usually after the second UTI in boys although some doctors order it after the first UTI. The child is unlikely to have a urinary tract infection because he does not have any symptoms of dysuria or fever, he does not appear septic on exam, and his urinalysis is negative for protein, leukocyte esterase, nitrites, and white cell count.

Urolithiasis (**choice E**) is unlikely mainly due to the lack of red blood cells in the urinalysis. Typically, the parent would describe the child having acutely severe abdominal pain with micturition (when the child is screaming). This would stop the moment micturition ends.

30. **The correct answer is B.** This patient most likely has hemolytic uremic syndrome. This is evidenced by the mild prodromal illness for 1 to 7 days often with vomiting, mild diarrhea, abdominal pain, and fever and then quite suddenly becoming severely ill and pale. There is coincident rapid hemolysis of red blood cells, renal insuf-

ficiency, decreased urine output, and thrombocytopenia. The confirmatory lab finding is microangiopathic hemolysis with burr and helmet cells and schistocytes. *Escherichia coli* 0157:H7 is a common cause.

Berger disease (**choice A**) typically runs a benign course in children. Gross hematuria occurs during or after an acute respiratory infection without evidence of azotemia, hypertension, or edema. Berger originally described IgA mesangial deposition. Recently there has been IgM deposition noted too. The child usually gets better and should not undergo recurrent invasive investigations.

Henoch-Schönlein syndrome (**choice C**) usually comprises a triad of gastrointestinal symptoms, purpura, and joint problems. The latter two are not seen in this patient. The additional presence of hematuria with or without proteinuria is indicative of glomerulonephritis.

Hirschprung disease (**choice D**) typically presents with constipation, abdominal bloating, vomiting, poor feeding, and weight loss. It is a problem of large bowel peristalsis related to an aganglionic colon (of the Auerbach plexus) which is diagnosed with a rectal biopsy, rectal manometry, or barium enema. Anemia and bloody stools are not typically seen.

Goodpasture syndrome (**choice E**) is rare in childhood and is composed of pulmonary hemorrhage, glomerulonephritis, and an anti-glomerular membrane antibody. Patients typically present with hemoptysis, proteinuria, and microscopic hematuria.

31. **The correct answer is A.** A CBC and platelet count will be the most helpful in making the diagnosis of idiopathic thrombocytopenic purpura (ITP). ITP is one of the most common pediatric bleeding disorders. It often follows a viral illness and nearly all patients have remission within a few months time. The physical examination may reveal ecchymoses and petechiae, especially over pressure-point areas of the body. Laboratory work reveals no anemia, red cell indices are normal, and the white cell count is normal. PT and PTT are normal and bleeding time may be increased if the platelet count is very low. The platelet count is frequently less than $20{,}000/mm^3$. A peripheral smear reveals a decreased number of enlarged platelets. If there is no concern based on history, physical, or abnormal CBC findings, a bone marrow is usually not indicated.

Renal studies should be done if one suspects conditions such as hemolytic uremic syndrome (HUS) or Henoch-Schönlein Purpura (HSP), but these are not indicated if ITP is suspected (**choice B**). HUS may follow an upper respiratory infection or gastroenteritislike illness. HUS is characterized by anemia, thrombocytopenia, and renal failure. Physical examination reveals edema and petechiae. HSP classically presents after an upper respiratory infection with palpable purpura, petechiae, and ecchymoses noted on the lower legs. HSP may be associated with glomerulonephritis.

Thrombocytopenia may be associated with many of the common viral infections of childhood, such as cytomegalovirus, Epstein-Barr virus, varicella, and rubella. Infectious mononucleosis in younger children may be asymptomatic and the Monospot is frequently unreliable. EBV titers, not a Monospot, should be done if history and physical suggest mononucleosis (**choice C**).

The rash alone is not sufficient to make a diagnosis of ITP (**choice D**).

Information is not given to suggest this is Kawasaki disease (**choice E**). An echocardiogram should be obtained in patients with Kawasaki disease because of the possible complication of coronary aneurysm. In Kawasaki disease clinical manifestations include fever, conjunctival injection, involvement of mucous membranes, peripheral extremity changes, rash, and cervical lymphadenopathy. A CBC usually reveals mild anemia and leukocytosis. After the first week of illness the platelet count is often increased, not decreased.

32. **The correct answer is D.** This patient exhibits several classic signs of cystic fibrosis (CF), a disorder that results from mutations in a gene encoding a chloride channel on the surface of epithelial cells. Dysfunction of this channel leads to a multisystem disease, which includes thickened secretions in the lungs with chronic pulmonary infections, failure to thrive due to malabsorption resulting from exocrine pancreas disease, meconium ileus at birth, and infertility. Inability to reabsorb chloride from sweat leads to an increased risk of dehydration and forms the basis of the major diagnostic test for CF. Increased sweat chloride in the setting of a suspicious clinical picture is a sensitive and specific test for CF.

The erythrocyte sedimentation rate (**choice A**) is a laboratory value that correlates with inflammatory processes. It is a useful marker to follow during the course of a long-standing disease, but would be of little value in this acute setting.

The diagnosis of pneumonia can be made on physical examination, with chest x-ray, or both. Even with appropriate antimicrobial therapy, the changes seen on chest x-ray can take weeks to resolve. Thus, a repeat chest x-ray (**choice B**) within that time frame is of little diagnostic utility.

Measurement of pulmonary function by spirometry, including the peak expiratory flow rate (**choice C**), can be a useful tool for the long-term follow-up of patients with obstructive or restrictive pulmonary disease. It is of value for monitoring the status of patients with CF, but is not of diagnostic utility in the workup of recurrent pneumonias.

Rectal biopsy (**choice E**) is the diagnostic test of choice for Hirschprung disease, aganglionosis of the distal colon. This entity is part of the differential diagnosis for delayed passage of meconium in the neonatal period, and manifests as dilated intestinal architecture proximal to the affected segment of bowel. However, there is no association with recurrent infections with Hirschprung disease.

33. **The correct answer is E.** This case scenario would be supportive of a diagnosis of anorexia nervosa (AN). The girl gives a history of amenorrhea before any significant weight loss. This is frequently seen with AN. Importantly, this girl is active in school, active in sports, and has been healthy for the past year. Her mother also suggests that she may be overly shy, hinting at possible self-image problems. Further information about her interpersonal relationships, especially with her parents, will be important to know. Her vital signs indicate bradycardia, low blood pressure, and decreased temperature. All these, taken together with a very low weight for height, must make one think of AN. Cold intolerance, overactivity, and constipation are common presenting symptoms in AN. Many of the physical signs in AN are related to the weight loss and have been reported in starvationlike states. Dry skin with yellow discoloration and hair loss may all be observed.

A history of headaches, polyuria, vomiting, and visual problems should be asked to rule out a CNS tumor, especially a tumor in the area of the hypothalamus or pituitary (**choice A**). Although weight loss and menstrual irregularities can be presenting symptoms of a CNS neoplasm it would not be the most likely diagnosis in this case scenario.

Hyperthyroidism should also be considered if review of system information reveals heat intolerance, fidgetiness, overactivity, and tremor (**choice B**). However, the reported vital signs would not be supportive of this diagnosis.

Possible infectious diseases such as tuberculosis or even HIV could lead to significant weight loss, and review of system questions about fever, cough, and rashes would be important to ask (**choice C**). Again, the additional information provided in this case makes the diagnosis seem unlikely.

Constipation, cold intolerance, inactivity, and dropping school grades might indicate hypothyroidism, but these symptoms could also indicate an underlying psychological disturbance such as depression (**choice D**).

34. **The correct answer is C.** Mild manipulation of the arm by flexing the elbow and supinating the forearm will treat the radial head subluxation (nursemaid elbow) and within minutes or right away the child will be moving her arm normally. When this is done many times you will feel a “click” sensation as the radial head pops back into place.

If this is a recurrent problem, other injuries are present, or the history seems otherwise, then child abuse might be suspected and child protective services (**choice A**) should be called.

Additional elbow and shoulder x-rays are not indicated (**choice B**). With a classic history of what happened, many times no x-rays are indicated.

Placing the arm in a cast or splint will not treat the underlying problem (**choice D**).

An orthopedic consult is unnecessary in this case (**choice E**). In some instances where the child does not move the arm well for an hour or so after manipulation, or when the injury may have occurred hours or days before any medical care is sought, then the orthopedist should be consulted.

35. **The correct answer is D.** The reticulocyte count should increase after 2 to 5 days of iron therapy for iron deficiency anemia.

A complete blood count will not indicate change so early (**choice A**). A small increase in the hemoglobin may occur after 7 to 10 days of therapy. If one is not in a hurry, the simple way to follow the patient would be to check another hemoglobin and hematocrit in a few months or several weeks after starting therapy.

Serum ferritin reflects the iron stores in the body and is the very last test to return to normal after iron therapy is completed (**choice B**).

The platelet count will not change after iron therapy (**choice C**).

The serum iron will not show early change (**choice E**).

36. **The correct answer is D.** Together the two abnormal findings in this newborn baby girl’s physical examination suggest the possibility of Turner syndrome. Edema of the hands and feet in a newborn infant girl might be

seen with Turner syndrome. Even though the heart exam is normal, the decreased femoral pulses suggest a coarctation of the aorta. It would be reasonable to get a cardiology consult in the near future, but this is not one of the choice answers. Therefore, the best answer is to obtain a karyotype to determine whether this infant has Turner syndrome (45,XO).

Digoxin (**choice A**) and furosemide (**choice B**) would be used for cardiac failure, but this is not evident in the newborn baby.

Simple observation of this infant is not the best answer (**choice C**). The abnormalities on exam need further workup.

Oxygen is not indicated in this infant who has a normal heart. There is no mention of respiratory problem or cyanosis (**choice E**).

37. **The correct answer is E.** He has pubic lice or *Phthirus pubis*. The best choice of therapy is to treat him with permethrin crème rinse. He may need to repeat this treatment in 4 to 5 days if it is not gone.

Clotrimazole (**choice A**) is used in candidiasis, not lice infestation.

Fluconazole (**choice B**) can be used to treat candidiasis, but is not effective against lice.

Griseofulvin (**choice C**) is an effective therapy for tinea infections that are unresponsive to topical therapy. It is not used to treat pubic lice.

Although lindane (**choice D**) might be considered as an acceptable choice of therapy, the better answer is permethrin because it has fewer side effects. Lindane has potential for neurotoxic effects and should be used with care.

38. **The correct answer is B.** Low-potency steroid creams such as 1% hydrocortisone cream should be very effective in treating these facial lesions, which are the typical findings of seborrheic dermatitis. The common areas affected with seborrhea are the face, eyebrows, behind the ears, and the perineum. She probably also has scalp involvement that would benefit from any of the various antiseborrheic shampoos, such as selenium sulfide, salicylic acid, or zinc pyrithione. This is a common skin condition seen at ages when hormonal stimulation of sebum production is high, namely during the first several weeks of life and at puberty.

Calcipotriene ointment (**choice A**) is a good choice for psoriasis; however, it is not typically used to treat seborrheic dermatitis.

Topical (e.g., mupirocin) or systemic antibiotics are not indicated in this case (**choice C**).

Permethrin crème rinse would be useful for lice (**choice D**).

TCA is used to treat condyloma acuminata, caused by the human papilloma virus (**choice E**). It is caustic and might well cause this young lady to never come back to see you.

39. **The correct answer is C.** Usually in cases of normal or familial obesity, children do not have growth delay. They enter puberty early and are frequently tall for their age. In cases where children are very short and very fat a possible endocrine disorder should be considered.

The fact that a boy has not entered puberty by age 13 is not necessarily a concern (**choice A**). His bone age that is 6 months less than his chronological age may be normal in this case.

If the boy is 13 years of age and his bone age is 1 year and 1 month advanced, this also appears to be normal because he has a pubertal development stage or SMR of 2 (**choice B**). The rate of bony maturation as determined by bone age corresponds better with physical and pubertal development than with chronological age.

As mentioned above, being tall and overweight is frequently normal and is seen commonly in familial obesity (**choice D**).

This boy is tall for his age and his SMR is 3, indicating that he may well be entering puberty earlier than many of his peers (**choice E**). For most males the peak growth spurt occurs during SMR 3 or 4.

40. **The correct answer is C.** This patient most likely has pertussis and should be treated with erythromycin. If identified early in the catarrhal stage, erythromycin will ameliorate the infection. However, it generally has little effect on the paroxysmal stage as seen in this case. Treatment in this case would be given to reduce the secondary transmission to family members.

Ampicillin (**choice A**) might be a possible choice of therapy in those patients who may not tolerate erythromycin, but it is not the drug of choice.

Ciprofloxacin (**choice B**) is also not recommended to treat pertussis. In vitro studies suggest that pertussis is susceptible to ciprofloxacin, but not enough clinical studies have been done.

Penicillin (**choice D**) is not the drug of choice and corticosteroids might help in reducing severe disease, but should be used with caution because of side effects.

Sulfonamide (**choice E**) is not the drug of choice for pertussis. Trimethoprim-sulfamethoxazole might be considered an alternative therapy for patients who do not tolerate erythromycin. Other alternative antibiotics include clarithromycin and azithromycin.

41. **The correct answer is D.** The ages of children in the sample population represents a skewed distribution of ages. With a skewed population the better measure of central tendency is the median.

An arithmetic spot is not an epidemiologic term (**choice A**).

The mean would give more weight to the outliers of age and would not be a good choice (**choice B**).

In this skewed population, the mean of the largest age group (**choice C**) would not be the best measure of central tendency. It would be misleading because it would not take into account the results of all the other age groups.

The mode refers to the age of a child that occurs more frequently. In this skewed population it would not be a good measure of central tendency (**choice E**).

42. **The correct choice is A.** The "slapped-cheek"-type rash together with the lacelike patterned rash on his arms point to a diagnosis of erythema infectiosum (Fifth disease). It is caused by parvovirus B19 and is no longer contagious to others after the appearance of the rash. He may attend school and the mother should not worry. However, if she is pregnant she should be told about its uncommon association with fetal death or hydrops fetalis.

As mentioned above, he is no longer contagious after the appearance of the rash (**choice B**).

This is an unlikely age for acne (**choice C**) and distinct papules or pustules are not described.

If this were mild acne (**choice D**) on the cheek, over-the-counter benzoyl peroxide might be a reasonable choice.

Topical antibiotics (**choice E**) would be an appropriate choice for mild papulopustular acne, but this is not acne.

43. **The correct choice is E.** In the majority of girls, breast development precedes the development of pubic hair. In this patient it is of concern that there is SMR 4 pubic hair development and only early SMR 2 breast development. Together with menstrual irregularities this would support a possible pubertal problem. Such a case may be seen with mosaic Turner syndrome. Mosaic cases often lack some of the Turner syndrome features, but short stature is usually present.

The 11-year-old female is appropriately prepubertal and not enough information is given to make anything of her past history of abdominal pain (**choice A**).

The 12-year-old male also appears to be in normal early puberty (**choice B**).

This 12-year-old male has features of early maturation with tall stature, obesity, and SMR 3 genitalia (**choice C**). More than 50% of adolescent males between 12 and 14 years of age may develop transient breast development, usually between SMR of 2 to 3.

The 14-year-old female who is assessed as SMR 4 has dysmenorrhea that is perfectly appropriate for her stage of development (**choice D**). Most girls do not experience dysmenorrhea until menses have become established for 1 to 2 years.

44. **The correct answer is A.** Early signs of copper deficiency include osteoporosis, neutropenia, and hypochromic anemia. Copper deficiency may be present in chronically malnourished children, preemies who are taking milks that do not have supplemental copper, and children who may be receiving total parenteral nutrition for extended periods of time without supplemental copper.

A serum ferritin would not be useful because you already know that if it is iron deficiency the anemia should have responded unless malabsorption or underlying diseases were present (**choice B**).

Lead deficiency is not associated with anemia (**choice C**). There is nothing in the history to suggest a lead toxicity situation. Lead poisoning is associated with hypochromic, microcytic anemia, but there would be no problem with neutropenia.

Selenium deficiency is not associated with anemia (**choice D**).

Zinc deficiency may be associated with anemia as with chronic disease states, but it does not cause neutropenia (**choice E**).

45. **The correct choice is D.** Diagnostic testing for mumps is indicated. Clinically, this boy has the symptoms and physical findings of parotitis, orchitis, and submandibular gland swelling suggestive of mumps, an RNA paramyxovirus. Acute and convalescent titers can be obtained.

This case is not very suggestive of cytomegalovirus (**choice A**). CMV is frequently asymptomatic in children or may present with an infectious mononucleosislike syndrome with several days of fever and mild hepatitis.

Epstein-Barr virus serology is not the best diagnostic test (**choice B**). EBV would frequently present in children with hepatosplenomegaly, tonsillitis, and malaise. Although it may present with nodes in the neck, patients characteristically have posterior cervical nodes.

HIV is another cause of parotitis, but the mumps testing is the best first step in this case (**choice C**).

Serum amylase would be increased with parotitis but would not help in differentiating possible underlying diagnoses (**choice E**). Coxsackie virus A, HIV, cytomegalovirus, and adenovirus can all cause parotitis.

46. **The correct choice is B.** In any male adolescents with gynecomastia it is important to complete the physical exam by examining the genitalia and assessing the Tanner staging or sexual maturity rating (SMR). Usually gynecomastia occurs during Tanner stage II to III. Particularly important in this very tall boy is to rule out any disorder such as Klinefelter syndrome. Characteristically, these patients have gonadal failure with small infantile testes and tall stature.

A bone age should not be done before assessing his height and weight together with the Tanner staging (**choice A**). A normal bone age will most closely correlate with the stage of pubertal development rather than the chronological age.

A serum testosterone is not the best next step in evaluating this boy (**choice C**).

Physiologic pubertal gynecomastia is very common during early puberty in most young males and a family history of gynecomastia is not very helpful (**choice D**). Knowing that close relatives may have had gynecomastia might make the emotional anguish of having "breasts" less of a worry to this boy, but it is definitely not the best next step.

Drug exposure to medications such as hormones (e.g., estrogen, testosterone, anabolic steroids) as well as drugs of abuse (marijuana, opioids, and other street drugs) may be the cause of breast symptoms including pain, gynecomastia, and galactorrhea. However, a urine screen for drugs is not the best next step in evaluation (**choice E**).

47. **The correct answer is B.** The child in the vignette has the classic features of congenital hypothyroidism or cretinism. This entity is rarely seen in the United States anymore due to the newborn screening program. These children can have growth retardation, myxedema, macroglossia, micrognathia, delayed fontanelle closure, jaundice, feeding problems, constipation, and a hoarse cry. The long-term sequelae of congenital hypothyroidism is severe mental retardation, which can be helped with the early initiation of treatment, which is why this disease entity is screened for as part of the routine newborn screening program in the United States.

Beckwith-Wiedemann syndrome (**choice A**) is a complex genetic syndrome that has some characteristics in common with hypothyroidism, namely macroglossia and abdominal wall defects. However, patients with this syndrome also have hemihyperplasia, ear anomalies, and renal anomalies.

Galactosemia (**choice C**) is an inborn error of metabolism. There is a deficiency of galactose-1-phosphate uridyltransferase. It is autosomal recessive and is associated with lethargy, hypotonia, hepatomegaly, and jaundice. These patients are more susceptible to gram-negative infections.

Infants with maple syrup urine disease (**choice D**) appear normal at birth and then develop poor feeding and vomiting during the first week of life, progressing to coma. There will be acidosis, hypoglycemia, and hyperammonemia and the urine will have a maple syrup odor.

Patients with a urea cycle defect (**choice E**) appear normal at birth and then have lethargy often proceeding to coma after a few days of protein in their diet. Labs reveal hyperammonemia.

48. **The correct answer is A.** The parents have the right to refuse immunizations for their children. No law forces parents to immunize their children. Of course, the child may not be able to attend public school without being immunized, but the parents are free to elect home schooling or other alternatives.

Immunizations are not harmless so you cannot assure the mother that the immunizations are harmless and tell her about the details of the diseases prevented by the immunizations (**choice B**). Although side effects and adverse reactions are relatively rare, they do occur.

The physician cannot proceed without parental consent (**choice C**). Failure to immunize does not place the child at risk of life or limb.

No law forces parents to immunize their children (**choice D**).

The public health department does not keep track of who accepts or refuses immunization (**choice E**).

Telling the mother you cannot continue to be the child's physician (**choice F**) constitutes abandonment, and is never acceptable.

49. **The correct answer is E.** The patient in question demonstrates a history that is consistent with children who have a reading disorder. To establish this diagnosis, however, the patient needs to demonstrate on standardized testing a proficiency in reading that is significantly lower than what should be expected given her age, education, and measured intelligence.

There is no indication for the routine use of electroencephalography (**choice A**) in the evaluation of learning disorders. A history of intermittent/episodic problems is clearly lacking in this patient, so the yield of an electroencephalogram to detect seizure activity is predictably low.

Given the absence of a history of head trauma or focal neurological signs, there is no indication for neuroimaging studies (**choice B**) in this patient in the diagnosis of a learning disorder.

The Minnesota Multiphasic Personality Inventory (**choice C**) is a useful battery of tests for the assessment of a wide variety of potential psychiatric conditions or when a patient's diagnosis and presentation are confusing (for example, due to the patient being a poor historian). It is not useful in the evaluation of learning disorders.

Projective psychologic testing (**choice D**) does not give information pertaining to the child's level of reading achievement relative to other academic areas. Given the absence of potential confounds such as depressive symptoms, it would be of limited utility in the establishment of the child's learning disorder.

50. **The correct answer is D.** This patient might have secondary syphilis. The presence of any body rash that is described as maculopapular, copper-colored, and involves the palms and soles should make you think of acquired syphilis. The secondary stage of syphilis begins 1 to 2 months after an indurated chancre may be seen. In addition to the rash, a patient may be ill with malaise and generalized lymphadenopathy. The presence of epitrochlear nodes may also be an important clue for syphilis because painless nodes at this location are rare. The RPR is likely to be positive in this young man.

A CBC would not be your next step with this rash (**choice A**). Results from a CBC would be nonspecific and not very helpful.

Tinea infections may possibly be confused with either the rash of pityriasis rosea or syphilis. A KOH wet prep might show hyphae in various types of tinea, but would not be helpful in identifying spirochetes (**choice B**). A KOH preparation of tinea versicolor scrapings would show short hyphae and spores in a "spaghetti and meatball" pattern.

Sometimes a rash accompanies streptococcal infection that may not look like the classic sandpaperlike rash we think of with scarlet fever. However, there is no good history for a sore throat or presence of tonsillar lymph nodes to warrant a rapid strep test or throat culture (**choice C**).

A Wood lamp exam would not be the best test to perform in this case (**choice E**). However, it may be helpful in identifying different types of tinea. *Microsporum canis* results in a green fluorescence and *Tinea versicolor* results in a yellow or gold fluorescence.

Pediatrics: **Test Two**

1. A 14-year-old African American girl comes to the office because of recurrent stomach cramps that typically occur after meals. Sometimes there is a bloating sensation and occasionally she has flatus. One of her brothers has problems when he drinks milk. She is not so sure milk is a problem for her, because she seldom drinks it. You suspect a diagnosis of lactose intolerance. The most appropriate next step in management to confirm the diagnosis is to

   (A) determine serum protein levels
   (B) order a breath hydrogen test
   (C) recommend dietary changes and reevaluate
   (D) send a stool specimen for analysis
   (E) test stool for occult blood

2. A 5-year-old boy is brought to the office by his parents because of a skin lesion on the face that suddenly developed 2 days ago. It started as a red pimple, but has grown to involve most of the cheek and is hot, red, and tense. The boy has no systemic symptoms, and all the parents remember was that he scratched his cheek several days earlier while playing with the neighborhood children. On physical examination, you find the boy to be well developed and well nourished, at the appropriate developmental level, and with height and weight in the fiftieth percentile for his age. He is not in acute distress and his vital signs are normal. On the right cheek there is a shiny, bright red, brawny, infiltrated plaque 5 × 6 centimeters in dimension with a distinct, well-marginated, and slightly elevated border. The periphery appears irregular because of projections of the inflammatory process. The lesion is tender and warm to palpation, and the right preauricular lymph nodes are enlarged and firm. The most likely causative agent of this boy's skin disease is

   (A) group A beta-hemolytic *Streptococcus*
   (B) *Haemophilus influenzae*
   (C) *Pityrosporum ovale*
   (D) *Pseudomonas aeruginosa*
   (E) *Staphylococcus aureus*

Items 3-4

The parents of one of your patients do not believe in additional immunizations. They believe that whatever they received when they were children was fine, but do not want any of these new and improved additional vaccines for their son. Their son has received the polio, DPT, MMR, Hepatitis B, but they had refused the varicella vaccine as recommended by the American Academy of Pediatrics. In mid-December the mother calls the office upset that her 10-year-old son seems to have chickenpox. He is fatigued and has a rash all over his body that consists of crops of red macules, some with water-blistered tops and others with pustular tops. His mother reports that his temperature is 38.3 C (101 F). You agree to see the boy in your office. An hour later he is ushered in the back door to avoid contact with other patients and you examine him in the back exam room. His vital signs are: temperature of 38.3 C (101 F), pulse of 83/min, and respirations of 25/min. Physical examination is fairly unremarkable except for a vesicular and papular rash in different stages of eruption. On his chest are groups of vesicles that have crusted over but are now oozing small amounts of pus. There also are wide areas of erythema around these chest lesions. The patient describes most of the lesions as itchy but the ones on his chest are also slightly painful.

3. The most appropriate next step in management is to

   (A) obtain a blood culture
   (B) obtain a complete blood count
   (C) order a chest x-ray
   (D) prescribe acyclovir
   (E) prescribe cephalexin
   (F) provide reassurance that no therapy is indicated

4. The appropriate steps are taken. The next day, the mother frantically calls your office asking for advice. She remembers what you said about the incubation time for chicken-pox being 10 to 21 days. In 2 weeks they are planning to travel out of town and visit her parents for Christmas. The grandmother is receiving chemotherapy for lung cancer. The mother is now concerned that her two younger unimmunized children at home may come down with chicken-pox because of the close contact with their brother, and she does not want to put her mother at risk. The most appropriate management is to

   (A) explain that she will likely have to cancel the trip
   (B) explain that the two younger siblings are unlikely to get chickenpox
   (C) perform varicella titers on her two children
   (D) suggest that the parents and siblings get varicella zoster immunoglobulin
   (E) suggest varicella zoster immunoglobulin for the two younger siblings

5. During the course of a physical examination for a 10-year-old girl you discover a firm, nontender nodule of the left lobe of the thyroid. There is no significant lymphadenopathy, and the rest of her examination is unremarkable. You know that a solitary thyroid nodule in a child warrants prompt evaluation. Current management recommendations suggest that the next best step for this girl is

   (A) a fine needle aspiration biopsy
   (B) a radionucleotide ^{123}I scan
   (C) serum T_4 and TSH
   (D) surgery
   (E) an ultrasound only

6. An 8-year-old is rushed to the emergency department by ambulance after sustaining multiple injuries during a bicycle accident. She is alert and cooperative and her vital signs are stable. Upon examination she is complaining of abdominal pain, and you note definite abdominal tenderness and absent bowel sounds. After determining that there are no spinal cord injuries, the most appropriate next step in management is to order

   (A) abdominal x-rays
   (B) a CT scan of the abdomen
   (C) a liver and spleen scan
   (D) peritoneal lavage
   (E) an ultrasound of the abdomen and pelvis

7. A 3-year-old boy is brought to the office for a routine well-child checkup. He has no significant past medical history, no allergies, takes no medications, and has been healthy over the past year. On physical examination you note pallor, but he has no significant lymphadenopathy or hepatosplenomegaly. You plot him on the growth chart and he is 50% for height and 40% for weight. His hematocrit is 26%. The most important history to obtain at this time is

   (A) birth history
   (B) developmental milestones
   (C) dietary history
   (D) family history of disease
   (E) history of trauma

8. A 9-year-old boy is brought to the office because of a 1-day history of diarrhea, vomiting, and low-grade fevers. The stool is loose and foul smelling, but there is no noticeable blood. He is drinking well but has no appetite. It seems to the mother that he has lost a bit of weight. His temperature in your office is 37.8 C (100 F). On physical examination his lips are dry and cracked, but his skin turgor is fine and mucus membranes are moist. There is no pharyngitis. His chest and abdominal examinations are benign. No rashes are noted, but there is redness with slight excoriation of his perianal area. You suspect he has a viral, not bacterial, gastroenteritis, and therefore the most appropriate management is to

   (A) do a stool exam for leukocytes
   (B) do a stool exam for mucus
   (C) observe the course of illness over the next few days
   (D) send a stool culture
   (E) test the stool for occult blood

9. You are called to the emergency department to see a 1-week-old male infant who has been vomiting over the past 2 to 3 days. His mother claims that he does not want to take his formula, and she has to spend time trying to coax him to eat. She is sure he has lost weight. On physical examination he is assessed to be mildly dehydrated. His genitourinary examination reveals hypospadias that the mother tells you has been there since birth. You are unable to feel either testis. The most appropriate next step in management is to order

   (A) an intravenous pyelogram
   (B) a karyotype
   (C) serum electrolytes
   (D) an ultrasound of his pelvis
   (E) an upper GI series

10. A 10-year-old boy is brought to the office complaining of frequent nosebleeds, joint pain, bleeding gums, shortness of breath, fatigue, and fever. His parents report that he has been especially susceptible to infections over the past 6 months. Subsequent examination and testing lead you to a diagnosis of acute lymphocytic leukemia. The oncologist and hematologist that you are working with believe that the boy is likely to die within 6 months, regardless of whatever treatment is initiated. Upon hearing the boy's diagnosis and prognosis, his parents appear visibly upset. With tears in her eyes, the boy's mother request that the boy be told nothing about the nature of his illness, nor how long he has to live. The best response to the parent's request is:

    (A) "I don't agree with your decision, but I will follow your wishes."
    (B) "I understand and agree with your decision."
    (C) "I'm afraid that I must insist on informing him of all the details if I am to remain as his physician."
    (D) "I'm sorry, but the child needs to know. Don't worry, I will tell him."
    (E) "I'm sorry, but the child needs to know; it would be best if you tell him."
    (F) "I'm sorry, but the child needs to know. Why don't we both go in and talk with him together?"
    (G) "Let's not make any decision now. Take some time to think about it and we can talk some more tomorrow."
    (H) "Tell me more about why you don't want the child to know."
    (I) "You do not want me to tell him because you have not yet accepted the reality of his condition."

11. A 3-year-old white boy is brought to the urgent care clinic by his parents because of a rapidly growing mole on his leg. They had noticed it 3 days earlier on the back of his lower leg and thought that it was just another one of many moles that have developed in the past year on his arms and legs; but this evening they were astonished to find that it had grown to be pea-sized and dark blue, almost black. The child is otherwise healthy and has no medical problems. He is a happy and thriving boy who spends most of his time outside, in the nearby park, weather permitting. On examination, the boy is a well-developed and well-nourished 3-year-old, merrily playing with his toy while you talk to the parents. He has no medical problems and takes no medication. He has multiple light to medium dark brown, 1- to 2-mm macules and papules on his trunk and extremities. On the posterior left leg, just below the popliteal fossae, there is a 5-mm bluish-black nodule with a 0.5-mm erythematous halo. You take your magnifying glass to confirm that, at the base of the lesion, several pairs of short, black legs are visible. After carefully removing the "mole" and ordering appropriate laboratory studies to be done, you tell the parents what they should watch for in their boy. The disease that the extracted organism transmits is

    (A) erythema ab igne
    (B) erythema chronicum migrans
    (C) erythema elevatum et diutinum
    (D) erythema infectiosum
    (E) erythema toxicum neonatorum

12. A 16-year-old girl is brought to the emergency department because of difficulty swallowing. Three days ago she started having a sore throat and fever. The following day she saw her pediatrician, who prescribed liquid amoxicillin for tonsillitis. This morning her throat was so sore that she could barely swallow the amoxicillin, and last night her temperature rose to 40.0 C (104.0 F). She denies any nausea or abdominal pain. She is otherwise healthy, although this is the third episode of tonsillitis that she's had in the past 6 months. Her temperature now is 39.1 C (102.4 F). She appears ill and is holding a cup into which she periodically spits saliva. She has moderate trismus and you have difficulty examining her oral cavity. With the help of two tongue blades, you manage to see that both tonsils are inflamed, but the right one appears significantly larger than the left. The soft palate is edematous on the right and the uvula is deviated to the left. Her neck is supple, although she has enlarged lymph nodes bilaterally. The most appropriate intervention at this time is to

(A) administer clindamycin intravenously and lactated Ringer solution in the emergency department and arrange follow-up with the child's pediatrician in the morning
(B) admit the child to the pediatric service for intravenous fluids and antibiotics
(C) consult otolaryngology for drainage of a peritonsillar abscess
(D) order a CT scan of the neck
(E) perform a throat culture, switch the antibiotic to amoxicillin clavulanate, and arrange followup with the child's pediatrician in the morning

13. A 14-day-old girl is brought to the clinic for a routine newborn checkup. She was born full term by normal spontaneous vaginal delivery. Her perinatal period was without complications, and she went home from the hospital on day 1 of life. She is breast-feeding well and has gained 2 pounds since birth. Her mother had an uneventful pregnancy, has no medical problems, and takes no medications. None of the infant's immediate relatives have any unusual health problems. On physical examination she weighs 10 lb, 3 oz. Her skin is clear and she has no gross deformities. She is breathing quietly and demonstrates a hearty cry when you pick her up. Examination of her oral cavity shows a strong suck reflex and no evidence of cleft palate. Upon palpation of her neck, you appreciate a firm, nonfluctuant mass at the lower third of the right sternocleidomastoid muscle. The mass feels fixed to the surface of the muscle and measures approximately 8 mm in diameter. Deep palpation does not seem to bother the child. The skin overlying the mass is normal. The child's neck is supple with no significant limitations in mobility. The remainder of the infant's physical examination is normal. You decide to do nothing at this time and see the infant back in 2 weeks. At her next visit, the mass is unchanged other than measuring approximately 12 mm in diameter. The most likely diagnosis is

(A) cervical teratoma
(B) cystic hygroma
(C) fibromatosis colli
(D) second branchial cleft cyst
(E) thyroglossal duct cyst

14. You receive a call from the principal of the local elementary school. The parents of one of the children enrolled in the school have just informed her that their son is HIV positive. The principal sounds upset and has called you to get some advice as to what she should do. Although the principal does not know it, you know the child to which the principal is referring and have been treating the child's HIV infection for the past year. The treatment has been effective at keeping the boy as healthy as possible without any opportunistic infections. At this point you should advise the principal that

(A) all children in the school should be tested for HIV
(B) HIV infection is not spread by casual contact and there is little risk to the other students
(C) the HIV-positive child should be assigned a separate bathroom to use to reduce the risks of contamination
(D) the HIV-positive child should be excluded from gym class so as to lower the risk to fellow students
(E) she should provide educational materials that explain HIV and associated risks to all of the parents of the children enrolled in the school
(F) there is a conflict of interest and you are unable to comment on this case
(G) tutoring should be arranged for the child, separate from the rest of the school's students
(H) you have been treating the boy and that he is responding well to treatment
(I) you should meet with her to discuss the case face-to-face

15. A 6-year-old girl from Haiti is brought to the office for an initial physical examination. She has no past history of illness and her shots are reportedly up-to-date. In fact, her mother reports that she received the Bacillus Calmette-Guerin (BCG) a few years before. Her past medical records reveal that she has already received the following immunizations: 3 hepatitis B, 5 DTaP, 4 IPV, 2 MMR, and 1 varicella. At this time the most appropriate next step in management is to administer

(A) DTaP, IPV, and PPD
(B) DTaP, IPV, and varicella
(C) IPV and PPD
(D) no vaccinations at this time
(E) PPD

16. An 18-year-old girl comes to the office for a well checkup before leaving for college. Her past medical history is unremarkable and her immunizations are up-to-date. Her 55-year-old father was diagnosed 6 months ago with early stage melanoma. She is concerned because she has many freckles and "moles". You review with her what she needs to know about any future changes in her "moles". To educate her about the ABCD or ABCDE signs of melanoma recognition, you tell her that these letters represent

(A) asymmetry, bleeding easily, color change or variegation, diameter >5 mm
(B) asymmetry, border irregular, central telangiectasia, deep and lobular
(C) asymmetry, border irregular, color change or variegation, diameter >4 mm
(D) asymmetry, border irregular, color change or variegation, diameter >6 mm
(E) asymmetry, border irregular, color change or variegation, deep, and exfoliating

17. An infant 3 months of age is brought to the emergency department with a high fever for 12 hours. The mother is very concerned as this is her first child and she has no experience with "such high fevers." The infant's temperature is 39.7 C (103.4 F), pulse is 145/min, and respirations are 30/min. She does not appear ill or toxic, and a complete physical examination is unremarkable. Since you want to be sure not to miss any form of sepsis or serious infection, the most appropriate next step in evaluation is to

(A) order a chest x-ray
(B) perform a lumbar puncture and send cerebrospinal fluid for culture
(C) send a stool specimen for culture
(D) send a throat culture
(E) send a urine culture

18. Both parents of a 6-year-old child schedule a visit to meet with you regarding their son's behavior. He has a problem with temper tantrums once or twice a week that are driving them crazy. They tried ignoring his behavior but it just gets worse, even in public. They have tried to be overly enthusiastic at other times and praise him when he behaves well, but this has not worked either. They state that he is very independent and exceedingly stubborn. The most appropriate advice to give these parents is to

(A) give him a harsh reprimand
(B) give him a "time out" for 30 minutes
(C) keep praising him at other times for good behavior
(D) repeatedly warn him that he will have a "time out" if he continues his behavior
(E) tell him he has two choices, he can stop it now and they can do a fun activity later, or he can persist with his tantrum and there will be a consequence for this unacceptable behavior

19. An 18-year-old patient who lives in the rainy, cloudy city of Seattle, Washington, is going to attend college in the fall in sunny California. She comes to the office for a precollege visit. A complete physical examination is normal. After counseling her about immunizations, she decides to receive a meningococcal meningitis vaccine. You also want to counsel her about the importance of sun protection. The best advice you can give her is that:

(A) Although it has not been shown to have a definite increase in risk for skin cancer, avoiding the tanning salon makes sense.
(B) Daily application of SPF 15 to 30 will ensure that she will not get sunburned.
(C) Sun protective factor (SPF) refers to the ratio of time that it will take to develop skin redness with an applied sunscreen versus the time to develop redness and burn with no sunscreen protection.
(D) Sunscreen with SPF 15 is best in preventing against ultraviolet-C (UVC).
(E) Sunscreen with SPF 35 or more is best in preventing against ultraviolet-B (UVB).

20. A 3-year-old girl is brought to the emergency department by her mother who reports that her daughter is "very ill." She had a runny nose, slight fatigue, and then suddenly she was burning with fever and became increasingly both irritable and lethargic. Physical examination shows petechiae on her distal extremities. A lumbar puncture reveals CSF pleocytosis. The child is admitted to the intensive care unit, and intravenous therapy with ceftriaxone and vancomycin is initiated. The next day her blood culture becomes positive for *Neisseria meningitidis*. After treating the patient appropriately, the next step in management is to provide prophylactic antibiotics to

(A) all her household contacts, including her parents and two siblings, only
(B) her parents, siblings, and also her aunt who came to the house for dinner the night before
(C) her parents, siblings, and the health care professionals with intimate exposure to her in the emergency department
(D) her parents, siblings, and the school friends of the siblings
(E) her parents, siblings, and the sibling's best friend who spent the night at the patient's house the weekend before the patient became ill

21. An 11-month-old infant is brought to the emergency department with breathing difficulty. He has had a number of episodes of "bronchitis" before, but this one is worse than usual. The boy is having both inspiratory and expiratory rales and rhonchi. His weight is just below the 3rd percentile and height is 20th percentile. His temperature is 37.8 C (100.0 F) and he is mildly tachypneic, but not cyanotic. Rhinorrhea is evident on physical examination and his throat is mildly erythremic, but ears are normal. Auscultation of the chest reveals rales, rhonchi, and occasional wheezing bilaterally, questionably right side greater than left. Cardiac examination reveals a systolic murmur, Grade 1/VI at the left lower sternal border. Abdominal examination is benign. Peripherally capillary refill is normal and there is no digital clubbing. The most appropriate next step in management is to order

(A) a chest x-ray
(B) a chest x-ray and complete blood count
(C) a chest x-ray, complete blood count, and sweat chloride concentration
(D) flexible bronchoscopy
(E) respiratory syncytial virus titers

22. A 3-year-old child is suspected to have mental retardation. He is very delayed in speech, displays no interactive game playing such as hide-and-go-seek, and he does not know his name. You elect to do further testing to help identify a possible etiology for this mental retardation. The diagnostic study that will most likely give the highest yield for such a case of mental retardation is

(A) chromosomal analysis
(B) a CT scan of the head
(C) a metabolic screen
(D) an MRI
(E) thyroid function tests

23. A 12-year-old girl has a vesicular skin eruption around the left eye. As you stare at it long enough you remember the anatomy and observe that the distribution of this rash is along the ophthalmic branch of the trigeminal nerve. In addition to sending her directly to an ophthalmologist, you tell her that treatment for this condition will most likely include

(A) oral acyclovir
(B) polymyxin-bacitracin
(C) topical steroids
(D) topical tobramycin
(E) varicella zoster immune globulin

24. A 16-year-old boy is brought to the office with a 7-day history of nausea, vomiting, and abdominal pain. Yesterday he noticed that his urine was dark in color, which prompted his visit to see you. He is generally healthy and is up-to-date on his immunizations. His temperature is 37.9 C (100.2 F). Physical examination reveals very mild scleral icterus and hepatomegaly that is slightly tender. There is no splenomegaly. Laboratory studies show

Anti-HAV IgM	positive
HBsAg	negative
Anti-HBs	positive
IgG Anti-HBc	negative
HBeAg	negative
Anti-HBe	negative

In counseling the patient, you should tell him that he

(A) may have caught this illness by eating contaminated food or drinking bad water and is at high risk for chronic liver disease
(B) most likely contracted this disease by blood transfusion or sexual relations and his risk for chronic hepatitis is low
(C) probably contracted this disease by blood transfusion and his risk for chronic hepatitis is low
(D) probably contracted this disease by contaminated food or water and his risk for chronic hepatitis is low
(E) probably contracted this disease through sexual contact and he will be contagious for 3 to 4 weeks

25. A 10-year-old boy comes to your office as a new patient because his parents recently changed health insurance policies. The boy's past medical history reveals that he has been in good health, but he has educational delay and attends a special school. The parents' real concern is that he still has temper tantrums at home and they feel he is too old for that. They want to know what is causing his problems. His height is 20th percentile, weight is 79th percentile, head circumference is 50th percentile, and blood pressure is 100/70 mm Hg. On examination he is noticeably obese and his hands and feet seem small in comparison. Neurologically, his muscle tone seems down, but his deep tendon reflexes are normal. He is Tanner stage 1 in development and his genitalia appear small. To help diagnose his condition you should refer him for

(A) behavioral counseling
(B) an endocrinology consultation
(C) genetic counseling
(D) a neurology consultation
(E) nutritional counseling

26. A 12-year-old previously healthy boy is brought to the emergency department late one evening. He had been seen by his private pediatrician the day before and was told he had an upper respiratory infection and an infection in his left ear. He was given a prescription for amoxicillin. He felt about the same when he went to school earlier in the day, but by the time he came home he was running a fever and his left eye looked red and "puffed up." He tells you that he has only taken one tablet of amoxicillin. On examination, he is calm and in no acute distress. His temperature is 37.8 C (101 F). The left upper eyelid is puffy and swollen with erythema tenderness and there is mild proptosis. There is bilateral conjunctivitis. His pupils react normally to light, and the anterior chambers of both eyes are clear. His throat is clear, there is no significant lymphadenopathy, and chest and cardiovascular examinations are normal. At this time the most appropriate next step in management is to

(A) change the antibiotic to amoxicillin clavulanate
(B) increase the dose of amoxicillin, and recommend use of warm soaks of topical ophthalmic antibiotic
(C) obtain a complete blood count and blood culture
(D) obtain an ophthalmologic consultation for first thing in the morning
(E) order a CT scan of the orbits and sinuses

27. A newborn infant has delayed passage of stool in the first 2 days of life. The parents are concerned because they remember that their two other children had "lots of stool in the early days of life." A workup reveals that he may have Hirschsprung disease. The most appropriate study to confirm this diagnosis is

(A) an abdominal x-ray
(B) anorectal manometry
(C) a barium enema
(D) radionuclide imaging using technetium [^{99m}Tc] pertechnetate
(E) a suction biopsy

28. You have been monitoring a 16-year-old girl during the last month of her pregnancy. Before that she had been without prenatal care, trying to hide the pregnancy from her parents and schoolmates. She goes into labor at full term but gives birth to a 2000-g, 16¾ inch baby boy with multiple bluish-red infiltrated macules measuring 2 to 8 mm in diameter widely dispersed over his entire skin. Many of the larger skin lesions are infiltrated and raised, and there are numerous petechiae that increase in number every time the baby cries. The neonate is also found to have congenital cataracts, deafness, hepatosplenomegaly, and a large anterior fontanel. You order radiographs of the long bones, which show small longitudinal areas of translucency in the metaphyses of the distal femur and proximal tibia. The infectious agent that is the most likely cause of this baby's congenital defects is

(A) herpes simplex virus
(B) human papilloma virus
(C) Rubivirus
(D) *Treponema pallidum*
(E) varicella zoster virus

29. A 6-year-old boy has a 14-day history of purulent nasal discharge and increasing problems with a nighttime cough. His cough awakens his older brother who sleeps in the same room. The boy continues to be active and has not missed school. His temperature is 37.9 C (100.2 F) and respirations are 28/min. Physical examination reveals boggy turbinates with yellow-green discharge noted in the left nostril. His mother suddenly offers that his eyes seem puffy in the morning, but you do not appreciate any swelling or edema of the lids. There is no facial tenderness. His throat and neck are otherwise normal. There are shoddy anterior cervical nodes. His chest is clear to auscultation and there is no hepatosplenomegaly appreciated. The next best step in management is to

(A) obtain a nasopharyngeal culture
(B) obtain sinus films
(C) prescribe amoxicillin
(D) provide reassurance and have them return if his symptoms do not resolve
(E) sinus aspiration
(F) transilluminate his sinuses

30. A previously healthy 15-year-old boy comes to the office because over the past few weeks he has had loose stools and the number of stools he has a day has increased. He occasionally has noted blood in his stool and sometimes has lower abdomen pain. He has not lost any weight and his appetite is unchanged. He had a well checkup with you 2 months ago and was found to be in great shape for his participation in basketball. You noted he was having a worsening problem of acne and had prescribed oral clindamycin. Physical examination is unremarkable except for mild abdominal pain on deep palpation. Sigmoidoscopy shows hyperemic, friable rectal mucosa with raised, yellowish plaques. In addition to discontinuing the clindamycin, to manage this patient's diarrhea you should prescribe

(A) acyclovir
(B) azithromycin
(C) chloramphenicol
(D) metronidazole
(E) trimethoprim-sulfamethoxazole

31. A 6-year-old boy with sickle cell disease is brought to the office because of fever, a headache, malaise, and anorexia for the past few days. You perform a thorough examination and send laboratory studies. The lab calls your office to report that the stool culture grew *Salmonella typhi*. The parents want to know more about their son's infection and how he might have gotten it. At this time the most correct statement about his condition is:

(A) No treatment is necessary.
(B) *Salmonella typhi* is a common diarrheal disease that needs therapy.
(C) The child may be at higher risk because he has sickle cell disease.
(D) The child may have gotten the infection from a pet at home.

32. A 13-year-old girl is referred to you for increasing behavior problems at home and at school and plummeting grades over the past year. Her parents report no significant past medical problems and her immunizations are up to date. Her menarche was 2 months ago. You examine her head to toe and note that head, neck, chest, and cardiovascular examinations are normal. Upon abdominal examination, however, you are surprised to find an enlarged, nontender liver. You think you also feel a spleen tip. While awaiting the results of the chemistry lab tests you decide to obtain a stat ophthalmology consultation. The ophthalmologist calls you that afternoon stating that your hunch was right, she has eye abnormalities! To best confirm the diagnosis you can order a(n)

(A) ammonia level
(B) drug screen
(C) liver biopsy
(D) serum α-1-antitrypsin
(E) 24-hour urinary copper level

33. A 2-month-old infant is brought to the office for a routine examination. She has been doing well, but the mother is overly concerned about everything, as this is her first child. She has many questions about the feeding and care of her baby. When providing anticipatory guidance, you should tell her that:

(A) Heating milk in the microwave is both safe and easy.
(B) Honey can be substituted for corn syrup sweetener.
(C) Hot water heater temperature should be no more than 120 to 130 F.
(D) She should use a front-facing infant car seat and place the baby in a supine sleeping position.
(E) She should use a rear-facing infant car seat and place the baby in a prone sleeping position.

34. A 13-year-old girl comes to the clinic for her annual checkup. She has been through a lot the past several years since she was diagnosed with a primitive neuroectodermal tumor of her hand at age 8. She underwent surgery and chemotherapy and has now survived past the 5-year mark. Her menarche was at age 11. Her weight is 30th percentile and height is 40th percentile. Vital signs are normal. Physical examination is normal except for the long linear scar along her right wrist. She smiles at you as you say "looking good." As you regroup with her mother who has been patiently waiting outside the examination room, you are asked what is her daughter's risk for developing osteoporosis. You explain that her risk for future problems with osteoporosis are most likely

(A) decreased because of her weight for height
(B) increased because of her early menarche
(C) increased because of her past bone tumor
(D) increased because she will likely experience premature ovarian failure
(E) increased because of the radiation treatments she received

35. A 12-year-old girl with Down syndrome wants to participate in a therapeutic horseback riding program that is aimed at self-building activities for disabled kids. Your routine examination reveals findings consistent with Down syndrome. Upon examination of her small ear canals you find it difficult to see the tympanic membranes, but the child has no ear complaints. Her chest is clear and there is no heart murmur. Abdominal examination reveals no hepatosplenomegaly or mass. She is Tanner stage 1. A complete blood count is normal and the urinalysis by dipstick reveals +1 protein. Before approving her participation in this horseback riding program the most appropriate next step is to

(A) determine serum thyroxine and thyroid stimulating hormone levels
(B) refer her for audiology evaluation
(C) obtain cervical spine films
(D) order an echocardiogram
(E) order a renal ultrasound

36. An 8-year-old boy is brought to the office by his mother because of a 1-day history of right knee pain that began after he fell in gym class 5 days ago. He is normally very healthy and is up to date with his immunizations. His temperature is 37.9 C (100.2 F), blood pressure is 100/50 mm Hg, pulse is 80/min, and respirations are 15/min. The patient's right knee is non-tender and appears unremarkable. His right hip is warm and tender to touch and to internal and external rotation. The remainder of the examination is unremarkable. Laboratory studies show a leukocyte count of 15,000/mm^3 and an erythrocyte sedimentation rate of 75 mm/hr. The most appropriate next step in the management of this patient is to

(A) administer antibiotics that cover *Neisseria gonorrhoeae*
(B) admit the patient to the hospital for surgical arthrotomy and drainage
(C) get an x-ray of the hip and give him a referral to an orthopedist within the next week
(D) obtain blood cultures and follow up in 48 hours to determine the best choice of antibiotics
(E) prescribe analgesics and reexamine in a week

37. A young child is brought to the clinic because of a diarrheal illness. He has not been well for a few days and the mother finally decided that he "must be really sick." He is generally very healthy and is up-to-date on his immunizations. Physical examination is unremarkable. A stool sample shows many fecal leukocytes. To establish a diagnosis, the initial best test is

(A) an abdominal x-ray
(B) a complete blood count
(C) a stool culture
(D) stool for ova and parasites
(E) a viral stool culture

38. A previously healthy 6-year-old boy is brought to the outpatient clinic with a "white spot" on his head. His mother tells you that 1 week ago she noticed this smooth bald area on the back of his scalp. He has no allergies and does not take any medications or vitamins. Physical examination is normal except for a perfectly round bald patch measuring 1 inch in diameter over the left occipital scalp. The skin is smooth and no hairs are evident. There is slight pallor of the area, but no discoloration, redness, or scaling. No other abnormalities of his scalp, nails, or body hair are noted. You decide that the best initial management is

(A) behavioral therapy
(B) a course of oral antibiotics for 10 to 14 days
(C) oral griseofulvin
(D) topical antifungal cream
(E) topical steroid cream

39. While conducting a newborn physical examination during the first day of life you notice that this first-born baby has a single transverse palmar crease on the palms of both hands. The rest of the examination is normal. In view of this finding your best plan of action is to

(A) do nothing
(B) obtain cardiac consultation including an echocardiogram
(C) perform cytogenetics on both parents
(D) perform cytogenetics on both parents and infant
(E) perform cytogenetics on only the infant

40. Late one evening a young mother brings her 2-month-old infant to the emergency department because he has become moderately ill over the past week. The infant went last week to the pediatrician's office for a well checkup. He received his first DTaP and the pediatrician noticed mild "pink eye." He gave the mother a prescription for antibiotic eye drops. His eyes are now fine, but ever since his checkup he has had a runny nose and increasingly bad cough. He wants to drink more than usual, is sometimes irritable, but he has no vomiting or rash. He is afebrile, pulse is 120/min, and respirations are 48/min. His color is good and mucus membranes are moist. There is dullness and slight retraction of his left tympanic membrane. There are scattered rales on inspiration, but no wheezing. A complete blood count reveals 8% eosinophils. A chest x-ray shows interstitial infiltrates bilaterally. At this time the most appropriate management is to

(A) admit to the hospital for observation and intravenous fluids
(B) obtain a surgical consult
(C) prescribe amoxicillin orally for 10 to 14 days
(D) prescribe erythromycin orally for 10 to 14 days
(E) recommend fluids and observation at home

41. A 4-year-old boy is rushed to the emergency department by his parents. They were having a New Year's Eve party and while the adult family members and friends were in one room having cocktails, the little boy was in the kitchen checking out the beautiful array of colored bottles of alcohol on the counter. You obtain a blood alcohol level, which shows that it is quite high. As you are starting an intravenous, you remember that the most important medical complication that you need to watch for in this child is

(A) abnormal bleeding
(B) hyperammonemia
(C) hypoglycemia
(D) hypocalcemia
(E) hypothermia

42. One fall day, shortly after school let out, an 11-year-old boy was approached by an eighth grader while walking home. The eighth-grade boy teased and bullied him around until a fight ensued. Blows were exchanged until all of a sudden the older boy bit the younger boy on the right shoulder. An adult neighbor intervened, breaking up the fight and took the younger boy home. His mother immediately used topical antiseptic and rushed him to your office. Besides a few scrapes and a very bruised ego, the boy has only an area of erythema with 4 teeth marks just below the right scapula. There is no dirt or loose skin, just puncture wounds. The most appropriate pharmacotherapy for this patient is

(A) amoxicillin
(B) amoxicillin clavulanate
(C) ciprofloxacin
(D) clarithromycin
(E) trimethoprim-sulfamethoxazole
(F) no antibiotic medication is indicated at this time

43. A 15-year-old diabetic girl is hospitalized for diabetic ketoacidosis (DKA). Over the past 24 hours she began having an increasing amount of abdominal pain and nausea, and felt very ill. Although she was beginning her menses she denied taking any acetaminophen or ibuprofen for pain. Her menarche was 3 months ago, and she has no history of previous menstrual cramp problems. She has not been ill over the past week. She denies drug use, but said she has tried alcohol before. She has never been hospitalized for her diabetes, except at the time of diagnosis when she was 9 years old. She reports perfect control of her diabetes for the past few weeks. She checks her glucose daily and reports they have been normal. Her glycosated hemoglobin is 18%. As you call her private pediatrician to inform him of her hospitalization, you suggest to him that the most likely reason she became so ill is probably due to

(A) alcohol ingestion
(B) changing needs of insulin because of puberty
(C) noncompliance
(D) renal disease related to her diabetes
(E) strep throat

44. A 19-year-old woman comes to see you for the first time for a well checkup. She reports that she is of previous good health. She attends a local college and has an A-average. She exercises a lot but does not participate in college sports. As you talk to her further you are concerned about some underlying behavioral or psychiatric problems. Her affect seems anxious and she appears distant and detached. You are hoping you will get a better understanding of all this during the physical examination. She is underweight, but otherwise you detect no abnormalities. But just as you are finishing you note some unusual abrasions on the back of her hand over the knuckles. These marks are most likely associated with

(A) abuse
(B) an anxiety disorder
(C) behavioral problems with excess fighting at school
(D) self-mutilating behavior
(E) weight loss and malnutrition

45. A 17-year-old boy comes to the emergency department because of the acute onset of right-sided scrotal pain. He wants your immediate diagnosis and help. He currently has a girlfriend, but claims he always uses a condom and has not had any sexually transmitted diseases, although he has never been tested. He does not have dysuria or penile discharge. He plays as point guard on the school basketball team. He recalls colliding with another player in a game 2 days ago, but does not remember significantly injuring himself. On examination his right scrotal area is enlarged, erythematous, and tender to palpation. As you carefully elevate the scrotum he states that there is no decrease in the pain. The cremasteric reflex is absent. The most appropriate next step in management is to

(A) obtain a complete blood count and erythrocyte sedimentation rate
(B) obtain a CT scan
(C) obtain an immediate surgical consult
(D) prescribe oral antibiotics
(E) recommend warm soaks and bedrest

46. A 9-year-old girl is brought to the office for an annual physical examination. Except for streptococcal pharyngitis a month ago, her past medical history is unremarkable. Review of systems is otherwise negative and immunizations are up-to-date. The child is afebrile and vital signs are normal. The examination is normal except for diffuse inflammation of the gingiva. The gums are mildly swollen and red. No ulcers or vesicles are noted. The most appropriate management at this time is to recommend

(A) fluoride supplementation
(B) nystatin suspension
(C) proper flossing and brushing of teeth
(D) supportive care with cool liquids and avoidance of spicy and salty foods
(E) vitamin C supplement

47. A 16-year-old boy comes to the office for his sports preparticipation examination. His past medical history is unremarkable and he takes no medications. He denies drug or alcohol use and sexual activity, and says that his school grades are "fine". Upon closer questioning you find he has a B- average. He was on the football team last year and thinks he may make varsity this year. The only complaint he mentions to you is that he keeps having a "runny" nose and it occasionally is bloody. He does not have a history of allergies, itchy eyes, sneezing, asthma, or eczema. His vital signs are normal and his weight and height are in the 60th percentile. He has significantly red, boggy turbinates with a slight amount of white discharge or mucus. The throat has mild erythema. There is no significant lymphadenopathy. Chest and abdomen are negative. Skin is clear. The best step in management is to

(A) counsel him regarding drug use
(B) do a rapid strep test and throat culture
(C) obtain a nasopharyngeal culture using a calcium alginate swab
(D) order sinus films
(E) prescribe a trial of fexofenadine

Items 48-49

You are called to the well-baby nursery to see a baby who was just born. The mother is a 29-year-old white woman who has no other children, although she has had one prior pregnancy that ended in a miscarriage at 11 weeks. During this pregnancy, the mother had no prenatal care because she was "too busy." On examination, the baby has a temperature of 37.3 C (99.1 F), a pulse of 136/min, and respirations of 42/min. You notice that she has triangular facies, edema of her hands and feet, and a webbed neck. Her heart, lungs, abdomen, and genitalia appear normal.

48. This patient is at greatest risk for

(A) coarctation of the aorta
(B) duodenal atresia
(C) endocardial cushion defect
(D) mental retardation
(E) primary amenorrhea

49. You wish to do a chromosome analysis on this baby. You should

(A) ask the nurse to talk to the mother because she seems to have a better relationship with her
(B) ask to speak to the father alone and discuss your concerns with him
(C) draw the blood and send it for the appropriate studies
(D) explain your concerns to the mother and get her consent to do the testing
(E) tell the mother her baby is okay and do not mention the test to her because you don't want to alarm her

50. A mother brings her 4-year-old daughter to the office because the child has developed multiple bruises over her body in the last few days. Her daughter has been "acting herself" and eating well. She was "pretty cranky" a couple of weeks ago when she had a cold. Physical examination shows petechiae on the lips and several ecchymoses on her abdomen, arms, and legs. Laboratory studies show:

Leukocyte count	$7000/mm^3$
Hemoglobin	12.0 g/dL
Hematocrit	36%
Platelets	$20,000/mm^3$

A peripheral blood smear shows large platelets. The most likely diagnosis is

(A) child abuse
(B) disseminated intravascular coagulation
(C) hemolytic uremic syndrome
(D) idiopathic thrombocytopenic purpura
(E) leukemia

Pediatrics Test Two: **Answers and Explanations**

ANSWER KEY

1. B
2. A
3. E
4. A
5. A
6. B
7. C
8. C
9. C
10. H
11. B
12. C
13. C
14. B
15. E
16. D
17. E
18. E
19. C
20. C
21. C
22. A
23. A
24. D
25. C
26. E
27. E
28. C
29. C
30. D
31. C
32. E
33. C
34. D
35. C
36. B
37. C
38. E
39. A
40. D
41. C
42. B
43. C
44. E
45. C
46. C
47. A
48. E
49. D
50. D

1. **The correct answer is B.** The lactose breath hydrogen test will show a rise in breath hydrogen after a test dose of lactose. The patient should be fasting overnight the evening before. The rise in hydrogen production results from the fermentation of the unabsorbed carbohydrate. Another confirmatory test would be to show that the blood glucose fails to increase more than 10mg/dL after ingesting a lactose dose of 1g/kg.

   Serum protein would be expected to be normal in this patient and it would not be a useful test to perform in this patient (**choice A**). Serum protein is part of an array of chemistry tests that should be performed in those patients suspected to have inflammatory bowel disease and enteropathies, such as celiac disease.

   Changing the diet would not prove the diagnosis (**choice C**). A change of diet may just happen to coincide with improvement in symptoms even though lactose intolerance may not be the underlying problem. Then the patient would be continuing a special restricted diet unnecessarily.

   Analysis of a stool specimen would not be specific enough to confirm the diagnosis (**choice D**). However, a frothy stool with an acid pH (less than 4.5) and positive for reducing substances would be supportive evidence for lactose intolerance.

   Testing the stools for occult blood is not the best answer (**choice E**). Blood in the stools could be due to a variety of diagnoses. For example, peptic ulcer disease would yield a positive occult blood test and also have a characteristic history of abdominal pains following meals.

2. **The correct answer is A.** This patient has erysipelas, a superficial cellulitis of the skin with marked lymphatic involvement, caused by group A beta-hemolytic *Streptococcus.*

   Erysipelas most commonly occurs in infants, very young children, and the elderly. In most cases, the organism gains access by direct inoculation through a break in the skin, but infrequently hematogenous infection may occur. After an incubation period of 2 to 5 days, a small area of redness develops and gradually enlarges to form the typical tense, painful, bright red, shiny, brawny, infiltrated plaque with a well demarcated, distinct, and slightly raised border (as opposed to deeper cellulitis that has no distinct border and is flush with surrounding skin). Projection of the inflammation by way of lymphatics produces an irregular outline, akin to pseudopods. Regional lymph nodes may be enlarged and firm. Systemic symptoms may develop with widespread infection in the form of malaise, weakness, fever, and chills. It is most commonly located on the scalp and face, but it may occur on any skin surface. Penicillin is the drug of choice for the treatment of erysipelas. In those allergic to penicillin, erythromycin or clindamycin are recommended.

   Haemophilus influenzae (**choice B**) is the most frequent cause of cellulitis in children 2 years of age and younger. Children with *Haemophilus influenzae* cellulitis may be very ill with signs of toxemia, upper respiratory tract symptoms, and an associated bacteremia or septicemia. Many of these children have a distinctive dusky red or bluish discoloration of the lesion. Treatment is with semisynthetic penicillins or cephalosporins.

   Pityrosporum ovale (**choice C**) is a yeast that causes Tinea versicolor, a superficial infection of the skin, most commonly on the upper trunk and proximal extremities of young adults who perspire freely. Hypo- or hyperpigmented, oval and round, slightly scaly patches are typical. Treatment is either with topical antifungal preparations or oral antifungals in persistent cases.

   Pseudomonas aeruginosa (**choice D**) is a gram-negative bacterium that causes a peculiar skin infection, ecthyma gangrenosum, on the skin of immunocompromised or debilitated patients. A necrotic, adherent eschar forms over a deep, rapidly enlarging ulcer with undermined borders. Treatment is with ciprofloxacin or other antibiotics with antipseudomonal activity, in addition to aggressive surgical debridement of the ulcer.

   Staphylococcus aureus (**choice E**) is a common cause of skin infections, but it does not cause acute erysipelas, such as the one seen in this patient. It more frequently causes a deeper cellulitis located in the subcutaneous tissues, and *Staphylococcus aureus* probably is the most common cause of deep cellulitis in children older than 2 years of age. Erythema, swelling, and tenderness develop over an ill-defined area of the affected body part, usually in the vicinity or around an existing wound or site of trauma. Constitutional symptoms frequently accompany the skin lesion. *Staphylococcus aureus* is penicillin-resistant, so it is appropriate to use semisynthetic penicillinase-resistant penicillins that should produce a rapid response.

3. **The correct answer is E.** Cephalexin is indicated to treat this boy's impetigo that is evident on examination. Some of the vesicles are pustular with widened areas of erythema underlying the papules. It is common in children to see impetigo occur when infection becomes superimposed on previously diseased or traumatized skin. This is frequently seen following bug bites, atopic dermatitis, and chickenpox.

Ordering a blood culture is unlikely to be helpful in this case (**choice A**). The patient is not toxic and unlikely to be septic or have a positive blood culture. It is not uncommon for patients with varicella to run fever in the early stages of the disease. If there were clinical evidence that this patient may be having more severe disease complicated by possible bacterial sepsis or pneumonia, then blood cultures might be indicated.

A CBC would not be nonspecific and not helpful in this case (**choice B**). Again, the boy does not appear very ill and a CBC would not add more to the management of varicella.

There is no indication to order a chest x-ray at this time (**choice C**). Pneumonia may be a complication seen in varicella, but in this case there is no history of cough, shortness of breath, or chest pain, and the respiratory rate is minimally elevated, consistent with his fever.

Oral acyclovir therapy should be reserved for severe varicella disease or unusual cases, such as immunocompetent patients who may be household contacts, siblings who have chronic disease, or older adolescents with varicella who may be at risk for severe disease (**choice D**). Even then, caution must be used and the risks versus the benefits weighed.

Since he most likely has chickenpox with a superimposed bacterial infection, he should be treated with antibiotics, and not reassured that no therapy is indicated (**choice F**).

4. **The correct answer is A.** With two more siblings at home who have been in close contact with their brother with chickenpox, the probability is very high that one and probably both will get chickenpox. It would be reasonable to cancel the trip because the time of break out will be at Christmas time. If they are ill with chickenpox they should certainly not expose their grandmother, who is immunocompromised by her cancer chemotherapy.

   The boy's siblings are very likely to get chickenpox, even more than schoolmates of the boy (**choice B**).

   There would be no point in ordering varicella titers on the siblings because they have not been immunized and they are surely susceptible (**choice C**). The parents will just have to wait to see who gets it and deal with it then.

   VZIG should not be given to the parents (**choice D**) or the siblings (**choice E**) unless they have immunodeficiencies or other significant chronic disease that would cause them significant risk for complications if they come down with the disease.

5. **The correct answer is A.** The fine needle aspiration generally will provide a diagnosis in solid lesions and "cure" cystic lesions.

   A radionucleotide scan will be helpful, but not the best answer (**choice B**). The scan will identify whether the thyroid gland is hyperfunctioning or not. A solitary nodule that is "cold" or shows decreased uptake is more suggestive of cancer, whereas a "hot" nodule or a nodule with increased uptake is frequently benign.

   Serum thyroid tests will not be so helpful in the initial workup of a thyroid nodule. One must first determine whether it may be cancerous or not (**choice C**).

   Surgery is not the next best step before further evaluation is done (**choice D**).

   Although an ultrasound (**choice E**) will help differentiate between a solid and cystic lesion of the thyroid, an ultrasound will not provide information about the functional state of the thyroid (e.g., whether the nodule is cold or hot). Frequently, the ultrasound may be used to guide the fine needle aspiration procedure.

6. **The correct answer is B.** CT scan of the abdomen would be the best test to perform in hemodynamically stable patients with significant injury. It would provide full anatomical detail. In blunt abdominal trauma cases it is particularly useful when there are signs of intra-abdominal injuries or gross hematuria. It is very useful in identifying the presence and extent of injuries to specific organs, including those in the retroperitoneum.

   Plain films of the abdomen have limited usefulness (**choice A**). However, they may be done in hemodynamically unstable patients. A cross-table lateral film may reveal free air and foreign bodies.

   A liver and spleen scan will not be helpful for injuries to other abdominal organs (**choice C**).

   Peritoneal lavage may be performed in unstable patients, but it is not the best management plan in this stable patient (**choice D**).

   An ultrasound of the abdomen and pelvis may be helpful where CT is not available, but CT is the better choice (**choice E**).

7. **The correct answer is C.** This child most likely has iron deficiency anemia. It is the most common cause of childhood anemia and usually relates to nutritional deficiency.

Obviously, a complete history is important, including a birth history. There is nothing to suggest the boy has had anemia before, and the more correct answer is dietary (**choice A**).

A developmental history is important as part of a complete history too. A delay might be suggestive of lead problems. If there is a history of pica or environmental exposures, lead poisoning might be more suggestive. Not enough history is given in this case to suggest lead as a cause of the anemia, but lead poisoning should always be kept in mind (**choice B**).

A family history should always be obtained, but the fact that this boy has been of previous good health points against a hereditary or congenital disease (**choice D**).

Without bruising or physical disability this is not the most important history to obtain first (**choice E**).

8. **The correct answer is C.** The patient is not dehydrated and not getting sicker by history. Also, his illness began with vomiting and then the diarrhea began. The best course of action is to observe how he does over the next few days and not to do any tests at this time.

   A stool revealing leukocytes is seen with *Salmonella* or *Shigella* dysentery. Looking for stool WBCs would not be so useful if you really suspect that it is a viral illness (**choice A**).

   Examining a stool for mucus is nonspecific and would not be worthwhile in this case (**choice B**).

   A stool culture would be obtained if you really suspect a bacterial etiology (**choice D**).

   A stool for occult blood would most likely be positive in this case because of the excoriated skin noted on examination (**choice E**). Therefore, it would not be helpful.

9. **The correct answer is C.** This is a very young infant who not only has hypospadias, but also has nonpalpable testes. Therefore, one should wonder if this case is really a baby girl who has adrenogenital syndrome. This very young infant is dehydrated. For all these reasons the first step in management would be to obtain serum electrolytes.

   Hypospadias may be an isolated anomaly or associated with other anomalies. Sometimes it may be associated with vesicoureteral reflux, but the reflux is usually low grade and an intravenous pyelogram is not recommended (**choice A**).

   A karyotype (**choice B**) might need to be ordered to rule out a chromosomal disorder, especially if this is a boy with hypospadias and one testis is absent. However, the physical exam seems to indicate otherwise.

   An ultrasound of his pelvis (**choice D**) is not indicated.

   An upper GI is unlikely to be helpful (**choice E**). There is no good history for bowel conditions, such as volvulus or pyloric stenosis.

10. **The correct answer is H.** The boy does need to be told. Telling him in words he understands gives him the cognitive tools to cope with what is happening to him and remove the deception that may inhibit him getting the support that he needs. Children generally know that something is wrong. However, before talking with the child, the physician must first work with the parents who are likely to also need help coping with the devastating news. It is best to try to understand why they do not want the child to know and to use the statement, "tell me more about why you don't want the child to know," as the start of that conversation.

    The child will cope best if he is given information and assisted in dealing with that information. Agreeing to keep information from the child (**choice A and B**), may seem kind at first, but ultimately makes caring for the child more difficult.

    Threatening to not continue as the physician (**choice C**) is a threat of abandonment and is always wrong.

    Forcing the issue with the parents is premature (**choice D, E, F**). It will take them time to come to grips with the hard news and learn to accept it. In a very real sense, the physician has two patients here: the child and the parents. The physician must provide guidance and support to the parents so that they can be the source of support and comfort the child will need. Before the child finds out about his condition, it is best to try to find out why the parents do not want him to know about it. There are many possibilities, but maybe he had a friend who suffered from a similar illness and died a horrible death. In this case, you can try to provide reassurance that you will do everything possible to try to make sure that he suffers as little as possible.

    Putting the conversation off until later (**choice G**) does not address the issue. The parents are there now, talk with them now.

    It is not the physician's job to analyze the parents' motives by suggesting that they have not accepted the condition (**choice I**). The parents must come to this insight on their own, not have it dictated by the physician.

11. **The correct answer is B.** This little boy has been bitten by a tick that has remained attached for blood feeding. Ticks are large, globular arachnoids with short legs and hard, leathery skin and mouthparts adaptable for sucking blood from mammals, birds, and reptiles. They are important vectors of diseases, such as erythema chronicum migrans, Lyme disease, relapsing fever, rickettsial infection, babesiosis, and tularemia. Ticks are found in grass, shrubs, vine, and bushes, from which they attach themselves to dogs, deer, cattle, and humans. The female tick attaches itself to the victim by sticking its proboscis into the skin to suck blood from the superficial dermal vessels. It will usually remain attached for days and then spontaneously fall off. The local bite is painless and innocuous, and often noted only days later, when the tick becomes engorged with blood and increases its size several fold. An infiltrated papule with an erythematous halo forms as a local inflammatory reaction to the tick bite and may persist for a couple of weeks. Often, the bites are followed by small, pruritic nodules that form as a foreign body reaction to the mouthparts remaining in the skin after improper removal of the tick. Ticks that carry the spirochete *Borrelia* transmit the bacterium during their attachment to the host and with it the risk of developing several diseases, namely erythema chronicum migrans (erythematous annular plaques that develop around the bite several weeks after inoculation has happened), Lyme disease (manifested by arthritic, cardiac, or neurological symptoms, depending on the species of *Borrelia*), and acrodermatitis chronica atrophicans (a late complication seen mostly in Europe in which the acral integument becomes atrophic and translucent). Prompt removal of the attached tick within the first 8 to 12 hours minimizes the chance of transmission of any of these diseases, but appropriate followup blood work should be done to evaluate if anti-*Borrelia* antibody titers are rising and treatment with antibiotics is necessary. In addition, the removed ticks can be analyzed to determine whether they carry any of the infectious microorganisms.

Erythema ab igne (**choice A**) is a reticulated brown network that develops on skin chronically exposed to high temperatures, such as repeated applications of a heating bottle to the same skin site or sitting close to a radiator with heat directed toward the skin from a very short distance. It is permanent and may undergo malignant transformation to squamous cell carcinoma many years later.

Erythema elevatum et diutinum (**choice C**) is a chronic vasculitis of the skin of unknown etiology. It manifests with flesh-colored to pink-red nodules and plaques most commonly located on the dorsal hands and feet, or on the elbows and knees.

Erythema infectiosum (**choice D**), also called fifth disease, is a viral infection caused by human parvovirus B19. It is mildly contagious and affects children 3 to 12 years of age. First an erythematous malar rash appears, followed by an erythematous maculopapular eruption on the extensor extremities the next day. When the rash fades, a few days later, areas of central clearing leave behind a reticulated, lacy-patterned rash that waxes and wanes for an average of 9 to 11 days.

Erythema toxicum neonatorum (**choice E**) is an asymptomatic, benign, self-limiting skin eruption of the neonatal period of unknown etiology. Erythematous macules, papules, and pustules occur anywhere on the body in the first two weeks of life and the individual lesions last an average of two days, after which they resolve completely.

12. **The correct answer is C.** The findings of trismus, unilateral soft palate edema, and uvular deviation are classic for peritonsillar abscess. The most appropriate management is to consult an otolaryngologist for drainage of the abscess. Most otolaryngologists would attempt intraoral incision and drainage in the emergency room; survey data indicate that only 14% would take the patient to the operating room for an abscess tonsillectomy. The other option is to attempt drainage with a 16-gauge needle. This will resolve a peritonsillar abscess in approximately 85% of patients.

Administering clindamycin intravenously and lactated Ringer solution in the emergency department and arranging followup with the child's pediatrician in the morning (**choice A**) would be appropriate for tonsillitis with borderline dehydration, but not for a peritonsillar abscess.

Admitting the child to the pediatric service for intravenous fluids and antibiotics (**choice B**) would be appropriate if the diagnosis of peritonsillar abscess were not absolute (e.g., peritonsillitis without abscess formation). An improvement in symptoms after 1 to 2 days of parental antibiotics would be suggestive of peritonsillitis, whereas failure to improve or progression of symptoms would be suggestive of peritonsillar abscess.

Ordering a CT scan of the neck (**choice D**) would be appropriate if examination of the oropharynx was not possible (e.g., patient refused examination) and a diagnosis could not be made.

Performing a throat culture, switching the antibiotic to amoxicillin clavulanate, and arranging followup with the child's pediatrician in the morning (**choice E**) would be appropriate for persistent tonsillitis that had not responded to first-line antibiotic therapy.

13. **The correct answer is C.** Fibromatosis colli, also known as congenital muscular torticollis, usually presents within the first 14 days of life as a nontender mass in the lower third of the sternocleidomastoid muscle. Over the next 2 to 4 weeks the mass typically increases in size. If left untreated, the muscle will become fibrotic and will contract, causing the head to tilt to the ipsilateral side and the chin to tilt to the contralateral side. The diagnosis can be confirmed with ultrasound. Initial treatment consists of passive stretching exercises of the sternocleidomastoid muscle. If the condition does not resolve with stretching, then surgery followed by splinting is necessary to prevent permanent contracture deformities.

    Cervical teratomas (**choice A**) and cystic hygromas (**choice B**) are typically diagnosed either in utero, in which they are often associated with maternal polyhydramnios, or within the neonatal period. They are frequently large enough to cause respiratory distress and eating difficulties, but size at presentation is variable. Regardless, both would present in the neck as compressible soft tissue masses, not clearly defined and not affixed to underlying muscle.

    A second branchial cleft cyst (**choice D**) would typically present as a soft mass high in the lateral neck deep to the anterior border of the sternocleidomastoid muscle.

    Thyroglossal duct cysts (**choice E**) normally are found in the midline of the neck and move with deglutition.

14. **The correct answer is B.** HIV is spread only by exchange of bodily fluids. You should help to discredit the myths of HIV transmission by telling the principal the facts. The principal called for information and the physician should give it to him.

    Testing all children for HIV (**choice A**) is excessive, invasive and, failing parental permission, illegal.

    Gym class (**choice D**) does not offer the opportunity for transmission of HIV, nor does bathroom sharing (**choice C**) transmit HIV.

    Launching an HIV information campaign (**choice E**), while part of a vital public health approach, is likely to raise community questions as to why this is happening now.

    The physician must respect the student's confidentiality and so should not reveal that the child is a patient, so there is a conflict of interest (**choice F**) or that he is under treatment (**choice H**) are both incorrect. However, you can comment on HIV in general without breaking confidentiality as to this patient's particulars.

    Sharing a schoolroom or even a playground does not place other children at any significant risk, so separate tutoring (**choice G**) is unnecessary.

    You are not going to discuss the case with the principal because of confidentiality issues and so have no reason for a face-to-face meeting (**choice I**).

15. **The correct answer is E.** Despite the fact that this girl received BCG, she will still need a PPD. A previous immunization with BCG is not a contraindication to PPD testing. A positive PPD in an asymptomatic child who had a prior BCG immunization should be evaluated with a chest x-ray. If the chest x-ray is negative, in general, treatment for latent tuberculosis infection should be initiated.

    This girl has received the appropriate number of DTaP and IPV vaccinations for her age. The fifth DTaP and the fourth IPV are given between 4 to 6 years of age (**choice A**). She only needs the PPD.

    This girl has received the appropriate number of DTaP and IPV vaccinations for her age. She also has received one varicella injection, which is all she needs for her age (**choice B**).

    A fourth IPV vaccination should be given between the ages of 4 to 6 years old. This girl has had her fourth shot and is up to date for polio (**choice C**). She does need a PPD.

    This girl needs to be checked for tuberculosis, so no vaccines (**choice D**) is incorrect. A PPD should be placed and read in 48 to 72 hours.

16. **The correct answer is D.** The letters of the alphabet, ABCD, refer to the important signs of skin lesions that are associated with melanoma, including: A = asymmetry; B = border is irregular; C = color change or variegation; and D = diameter is >6 mm. Asymmetry of pigmented skin lesions is an important indicator of possible malignant melanoma. However it should be remembered there are always exceptions to this alphabetic rule and that some melanomas may lack many of these defined features.

    While it is true that a symptom of melanoma could include bleeding, the B that is to be remembered is irregular border (**choice A**).

    Central telangiectasia may be an initial finding in a hemangioma (**choice B**). Deep and lobular findings do not suggest melanoma.

    Asymmetry, border, color change, and diameter over 6 mm, not 4 mm, are the important ABCD features of melanoma to remember (**choice C**).

If the nevus or skin lesion is deep and exfoliating, this is not necessarily indicative of melanoma. Melanoma-like lesions may be crusty and bleed (**choice E**). Some dermatologists may use an "ABCDE" guide for the signs of early melanoma. Here the E stands for either elevation or enlargement. However, all melanomas are not elevated. Some small melanomas may be flat and clinically impalpable.

17. **The correct answer is E.** In males <6 months or girls <2 years of age who are ill with high fever and there is no apparent cause, a urine culture should be obtained to rule out a urinary tract infection or even urosepsis. This should be done even in the absence of urinary symptoms. A urine specimen is collected by catheterization or suprapubic tap.

A chest x-ray is not the best first test, especially in this vignette where the infant is described to be nontoxic and does not have a high respiratory rate for the degree of temperature elevation (**choice A**). There is no history of cough or wheezing that might lead one to think about the possibility of pneumonia.

Performing a lumbar puncture and sending a cerebrospinal fluid for culture would be useful if the child appears very ill or toxic or there is a history to suggest that the child may have meningitis (**choice B**). If this child were less than 4 to 6 weeks of age, a lumbar puncture should also be performed.

A stool culture is not indicated without a history of diarrhea or other symptoms (**choice C**).

A throat culture is not indicated in this young infant (**choice D**). Streptococcal disease usually occurs in older children. There is also no history of illness in the family.

18. **The correct answer is E.** Giving the child a forced choice between stopping the tantrum or continuing it (and experience a consequence) is a good method to stop the temper tantrums. Parents should emphasize the positive if he chooses to stop the unacceptable behavior. They may want to say if he stops it they can have a snack or they will go somewhere after they are finished. The other choice (not to stop the tantrum) is the negative one where there will be a consequence if he continues.

Giving him a harsh reprimand is not usually effective and may make things worse (**choice A**).

Setting a "time out" for 30 minutes is too long. "Time outs" should be brief, for 3 to 5 minutes (**choice B**).

To keep praising him for good behavior will unlikely correct the problem because the parents have told you that it has not worked for them (**choice C**).

Warning him of a future "time out" if he does not stop will just prolong the behavior. A parent should just give him a "time out", not just keep warning him that he will receive one (**choice D**).

19. **The correct answer is C.** If a person burns after 15 minutes in the sun without sunscreen, then after applying sunscreen with SPF 15, it should take 30 minutes before burning in the sun.

Tanning salons are known to increase the risk for skin cancer (**choice A**).

Sunscreen does not assure that someone will not get sunburned (**choice B**). Best protection is sun avoidance, protective clothing, hats, and sunglasses.

Sunscreen is applied to prevent sunburn caused by UVB (**choice D**). UVC is cytotoxic and might cause retinal injury. Most UVC is absorbed by the ozone.

SPF of 15 to 30 is the usual recommendation for sunscreen (**choice E**).

20. **The correct answer is C.** All close contacts, including the staff at the hospital who had intimate contact with the child before therapy, must be treated. Intimate contact would include exposure such as unprotected mouth-to-mouth resuscitation, intubation, and suctioning.

While the household contacts should be treated, choice C is the best answer (**choice A**).

The aunt who had dinner at their house the night before does not need prophylactic treatment (**choice B**).

The school friends of the patient and those of her siblings do not need prophylactic treatment unless they had very close contact (**choice D**).

For the same reasons as above, the sibling's best friend who spent the weekend at the house does not need therapy (**choice E**).

21. **The correct answer is C.** There is enough information here to suggest that this child could have cystic fibrosis. He is very underweight for height (less than 3rd percentile) and has had recurrent episodes of bronchitis with inspiratory and expiratory rales and rhonchi. Although a chest x-ray and CBC would be appropriate, given the growth data on this child, including a sweat

chloride seems to be the best answer. It should be remembered that digital clubbing is frequently not present before one year of age.

If the sweat chloride test is negative in this child, alternative diagnoses such as gastroesophageal reflux or asthma should be considered.

In this case the provided information suggests the patient needs more than a chest x-ray (**choice A**).

More tests than a chest x-ray and CBC (**choice B**) are indicated.

Inhaled or ingested foreign bodies occur especially between the ages of 0 to 18 months, and they can present with recurrent episodes of pneumonia or bronchitis. However, this child would first need a chest x-ray if there is a question of a foreign body. Inspiratory and expiratory films are frequently helpful in identifying locations of foreign bodies. A flexible bronchoscopy would not be a first choice procedure (**choice D**).

Respiratory syncytial virus (RSV) (**choice E**) can cause upper respiratory infection, pneumonia, and bronchiolitis. An RSV titer might be helpful and important to know whether this child has RSV (e.g., high risk patients, high risk household contacts, hospitalized patients), but in this case scenario it would not be the best choice.

22. **The correct answer is A.** Chromosomal abnormalities may be present in up to 25% of cases of mental retardation. Many times, anomalies may be a tip-off to an underlying chromosomal disorder, but not necessarily.

A CT is helpful when mental retardation is associated with craniosynostosis or intracranial calcifications, but not in this case (**choice B**).

Metabolic screening is done routinely in the newborn nursery to rule out certain diseases such as phenylketonuria, and other times it is performed when newborns are quite ill. Many metabolic diseases are associated with mental retardation, especially phenylketonuria and galactosemia. However, in this case scenario these tests would be relatively low yield in the workup without other symptoms (**choice C**).

An MRI might be a good test when a child not only has mental retardation, but also has neurocutaneous signs, seizures, or an unusually shaped head. In this case, without further findings, the best test would be chromosomal studies (**choice D**).

Worldwide iodine deficiency is a leading cause of severe hypothyroidism, and mental retardation may result (**choice E**). However, in this case scenario, without further information, thyroid screening would not be the best test to order.

23. **The correct answer is A.** Acyclovir is the preferred drug choice for herpes zoster. Supportive therapies may include soaks and topical antibiotics; however, a referral to an ophthalmologist is indicated at this time to ensure the proper management.

Polymyxin-bacitracin can be used as an adjunct to help prevent or treat secondary bacterial infection, but the antiviral therapy is the best choice (**choice B**).

Topical steroids (**choice C**) are not first-line therapy for herpes zoster. If anterior uveitis is present, it is typically used; however, if a dendritic ulcer from herpes simplex is present, topical corticosteroids should not be used. Referral to an ophthalmologist is very important to ensure the proper management.

Topical tobramycin (**choice D**) is another antibiotic that can be used topically in bacterial conjunctivitis, but is not the drug of choice for herpes zoster.

Varicella zoster immune globulin (**choice E**) is not helpful once a patient has the disease.

24. **The correct answer is D.** This patient has the hepatitis A virus that can result from contact with affected individuals or by transmission from contaminated food or water supplies. The risk of chronic hepatitis is low. Note that an individual who receives the full series of the hepatitis B vaccine will be hepatitis B surface antibody positive, which indicates immunity.

Transmission of hepatitis A through contaminated food or water is common; however, there is a very low risk for chronic hepatitis (**choice A**).

Transmission of hepatitis A through blood products or by sexual relations is very rare (**choice B**). It is usually spread by the fecal-oral route. It may help explain where the person contracted the virus if they know of anyone who was jaundiced (incubation is usually 2 to 5 weeks), but frequently many affected persons are anicteric and their illness is not discovered.

Transmission of hepatitis A through blood products is rare (**choice C**).

Hepatitis A is usually spread by the fecal-oral route. A patient is frequently noncontagious when he becomes jaundiced (**choice E**). Most children recover without sequelae.

25. **The correct answer is C.** This boy has the characteristic features of Prader-Willi syndrome, including short stature, obesity, muscular hypotonia, mental retardation, and hypogonadism. These children frequently have problems with temper tantrums and excessive appetite. In most cases this is due to a cytogenetic abnormality, resulting from an alteration of the imprinting process with loss of function of a paternally inherited gene cluster on chromosome 15q11.2.

Behavioral counseling may be helpful with the management of temper tantrums, but does not address the underlying condition (**choice A**).

Prader-Willi syndrome is a genetic disorder that includes endocrine dysfunction with hypogonadism, and most people with the condition have decreased secretion of growth hormone and require hormone replacements (**choice B**). The first step, however, would be to obtain a genetic evaluation to make the definitive diagnosis.

Although the hypotonia might suggest an underlying muscular disease, with Prader-Willi one would expect normal reflexes and the hypotonia is felt to be due to a central cause (**choice D**).

Nutritional counseling is unlikely to be helpful in this case until behavioral issues are addressed and the genetic diagnosis of Prader-Willi is established (**choice E**).

26. **The correct answer is E.** The patient with an erythematous, swollen eyelid represents a complex clinical challenge. Does the child have a bad case of conjunctivitis, or is it a case of periorbital or orbital cellulitis? Importantly, this child has a swollen red eyelid with proptosis. Proptosis and limited range of movement of the eye or ophthalmoplegia would support a diagnosis of orbital cellulitis. A CT is the method of choice to confirm clinical diagnosis and to determine the extent of any complications. Parenteral antibiotics with or without surgery may be necessary. An immediate ophthalmologist consultation should be sought and should not be delayed until the next morning (**choice D**).

Further diagnostic workup to rule out orbital cellulitis is necessary before continuing antibiotics. If this were a case of sinusitis or early periorbital cellulitis, amoxicillin clavulanate would be a proper antibiotic choice (**choice A**).

Increasing the amoxicillin dosage and using local therapy with warm soaks and topical antibiotics would be appropriate if this were an early stage of periorbital or preseptal cellulitis (**choice B**). However, the first step in management must be to determine if this is orbital cellulitis.

In the described case, obtaining a CBC and blood culture will probably be necessary, but is not the first best action (**choice C**).

27. **The correct answer is E.** A biopsy of the distal rectum will reveal the absence of ganglion cells in the mucosal and submucosal layers of bowel, thus confirming a diagnosis of Hirschsprung disease.

An abdominal x-ray may show a dilated proximal colon and absence of air in the rectum. This alone is not the confirmatory test (**choice A**).

Manometry will show abnormal contraction of the internal anal sphincter, but by itself is not diagnostic (**choice B**).

Barium enema will usually demonstrate a contracted distal segment of the affected bowel (**choice C**). This is not diagnostic for Hirschsprung disease.

A technetium scan (also referred to as a Meckel scan) is performed to diagnose Meckel diverticulum, not Hirschsprung disease (**choice D**).

28. **The correct answer is C.** This baby has congenital rubella syndrome caused by Rubivirus, family Togaviridae. Infants of mothers with rubella infection early in pregnancy may have developed systemic involvement in addition to the classic triad of congenital cataracts, deafness, and congenital malformations of the heart. Infected infants are usually born at term but with low birth weight. They may show only a few manifestations at birth or be asymptomatic, with consequences of the infection manifesting in the subsequent months, or they may have widespread involvement with growth retardation, thrombocytopenic purpura, hyperbilirubinemia, hepatosplenomegaly, pneumonia, cardiac defects, osseous defects, and meningoencephalitis. The most prominent cutaneous features are thrombocytopenic purpura and bluish-red infiltrated macules measuring 2 to 8 mm in diameter, the so-called "blueberry muffin lesions," usually noted at birth or within 24 hours. They are widespread on the head, neck, trunk, and extremities, and the larger ones tend to be raised. Blueberry muffin lesions tend to disappear in 3 to 6 weeks. They are sites of extramedullary hematopoiesis and may be seen in other disorders of the fetus, such as congenital toxoplasmosis, cytomegalic inclusion disease, neuroblastoma, congenital leukemia, erythroblastosis fetalis, and twin transfusion syndrome. Congenital rubella should be suspected in infants with intrauterine growth retardation and the above listed congenital malformations. Bony abnormalities are seen in up to 80% of these infants and include a

large anterior fontanel and characteristic small longitudinal translucent areas in the metaphyses of the long bones, especially the distal, femur, and proximal tibia, during the first 2 to 3 months of life. The diagnosis may be confirmed by isolation of the virus from tissue or secretions and identification of antibodies in the newborn (IgM or persistent IgG antibodies).

Early intrauterine herpes simplex virus (**choice A**) infection with disturbance of embryogenesis occurs during the first 8 weeks of gestation. It may result in abortion, cutaneous scarring, or the following severe congenital malformations: intrauterine growth retardation, severe brain damage, intracranial calcification, microcephaly, hydranencephaly, microphthalmia, chorioretinitis, retinal dysplasia, cardiac abnormalities, and short digits.

Human papilloma virus (**choice B**) is not a known cause of congenital malformations in newborns. Infection with these viruses may, however, occur during birth by passage through an infected birth canal and these babies are at risk of developing laryngeal papillomatosis or cutaneous/genital warts during the first 2 years of life.

Congenital syphilis develops when a fetus becomes infected with the spirochete *Treponema pallidum* (**choice D**) sometime after the 16th week of pregnancy. It can be divided clinically into early congenital syphilis (appearing before age 2) and late congenital syphilis (appearing after age 2). The manifestations of early congenital syphilis are generally infectious (rhinitis, maculopapular exanthem, lymphadenopathy, hepatosplenomegaly, osteochondritis), and because there is no primary stage, may resemble those of acquired secondary syphilis, but are more widely distributed, more severe, and last longer. The lesions of late congenital syphilis are either a hypersensitivity reaction of the host or scars and deformities resulting from the infection.

Congenital varicella zoster syndrome is caused by in utero infection of the fetus by varicella zoster virus (**choice E**) during an episode of maternal varicella. It manifests with low birth weight, congenital eye defects (microphthalmia, cataracts, and chorioretinitis), encephalomyelitis, often with severe brain damage, hypoplastic limbs with flexion contractures, cutaneous scars, micrognathia, pneumonitis, and increased susceptibility to infection.

29. **The correct answer is C.** This child has many of the features of sinusitis, including nasal discharge for more than 10 days, low-grade fever, eye swelling, malodorous breath, and cough during the day (that may worsen at night). The best course of action is to treat the child and followup his response to antibiotics. Amoxicillin is the drug of choice for most sinusitis. Amoxicillin clavulanate may also be used, especially if one is worried about resistant organisms. Most infections in younger children involve the ethmoid and maxillary sinuses. Adolescents more frequently have infections involving the frontal sinuses.

Obtaining a nasopharyngeal culture would not be important or clinically significant in this case (**choice A**).

Sinus films may confirm a diagnosis, revealing opacification of the sinuses and increased mucosal thickening (**choice B**). However, in pediatrics, radiographs are not usually performed to make a diagnosis of acute sinusitis. Their interpretation is sometimes difficult in younger children.

Reassurance (**choice D**) is inappropriate as he has many of the features of sinusitis including nasal discharge for more than 10 days, low-grade fever, eye swelling, malodorous breath, and cough during the day (that may worsen at night) and therefore should be treated with an antibiotic.

Aspiration of the sinuses may be performed by an otolaryngologist, but this procedure is usually only performed in cases when a patient has failed antibiotics, has severe facial pain, has orbital or other complications, or has underlying problems with immunodeficiency (**choice E**).

Transillumination of the sinuses is not very helpful in diagnosing acute sinus infections in children. The sinuses are not well developed before the age 10 (**choice F**).

30. **The correct answer is D.** Metronidazole and vancomycin are the drugs of choice to treat pseudomembranous colitis due to *Clostridium difficile.*

Acyclovir is an antiviral drug and not used to treat *Clostridium difficile* (**choice A**).

Azithromycin is also an antibiotic that is commonly associated with the development of antibiotic-associated diarrhea due to *Clostridium difficile* (**choice B**). Therefore, it would not be a good choice.

Chloramphenicol is not a drug of choice against *Clostridium difficile* (**choice C**).

Trimethoprim-sulfamethoxazole is not used to treat *Clostridium difficile*. In fact, it is one of the more common antibiotics responsible for the development of pseudomembranous colitis (**choice E**).

31. **The correct answer is C.** Children with sickle cell disease and underlying immune disorders may be at higher risk for *Salmonella typhi* infections, and may have complicated disease with osteomyelitis, meningitis, and sepsis.

    Salmonella typhi can be quite serious and usually needs therapy, especially in the young child (**choice A**).

    Salmonella typhi rarely gives problematic diarrhea. It does cause invasive disease invading the small bowel wall (**choice B**).

    Salmonella typhi is a human disease. Other types of salmonella may be transmitted by pets (**choice D**), such as turtles.

32. **The correct answer is E.** This patient most likely has Wilson disease. She has neuropsychiatric symptoms as well as hepatomegaly. The ophthalmologist reports abnormal eye findings, which in this case is surely the presence of Kayser-Fleischer rings seen on slit lamp examination. Wilson's disease is an autosomal recessive disorder that may present during late childhood or early adolescence with hepatic symptoms. Many times it is difficult to arrive at the diagnosis without doing several different tests. Measurement of liver copper levels, 24-hour collection for urinary copper, and serum ceruloplasmin levels are particularly helpful.

    Elevated ammonia levels may be high in many liver diseases (e.g., Reye syndrome) (**choice A**). Serum ammonia may be helpful in the workup of a patient who presents with acute liver disease, but in and of itself is not specific.

    A drug screen is an important test to consider ordering in any adolescent with altered personality, behavior problems, truancy, or poor grades. It would not explain the multiple signs and symptoms in this patient (**choice B**).

    A liver biopsy will be helpful, but is frequently not diagnostic in Wilson disease (**choice C**).

    A serum α-1-antitrypsin level would help make the diagnosis of α-1-antitrypsin deficiency. This disease may present with pulmonary and liver disease, but not neurological or psychiatric symptoms (**choice D**).

33. **The correct answer is C.** Setting hot water heater temperature less than 120 to 130 F will help prevent many scalding burn injuries in children.

    Parents should be advised about the risks of using a microwave to heat milk for their child. It can heat the milk unevenly (**choice A**). Burn injuries of the trachea and other areas have been reported.

    Honey is not recommended for young infants because of the risk for infant botulism (**choice B**).

    In the first few months of life until he achieves a weight of 20 pounds, an infant should be placed in a rear-facing, not front-facing, infant car seat (**choice D**). The risk for sudden infant death syndrome (SIDS) in infants has been reduced by laying the infant to sleep on his back or in a supine position.

    A rear-facing infant car seat is appropriate for the first few months of life, but by placing the baby on his stomach to sleep there would be an increased risk of SIDS (**choice E**).

34. **The correct answer is D.** Children who received chemotherapy for cancer are at increased risk for developing premature ovarian failure. This would be the most important risk factor for later problems with deficient bone mass and osteoporosis.

    Her overall thinness is not extreme or of major concern (**choice A**).

    Adolescent girls who experience an early menarche may have a higher bone mineral density and thus have a decreased, not increased, risk for later development of osteoporosis (**choice B**). However, further ongoing studies are researching this area and the answers are not all in. There is increasing scientific evidence promoting higher levels of calcium intake during the years of adolescent growth.

    Although chronic illness may contribute to poor bone mineral density and later osteoporosis, this case describes a very localized tumor, and her chemotherapy treatments are more important as a risk factor for osteoporosis (**choice C**).

    There may be diminished skeletal resistance to fractures later in life at the site of radiation and/or surgery for this tumor; however, the overall impact of chemotherapy-induced premature ovarian failure is most important (**choice E**).

35. **The correct answer is C.** Down syndrome is commonly associated with joint laxity. Importantly, atlantoaxial and atlantooccipital instability can be detected on x-ray. Head trauma and significant falls particularly can occur while horseback riding and these Down syndrome children with cervical instability are at high risk for dislocation and other serious spinal injuries.

Health maintenance is important for children with Down syndrome because they are more likely to have conditions such as thyroid disease. All children with Down syndrome should be screened for thyroid disease. Could this girl have some delay in puberty due to hypothyroidism? Possibly. There is not enough information given regarding her growth and review of system for thyroid disease. Thyroid screening is worthwhile, but not the best answer for this pre-participation exam (**choice A**).

Down syndrome children may frequently have conductive hearing loss and language disorders. If a history is suggestive of problems, further evaluation is advised. But this is not so important in the described case (**choice B**).

While it is true that Down syndrome may be associated with a variety of cardiac defects, particularly of the atrioventricular canal, there is no history of past problems. Without a murmur, a referral to a cardiologist and obtaining an echocardiogram would not be in order (**choice D**).

A renal ultrasound is not indicated either because there is +1 proteinuria or on the basis of the Down syndrome diagnosis. It is not documented that persons with Down syndrome have an increased risk for renal disease or renal anomalies (**choice E**).

36. **The correct answer is B.** This patient has a clinically septic arthritis of the hip until proven otherwise. This is a surgical emergency that requires admission to the hospital for surgical drainage and IV antibiotics. The hip is the most common location in children and occurs usually secondary to hematogenous spread from distal infection sites like the pharynx or middle ear. The treatment of septic arthritis is primarily surgical drainage and lavage due to the difficult access of this joint to simple needle arthrocentesis.

Neisseria gonorrhoeae (**choice A**) is a common organism in sexually active, young adults. However, the choice of antibiotics in this young child should aim at *Staphylococcus* and *Streptococcus* coverage with additional gram-negative coverage. Naficillin with gentamycin would be an appropriate choice.

Plain film of the hip (**choice C**) is useful to rule out any fracture, foreign body, or concomitant osteomyelitis of the femur. It should not, however, distract the physician from recognizing the emergency and need for hospital admission if it is normal. Some helpful radiological modalities include ultrasonography for the guidance of needle arthrocentesis, magnetic resonance imaging of joints, and bone scans that recognize adjacent osteomyelitis.

Blood cultures (**choice D**) are only positive in 50% of cases and should not delay treatment. Other sites should also be cultured, such as urine or the pharynx, especially if patients are displaying symptoms.

Failure to recognize this disease and delay in treatment (**choice E**) will result in joint destruction and several complications including, in the case of the hip, avascular necrosis.

37. **The correct answer is C.** The stool sample with many fecal leukocytes suggests an inflammatory type of diarrhea. Common pathogens such as *Shigella*, *Salmonella*, and invasive *E. coli* would be detected by a stool culture.

A complete blood count (CBC) would not be helpful in sorting out the different diagnoses of diarrhea (**choice A**).

Abdominal x-rays usually are not indicated in the early evaluation of diarrheal illness (**choice B**).

Intestinal parasites (such as Giardia) may cause diarrhea, but they are not associated with mucus or leukocytes in the stool (**choice D**).

Diarrheal illness caused by common viruses, such as rotavirus or adenovirus, are not associated with the finding of fecal leukocytes (**choice E**).

38. **The correct answer is E.** The bald area is most likely alopecia areata. Alopecia areata usually presents as one or more patches of smooth bald spots on the scalp. It can be treated with high potency topical steroids. If this therapy does not work, then intralesional corticosteroids may be used. Alopecia areata can be a difficult condition to treat.

Behavioral therapy might be helpful if this were a case of trichotillomania. However, with hair pulling or excess rubbing there would most likely be evidence of many broken hairs (**choice A**).

Oral antibiotics can be used for impetigo or infected scalp areas, but this child has no evidence of inflammation or infection (**choice B**).

Griseofulvin is appropriate therapy for tinea capitis, but with tinea there is scaling. Frequently, black dots are evident in the balding area where hairs have completely broken off (**choice C**).

Topical steroid creams are typically used for tinea corporis, but there is no evidence for tinea on the non-scalp areas of this child (**choice D**).

39. **The correct answer is A.** Simian creases are found in nearly 5% of the normal population. Without finding other anomalies or stigmata suggesting Trisomy 21 or other syndromes, no further workup is necessary. If there were other findings present that are consistent with Down syndrome, then cytogenetics on the infant should be performed (**choice E**). However, this is not indicated at this time.

If signs or symptoms suggest a congenital heart disease or other cardiac lesion, or if the infant has Down syndrome or another condition associated with heart disease in the newborn period, then a cardiac consultation may be sought (**choice B**).

Cytogenetic testing on the parents is not indicated at this time (**choice C**).

Cytogenetic testing is not indicated for the parents or infant (**choice D**). If an infant has Down syndrome, a karyotype needs to be performed. If it reveals translocation, then further karyotyping of the parents and even other family members may need to be performed.

40. **The correct answer is D.** This 2-month-old infant has the signs and symptoms of *Chlamydia trachomatis* pneumonia including a cough, no fever, tachypnea, rales, eosinophilia, and a chest x-ray with interstitial infiltrates. As in this case, *Chlamydia trachomatis* may be associated with conjunctivitis. Oral erythromycin is the appropriate therapy.

Admission to the hospital is probably unnecessary and the best outpatient management is antibiotic therapy with erythromycin (**choice A**).

There is no indication that this infant has a lung anomaly or other problem that would warrant surgical consultation (**choice B**).

Amoxicillin is not the drug of choice for *Chlamydia trachomatis*. Amoxicillin is frequently used to treat first-time otitis media, but is not the proper choice in this case (**choice C**).

The infant is well hydrated and afebrile, but has pneumonia that needs medication (**choice E**). Without further history of lethargy, retractions, cyanosis, or problems drinking, he appears to be fine to receive antibiotics and followup at home.

41. **The correct answer is C.** Primary problems associated with alcohol poisoning are hypoglycemia and metabolic acidosis. Starting D_5W or even $D_{10}W$ if the glucose is low (<60 mg/dL) is important. In severe cases, cerebral edema and seizures can be problematic.

Abnormal bleeding problems can be seen in chronic liver disease due to the decreased absorption of vitamin K or the poor utilization of vitamin K. These are not found in acute alcohol poisonings (**choice A**).

Hyperammonemia is associated with severe hepatic diseases such as Reye syndrome, but not with acute alcohol poisoning or ingestion (**choice B**).

Hypocalcemia does not result from acute ethanol poisoning (**choice D**). However, in poisonings of ethylene glycol there can be kidney damage due to calcium oxylate crystals that precipitate in the renal parenchyma. This may be associated with hypocalcemia.

Hypothermia is not associated with acute alcohol or ethanol poisoning (**choice E**).

42. **The correct answer is B.** Human bites are at high risk for infection and prophylactic antibiotics are commonly prescribed. Organisms that may result from human bites are those from the normal mouth flora, including such organisms as *Streptococcus viridans*, *Eikenella corrodens*, *Haemophilus influenza*, *Staphylococcus aureus*, and various oral anaerobes, many of which are beta-lactamase producing. Therefore amoxicillin clavulanate is the antibiotic of choice.

Amoxicillin would not be effective against the beta-lactamase producing organisms (**choice A**).

Ciprofloxacin is not a drug of choice to treat human bites (**choice C**).

Clarithromycin does not offer proper coverage of the gram-negative organisms commonly found in human bites (**choice D**).

Trimethoprim-sulfamethoxazole is not an alternative drug to be used to treat human bites unless used in combination with clindamycin (**choice E**).

As stated above, human bites are a high risk of an infection and therefore it is inappropriate to not prescribe antibiotics (**choice F**).

43. **The correct answer is C.** The most likely cause of this girl's DKA is noncompliance with her diabetic management plan. Her history of normal glucose readings and the elevated hemoglobin A1C do not jibe. Most episodes of DKA during adolescence are most often due to issues of noncompliance in which patients have stopped insulin therapy whether because they lacked money to buy the insulin and supplies or it was a control issue. Many episodes of DKA can be prevented by improving patient education and access to continuity of care, and addressing behavioral issues involved with having a chronic illness.

The girl is most likely to have problems with hypoglycemia when she drinks alcohol. She needs to be counseled regarding the problems of alcohol that are particularly important to diabetic management (**choice A**).

This girl has a history of menarche a few months before; therefore, most of her growth in stature is complete and insulin needs are unlikely to be due to puberty (**choice B**).

There is no history to suggest she may have underlying renal disease and that this would relate to her acute episode of DKA (**choice D**).

Not enough findings on physical exam or by family history are given to suggest that she has streptococcal disease (**choice E**).

44. **The correct answer is E.** The abrasions over the dorsal aspects of the hand (Russell's sign) are a consequence of self-induced vomiting with resultant trauma to the hand from scraping against the teeth. This woman has an underlying eating disorder of anorexia nervosa, leading to weight loss and malnutrition. Her excellent grades and history of exercising a lot also are consistent with this disorder.

The abrasions on the back of her hand would not necessarily be consistent with any type of physical abuse (**choice A**).

The woman might have an anxiety disorder in association with her underlying eating disorder but this is not the best answer (**choice B**). Comorbid diagnoses of anxiety, depression, and obsessive-compulsive disorders are associated with eating disorders.

This woman might have problems with anger control or an underlying personality disorder that would result in fist fighting and thereby account for such abrasions on her hand (**choice C**). However, this is not the best explanation.

In some seriously depressed and/or psychiatrically disturbed adolescents there may be problems with excessive self-mutilation or self-inflicted wounds. Body piercing, burning, or stabbing oneself may be evident. This does not seem to be the case in this woman (**choice D**).

45. **The correct answer is C.** Testicular torsion has the classic signs and symptoms of acute onset of testicular pain, with typically no relief of pain with scrotal elevation, and negative or absent cremasteric reflex, and the testicle is usually high in the scrotum in a horizontal and rotated position. Treatment is surgical and a testicular scan may be performed before surgery (but typically should not delay consulting the surgeons) to identify the decreased or absent blood flow to the affected testes. Testicular torsion may be confused with other conditions such as epididymitis, incarcerated hernia, prostatitis, and varicocele.

Obtaining a complete blood count (CBC) and erythrocyte sedimentation rate is not the most important initial step (**choice A**) as this is likely a surgical emergency.

A Doppler ultrasound or radionuclide testicular scan may be used if the diagnosis is uncertain; however, a CT scan is not the scan to order (**choice B**).

If this boy appeared to have orchitis or epididymitis, then the appropriate care would be to obtain cultures for chlamydia and gonorrhea and to empirically treat with antibiotics. However, in this case he had an absent cremasteric reflex and no relief of pain with scrotal elevation, which instead suggests a diagnosis of testicular torsion (**choice D**).

To treat this boy with soaks and bedrest would delay the urgent need for diagnosis and treatment (**choice E**).

46. **The correct answer is C.** This child has mild gingivitis. There is no evidence of herpes or other infection, and preventive dental and gum care should be advised with proper oral hygiene including daily flossing and brushing of teeth.

Fluoridated water and toothpaste and tooth sealant applications have been used to help eliminate dental caries in children. Additional fluoride in this child is not the best management for gingivitis (**choice A**).

Although this child was most likely treated with antibiotics for strep throat, there is not enough clinical information to suggest that the gum inflammation is due to candidiasis. Nystatin is not the best answer (**choice B**).

It is not stated in this vignette that this child is symptomatic. Gingivitis is a common pediatric problem that is usually asymptomatic and results from poor oral hygiene. Proper preventive care is important. Supportive therapy to relieve symptoms of painful gums can include cool fluids and mildly seasoned foods, but this is not the best answer (**choice D**).

A deficiency in vitamin C can result in bleeding gums and other signs such as angular stomatitis of the lips, glossitis, and bruising. Full-blown cases of scurvy are rare, but many children may be somewhat deficient in vitamin C by not getting enough fruits and vegetables in their diets. There is not sufficient information in this case to suggest an underlying vitamin C deficiency (**choice E**).

47. **The correct answer is A.** This young man may have a problem of chronic cocaine use. He has a history of chronic rhinitis with no good history for it being related to allergies or upper respiratory infection. The fact that he denies drug use is not unusual. Cocaine not only would give red boggy turbinates and discharge, but could also present with problems of nasal crusting, bleeding, and septal perforation.

A rapid strep test and throat culture are not indicated (**choice B**). The mild red throat without significant lymphadenopathy is not clinically important.

Although a calcium alginate swab is the better type of applicator to collect mucus for culture, a nasopharyngeal culture is unnecessary (**choice C**).

There is insufficient history to suggest that there is sinusitis or other sinus abnormality (**choice D**). Sinus films are not warranted.

Fexofenadine is a less sedating type of antihistamine. There is no good history that this boy has allergies or upper respiratory inflammation. Prescribing an antihistamine would not be a good choice in management (**choice E**).

48. **The correct answer is E.** The above case describes a baby that has the typical characteristics of a baby with Turner syndrome. Other features that you may see are a shield shaped chest, widely space hypoplastic nipples, a low hairline, increased carrying angle, short stature, and multiple pigmented nevi. Due to the fact that several genotypes can result in Turner syndrome (45X,O, 46X,X with a deletion on the short arm of one of the X chromosomes), the phenotype may vary significantly. Even with variability in genotype, gonadal dysgenesis is found in 100% of patients and is associated with primary amenorrhea and a lack of pubertal development due to a loss of ovarian hormones.

Coarctation of the aorta (**choice A**) is also associated with Turner syndrome. As opposed to amenorrhea, which is seen in 100% of the cases, coarctation is only seen in about 20% of patients with Turner syndrome. It should be noted that in any girl with coarctation of the aorta, Turner syndrome should be considered.

Both endocardial cushion defect (**choice C**) and duodenal atresia (**choice B**) are associated with trisomy 21 (Down syndrome). Common dysmorphic features in these children include flat facial profile, up-slanted palpebral fissures, flat nasal bridge with epicanthal folds, small mouth with protruding tongue, short stature, single palmar crease (simian crease), short broad hands, incurved fifth finger, small genitalia, a gap between the first and second toes, and hypotonia. Cardiac defects are seen in about 50% of children with trisomy 21.

Intellectual functioning is almost always normal in patients with Turner syndrome, although they may have impaired spatial relations and perceptual motor organization. Therefore, even though mental retardation (**choice D**) is not a concern, they may have a lower nonverbal IQ. Also, it is important to keep in mind that they may have psychological problems arising from both their perceptual motor difficulties and from their sexual infantilism.

49. **The correct answer is D.** Not only is it important to let the mother know as soon as possible that there are some concerns with the baby, but it is necessary to get informed written consent in order to perform chromosome testing. When you talk to the mother, it is important to let her know that the diagnosis is not certain and in order to get a definitive diagnosis you need to do the testing. You should also discuss with her a little bit about Turner syndrome and answer any questions she might have.

Oftentimes the nurses have good relations with the mothers. Therefore, it is often helpful when going to talk to a parent about a sensitive issue to bring the nurse with you into the room. It is not the responsibility of the nurse to explain to the mother about your concerns (**choice A**) even if she does have a better relationship. You will probably be better able to answer any questions that the mother may have, and you are the one doing the testing, so you need to get consent.

Although the father should also be involved in the decision, he should not be approached alone (**choice B**). Depending on the involvement of the father, he should be approached together with the mother, or the mother should be approached first and asked what she wants the father to know. Especially if the parents are not married, the mother is the one who has to sign consent for the testing.

As above, drawing the blood and not telling the mother (**choice C**) is inappropriate. Because of the future implications (for insurance purposes, etc.), the mother must sign consent for the genetic testing.

By telling the mother that her baby is okay and not mentioning the test (**choice E**), you are lying to the mother. When you explain your suspicions to her, you can emphasize that the baby is doing well, but there still is something that you are concerned about and you need to let her know too. In order to perform chromosome testing you need parental consent, so you have to tell her about the test.

50. **The correct answer is D.** Acute ITP is the most common bleeding disorder of childhood, most frequently occurring between the ages of 2 and 5. The most common presentation is that of an otherwise healthy child with the acute onset of ecchymoses and petechiae and sometimes epistaxis. The child usually has a history of a viral infection 1 to 4 weeks prior to the onset of ITP. Apart from a markedly decreased platelet count (sometimes even less than $10,000/mm^3$), the complete blood count is normal. The peripheral smear will show a normal differential and large platelets. The disease results from autoimmune antibody formation against self-platelets, and approximately 80% of cases resolve spontaneously within 6 months. Although most children require no therapy, those with significant bleeding, or a platelet count less than approximately $10,000/mm^3$ may receive steroids, intravenous immune globulin, or Rh (D) immune globulin.

Child abuse (**choice A**) can sometimes present with multiple ecchymoses. The difference in this case is that this child has an extremely low platelet count to explain the bruising. A normal, active child may come in to your office with multiple bruises, but these should be seen on extensor surfaces like the shins and in places that you would expect a child to bump himself. Any bruising on a soft, non-exposed area should raise the idea of abuse, and further questioning of the caregiver and child as to how the bruises were acquired is indicated.

Disseminated intravascular coagulation (DIC) (**choice B**) is a disorder characterized by activation of both the coagulation and fibrinolysis pathways. Therefore, both the coagulation elements, such as the clotting factors and platelets, and anticoagulant proteins, such as antithrombin III and plasminogen, are consumed. It can be associated with acute conditions such as sepsis, trauma, shock, and burns, or chronic conditions such as malignancy, cirrhosis, and pre-eclampsia. Laboratory studies are significant for prolonged prothrombin time, prolonged partial thromboplastin time, low fibrinogen, elevated fibrin split products and d-dimers, and schistocytes on peripheral smear. DIC can be a life-threatening illness, so diagnosis and prompt treatment of the underlying condition that caused DIC are of the utmost importance.

Hemolytic uremic syndrome (HUS) (**choice C**) is a syndrome characterized by the triad of anemia, thrombocytopenia, and renal failure secondary to a disorder of immunoregulation precipitated by infection with *E. coli O157* or with pneumococcal infection. It is most commonly seen in children under 2 years of age, although older children can be affected. The illness is preceded by a prodrome of abdominal pain, vomiting, and diarrhea. This is followed by oliguria, pallor, and bleeding manifestations. Some children may develop hypertension and seizures or other significant central nervous system involvement. The anemia in HUS is usually severe and red cell fragments are seen on peripheral smear. This is a very serious illness that requires immediate attention although with the right care may completely resolve within 2 to 3 weeks with no residual defects.

Although leukemia (**choice E**) may present with ecchymoses, you would expect to see other cell lines affected on a complete blood count. For example, anemia might be present due to the crowding of the bone marrow with malignant cells and therefore an inability to produce red cell precursors. Also, a markedly elevated white cell count (due to blasts) might be found, or a decreased white cell count (again due to bone marrow crowding). In fact, if the picture is not typical for ITP, a bone marrow aspirate should be performed to rule out leukemia as a cause of thrombocytopenia.

Pediatrics: Test Three

1. A 4½-year-old girl is brought to the office complaining of bilateral ear pain and drainage. She has a long history of ear infections, with ear tubes placed at the age of 9 months and then again at the age of 4 years. She has had a runny nose for the past week and, as this is the usual pattern for her, now has ear pain and drainage. Her past medical history is otherwise unremarkable. She takes no medications and has no medication allergies. Her temperature is 38.1 C (101.6 F). Physical examination shows that the ear canals are both filled with thick yellow drainage. She is uncomfortable and finds it difficult to let you look in her ears. The next best step in her management would be to

   (A) refer her for reevaluation by her otolaryngologist, as her tubes do not seem to be working well
   (B) treat with antibiotic eardrops alone
   (C) treat with intravenous antibiotics given her history of recurrent infections, in an attempt to clear the infection
   (D) treat with oral antibiotics alone

2. A 5-week-old, breast-fed, full-term boy is brought to your office by his parents. They state that the baby was doing well when he came home from the hospital, after an uncomplicated delivery, until about 3 days ago when he began getting fussy and started to vomit. Over the past 36 hours his vomiting has become projectile. There is no "green color" to the vomitus. It has now gotten to the point where the baby can no longer keep down any breast milk and the family is quite concerned. He had normal bowel movements yesterday but his diaper has been dry for the past 12 hours. This is the first child for both parents. The patient is afebrile but tachycardic. His anterior fontanelle is sunken and there is tenting of his skin. His abdomen is nondistended and soft. There is a nontender, bulging mass in the mid-epigastric area. Stool is guaiac-negative. Serum electrolytes show a hypokalemic, hypochloremic metabolic alkalosis. You should tell the parents that the baby

   (A) can be managed at home
   (B) probably has cancer
   (C) should be admitted to the hospital for observation
   (D) should be given medication to correct the problem
   (E) will need surgery

3. A 2-year-old girl is brought to the clinic because of a 7-day history of fever and vomiting followed by watery diarrhea. The mother tells you that the child was very dehydrated earlier in the week, but she seems to be improving. The number of diaper changes that she requires have been decreasing in the past few days and the stool is more formed and "never spills out of the diaper anymore." She attends day care 3 days a week, and two other children have had similar symptoms over the past 3 weeks. The mother is concerned because this "outbreak" has occurred a few other times and now she is considering switching day care centers because they "obviously have poor sanitation practices." She is very upset because she cannot miss any more days at work, so she really needs to drop her daughter off at day care after this visit. She has not traveled lately. The patient appears well hydrated and has normal vital signs. When you examine her you notice that there is a moderate amount of soft stool in the diaper, but it is completely contained. You advise the mother to provide plenty of fluids to the patient. You should also tell her that:

(A) Antibiotic therapy for all affected children is indicated at this time.

(B) As long as the stool can be contained within diapers, the patient can attend day care.

(C) Boiling all drinking water at the day care center will eliminate future outbreaks of this infection.

(D) Careful handwashing of the caregivers and children does not prevent the spread of infection.

(E) Immunization of the children and staff at the center should be performed to decrease the number of infections.

(F) Meticulous laundering of the bedding and clothing of the caregivers and children will stop the spread of infection.

(G) Unfortunately, the patient must be kept at home from day care, until a few days after the diarrhea ceases.

4. A 7-year-old boy is brought to the office because of constipation that began 3 months ago, after school began in the fall. His mother tells you that he only has one bowel movement every 4 to 5 days, and when it finally does occur, he is in an "awful lot of pain." She can usually hear "hollering" coming from the bathroom as she prepares dinner in the kitchen. She tells you that he has always been an "unusual boy," very fussy and neat, always cleaning up his room and straightening things around the house. The teachers at school call home to tell her "what a good helper" she is raising. He is very particular about cleanliness. He does not take any medications and has no other medical illnesses. His family history is unremarkable. His temperature is 37.0 C (98.6 F). Physical examination shows mild abdominal tenderness, a hard mass in the lower abdomen, and a dilated rectum filled with a large amount of hard, guaiac-negative, brown stool. The most appropriate next step is to

(A) ask him if he uses the school bathrooms

(B) obtain a consult with a pediatric gastroenterologist

(C) obtain an x-ray of the abdomen

(D) recommend a balanced diet containing whole grains, fruits, and vegetables

(E) schedule an anal manometry

5. A 12-year-old boy with asthma and seasonal allergies is brought to the office complaining of left-foot-pain that is around his heel, and that worsens after soccer games. Last year during the soccer season, he sustained a left tibial stress fracture that went on to heal with nonsurgical management. The athletic trainer informed his mother that he has "weak ankles and requires a physical therapy prescription." There is no history of trauma. Physical examination reveals an otherwise healthy boy at the 60th percentile for height and weight. There is no leg length discrepancy. Inspection of the left foot reveals the skin to be intact, no swelling, and a slightly tender bump at the distal medial malleolus. Neurovascular examination of the left lower extremity is unremarkable. Passive and active inversion and eversion motion is significantly less than the opposite foot. The patient states this motion elicits foot pain. X-rays completed 1 month ago for the same complaint were negative. The most appropriate next step in management is to

(A) recommend activity modification and do not repeat the foot x-rays, but instead order a CT scan of the hind-foot region
(B) recommend activity modification and do not repeat the foot x-rays, but instead order an MRI of the hind-foot region
(C) recommend activity modification and give him a prescription for physical therapy that should emphasize plantar fascia stretching and peroneal muscle strengthening
(D) repeat the foot x-rays and include stress views of the ankle to rule out ankle instability secondary to ligamentous and tendon insufficiency
(E) repeat left leg x-rays to rule out recurrence of the previous stress fracture and the possibility of referred pain as the source of foot discomfort

6. You are seeing a 5-year-old boy in your office for a rash. He attends both school and day care, and his parents are concerned about whether he should be staying home because of the rash. The parents first noticed the rash last night on the child's cheeks. It was bright red. The child had a low-grade fever the week prior and some decreased activity, but was otherwise well. When they awakened this morning the rash had spread to his entire body. The child complains of mild pruritus. There are no apparent new environmental exposures. The child has no history of any chronic medical problems. His temperature is 38.2 C (100.7 F), blood pressure is 95/50 mm Hg, pulse is 85/min, and respirations are 18/min. The child appears well. His examination is remarkable only for a macular, erythematous, generalized lacy rash. There are no vesicles. At this time the most correct statement about his condition is:

(A) Administration of ceftriaxone is indicated.
(B) Admission to the hospital for further testing is indicated.
(C) He cannot return to school or day care until the rash resolves.
(D) Pregnant contacts should be referred for evaluation.
(E) Treatment with prednisone for severe allergic reaction is indicated.

7. A previously healthy 8-year-old boy is brought to the urgent care clinic because of the abrupt onset of facial swelling, edema, and "foamy urine." His blood pressure is 110/60 mm Hg and pulse is 85/min. He has periorbital and facial swelling. Examination of the urine is normal, except for the presence of protein. His blood urea nitrogen and creatinine levels are normal. The most appropriate next step in management is to

(A) check antistreptolysin O titers
(B) check fasting glucose level
(C) perform a kidney biopsy
(D) start the patient on cyclophosphamide
(E) start the patient on steroids

8. A 27-year-old African American woman who is a mother of two comes to the office concerned about "birthmarks" present on her younger child that seem to be increasing in number as he is getting older. She has no significant medical history and both pregnancies were uneventful. Her firstborn is now a healthy 3-year-old girl who is developing normally. Her son just celebrated his first birthday and has reached all the predicted milestones. Both children are at the 90th percentile for height and weight. They are playing together happily while you talk to the mother. As you examine the boy, you notice that he has three well-demarcated, oval, dark brown patches from 2 to 5 mm in diameter on the back. The mother confirms that only two of them were present at birth. It is appropriate to advise the mother that:

   (A) An extensive laboratory and imaging workup should be done for the sake of the mother's peace of mind.
   (B) It is very peculiar that her son is developing new lesions, and a biopsy should be taken to exclude melanoma.
   (C) Surgical excision of the existing "birthmarks" is warranted to prevent malignant transformation later on in life.
   (D) The boy does not have neurofibromatosis because there is no family history of the disease.
   (E) These "birthmarks" are not infrequent in African American children and, close to one in five newborn babies will have at least one.

9. A concerned mother brings her 8-year-old daughter to the emergency department because of a new onset rash that started with faint pink spots on her trunk, but has developed into drop-sized, red, scaly lesions all over her body over the course of 3 to 4 days. She is scared that her daughter might be developing the same skin disease her husband has had on his elbows and knees since he was a child. You inquire if the girl had any recent upper respiratory tract infections and the mother recalls a short-lived episode of sore throat and fever 10 days ago that resolved with a couple of doses of acetaminophen. On examination, she is a well developed, well nourished girl in no acute distress. She has diffuse erythematous papules with fine silvery scales on her trunk and extremities. There is also coarse pitting on her fingernails. The most appropriate diagnostic study at this time is

   (A) diascopy
   (B) a KOH test
   (C) a monospot test
   (D) a rapid strep test and ASO titer
   (E) a Wood light examination

10. You are finishing your morning rounds in the hospital when the parents of a 2-year-old boy call you. You saw him in the office 2 days ago and concluded that he probably had a viral infection because the physical examination was unrevealing except for a fever of 39.0 C (102.2 F) and mild lymphadenopathy. You sent the family home with instructions to use acetaminophen for fever reduction, give him lots of fluids, and as much rest as a 2-year-old could handle. They tell you that their child has had a fever between 38.0 C and 39.0 C (100-102 F) for 3 days straight, despite the regular use of acetaminophen, but it miraculously subsided during the night and this morning it is 36.5 C (97.7 F). Now, though, he has a head-to-toe skin rash. You agree to see them in the emergency department and when they arrive you note that the child is playful, giggling, and smiling at all the staff, but has a diffuse, erythematous, macular exanthem on the neck, trunk, buttocks, and extremities. The examination is otherwise unremarkable at this time. The most likely causative agent of this child's disease is

   (A) herpes simplex virus type 1
   (B) human herpes virus type 6
   (C) human herpes virus type 8
   (D) human papillomavirus type 6
   (E) parvovirus B-19

11. An 8-year-old is brought to the office for a fever and a sore throat. You advise the mother to provide symptomatic therapy, and 3 days later, she calls you to say that the fever and sore throat are a little improved, but the daughter has developed red spots, first on the neck, and then on the trunk. Today, she is starting to get widespread scaling. You agree to see her the next morning. When they arrive you note diffuse fine scales on her trunk and extremities. There are also a few petechiae in her antecubital fossae. Her tongue has a diffuse white-coating and prominent red papillae. Cervical and submandibular tender lymphadenopathy is present and her temperature is 38.2 C (100.7 F). The most appropriate treatment for this child is

(A) intravenous acyclovir for 7 days
(B) intravenous penicillin for 4 weeks
(C) oral ciprofloxacin for 10 days
(D) oral penicillin for 10 days
(E) topical steroids until the rash resolves

12. A 5-year-old African American boy is brought to the office for a well-child check-up. The mother states that the boy is current with respect to his immunizations and is doing well in school. She has no concerns except for the fact that he is a very picky eater who eats mostly candy and meat (hot dogs and hamburgers), and drinks only carbonated colas. He is a thin child with his height and weight in the 10th percentile. Vital signs are within the age-appropriate values. The examination is only remarkable for pronounced genu varum. You then ask the patient's mother if she has noticed this and she states that she thinks it is actually getting worse. The most appropriate next step in management is to

(A) inform the patient and his mother that genu varum in children is normal and he will likely grow out of it over time
(B) obtain a dietary consult and recommend calcium supplements and expect the deformities to resolve
(C) obtain an emergency serum calcium level and prepare to admit this child for calcium supplementation
(D) obtain an orthopedic surgery consult and recommend long-leg weight-bearing radiographs
(E) tell the child protective services that you suspect physical abuse and neglect of this child and have him placed in protective custody

13. A 21-month-old boy is brought to the clinic because he has not been using his right arm since early this morning. The mother denies any history of trauma and does not think that he fell or was left alone for any appreciable time period. When you ask her to review her son's morning she begins by telling you that the boy's father was responsible for waking the child up, and that every morning they have about 30 minutes of playtime. She does recall that this morning's play was a little rough, and that the boy did cry for a few minutes after his father picked him up by the forearms and spun him around, but that they usually did this. On further history taking, the boy has met all developmental milestones, is current on his immunizations, and is in the 50th percentile for both height and weight. On examination, the boy is a clean, quiet, well-nourished 18-month-old. Fundoscopic examination reveals no retinal hemorrhages and with the exception of the boy's right upper extremity, you note no abnormalities on examination. The right shoulder and arm are not tender to palpation and do not appear deformed, but the right elbow is very tender and appears slightly swollen. The boy will not flex or extend at the elbow. The forearm has no gross deformity, distally the boy has a 2+ radial pulse, and it appears the sensation and motor function distally (wrist/hand) are intact. The mother is very concerned and asks you what to do next. You should

(A) inform the boy's mother to take her son home and advise that he will start using the arm in the next few days because he has likely bruised it while playing with his father
(B) obtain radiographs of the right elbow, as the boy has likely sustained a radial head dislocation, and rule out any other fractures
(C) place the boy's arm into a sling because he has dislocated his right shoulder, and obtain a referral to the local pediatric orthopedic surgeon
(D) tell the patient's mother that you are contacting child protective services because this is likely a case of child abuse
(E) tell the patient's mother that you are going to forcibly reduce the boy's dislocated elbow and that she may want to leave the room for this procedure

14. An 8-year-old boy is brought to the clinic by his mother because of fecal soiling of his underwear that has been an intermittent problem since he began using the bathroom by himself. The patient has no complaints himself and remains quiet during the interview. The patient and his mother deny any prominent family stressors, and the patient is popular with his peer group and a good and well-behaved student. On physical examination, the patient is found to have a slightly distended abdomen with hyperactive bowel sounds. On rectal examination, there is watery stool leaking from the patient's anus. The most appropriate next step in the management of this patient is to

(A) perform a sleep study
(B) prescribe an antidepressant medication
(C) prescribe an antipsychotic medication
(D) recommend special education placement
(E) remove stool from the patient's rectal vault

15. A 6-year-old girl is brought to the urgent care clinic because of a 1-day history of compulsive hand-washing, checking the family's front door repeatedly to ensure that it is locked, and subtle, though repetitive, facial tics. The patient's parents state that they have never seen her behave in this manner before. Her vital signs are stable and physical examination is unremarkable except for a perceptible, repetitive facial tic. The patient's review of systems is negative, except for the fact that she was kept from school for 1 week approximately 3 weeks ago because of a sore throat and fevers. Based on her current condition and past history, it is possible that she has

(A) disseminated fungemia
(B) erythema nodosum
(C) influenza A
(D) mononucleosis
(E) a streptococcal infection

16. A 19-year-old mother brings her 4-week-old firstborn girl to the office for immunizations and tells you about a scalp problem her baby has developed in the past 2 weeks. Otherwise, the baby is doing well. She is breast-feeding every 3 hours and sleeps most of the time in between. The parents give her a bath every night with mild baby soap and luke warm water. They do not rub the scalp too hard in fear that they may hurt her head. The scaling started about 2 weeks ago on the top of her scalp and has been progressively getting worse. Over the past 3 days, she noticed that some scaling appeared on her eyelids, too. The baby has diffuse faint erythema on the parietal scalp and vertex covered by thick yellow scales that are adhering to the hair and tufting on the vertex. The rims of both eyelids also have fine, yellow scales. The most appropriate treatment for this patient is

(A) avoidance of washing until the lesions resolve
(B) daily washing only with water
(C) daily washing with mild baby shampoo after applying topical betamethasone cream
(D) daily washing with mild baby shampoo after applying topical permethrin cream
(E) daily washing with mild baby shampoo after soaking the scalp with baby oil for 1 to 2 hours

17. A 14-year-old boy is brought to the emergency department by his parents with pain and redness on the forearm that has developed in the past 24 hours after a bite by an aggressive dog. The boy appears somewhat ill. His body temperature is 38.5 C (101.3 F) and he has a pulse of 100/min. There is a purulent bite wound on his medial right forearm with an ascending lymphangitis. His leukocyte count is $12,000/mm^3$ with a marked left shift. The most likely causative microorganism is

(A) group A streptococcus
(B) *Pasteurella multocida*
(C) *Pseudomonas aeruginosa*
(D) *Salmonella typhi*
(E) *Staphylococcus aureus*

18. You have been taking care of a 32-year-old woman with HLA-DR3 positive lupus erythematosus and anti-Ro/SSA antibodies for the past 2 years. Her disease has been well controlled with hydroxychloroquine, but she discontinued the medication when she became pregnant 9 months earlier. The pregnancy was uneventful and she gave birth to a baby girl who had multiple annular, scaling, erythematous macules and plaques on the head and extremities. You explain to the mother that her child has neonatal lupus and that the skin lesions will probably spontaneously resolve over 6 months or so. Unfortunately, you tell her, there is a 50% chance that the disease caused a more serious, permanent defect for which you will have the baby checked by a specialized neonatologist. The permanent sequelae of neonatal lupus that you are referring to is

(A) lupus panniculitis
(B) photosensitivity
(C) scarring alopecia
(D) third-degree heart block
(E) ulcerations of the hard palate

19. A 27-year-old mother brings her two children, a 5-year-old boy and a 3-year-old girl, to your office for what she calls "pimples" that started appearing on their skin. They moved into the area 6 months ago and, after settling down, she enrolled them into a day care center in preparation of searching for a job. The "pimples" began appearing on their neck shortly after they enrolled into day care, about 2 months ago, and are steadily increasing in number. Even though some resolve on their own, she thinks more come up in the meantime. She tells you that they have both been healthy in the past year or two, except for mild childhood eczema present since they were infants. You ask her how she takes care of their skin and she tells you that she does not allow bubble baths and regularly lubricates their skin with a thick emollient cream every day after they shower. All immunizations are up-to-date. The family history is positive for hay fever in the father, and the mother herself had childhood eczema until school age when it resolved spontaneously. You examine the children to find that they are both well developed, well nourished, and at the appropriate stage of development. The boy has dry skin and a few scaly pink patches on his arms and legs. There are 10 to 12 flesh-colored, pearly, umbilicated 2 to 3 mm papules with a scaly, erythematous halo in his right axilla and on the neck. The girl has keratotic follicular papules on the extensor upper arms and thighs with some dry patches on the legs. She has 6 to 7 similar looking pearly, flesh-colored, 1 to 3 mm umbilicated papules on the neck. The most likely causative agent of their skin infection is

(A) *Cryptococcus neoformans*
(B) *Histoplasma capsulatum*
(C) human papillomavirus
(D) Molluscipoxvirus
(E) Orthopoxvirus

20. A 15-year-old African American boy with sickle cell disease is admitted to the hospital with fever, chills, and mild leg pain. He developed pain in the middle third of his right anterior thigh 14 days following a bacterial gastroenteritis from which he is recovering. He denies trauma to the area despite the fact that his right thigh is swollen and tender. His temperature is 38.5 C (101.3 F), blood pressure is 132/90 mm Hg, pulse 88/min, and respirations are 18/min. There is swelling and erythema over his right thigh. No definite fluctuance is felt. His erythrocyte sedimentation rate is 98 seconds, hematocrit is 30% (which is slightly below his baseline), and leukocyte count is 15,000/mm^3. A duplex Doppler ultrasound examination of the right lower extremity is limited due to pain, but negative for deep vein thrombosis. The most important management of his condition is

(A) blood cultures and a needle biopsy of the bone, followed by 4 to 6 weeks of organism-specific intravenous antibiotics
(B) despite the ultrasound examination, begin a heparin drip until an MRI can be obtained
(C) ibuprofen and discharge
(D) meperidine and promethazine for his acute sickle cell pain crisis
(E) a radionuclide bone scan

21. A 4-year-old girl is brought to the emergency department by her parents after an accidental fall from the bed during which she injured her arm. She is in obvious pain and is sitting in her father's lap, holding her teddy bear in her other hand. The resident asks the parents to leave the room so that he can talk to and examine the child alone. The parents refuse to do so, stating that their daughter is already upset and scared. The nursing staff seems upset with the attitude of the parents and some of them already suspect abuse. In order to avoid further problems they call you at home for advice. You should advise them that the best intervention at this time is to

(A) call a psychiatry consult to mediate the conflict resolution between the parents and staff
(B) immediately drive to the hospital to see the case personally and discuss it with the parents
(C) immediately report the suspected child abuse to the appropriate authorities
(D) suggest that the presence of parents may facilitate the examination and minimize the stress the child is experiencing related to the trauma and the visit to the hospital
(E) support the resident and staff in their intent to see the child alone

22. A 16-year-old boy comes to your office for an examination prior to joining his school's basketball team. He says that he is generally healthy but does sometimes experience mild shortness of breath on exertion. He thinks that these symptoms are occurring because he is "out of shape." His parents are both alive and well, as are his brother and sister. He had an uncle that died suddenly at 27 years of age, but does not know any of the circumstances involving his death. His temperature is 37.0 C (98.6 F), blood pressure is 110/70 mm Hg, pulse is 63/min, and respirations are 14/min. He is a well-developed, well-nourished young man who appears properly developed for his age. There is an audible S4 and a nonradiating systolic ejection murmur that increases in intensity with standing up. You send the patient for an echocardiogram, which confirms your diagnosis. At this time the most appropriate management of this patient is

(A) reassurance, no activity restrictions are necessary
(B) referral for a dual-chambered pacer
(C) referral for myomectomy
(D) treatment with digoxin
(E) treatment with verapamil

23. A 13-year-old girl with no significant medical or surgical history comes to the clinic for evaluation before attending a local junior high and participating in extracurricular activities. During your physical examination you notice an abnormal curvature of the patient's spine with the presence of a prominent rib hump during a forward bend test. You mention this to your patient and her mother. The patient denies any back or leg pain but now does note that she feels that one of her shoulders is higher than the other. Her mother has noticed this curvature ever since a recent vacation to the beach. The patient's mother also remembers that her two sisters also had "curved spines" when they were growing up. The patient's mother tells you her daughter is normal and wants you to sign the examination card as "normal" so that she can participate in cheerleading. The most appropriate next step in management is to

    (A) direct the patient and her mother to go to the local emergency department, as the patient likely has a life-threatening neurological condition
    (B) order an MRI of the patient's brain and spinal column
    (C) perform a comprehensive neurological examination that includes motor strength, sensation, and deep tendon reflexes
    (D) send the patient to a local shop that will make her a back brace to straighten her out
    (E) tell the patient and her mother to see one of your orthopedic surgery colleagues because the patient needs a spinal fusion

24. A 5-year-old boy is brought to the office by his parents who are concerned about their child's frequent ear infections. The child had his first ear infection 18 months ago and has had eight ear infections in the last 12 months. These ear infections have all been treated with antibiotics and have resolved with 10 to 14 days of therapy. The parents have noticed that the child turns the volume way up when watching television and sits very close to the television set. The child has no other significant medical history and has no drug allergies. His immunizations are up-to-date. Otoscopic examination reveals dull, immobile tympanic membranes bilaterally. There is no erythema of the tympanic membrane. The remainder of the examination is normal. The most appropriate next step is to

    (A) prescribe antibiotic drops to be used in each ear three times per day for 3 weeks and reexamine the child at the conclusion of therapy
    (B) prescribe oral antibiotics for acute otitis media
    (C) reassure the parents that the child will grow out of the ear infections in the next few years
    (D) refer the patient to an otolaryngologist for a hearing test and evaluation for myringotomy tubes
    (E) send the child for a CT scan of the temporal bones to evaluate for middle ear and mastoid problems

25. A previously healthy 7-year-old girl is brought to the urgent care clinic because of fever and a rash for 8 weeks. The rash began on the left flank and then spread to all areas of the body. Initially, it was erythematous and intermittently pruritic, usually at night. At that time the patient was seen by her physician, who diagnosed fifth disease. She was sent home with supportive treatment but the symptoms continued. She is usually afebrile during the day and has fevers and chills at night. The rash becomes more prominent when the child is febrile. Two weeks after the initial doctor's visit the child began complaining of joint pain of the left knee and wrist with stiffening. She is having trouble with her daily activities and gets "wiped out" in the evening hours. There is no nausea, diarrhea, vomiting, or allergies. Her vision is normal and she denies dysuria. Her temperature is 37.2 C (99 F). She has a palpable spleen and a diffuse macular rash with each about 7 mm in size. The macules are diffusely present on the torso, abdomen, and extremities but not on the palms and soles. The mother requests that her child be tested for Lyme disease. The most appropriate response to the mother's request is which of the following:

(A) "A Lyme titer will probably be negative because Lyme disease is not the diagnosis."
(B) "It is possible that your daughter has Lyme disease and we will work this up along with some other possible conditions that might explain her symptoms."
(C) "The diagnosis is juvenile rheumatoid arthritis, and the Lyme titer would probably be negative."
(D) "Your daughter does not fit the correct age group for the diagnosis to be Lyme disease."
(E) "Your daughter does not fit the correct age group for Lyme disease, but we will do a Lyme titer just to be sure."

26. A 12-year-old Hispanic boy is brought to the clinic by his mother because she and the boy's father both have type 2 diabetes and she is concerned about the likelihood of her son developing it. You notice when reading his chart that the child has height and weight percentiles above the 85th percentile and that his last serum glucose was in the normal range. At this time, the most appropriate advice is:

(A) "I understand your concern and in view of his obesity your son should be enrolled in a weight loss program involving low-calorie and high-protein diets."
(B) "I understand your concern and in view of his obesity your son would benefit from participating in his favorite sport at school."
(C) "I understand your concern and in view of his obesity your son would benefit from a treatment program that includes exercise, diet, and behavior modification."
(D) "I understand your concern. Your child is obese and he should start taking an antiobesity agent now to reduce the risks of diabetes."
(E) "Your child's last serum glucose was normal so we do not need to do very much right now besides measuring his glucose again in 6 months."

27. A 7-year-old African American boy is brought to the emergency department by his mother after he rode his bicycle into the garbage bins on the side of the house. He was hurled forward and landed on the ground. The child did not lose consciousness and began crying immediately. He was able to get up without difficulty and he was walking normally, but began complaining of pain in his shoulder. His blood pressure is 100/70 mm Hg, pulse is 80/min, and respirations are 18/min. On physical examination, there are no obvious lacerations or abrasions on his body. His extremities are normal but you note a small, tender swelling over the right clavicle. The overlying skin appears unaffected. An x-ray is shown:

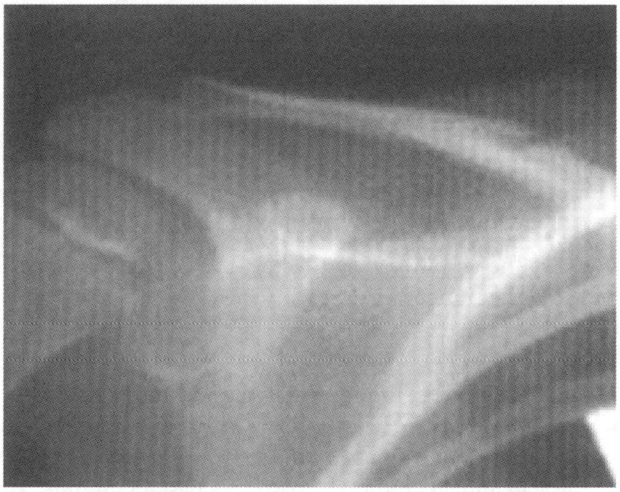

The most appropriate management for this injury is to

(A) admit the patient to the hospital for observation and immediately call child protective services
(B) admit the patient to the hospital for vital sign observation
(C) admit the patient to the hospital for open reduction and internal fixation of the injury under general anesthesia the following morning
(D) immediately take the patient to the operating room for an internal fixation of the injury under general anesthesia provided he has not eaten anything for the past 12 hours
(E) send the patient home in a collar splint and arrange an outpatient appointment with orthopedics

28. You are called to evaluate a 1-day-old white baby boy in the newborn nursery because the mother is concerned about his head. The delivery of the child was prolonged but was an otherwise uncomplicated vaginal delivery. The nurses report that he has voided and passed meconium. As part of the clinical examination you note that the child is pink and all pulses are present and equal. His fingernails are normal. He has no neck or clavicular masses. His red reflex of the eyes is normal. His heart and breath sounds are normal. His abdomen is negative for hepatosplenomegaly. His testes are descended, urethral meatus is patent, and the foreskin appears normal. His hip examination is negative for clicks. His Morrow, suck, grasp, and plantar reflexes are normal. Examination of the head reveals a poorly demarcated soft tissue swelling that crosses suture lines with some pitting edema. There is no evidence of depression fractures. A photograph of the head is shown:

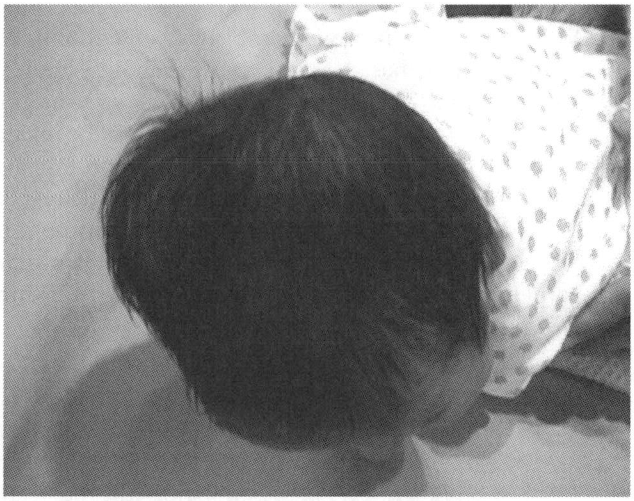

The most appropriate response to the mother's expressed concern is:

(A) "Did you leave your child unattended?"
(B) "I understand your concern about the child's head and I will order a CT scan of the head to evaluate for any bone or soft tissue injury."
(C) "I understand your concern about your child's head and I want to reassure you that it will resolve within days and only observation is indicated at this time."
(D) "I understand your concern about your child's head and I will obtain a consultation with a neurosurgeon for immediate evaluation."
(E) "Is there any history of babies with large heads in your family?"

29. A 2-year-old white boy is brought to the clinic because of a 24-hour history of diarrhea. He is still breast-feeding. On physical examination he is alert, his mucous membranes are moist, and skin turgor is good. You note that he has liquid stool in his diaper. The mother asks what she should do about feedings. You should advice her that

(A) oral intake should be limited to clear fluids, bananas, rice, applesauce, and toast
(B) the child should eat an age-appropriate diet and gradually discontinue breast-feeding
(C) the child should eat an age-appropriate diet and continue breast-feeding
(D) the child should discontinue breast-feeding immediately
(E) the mother should temporarily withhold breast-feeding to promote intestinal recovery

30. An African American woman brings her 2-month-old son to the clinic because she is worried about a lump on his abdomen. "That thing sticks out whenever he cries and strains," says the mother as she points to the infant's abdomen. The child has not had any symptoms since birth and has been gaining weight and height along the 80th percentile. On physical examination you notice a mass located at the site of the umbilicus that protrudes as the child begins crying. It is reducible. At this time the most appropriate management is

(A) observation on an outpatient basis
(B) strapping
(C) surgical reduction
(D) transcutaneous nerve stimulation of the rectus abdominis
(E) ultrasound of the abdomen

31. A 9-month-old white boy is brought to the clinic by his mother who is concerned that the child appears "paler than his normal self" and has become irritable. When reviewing his charts you note that he was delivered by a spontaneous vaginal delivery at 37 weeks' gestation and had a cephalohematoma. He had regularly scheduled visits at 2 and 4 months of age, when he was immunized. He is bottle-feeding well with cow's milk and has a good appetite and can tolerate over a pint a day. He appears pale. His vital signs are: temperature 37.0 C (98.6 F), blood pressure 90/65 mm Hg, pulse 84/min, and respirations 18/min. His height and weight are in the 95th percentile. His hematocrit is 28% and you suspect an iron deficiency anemia. The best explanation for his current condition is

(A) cephalohematoma formation in the child at the time of birth
(B) cow's milk
(C) excessive maternal blood loss at the time of birth
(D) maternal iron deficiency anemia during pregnancy, with hemoglobin of 10 g/dL and hematocrit of 32%
(E) the gestational age of the child being 37 weeks at the time of birth

32. You are called to see a 5-year-old girl in the emergency department who was brought in by her mother who became gravely concerned when her daughter became flaccid and less responsive over the past 45 minutes. Her temperature is 39.4 C (103 F), blood pressure is 70/30 mm Hg, pulse is 110/min, and respirations are 12/min. Her skin is pink and very warm and she is flaccid with a flat affect. You suspect that she may be going into septic shock and manage her appropriately. Three attempts at peripheral venous cannulation over 90 seconds are unsuccessful. The most appropriate next access method that should be attempted is

(A) a further attempt at a peripheral venous cannulation
(B) an intraosseous cannulation without local anesthetic
(C) saphenous vein cutdown preceded by local anesthetic
(D) scalp vein cannulation
(E) subclavian vein cannulation

33. You are the only physician in the office today and it seems that most of the presenting complaints are orthopedic issues. Throughout the afternoon you see a variety of orthopedic problems. The child that requires a referral to an orthopedic surgeon for further evaluation is

(A) an 18-month-old boy with a dorsiflexed foot that can be plantar flexed to neutral
(B) a 5-year-old boy with flatfeet
(C) a 3-month-old boy with metatarsus adductus whose foot can be stretched to neutral
(D) a 3-year-old girl with overriding fourth toes
(E) a 20-month-old girl who usually walks on her toes, although she is able to dorsiflex her foot past the neutral position

34. While working at the urban urgent care center you are visited by a mother and her 16-month-old son. The boy's mother states that she has noticed her son will not step on his left leg. She says that he fell off a chair at home and landed on his left foot awkwardly. The patient's mother states the patient lives with her in a small one-room apartment and that her boyfriend frequently stays over as well. The boy's mother denies any previous injuries or fractures. On physical examination, the boy is wearing dirty clothes and is very thin. His vital signs are unremarkable. The patient has a swollen left thigh and has pain with palpation of his thigh. You also notice well-healed circular scars on the patient's abdomen. You obtain radiographs of the boy's leg, and a spiral mid-shaft femur fracture is noted. The left knee is also included in the radiograph, and it appears to show a healed proximal tibia fracture as well. At this time you should

(A) give the patient's mother a prescription for crutches and pain medicine for her son and tell her the fracture will heal in 2 to 3 weeks because her son is very young and these fractures heal well
(B) physically take the child away from his mother and call the police because you know that these injuries were inflicted by his mother
(C) place a long-leg cast for the proximal femur fracture and refer them to the local pediatric orthopedic surgeon so that the patient will have proper followup
(D) suggest a complete metabolic workup and a bone biopsy, as this patient likely has osteogenesis imperfecta and is at risk for many other serious fractures
(E) tell the patient's mother that this fracture is not common after a fall and that you are concerned her son's injury is a result of abuse; contact Child Protective Services and order a skeletal survey to look for other previous fractures

35. A 4-day-old boy is brought to the urgent care clinic because of a 24-hour history of red eyes. The mother tells you that she had an uneventful pregnancy and her son had no problems at birth. On examination, the baby's eyes are shut and there is a mucopurulent discharge on the lashes. You gently open his eyes and note conjunctival hyperemia and a mucopurulent discharge in the fornices. The corneas are clear and pupils are round and reactive. A Gram stain of the discharge shows gram-negative organisms. At this time the most correct statement about his condition is

(A) Treatment with topical bacitracin or erythromycin is not indicated
(B) Irrigation of the eyes with saline is contraindicated
(C) Treat with topical antibiotics for a gonococcal infection will treat the infection
(D) Systemic antibiotics for suspected gonococcal and chlamydial infections are indicated

36. A 4-year-old boy is brought to the emergency department by his parents who report that he has been crying and pulling at his right ear for a week and has had temperatures to 39.1 C (102.4 F). Over the last few hours they have noted that the child has become lethargic. They had visited the emergency department several days ago because of an "ear infection" in the same ear and were prescribed amoxicillin-clavulanate. However, they reluctantly admit that they did not fill the prescription because they have no insurance and could not afford the medication. The child has had one previous ear infection 6 months ago. He has no other medical history and no drug allergies. On examination, the patient is lethargic and febrile with a temperature of 40.0 C (104 F). Otoscopic examination reveals a red, immobile, bulging tympanic membrane on the right side. Examination of the neck reveals nuchal rigidity. The child is unable to extend the leg when the thigh is fully flexed. Ophthalmologic examination is difficult as the child complains of pain due to the light, but there is no papilledema. The most important next step in the management of this child is to

(A) call Child Protective Services to report child neglect and perform a lumbar puncture to obtain CSF for culture and Gram stain
(B) call social work to obtain emergency insurance for the child so that he can get prescription medications
(C) perform a lumbar puncture to obtain CSF for culture and Gram stain
(D) start intravenous antibiotics immediately
(E) send the child for a CT scan prior to performing lumbar puncture

37. A 1-day-old boy is in the intensive care nursery with renal and respiratory failure. On prenatal ultrasound, he has severe hydroureteronephrosis and a large bladder. Late in the prenatal course, oligohydramnios developed, prompting a premature delivery. He is placed on mechanical ventilation and on 100% oxygen; he has an oxygen saturation of 82%. On physical examination, there is a palpable mass in the lower abdomen, presumed to be the bladder seen on prior ultrasound examination. Laboratory studies show a creatinine of 2.4 mg/dL and blood urea nitrogen of 42 mg/dL. A portable ultrasound confirms the prenatal scan, and a diagnosis of posterior urethral valves is postulated. Despite placing a suprapubic catheter, on day 5 of life, the patient continues to require 100% oxygen with jet ventilation and is requiring 3 high-level vasopressors to maintain a systolic blood pressure of 82 mm Hg. There is no sign of brain activity. You approach the parents to suggest withdrawal of care. The parents are vehemently opposed. The most appropriate action is to

(A) discuss why you think it is the appropriate decision and tell the parents that you ultimately have the final say, but you are willing to listen to their ideas
(B) discuss why you think it is the appropriate decision; however, tell the parents that it should be an open conversation and you are willing to listen to their ideas
(C) have one of the parents' family members convince them that they must withdraw care
(D) tell the parents that this situation is medically futile and that they are prolonging their own suffering and wasting money at this point
(E) withdraw life support despite the parents' wishes

38. A 5-year-old previously healthy child is brought to the emergency department by her mother after ingesting some unknown pills at her baby-sitter's house. She received a phone call from the baby-sitter today to pick the child up because "she wasn't acting like herself." When the mother got to the baby-sitter's home, the baby-sitter explained that she found some pills scattered on the floor of the room where the child had been playing; she did not know what kind of pills they were. At this time, the mother noted that her child appeared flushed and felt very warm. She was also complaining that she was very thirsty. Her temperature is 39.0 C (102.2 F), pulse is 138/min, and respirations are 24/min. She appears slightly drowsy. She knows her name, but does not know where she is or what day it is. Her skin is warm, dry, and flushed and you note mydriasis on her ophthalmologic examination. The pills that she most likely ingested are

(A) anticholinergics
(B) cholinergics
(C) narcotics
(D) salicylates
(E) sympathomimetics

39. You are asked to see a 14-year-old boy for short stature. He is not complaining of any other symptoms, though the fact that he is so much shorter than the rest of his classmates is distressing to him. He has never been hospitalized before and has had no major surgeries. On examination, he is 150 cm tall (<5 percentile) and his weight is 40 kg (5th percentile). His parents are of normal height, with his mother standing 163 cm and his father standing 176 cm. His father recalls finishing his growth after starting college. Previous height measurements from well-child visits show a normal height velocity of 8 cm/year. Examination of his fundi are normal and there are no deficiencies in his visual fields. He has Tanner stage II pubic hair and there is no axillary hair present. His testicles are 5 cc bilaterally. The most appropriate next step in the management is to

(A) begin monthly testosterone injections to increase growth velocity
(B) get an MRI of the head to exclude a pituitary tumor
(C) measure inducible growth hormone secretion
(D) measure morning serum cortisol levels
(E) obtain a PA hand/wrist x-ray

40. You are seeing a 6-week-old girl in the emergency department because of emesis for 1 day. She has had no fever or diarrhea. She has vomited five times over the last day; the last episode was bilious. Her birth history is notable for being born by cesarean section at 38 weeks. She left the hospital after 3 days with her mother. She was slightly jaundiced in her first few days, but this resolved without therapy. No one else in the household is sick, and she lives at home with her mother, father, and a well 4-year-old brother. On examination, she is fussy and poorly interactive. Her temperature is 37.3 C (99.2 F), blood pressure is 90/30 mm Hg, pulse is 170/min, and respirations are 65/min. Her skin is somewhat cool and pale, with a capillary refill time of 4 seconds. Her heart sounds are normal, but her abdomen is somewhat full. Her liver and spleen cannot be felt. There are no evident hernias. The most appropriate next step in the management is to

(A) admit her for intravenous rehydration and evaluation for bacterial gastroenteritis
(B) begin fluid resuscitation, and prepare her for an emergent laparotomy
(C) begin oral rehydration and give her a close followup
(D) order an abdominal CT without contrast
(E) order an abdominal ultrasound

41. You are asked to see a 7-year-old boy in the office because of multiple bruises. The parents are not aware of any unusual trauma, though he is active and is often running into things. The bruises are mostly over his arms and legs. There are no bruises on his back, abdomen, or buttocks. He has not had any nosebleeds or gum bleeding. He has not had any fevers or sweats and, as far as his parents are aware, he has been growing normally. There is no history of malignancies in his family and he has one healthy 3-year-old brother. He is not taking any medications or vitamin or herbal supplements. He had a cold about 3 weeks ago, but has never been hospitalized before. On examination, he is 10th percentile for height and weight. He has several ecchymoses over his arms and legs ranging from about 1 cm in diameter to 7 to 8 cm. There are a few scattered petechiae over his chest and abdomen. His cardiac and lung examinations are normal. His abdomen is soft and the spleen cannot be felt. His neurologic examination is normal. Preliminary laboratory studies show:

Leukocyte count	$10.5 \times 10^3/mm^3$
Hemoglobin	12.0 g/dL
Hematocrit	36%
Platelets	$3 \times 10^3/mm^3$
Neutrophils	53%
Lymphocytes	24%
Monocytes	14%
Eosinophils	8%
Basophils	1%
Morphology	normal erythrocytes, extremely rare large platelets, normal lymphocyte morphology

The most appropriate next step in the management is to

(A) admit him for bone marrow biopsy
(B) give him 2 gm/kg of intravenous immune globulin and recheck the platelet count
(C) obtain an MRI of the head
(D) transfuse 2 units of platelets and recheck the platelet count

42. You are examining a well newborn baby in the nursery. He was born 12 hours ago to a 28-year-old white mother who had excellent prenatal care. He was born at term, though delivery was complicated by a breech presentation. As a result, he was delivered by cesarean section. The delivery was otherwise uncomplicated. He required only warming, drying, and suction after delivery, and his Apgar scores were 9 at 1 minute and 9 at 5 minutes. There is no significant family history. The mother is a freelance writer and the father is not involved. The mother feels her financial situation is adequate to care for the child, and her parents live nearby and are excited about and supportive of their new grandchild. On examination of the infant you find a vigorous, crying baby, weight 3828 g. He is pink and well perfused and his overall tone is normal. He has a red reflex present bilaterally, his lung and heart sounds are normal, and his abdominal examination is normal. While performing the Barlow maneuver, a palpable clunk is felt in the left hip. Ortolani maneuver is also positive. The feet are normally formed and there is no evidence of spinal dysraphism. The most important next step in management is to

    (A) follow the hip examination weekly and if still positive at 4 months place the child in a Pavlik harness
    (B) obtain a screening ultrasound of the hip
    (C) obtain x-rays, AP and frog leg views, of the hips
    (D) place the child in a Pavlik harness and arrange for prompt orthopedic evaluation
    (E) recheck the hip examination at the 2-week visit

43. A previously healthy 3-year-old boy is brought to the emergency department by his parents after swallowing a disk battery 1 hour ago. He coughed for about the first 10 minutes after ingestion, but has been behaving like his normal self since then. His vital signs are stable and physical examination is unremarkable. A chest x-ray shows the battery in the distal 1/3 of the esophagus. The most appropriate next step in management is to

    (A) admit the child to the hospital overnight for observation
    (B) discharge the patient home to followup with his pediatrician in 1 week
    (C) discharge the patient home to followup with a gastroenterologist in the morning
    (D) prepare the child for emergent removal of the battery by esophagoscopy
    (E) schedule the child for a followup chest x-ray in 24 hours

44. You are assigned to a 3-year-old girl with terminal leukemia on the pediatric oncology floor. She is very pleasant and inquisitive by nature. One day while seeing her alone she tells you that she is very afraid and is wondering what will happen to her. You should

    (A) explain that you can only discuss this with her parents present
    (B) reassure her that as long as she remains well behaved nothing bad will happen to her
    (C) reassure her that she will have people taking care of her in case she does not feel well
    (D) tell her that she is going to die soon because of her illness
    (E) tell her that you will discuss the matter later with the hope that she will forget that she asked this question

45. You are making rounds in the well-baby nursery one morning and you go to examine a baby born 6 hours ago to a 38-year-old mother. There were no complications prenatally or at the time of delivery, and the baby's mother did not have an amniocentesis for religious reasons. The nurse mentions to you that the baby has seemed "floppy" since arrival to the nursery and has not been feeding well. She has had her first void and her first stool. On your examination, you observe a hypotonic baby with a flat face, epicanthal folds, upslanting palpebral fissures, a downturned mouth, and a protruding tongue. Her anterior fontanelle is enlarged. Her right hand has a single palmar crease and she has shortened fifth fingers. Cardiac auscultation reveals a 3/6 nonradiating, holosystolic murmur at the left lower sternal border. Her peripheral pulses are strong and she is acyanotic. You are most concerned that this newborn most likely has

    (A) Beckwith-Wiedemann syndrome
    (B) hypothyroidism
    (C) trisomy 13
    (D) trisomy 18
    (E) trisomy 21

46. A mother brings her 2-week-old infant to the office for her initial well-child visit. The baby was born full-term via normal spontaneous vaginal delivery and her birth weight was 2.5 kg (5th percentile). Further history from the mother reveals that she did not receive prenatal care until her third trimester; her reason for this was that she has three other kids so she "knew what to do." She is formula feeding the infant appropriately. The baby's weight today is 2.6 kg (5th percentile) and her head circumference is 34 cm (10th percentile). On examination you note a small baby with a thin vermilion border and a flat philtrum. The rest of the examination is unremarkable. On the basis of your findings, you should further question the mother about her

(A) intake of folic acid during pregnancy
(B) seizure history
(C) use of alcohol during pregnancy
(D) use of cocaine during pregnancy
(E) use of isotretinoin during pregnancy

47. A 2-year-old girl is brought to the emergency department by her mother because she has been vomiting for the past 2 hours and is "not acting like herself." She has otherwise been healthy. Her mother denies trauma, but she did state that the child was alone, playing near the bathroom for about 5 minutes earlier today while she answered the phone. Her temperature is 39.0 C (102.2 F) and respirations are 38/min. She is a lethargic-appearing toddler who is diaphoretic and in mild respiratory distress. Besides a minty smell on her breath, her examination is otherwise within normal limits. You suspect a toxic ingestion of

(A) acetaminophen
(B) ethylene glycol
(C) iron
(D) methanol
(E) salicylate

48. A mother brings her 22-month-old son to the office because of an 8-day history of "extremely high fevers." She has also noted for the past 2 days that he looks like he has "pink eye" and his hands have been "big and puffy." His temperature is 40.1 C (104.2 F) and pulse is 116/min. Physical examination shows bilateral conjunctivitis without discharge, edema of the hands with periungual desquamation, a strawberry tongue, and cervical lymphadenopathy, with the largest lymph node measuring approximately 1.9 cm. Laboratory studies will most likely show

(A) hematuria
(B) neutropenia
(C) a positive antinuclear antibody
(D) a positive rheumatoid factor
(E) thrombocytosis

49. A previously healthy 22-month-old boy is brought to the clinic because he has been coughing for the past 4 days. There is no associated fever or rhinorrhea. He is developmentally appropriate and "very inquisitive." His vital signs are normal. On examination, you note a well-nourished boy in no acute distress. Auscultation of his chest reveals wheezing on the right, but good breath sounds on the left. There are no retractions. The rest of the examination is within normal limits. Anteroposterior and lateral chest films appear normal; a right lateral decubitus film shows hyperinflation on the right side. The most likely diagnosis is

(A) cough-variant asthma
(B) croup
(C) epiglottis
(D) foreign body aspiration
(E) vascular web

50. A 4-month-old baby girl is brought to the emergency department because her mother feels that she is having "difficulty breathing." The baby has had a runny nose and mild cough for the past 2 days, and everyone at home has a cold. Her temperature is 37.0 C (98.6 F), respirations are 64/minute, and oxygen saturation is 91% on room air. On examination, you note a well-developed baby girl in moderate respiratory distress with nasal flaring and subcostal retractions. Auscultation of the lungs reveals scattered wheezing bilaterally. The remainder of the examination is within normal limits. A nasopharyngeal washing is sent to pathology and the enzyme immunoassay reveals respiratory syncytial virus. The most appropriate treatment at this time is

(A) albuterol nebulizers
(B) ampicillin
(C) dexamethasone
(D) normal saline nebulizers
(E) ribavirin

Pediatrics Test Three: **Answers and Explanations**

ANSWER KEY

1. B
2. E
3. B
4. A
5. A
6. D
7. E
8. E
9. D
10. B
11. D
12. D
13. B
14. E
15. E
16. E
17. B
18. D
19. D
20. A
21. D
22. E
23. C
24. D
25. B
26. C
27. E
28. C
29. C
30. A
31. B
32. B
33. A
34. E
35. D
36. D
37. B
38. A
39. E
40. B
41. B
42. D
43. D
44. C
45. E
46. C
47. E
48. E
49. D
50. A

1. **The correct answer is B.** Recurrent otitis media is defined by the occurrence of at least three episodes of otitis media within a 6-month period. This is just one indication for placement of myringotomy tubes. A common misconception is that ear tubes should prevent otitis media. While they may reduce the frequency (studies show that they can reduce the frequency by 50%), they appear to reduce the severity of infections and make them easier to treat. The best treatment of otitis media is delivery of antibiotics to the area of infection in the simplest manner. One of the benefits of myringotomy tubes is that topical eardrops delivered through the ear canal can reach the site of infection. It allows these infections to be cleared without repeated use of oral or intravenous (almost never indicated for otitis media) antibiotics.

   Myringotomy tubes allow infected material to exit the middle ear and drain through the ear canal. Therefore, the tubes appear to be working well, and reevaluation (**choice A**) is not necessary unless the patient has an infection that does not respond to antibiotic drops and (if unsuccessful) the addition of oral antibiotics.

   Intravenous antibiotics (**choice C**) are almost never indicated for uncomplicated otitis media.

   The simplest, most direct delivery of antibiotics to the site of infection is eardrops. Therefore, oral antibiotics (**choice D**) are not indicated unless the infection does not respond to antibiotic eardrops.

2. **The correct answer is E.** This baby is suffering from hypertrophic pyloric stenosis. This syndrome is four times more common in male infants than females. It is also more common in first-born sons and in mothers who may have had the disease as a child. Typical presentation is at about 1 month of age with increasing vomiting that ultimately progresses to projectile vomiting. Vomitus is nonbilious because the obstruction is proximal to the ampulla of Vater. The emesis leads to dehydration and electrolyte imbalances, specifically a hypochloremic contraction alkalosis. This is the result of the kidneys attempting to retain sodium and water at the expense of hydrogen and potassium. The treatment for this condition is a pyloromyotomy. This is the surgical release of the hypertrophic pylorus muscle. The procedure is well tolerated and patients resume feedings relatively soon after surgery.

   It would be inappropriate to send home a baby (**choice A**) who is clearly dehydrated and unable to tolerate oral feedings.

   This condition is not related to cancer (**choice B**), and therefore the parents should not be informed that it is.

   Admitting this child strictly for observation (**choice C**) will delay the necessary surgical intervention. At the minimum, the child should be brought in for hydration and surgical evaluation.

   There is no medical treatment for this condition (**choice D**).

3. **The correct answer is B.** This patient most likely has a rotavirus infection, which is one of the most common causes of infectious diarrhea in infants and young children. The infection has a fecal-oral mode of transmission, which makes it a serious problem in day care centers. The infection can be spread before and after individuals become sick with diarrhea. According to the Committee of Infectious Disease of the American Academy of Pediatrics in the year 2000, a child with a rotavirus infection in whom stool cannot be contained by diapers or toilet use should be excluded from childcare centers until diarrhea ceases. This child's stool is contained within the diaper so she can attend day care.

   Antibiotics (**choice A**) are not given to children with a rotavirus infection because it is a viral infection.

   Boiling all drinking water (**choice C**) is not helpful because the rotavirus is shed in the stool of infected individuals and is easily spread on contaminated hands and objects.

   The current recommendation to prevent the spread of rotavirus is careful handwashing (**choice D**). A 70% ethanol solution is also recommended to inactivate the rotavirus.

   A recommended, approved vaccine is not currently available in the United States (**choice E**). A vaccine is available, but it has been associated with intussusception, and it is therefore recommended that administration be suspended until further studies are done.

   Meticulous laundering of the bedding and clothing (**choice F**) is used to prevent reinfestation in a scabies or lice infestation and is not the recommended method of prevention of a rotavirus infection.

   Saying that the patient must be kept home from day care until the diarrhea completely ceases (**choice G**) is incorrect because according to the Infectious Disease Committee of the American Academy of Pediatrics she can attend day care if the stool can be contained by diapers or toilet use.

4. **The correct answer is A.** In evaluating a child for constipation, a detailed history is often very helpful in establishing the underlying cause of the condition. School bathroom avoidance is not all that uncommon and should definitely be asked about, especially in this type of child who is a "neat freak." If he tells you that he does not use the school bathroom, you should find out the reason. He now has fecal impaction, which can be determined by finding a hard mass in the lower abdomen and a dilated rectum filled with a large amount of hard stool. This often occurs because of fecal stasis in the colon leading to an increased absorption of fluids, which in turn leads to the accumulation of large, hard stools that are painful to pass. This pain often leads to avoidance of defecation, even if the child is at home. The treatment includes disimpaction by oral or rectal medications and dietary and behavior modification.

   A consult with a pediatric gastroenterologist (**choice B**) is usually only necessary after the child fails therapy, when an organic disease is suspected, or when there is complex management. A detailed history needs to be obtained to determine if this case is a straightforward case of impaction caused by fecal withholding. After this is done, it can be determined if a consult is necessary.

   An x-ray of the abdomen (**choice C**) is not necessary to establish the diagnosis of fecal impaction if the physical examination reveals a hard mass in the lower abdomen and a dilated rectum filled with a large amount of hard brown stool. It may be necessary if the child refuses a rectal examination.

   After a thorough history, physical examination, and disimpaction, you should recommend a balanced diet containing whole grains, fruits, and vegetables (**choice D**) and behavior modification to promote healthy bowel habits.

   Anal manometry (**choice E**) is used in the evaluation of Hirschsprung disease, which is a cause of constipation in infants and rarely in school-age children. It is caused by a lack of colonic ganglion cells. Physical examination usually reveals a distended abdomen, a contracted anal sphincter, and a rectum devoid of stool. A thorough history needs to be obtained before this diagnosis is considered and diagnostic studies are ordered. The physical examination of the child in this case is inconsistent with Hirschsprung disease.

5. **The correct answer is A.** This patient has the classic presentation of a talocalcaneal (TC) coalition. A coalition is a connection or bar between two bones. The incidence is approximately 5%, and calcaneonavicular (CN) and talocalcaneal coalitions are the most common types. During childhood the bar is unossified, flexible, and typically asymptomatic. During adolescence the coalition goes on to ossify, become rigid, limit subtalar motion, and cause heel pain. Often misdiagnosed as recurrent ankle sprains, patients may experience months to years of pain before proper diagnosis. Clinically the presence of a bump distal to the medial malleolus, and limited subtalar motion demonstrated by limited eversion and inversion are typical of TC coalition. An oblique foot x-ray will reveal a CN coalition. TC coalitions are difficult to appreciate on x-ray, and a CT scan is often necessary. (One way to remember which study to order for a TC coalition is to reverse the letters TC to obtain "CT" for CT scan.) Treatment in symptomatic patients involves bar resection and interposition of a substance to inhibit regrowth of the bony bar. Subcutaneous fat from the foot is a common interposition material. Differential diagnosis includes arthritis and tumor, such as an osteoid osteoma.

   MRI (**choice B**) is best for soft tissue such as tendons, ligaments, nerves, etc. A CT scan is the best diagnostic modality for TC coalitions.

   Activity modification will likely decrease his symptoms, but this patient wants to be physically active. Medical management (**choice C**) targeted at an unstable ankle will not improve this patient's symptoms.

   TC coalitions are best seen on CT scans. Repeat x-rays (**choice D**) will not be informative. Stress views are also not helpful in diagnosing coalitions.

   The stress fracture (**choice E**) in the same leg is an insignificant part of the history and physical examination of this patient.

6. **The correct answer is D.** This patient has the classic findings of parvovirus B-19 infection (fifth disease). Infection during pregnancy increases the risk of fetal loss or hydrops fetalis. Pregnant women should be evaluated to determine if they are susceptible to infection when they are exposed to others with acute infection. It may be necessary to do antibody titers to establish the risk of infection.

   There is no indication for antibiotic treatment (**choice A**) in parvovirus infections. The patient should be treated for symptomatic relief of fever with antipyretics.

Admission to the hospital (**choice B**) is not necessary in this patient, as he has no signs of serious illness or complication of this infection. Complications of this infection do include chronic bone marrow failure in patients with persistent infections. This may occur in immunocompromised patients.

The patient is only "contagious" in the prodromal stage of illness. Now that the rash is apparent, there is no further risk of transmission and he can safely return to school and day care. Therefore, telling him that he cannot return to school or day care until the rash resolves (**choice C**) is incorrect.

This rash is not typical of the rash seen in allergic reactions (**choice E**). There is also no history to suggest exposure to a new allergen. Also, severe pruritus usually is associated with allergic reactions.

7. **The correct answer is E.** This patient has nephrotic syndrome. Given the patient's age and clinical presentation, the most likely cause is minimal change disease (MCD). MCD is characterized by the abrupt onset of edema, proteinuria, benign urinary sediment, normal renal function, and normotension. It is the most common cause of nephrotic syndrome in children. Diagnosis is confirmed by a therapeutic trial of steroids. If steroid treatment fails, diagnosis is made by a renal biopsy (**choice C**). Patients with MCD who don't respond to steroids or those who have frequent relapses should be given cyclophosphamide (**choice D**) to induce prolonged remissions.

   Poststreptococcal glomerulonephritis occurs after an infection with group A beta hemolytic streptococci and usually presents with hematuria, proteinuria, edema, hypertension, and renal insufficiency. Antistreptolysin O (**choice A**) indicates a prior streptococcal infection.

   Although diabetes mellitus (**choice B**) is the major cause of nephrotic syndrome in adults, it rarely causes nephrotic syndrome in children.

8. **The correct answer is E.** This child has multiple café au lait spots. A cafe au lait spot is a uniformly pigmented light to dark brown macule, unevenly round or oval, up to 15 cm in diameter, most often present at birth and almost always present by the age of one. In the U.S., solitary café au lait spots are present at birth in 0.3% of Caucasians, 3% of Hispanic, and in 18% of African American babies. In childhood, solitary café au lait spots occur in 13% of Caucasians and 27% of African Americans, whereas multiple occur in 8% of African Americans. The finding of six or more of these lesions at least 1.5 cm in diameter (0.5 cm in prepubertal children) is diagnostic of neurofibromatosis, usually type I, and these children may also have pseudarthroses, congenital glaucoma, and sphenoid wing dysplasia present at birth.

   Since this child does not satisfy the criteria for the diagnosis of neurofibromatosis, an extensive laboratory and imaging workup (**choice A**) is not indicated. For patients with diagnosed neurofibromatosis, annual clinical examinations and a problem-focused approach are the recommended monitoring guidelines at this time.

   Café au lait macules may be observed at birth, though typically they are very light at this age and may be difficult to appreciate. The skin lesions continue to develop in early infancy. They may enlarge in size and become obvious after age 2 years. Thus, it is not peculiar that her son is developing new lesions (**choice B**) and a biopsy is not warranted.

   Café au lait spots are caused by an increase in melanin content with the presence of giant melanosomes. Melanocytes are not increased in number and malignant transformation does not occur, so surgical excision of these lesions (**choice C**) should not be performed.

   Even though neurofibromatosis is an autosomal dominant disorder, about 50% of individuals with neurofibromatosis type I have a spontaneous mutation. The high incidence of new mutations is thought to result from the large size of the gene, which increases the likelihood of spontaneous mutations. When inherited, it can be very heterogenous, with members in the same family showing differing degrees of severity. Therefore, it would be incorrect to say that the boy doesn't have neurofibromatosis, because there is no family history (**choice D**).

9. **The correct answer is D.** This girl has guttate psoriasis, a form of psoriasis that is most commonly seen in children and young adults 1 to 2 weeks after an acute streptococcal pharyngitis. Typical lesions are the size of water drops (guttate), 2 to 5 mm in diameter. They are usually responsive to topical steroids or ultraviolet B therapy, but tend to recur due to pharyngeal carriage of the responsible streptococcus. The rapid strep test and antistreptolysin O (ASO) titer would be the tests of choice to determine the cause of this acute episode. Treatment with a penicillin or cephalosporin antibiotic is indicated, and eradication of the streptococcus will aid in the resolution of the guttate psoriasis as well. Psoriasis may be inherited in a multifactorial manner and with variable expression. The child's father most probably has chronic stable plaque psoriasis based on

the above description and the fact that the child has coarse pitting of the nails indicates a psoriatic diathesis she has inherited from him.

Diascopy (**choice A**) is a diagnostic tool that is frequently utilized to determine whether skin lesions that are red in color are cause by vasodilatation or extravasation of red blood cells. A clear plastic or glass slide is pressed over the skin lesion. If the red color disappears (the lesion blanches) it is caused by vasodilatation (pressure on blood vessels will cause collapse of dilated blood vessels and disappearance of the red color). If the lesion persists under diascopy it has been caused by extravasation of red blood cells that cannot be removed from the tissue by applying transient pressure. The most common application of this method is to differentiate lesions caused by vasculitis in the skin, where extravasation of erythrocytes via damaged blood vessels occurs.

A KOH test (**choice B**) is performed when fungal infection of the skin is suspected. Microscopic examination of skin scrapings treated with potassium hydroxide will reveal presence of fungal elements in skin lesions caused by dermatophytes. The clinical presentation of this child does not warrant a KOH test because fungal infection of the skin (ringworm) in immunocompetent individuals does not present as a diffuse, red, scaly, papular eruption.

A monospot test (**choice C**) is utilized to diagnose Epstein-Barr virus infection when infectious mononucleosis is suspected. This child's upper respiratory symptoms are very mild and do not support a diagnosis of infectious mononucleosis.

A Wood light examination (**choice E**) is performed to diagnose certain infections of the skin caused by yeast (*Pityrosporum ovale* will fluoresce yellow), bacteria (*Corynebacterium minutissimum* will fluoresce red), or dermatophytes (*Microsporum canis* will fluoresce green). It can also be used to determine localization of abnormal pigment in the skin: epidermal pigment will be accentuated by it, while dermal pigment will not.

10. **The correct answer is B.** This is the typical clinical picture of exanthema subitum (roseola infantum) caused by human herpes virus type 6. Roseola infantum is a common cause of sudden, unexplained high fever in children between 6 and 36 months of age. Prodromal fever is usually high; convulsions and lymphadenopathy may accompany it. Suddenly, on about the fourth day, the fever drops, and a morbilliform erythema consisting of rose-colored discrete macules appears on the neck, trunk, and buttocks, and sometimes on the face and extremities. The mucous membranes are spared. Complete resolution occurs in 1 to 2 days. Infection with human herpes virus type 6 is almost universal in adults, with seropositivity in the 80 to 85% range in the United States and seroprevalence almost 100% in children. Primary infection with human herpes virus type 6 is associated with roseola only 9% of the time. Other common findings include otitis media, diarrhea, and bulging fontanelles, sometimes with findings of meningo-encephalitis.

Herpes simplex type 1 (**choice A**) is the cause of orolabial herpes simplex ("cold sore"). Although initial infection is usually asymptomatic, a vesicular gingivostomatitis may develop in up to 1%, chiefly in children and young adults.

Human herpes virus type 8 (**choice C**) has been detected in virtually all patients with Kaposi sarcoma, including those with AIDS. It has also been associated with body cavity-based B-cell lymphoma and Castleman disease.

Human papillomavirus type 6 (**choice D**) is the cause of anogenital warts. Albeit infrequently, it can cause laryngeal papillomatosis in children born vaginally to mothers who have either viral shedding or overt genital warts at the time of delivery.

Parvovirus B-19 (**choice E**) causes erythema infectiosum (fifth disease), a worldwide benign infectious exanthem that occurs in epidemics in the winter and early spring. Erythema infectiosum has three phases. It begins abruptly with an asymptomatic erythema of the cheeks, giving the child a "slapped cheek" appearance. One to four days later discrete erythematous macules and papules appear on the proximal extremities, and then on the trunk. This evolves into a reticulated or lacy pattern. A characteristic third phase is the recurring stage. The eruption is markedly reduced or resolved, only to reappear when the patient is exposed to heat or sunlight, or in response to crying or exercise.

11. **The correct answer is D.** This young girl has scarlet fever. Prompt antibiotic treatment is critical and penicillin for 10 days is currently recommended as first-line therapy. Penicillin treatment failures are common if the patient was recently treated with the drug, in which case cephalosporins or azithromycin should be administered. Pyrogenic exotoxins produced by beta-hemolytic streptococcus group A are responsible for most cases of scarlet fever. Fever and sore throat precede the skin eruption by several days. The rash begins on the face and neck and spreads downward, sparing palms, soles, and the perioral area (circumoral pallor). Tiny scaly

papules appear on the trunk, giving the skin the texture of sandpaper. Fine desquamation occurs from the face and neck down. The palms and soles may desquamate in a "gloves and socks" fashion. The erythema is accentuated in skin folds, where petechiae may also occur. The most characteristic mucosal lesion is the strawberry tongue: protruding, enlarged, erythematous papillae and a thick white coating. The diagnosis may be made clinically and is supported by throat cultures and a rising antistreptolysin O titer. The primary objective of treatment is prevention of rheumatic fever, although it also accelerates clinical improvement. Treatment does not influence the incidence of post-streptococcal glomerulonephritis, and a followup urinalysis several months after the acute illness has resolved should be done to search for microscopic hematuria.

Acyclovir (**choice A**) is an antiviral drug used in the treatment of herpes simplex and varicella zoster virus infections, usually orally.

Intravenous penicillin for 4 weeks (**choice B**) would be overkill in treating an acute, uncomplicated streptococcal infection in a child who is otherwise in good health.

Oral ciprofloxacin for 10 days (**choice C**) is not the recommended treatment of choice for infection caused by beta-hemolytic streptococcus group A. It is also a very expensive drug that is useful in the treatment of some rare and resistant bacteria, so it would not be prudent to use it to treat a strep throat with scarlet fever.

Topical steroids (**choice E**) are not indicated in the treatment of the rash of scarlet fever because an exfoliating toxin and not an inflammatory reaction causes it.

12. **The correct answer is D.** This patient likely has dietary calcium insufficiency (one type of rickets). Tibial bowing is a common deformity in these patients which can lead to permanent deformity and impairment if not correctly diagnosed and treated. Of all of these choices, an orthopedic surgery consult and long-leg weight-bearing radiographs is the most appropriate management.

Although some children have a moderate degree of physiologic genu varum, this patient has the dietary history and physical findings concerning for dietary rickets. Thus, if his calcium deficiency and deformities are not addressed, serious long-term complications will result and it is unlikely that he will grow out of it (**choice A**).

This patient does need a dietary evaluation and some form of calcium introduced into his diet but neither will resolve his already pronounced genu varum (**choice B**), and thus a consult is required.

It is unlikely that this patient's serum calcium is dangerously low, and emergency blood draws and IV calcium are seldom, if ever, required in chronic dietary calcium deficiency (**choice C**).

There is no reason to suspect physical abuse (**choice E**) in this case, but the question of neglect may be valid due to this child's diet; however, the patient's mother is concerned about his diet and is turning to you for suggestions.

13. **The correct answer is B.** Although this patient has the classic history and examination for a radial head dislocation and some physicians would simply perform a gentle reduction maneuver, it is often best to document that no other fractures (supracondylar humerus or physeal separation) have occurred. A "nursemaid elbow" occurs when the radial head is pulled out of it's normal position because of a torn or stretched annular ligament. These are generally easy to reduce and the child will often start using their elbow immediately after the reduction. Missing a radial head dislocation can lead to a chronic dislocation of the radial head with significant loss of motion about the elbow as well as loss of supination/pronation of the forearm.

The child clearly does not have a simple bruise and no mention of such a finding on examination was noted. A child who is not using an extremity needs a complete work up to find the source of the problem and should not simply be sent home (**choice A**).

Shoulder dislocations (**choice C**) are rare in this age group, this boy will let you move his shoulder, and you noticed no gross abnormalities about the appearance of the shoulder.

Although you must always be concerned about abuse (**choice D**), a radial head dislocation is common and does not have to be sustained by violent trauma like femur fractures or rib fractures. There is no indication on examination of abuse (no retinal hemorrhages or other bruises or skin lesions were noted).

If you were completely confident in your diagnosis of a dislocated radial head, then a reduction would be appropriate; however, it is always a good idea to document that no other fractures or dislocations were present by radiographic means. The reduction maneuver for a "nursemaid elbow" is a gentle reduction and should not be performed "forcibly" (**choice E**).

14. **The correct answer is E.** The patient in question has evidence from physical examination to indicate that he has stool that has become impacted in his rectal vault. To prevent further complications, the patient should have the stool disimpacted as soon as possible.

There is no indication for a sleep study (**choice A**) in the evaluation of primary or secondary encopresis.

The patient does not give clinical signs indicating that he is depressed. Therefore, an antidepressant (**choice B**) is not indicated.

The patient manifests no signs of psychotic illness. There would be no benefit in this patient of having treatment with an antipsychotic (**choice C**).

The patient performs well in school in spite of having an elimination disorder. There is no indication to remove him from his regular education placement to special education (**choice D**) solely on the basis of having an elimination disorder.

15. **The correct answer is E.** Pediatric autoimmune neuropsychiatric disorder associated with streptococcal infection (PANDAS) is associated with the abrupt onset of obsessive-compulsive-disorder-like symptoms and tics in prepubertal children. The abruptness of onset of compulsive behavior and tics in this patient and the presence of a prodromal illness consistent with streptococcal pharyngitis are cues to the diagnosis in this patient. Treatment may involve parenteral antibiotics and immunoglobulin.

The patient's presentation is not consistent with a disseminated fungal infection (**choice A**). The patient appears otherwise healthy and has no history of autoimmune disease or immunocompromise. Regardless, a literature on obsessive-compulsive symptoms and fungemia is not established.

Erythema nodosum (**choice B**) can be associated with other multisystem and autoimmune disorders with psychiatric manifestations. However, obsessive-compulsive symptoms and tics are not associated with erythema nodosum per se.

Influenza A (**choice C**) has not been associated with the development of obsessive-compulsive symptoms in children.

Mononucleosis (**choice D**) most typically presents with psychiatric symptoms that mimic depressive illness, most specifically fatigue and loss of interest. Obsessive-compulsive symptoms are not typically associated with mononucleosis.

16. **The correct answer is E.** This baby has "cradle cap," a type of seborrheic dermatitis that appears in infants in the form of yellow or brown scaling lesions on the scalp with accumulated epithelial debris. The supraorbital region as well as the eyelids may be erythematous and with flaky yellow scale. It is a very common condition that appears within the first few weeks of life and tends to last only a few weeks to months. Parents are instructed to brush the baby's hair with a soft toothbrush to eliminate the scale and to wash daily with mild baby shampoo. If there is abundant scale and debris adherent to the hair, applying baby oil or an antibiotic ointment for an hour or two before washing the hair helps loosen the accumulations. Scale on the eyelids can be removed with a cotton tip applicator dipped into baby shampoo diluted in water and rinsed with clean water.

Avoidance of washing (**choice A**) would cause further accumulation of scale and debris and worsening of the cradle cap. This may then be complicated by bacterial superinfection, which could lead to other, more serious, complications.

Daily washing only with water (**choice B**) would not be sufficient to eliminate the scale and debris that accumulates on the scalp in cradle cap. Shampoo has surfactants that help loosen scale and separate it from the skin and hair. There are certain skin conditions, such as atopic dermatitis or severe xerosis, where it is suggested that washing be done only with water whenever possible, because soaps and shampoos eliminate the skin's natural lipids and dry it out, predisposing to worsening of the disorder.

Topical betamethasone cream (**choice C**) is a high potency, category I corticosteroid that should not be used in infants because of potentially serious side effects such as atrophy, telangiectasis, steroid acne, glaucoma, cataracts, and potential of systemic absorption due to a very high skin surface-to-volume ratio.

Topical permethrin cream (**choice D**) is used for the treatment of pediculosis and scabies and has no place in the treatment of seborrheic dermatitis/cradle cap.

17. **The correct answer is B.** The nasopharynx of cats and dogs is colonized by a small, gram-negative coccobacillus, *Pasteurella multocida*. Cats have the highest colonization rate, followed by dogs, swine, and rats. *Pasteurella multocida* causes a localized soft tissue infection (cellulitis) after the animal bite. Infection typically manifests 8 to 24 hours after the bite as pain at the site of injury with cellulitis accompanied by purulent, sometimes foul-smelling discharge. Septic arthritis and

osteomyelitis may develop if the canine tooth penetrates synovium or bone. About 25% of the affected patients will also develop lymphangitis. The treatment of choice is penicillin, or doxycycline for penicillin-allergic patients. Surgical debridement is often necessary. Complications include septicemia, pneumonia, meningitis, and deeper pelvic and abdominal infections. Each year in the United States, between 1 and 2 million animal-bite wounds are sustained; the vast majority are inflicted by pet dogs and cats, which number more than 100 million. Dogs are responsible for approximately 80% of bite wounds, an estimated 15-20% of which become infected. A study for the period 1992 through 1994 found that dog bites resulted in more than 900 emergency department visits each day in the United States. Most dog bites are provoked and are inflicted by the victim's pet or by a dog known to the victim. These bites frequently occur during efforts to break up a dogfight. Victims tend to be male, and bites most often involve a lower extremity.

Group A streptococcus (**choice A**), or *Streptococcus pyogenes*, is responsible for streptococcal pharyngitis, one of the most common bacterial infections of school-age children, and for the postinfectious syndromes of acute rheumatic fever and poststreptococcal glomerulonephritis.

Pseudomonas aeruginosa (**choice C**) is widespread in nature, inhabiting soil, water, plants, and animals (including humans). It has a predilection for moist environments. This organism occasionally colonizes the skin, external ear, upper respiratory tract, or large bowel of healthy humans. Rates of carriage are relatively low, however, except among patients who have serious underlying disease, whose host defenses have been naturally or iatrogenically compromised, who have previously received antibiotic therapy, and/or who have been exposed to the hospital environment.

Salmonella typhi (**choice D**) causes inflammatory diarrhea by invasion of the bowel mucosa, but generally is not associated with the destruction of enterocytes or the full clinical syndrome of dysentery. *Salmonella typhi* can penetrate intact intestinal mucosa, multiply intracellularly in Peyer patches and intestinal lymph nodes, and then disseminate through the bloodstream to cause enteric fever, a syndrome characterized by fever, headache, relative bradycardia, abdominal pain, splenomegaly, and leukopenia.

Staphylococcus aureus (**choice E**) causes two types of syndrome: intoxications and infections. The clinical manifestations of intoxications are attributable to the action of one or a few secreted products of the micro-organism (toxins), and these clinical features can be reproduced by administration of the toxin(s) in the absence of the micro-organism. The toxin can be produced either in vivo (as in toxic shock syndrome or staphylococcal scalded skin syndrome) or in a suitable vector that subsequently delivers it to the host (as in staphylococcal food poisoning). Infections, in contrast, involve bacterial proliferation, invasion or destruction of host tissues, and in most cases local and systemic inflammatory responses by the host to these events. Hosts at particular risk for staphylococcal infection include those with frequent or chronic disruptions in epithelial or mucosal integrity; those with disordered leukocyte chemotaxis, such as patients with the Chédiak-Higashi or Wiskott-Aldrich syndrome; those whose phagocytes are defective in oxidative killing, as in chronic granulomatous disease; those with neutropenia or acquired functional deficiencies (e.g., deficiencies induced by exogenous glucocorticoids); and those with indwelling foreign bodies, which provide a matrix for staphylococcal adherence and biofilm formation and seriously impair phagocytic function. Patients with disorders of immunoglobulin or complement (especially C1-C4 deficiencies) are also at increased risk for *Staphylococcus aureus* infection.

18. **The correct answer is D.** This woman had subacute cutaneous lupus erythematosus, a clinically distinct subset of patients with lupus erythematosus that most often affects white women aged 15 to 40. The majority of cases have antibodies to Ro/SSA autoantigen, and a comparable number are HLA-DR3-positive. The disease generally runs a mild course, and renal, central nervous system, and vascular complications are rare. It responds well to antimalarials with short courses of oral steroids and photoprotection. Hydroxychlorothiazide has been reported to induce this type of lupus erythematosus, as well as piroxicam, glyburide, penicillamine, griseofulvin, and spironolactone. Annular, scaling, erythematous macules and papules may appear on the head and extremities of babies born to mothers with lupus erythematosus, rheumatic disease, or other connective tissue disorders. Half of the mothers are asymptomatic at the time of delivery. The children's lesions usually resolve spontaneously by the age of 6 months, and usually heal without scarring. Photosensitivity may be prominent. Seventy five percent of patients with neonatal lupus are female. Although the skin lesions are transient, half of the patients will have an isolated congenital heart block, usually of the third degree, which is permanent. As with other forms of subacute cutaneous lupus erythematosus, there is a strong association with Ro/SSA autoantibodies. Nearly all the mothers, and

therefore, nearly all the babies born to them, are Ro/SSA autoantibody positive. There is also a linkage to HLA-DR3-positivity in the mother.

Lupus panniculitis (**choice A**) is a subtype of chronic cutaneous lupus erythematosus that is usually seen in middle-aged female patients and resolves leaving atrophic, depressed scars on the cheeks, upper arms, and buttocks most commonly. It does not affect infants with neonatal lupus.

Photosensitivity (**choice B**) may be seen in neonatal lupus but it resolves by the age of 6 months, along with any skin lesions that were present. This coincides with elimination of Ro/SSA autoantibodies of maternal origin. Clinically, photosensitivity is manifested with appearance or worsening of the lupus dermatitis after exposure to natural or artificial ultraviolet light.

Scarring alopecia (**choice C**) is encountered in patients who have chronic cutaneous lupus erythematosus of the scalp; the inflammatory process destroys appendages and leaves a permanent scar in affected areas. Subacute cutaneous lupus erythematous is clinically characterized by erythematous papules and plaques that resolve without scarring.

Ulcerations of the hard palate (**choice E**) are one of the 11 criteria set forth by the American Rheumatological Association for the diagnosis of systemic lupus erythematosus. They are extremely uncommon in patients with neonatal lupus, and are not permanent (ulcerations heal over time and with appropriate treatment without sequelae).

19. **The correct answer is D.** These two children most likely have molluscum contagiosum, an infection caused by Molluscipoxvirus, a virus of the poxvirus family. Typical lesions are small, firm, umbilicated papules with a shiny, waxy, or pearly surface and central umbilication. The base may or may not be erythematous or eczematous ("molluscum dermatitis"). An average patient has 10-20 lesions 1 to 10 mm in size. Individual lesions last 2 months or more before they spontaneously resolve, and the average case clears in 2 years or less. It affects only humans, and skin-to-skin transmission and contact with fomites are the method of spread. It is most commonly seen in children. Autoinoculation frequently happens, especially when the lesions are pruritic and the child scratches them. Sites of predilection are the axillae, antecubital and popliteal fossae, and the crural folds, but lesions may appear anywhere on the skin. In adults, molluscum contagiosum is often acquired as a sexually transmitted disease, and the lesions appear in the genital and perigenital area. Atopic dermatitis (childhood eczema) and compromise of skin integrity can increase the risk of infection. A widespread eruption, especially on the face, is seen in immunocompromised patients, particularly those with AIDS. These are very resistant to treatment. The diagnosis of molluscum contagiosum can be made by histologic demonstration of cytoplasmic eosinophilic inclusions characteristic of poxvirus replication. This virus cannot be propagated in vitro, but electron microscopy and molecular studies can be used for its identification. There is no specific systemic treatment for molluscum contagiosum, but a variety of techniques for physical ablation have been used, such as liquid nitrogen, curettage, cantharidin, podophyllotoxin, tretinoin, silver nitrate, and others. Molluscum contagiosum may respond to effective control of HIV infection with highly active antiretroviral therapy. Cidofovir is also being investigated for potential clinical use against molluscum contagiosum.

Cryptococcus neoformans (**choice A**) causes cryptococcosis, primarily a pulmonary infection that remains localized to the lung in about 90% of the cases. In the remaining 10%, dissemination to other organs occurs, the central nervous system and the skin being the most common secondary sites. The latter is usually seen in debilitated or immunocompromised patients. Skin infection occurs most commonly on the head and neck, with swelling, abscesses, blisters, tumorlike masses, large umbilicated papules and nodules, ulcers, and other nonspecific lesions. Primary inoculation of the skin is extremely rare. For all practical purposes, identification of cryptococci in skin lesions indicates disseminated disease with a poor prognosis and it requires a search for other organ involvement.

Histoplasma capsulatum (**choice B**) causes primary cutaneous histoplasmosis, a rare entity characterized by a chancre-type lesion and regional lymphadenopathy, most frequently located on the penis. In immunocompromised patients it may cause progressive disseminated histoplasmosis with skin lesions, such as umbilicated nodules, papules, and ulcers, present in about 6% of cases.

Human papillomavirus (**choice C**) includes more than 80 types, most of which cause specific types of warts and favor certain anatomic locations, such as plantar warts, common warts, genital warts, and so on.

The orthopoxvirus genus (**choice E**) causes the following infections: vaccinia, cowpox, variola, and monkeypox.

20. **The correct answer is A.** Patients with sickle cell anemia are prone to osteomyelitis with the usual organisms such as *Staphylococcus aureus* but are also at risk for unusual organisms such as *Salmonella*. They require rapid diagnosis and a long course of organism-specific intravenous antibiotics.

The ultrasound examination was negative, although limited. This patient is presenting with signs of leg infection, and not deep vein thrombus (DVT). He may benefit from subcutaneous heparin for prophylaxis of DVT; however, a heparin drip (**choice B**) is not required.

Meperidine and promethazine (**choice D**) constitute appropriate medications for sickle pain crises; however, this patient has signs and symptoms of a potentially severe infection of the lower extremity that require immediate evaluation. Pain medication is important; the case says "mild pain" and therefore the most important step in management of this patient is blood cultures and needle biopsy of the bone, followed by 4 to 6 weeks of organism-specific intravenous antibiotics. Ibuprofen and discharge (**choice C**) is similarly incorrect.

Radionuclide bone scans (**choice E**) help in the diagnostic workup of osteomyelitis, but do not help in discovering the pathogen and organism-specific treatment.

21. **The correct answer is D.** At this point it is easier for both parents and child, who are stressed about the situation, to have the parents present for the examination. It would comfort the child and facilitate the examination. Only after the examination and diagnostic tests are done should one proceed with further steps if there is a concern about abuse.

Calling psychiatry (**choice A**) is appropriate if there is an issue related to the child or parents that needs to be evaluated. A psychiatrist's consultant role should not be one of mediator between the conflicted parties, even though it is possible sometimes. Calling a psychiatrist might upset the parents even more.

Immediately driving to the hospital to see the case personally and discussing it with the parents (**choice B**) may not be necessary unless the parents are so upset with the attitude of resident and staff that they refuse any intervention. It will also only delay the appropriate care.

Immediately reporting child abuse (**choice C**) based only on the refusal of parents to leave the child is not appropriate. It may be seen as a punishment because of their behavior rather than an act of real concern for the child's well being. If there is a reasonable suspicion based on the mental and physical examination of the child, one should proceed with that.

Supporting (**choice E**) the staff will only worsen the situation and implies that the power struggle between parents and child seems more important than the child's well being.

22. **The correct answer is E.** This patient has idiopathic hypertrophic subaortic stenosis (IHSS). Evidence for this is a patient with a nonradiating systolic mummer that increases with intensity as preload is decreased (standing and Valsalva). An S4 can sometimes be heard in younger patients with this condition. A family history of sudden death at a young age should make you suspect the diagnosis. Patients with IHSS may be asymptomatic, but if they have symptoms, treatment with negative inotropic drugs such as verapamil or a beta-blocker is indicated. This will both slow the heart rate, which allows for increased left ventricular filling, and decrease the force of contraction, which decreases flow velocity and therefore decreases the degree of obstruction.

Patients that are asymptomatic do not require treatment with medications. Some of the patients will never develop problems from their disease. Others will become symptomatic later in life. Since this patient is symptomatic, medical management is indicated rather than reassurance (**choice A**). Advice on participation in sports should probably be deferred to a cardiologist.

Pacemaker implantation (**choice B**) may be beneficial in patients with IHSS by altering the sequence of atrial and ventricular contractions and thereby reducing with outflow obstruction. Medical management should be attempted prior to surgical intervention. If patients continue to have symptoms of IHSS after medical management or cannot tolerate medications, more invasive measures such as pacing can be considered.

Myomectomy (**choice C**) is indicated in patients with severe heart failure (class III or IV) who have failed trials of medications. In this surgery, part of the septum is removed surgically to relieve the outflow obstruction. This patient does not have severe heart failure and has not been tried on medications yet, so he is not a surgical candidate.

Digoxin (**choice D**) is contraindicated in the hyperdynamic stages of IHSS since it increases the force of ventricular contraction, thereby increasing the amount of outflow obstruction.

23. **The correct answer is C.** This patient likely has adolescent idiopathic scoliosis. Scoliosis is defined as an abnormal curvature of the spine. Estimates of the prevalence of scoliosis depend on the threshold for

definition. While 1.5 to 3% of the population have curves over 10 degrees, only 0.5% have curves greater than 25%. Regardless of definition, most physicians will encounter a patient who has concerns over a possible curvature of their spine. It is important to document the neurologic status of all patients with scoliosis. In most cases of adolescent scoliosis the neurologic examination will be unremarkable. Some potential known causes of scoliosis include tumors and infection in the spine; often these patients will present with pain or an abnormal neurologic examination.

Until a neurologic examination is performed there is no reason to suspect that this patient has any life-threatening neurologic condition (**choice A**).

An MRI would be useful in only certain cases of scoliosis (if a spinal cord anomaly is suspected, tumor, or infection are suspected). Before an MRI is ordered, one should obtain standing PA radiographs of the spine to document the degree of spinal curvature (**choice B**).

Although bracing may be an option in the treatment of adolescent idiopathic scoliosis, many factors, such as degree of curvature, skeletal maturity, and likelihood of compliance, need to be determined before any brace is made (**choice D**). It should also be noted that bracing usually retards the progression of curvature and does not straighten the spine.

Scoliosis is a diagnosis that carries many different images for patients and their families. Spine surgery is generally considered major surgery, and no indication should be given to the patient and their family that surgery is required until they have had a chance to discuss and understand the diagnosis of scoliosis. Most cases of adolescent scoliosis do not require spinal fusion, only those that have documented progression and curves generally greater than 40 to 50 degrees (**choice E**).

24. **The correct answer is D.** This child has serous otitis media and probably has hearing loss due to the fluid in the middle ears. Serous otitis media is a collection of fluid in the middle ear without obvious infection. Symptoms include hearing loss, and examination reveals a dull, immobile tympanic membrane. The most appropriate next step is to refer the child for a hearing test and possible drainage of the fluid. Serous otitis media results in part due to eustachian tube dysfunction. While it is true that older children have less risk of serous otitis media and acute otitis media, the hearing loss and frequent episodes of acute otitis in this patient need to be addressed. Therefore, reassurance to the parents that the child will grow out of the ear infections in the next few years (**choice C**) is incorrect.

Antibiotic drops (**choice A**) are prescribed for processes involving the external ear canal or in patients with a perforated tympanic membrane. They have no role in the treatment of serous otitis media.

The symptoms of acute otitis include a bulging, red, inflamed tympanic membrane with symptoms of pain and, frequently, a fever. This patient does not have acute otitis media, therefore prescribing oral antibiotics (**choice B**) is incorrect.

A CT scan is not indicated for obvious serous otitis media. The middle ear and mastoid air cells will be filled with fluid, which cannot be distinguished on CT from other soft tissue masses. As there is no suspicion of cholesteatoma or other soft tissue mass in this case, a CT scan (**choice E**) is incorrect.

25. **The correct answer is B.** This is a difficult and common scenario. The differential diagnosis of pediatric syndromes in an initial encounter is large, and not enough information in this history and physical examination can confirm or exclude Lyme disease as a diagnosis. Your response would be the one that is least confrontational and introduces to the mother the need to investigate for other possibilities. The differential would include systemic lupus erythematosus, rheumatic fever, juvenile rheumatoid arthritis, Lyme disease, and leukemia. Laboratory studies would include WBC, platelet count, antinuclear antibody levels, rheumatoid factor, complement levels, and a bone marrow evaluation.

"A Lyme titer will probably be negative because Lyme disease is not the diagnosis" (**choice A**) is confrontational and falsely presumes that Lyme disease is not the diagnosis. It may still be possible in view of the arthralgia, rash, and fevers. The small joints were not affected, which also does not rule out Lyme disease yet.

"The diagnosis is juvenile rheumatoid arthritis and the Lyme titer would probably be negative" (**choice C**) is incorrect at this stage. Juvenile rheumatoid arthritis is a diagnosis of exclusion, and there are no tests that are specific to its diagnosis. In fact, no blood tests are available yet to confirm any diagnosis. In addition, one should never prematurely label a child with a diagnosis of arthritis since it would cause much distress to any parent.

"Your daughter does not fit the correct age group for the diagnosis to be Lyme disease" (**choice D**) and "Your daughter does not fit the correct age group for Lyme disease but we will do a Lyme titer just to be sure" (**choice E**) are incorrect because Lyme disease can occur in people from age 2 to 20 years of age. Since the girl is 7 years old she would still fall into the age category consistent with Lyme disease.

26. **The correct answer is C.** Primary care doctors have an obligation to encourage lifestyle modifications that might delay or prevent the onset of type 2 diabetes in children at high risk. Lifestyle changes focusing on weight management and increasing physical activity should be promoted in all children at high risk. Weight loss programs with the best results have been those combining exercise, diet, and behavioral modification. A dietitian would advise on reducing readily digested starches and saturated fats and encourage diets high in fiber and monounsaturated fatty acids.

Use of low-calorie or high-protein diets (**choice A**) is not recommended and dieting alone may be unsafe and rarely results in long-term weight control. They do not promote long-term healthy eating behavior either.

Participating in school sports is an ideal way to promote exercise (**choice B**) but would be better in combination with healthier eating habits, too. It is not as good an answer as choice C.

Drug therapy to reduce weight (i.e., antiobesity agents) (**choice D**) is not recommended in children and usually would begin at the age of 16 years of age only when exercise and balanced dieting have not worked.

Prevention of type 2 diabetes should be considered at two stages in the condition's natural history. Intervention can take place at an early stage when blood glucose levels are still normal or at the stage of impaired glucose tolerance when glucose levels are elevated but not yet diagnostic of diabetes. Thus, telling the mother that there is no reason to do very much right now since his glucose is normal (**choice E**) is inappropriate and also the least proactive response to give the boy's mother.

27. **The correct answer is E.** This patient has a fracture of the medial third of the clavicle after a bicycle accident. The fracture will heal satisfactorily with remodeling at this age without the need for surgical intervention. This typically takes about 4 to 6 weeks and is aided by the absence of displacement of the proximal and distal components of the fracture. A figure 8 splint or collar splint will provide adequate support and inhibit the child from aggressive activity. Followup with serial x-rays to document remodeling will be appropriate.

The probability of child abuse (**choice A**) is very low. This is because the child was brought in quickly and there is no discrepancy between mother's witnessed account and the physical/x-ray findings. If abuse were suspected one would admit the child for a bone scan to evaluate for old fractures and occult fractures.

There is no evidence in the history or physical examination to suggest a head injury since the child did not lose consciousness (he cried immediately), was able to pick himself up and walk without difficulty, and he was neurologically intact in the emergency department. Admitting him for vital sign observation (**choice B**) would therefore be inappropriate.

Unless there is neurovascular injury or an open fracture, there is no indication for an open reduction and internal fixation of the clavicle in this child (**choice C**). If surgical intervention is required, it would still not be deemed a surgical emergency (**choice D**) to warrant an urgent operating room visit.

28. **The correct answer is C.** The newborn examination is normal and the child has already voided and passed meconium, which is reassuring. He most likely has a caput succedaneum, which is a common form of head trauma seen in newborns after prolonged labor. It is secondary to an accumulation of edema above the periosteum that crosses the suture lines. No treatment is required because the condition typically resolves within days.

Caput succedaneum is a common form of head trauma seen in newborns after prolonged labor and instrumentation. The mother should be reassured about this instead of being faced with an accusatory question such as "Did you leave your child unattended?" (**choice A**).

A CT scan is not needed at this time (**choice B**) since it will not change your conservative management. A skull fracture is unlikely. Where there is a minor possibility of a skull fracture there is usually a fluctuant swelling that does not cross the suture (a cephalhematoma). If this were the case, a plain skull film would be appropriate, which may be repeated in 4 weeks to ensure closure of a linear fracture.

A neurosurgic consult (**choice D**) would be required if a depression fracture is suspected on examination or noted on the plain film; however, at this time it would be inappropriate.

"Is there any history of babies with large heads in your family?" (**choice E**) is inappropriate. It addresses a family history of macrocephaly, which is a familial anomaly with autosomal dominant or recessive inheritance. There is nothing to suggest macrocephaly on physical examination. Macrocephaly is defined as a measurement of the distance around the widest part of the skull that is larger than expected for the age and background of the child.

29. **The correct answer is C.** Current recommendations for the appropriate management of children with acute diarrhea are to give an age-appropriate diet and that breast-fed infants should continue at the breast.

Bananas, Rice, Applesauce, and Toast (**choice A**) was once a popular dietary recommendation for children of this age group (BRAT diet). It has been shown to be ineffective. In addition, there is no evidence that changing the child's diet will reduce the diarrhea.

There is no valid evidence recommending the restriction of the diet of a child with acute diarrhea. Thus, there is no reason to withhold breast-feeding even on a temporary basis. Thus, advising that he eat an age-appropriate diet and gradually discontinue breast-feeding (**choice B**), and stop breast-feeding immediately (**choice D**), are incorrect.

Current evidence suggests that continued feeding during acute diarrhea promotes mucosal recovery (**choice E**).

30. **The correct answer is A.** Most umbilical hernias that appear before the age of 6 months disappear spontaneously by 1 year of age. Even large hernias have been known to close by age 5. Therefore, observation on an outpatient is the appropriate management at this time.

Strapping (**choice B**) consists of wrapping a beltlike cloth around the waist at the level of the belly button to "push" the hernia back in. Today, strapping is considered ineffective and is not recommended.

Surgery (**choice C**) is indicated if there is evidence in the history and physical examination of strangulation (e.g., abdominal pain, fever, vomiting, weight loss). It is also indicated if the hernia enlarges after 1 to 2 years of age.

There is absolutely no indication for transcutaneous stimulation in this child (**choice D**).

An ultrasound (**choice E**) will not change any conservative or surgical management and is therefore unnecessary.

31. **The correct answer is B.** Risk factors for iron deficiency anemia in the infant include rapid weight gain from excessive consumption of cow's milk. Dietary instruction is necessary and the amount of cow's milk consumed should be reduced to 1 pint a day or less. It need not be completely eliminated. Iron supplementation (and then iron-containing foods) should be started no later than 4 months of age, when iron stores are no longer sufficient.

A cephalhematoma (**choice A**) is typically seen in prolonged labors and often with instrumentation. It would also have to be very large to cause an anemia in the child, which would resolve after a few weeks with the resolution of the cephalhematoma. Also, cephalhematomas are often associated with hyperbilirubinemia.

There is no evidence in the history suggesting a vaginal delivery complicated by severe maternal blood loss (**choice C**), which is defined as maternal hemoglobin of 6 g/dL or less.

The infant's iron stores do not correlate to maternal iron states unless the maternal hemoglobin is less than 6g/dL; therefore, maternal iron deficiency anemia during pregnancy with hemoglobin of 10 g/dL and hematocrit of 32% (**choice D**) is incorrect.

A premature baby is one born at 36 weeks' gestation or less and would be at risk of iron deficiency anemia. This infant does not fit the definition of a premature baby and therefore the gestational age of the child being 37 weeks at the time of birth (**choice E**) is incorrect.

32. **The correct answer is B.** This urgent situation (septic shock) requires the immediacy of intravenous access in order to provide aggressive fluid hydration and antibiotics. The fastest, safest, and most reliable route for intravenous access is intraosseous access. It is unlikely to interfere with resuscitation either.

Further peripheral venous cannulation (**choice A**) should not be pursued if three attempts at venipuncture are unsuccessful or are not done within 90 seconds, whichever comes first.

A saphenous vein cutdown (**choice C**) takes longer than 10 minutes, has a greater rate of infection, and should only be attempted when peripheral, central, and intraosseous cannulation fail. Local anesthetic is not indicated in this emergency.

A scalp vein cannulation (**choice D**) in this child who is unstable is more difficult to do and should be avoided.

A subclavian vein cannulation (**choice E**) could take longer than 10 minutes, and other methods of accessing the central veins may be preferred.

33. **The correct answer is A.** An 18-month-old boy with a dorsiflexed foot that can be plantar flexed to neutral describes a calcaneovalgus foot that would normally resolve spontaneously in a newborn. At age 18 months the child would benefit from an orthopedic referral for a tendon release procedure.

Flatfeet (**choice B**) rarely cause disability or pain.

Flexible metatarsus adductus (**choice C**) usually resolves without treatment.

Overriding toes (**choice D**) rarely cause anything more than a cosmetic deformity.

If the foot of a child who toe walks (**choice E**) can be brought back to neutral then the condition usually resolves.

34. **The correct answer is E.** This unfortunate clinical scenario is very common with pediatric fractures. A spiral fracture of the femur without the appropriate mechanism of injury (a violent twisting injury is usually required to create this fracture pattern) must raise suspicions of abuse. Physicians are required in all states to notify Child Protective Services who will then investigate the events surrounding the injury as well as the environment of the child. A skeletal survey is appropriate to look for other previously healed long-bone fractures.

As discussed previously, the physician who suspects abuse must report their suspicion to the proper authorities. Sending this patient out of your clinic without doing so is inappropriate treatment and is illegal. Another part of this answer is incorrect because, in general, children under 4 years of age have difficulty using crutches and a femur fracture will not be completely healed in 2 weeks (**choice A**).

It is not wise to physically separate a mother from her child, and in this case it is very possible the mother's boyfriend is the perpetrator of the abuse (**choice B**).

Placement of a long-leg cast for the proximal femur fracture and a referral to the local pediatric orthopedic surgeon so that the patient will have proper followup (**choice C**) is not correct for several reasons. Again, the proper authorities must be notified and a proximal femur fracture in young patients should be treated with a hip spica cast, not a long-leg cast.

Osteogenesis imperfecta (OI) is a possible cause for multiple fractures in children. OI fractures are generally *not* spiral in nature, and the diagnosis of OI is generally a clinical one (**choice D**).

35. **The correct answer is D.** Neonatal conjunctivitis with *Neisseria gonorrhoeae* is a very serious eye infection. *Gonorrhoeae* is one of the few organisms that can penetrate an intact corneal epithelium, leading to a high risk of a corneal ulcer. That is why irrigation of the eyes with saline is recommended, not contraindicated (**choice B**). Conjunctivitis caused by gonorrhea usually presents between days 3 to 5 of life with a unilateral or bilateral conjunctivitis. The discharge is usually purulent. A neonate with gonococcal conjunctivitis should be thoroughly evaluated for disseminated infection with a careful physical examination. Antibiotics should be administered both topically and systemically (**choice A**), not just topically (**choice C**). All neonates with gonorrhea should also be treated for chlamydia with erythromycin elixir.

36. **The correct answer is D.** This patient obviously has meningitis due to untreated bacterial otitis media. The signs and symptoms of meningitis include change in mental status (lethargy), nuchal rigidity, photophobia, inability to extend the leg with the thigh flexed (Kernig sign), flexion of the hip and knee with neck turning (Brudzinski sign), and headache. The single most important intervention in a patient with suspected bacterial meningitis is to start intravenous antibiotics immediately. Without appropriate antibiotic therapy, bacterial meningitis can result in death in hours. Antibiotics should be initiated prior to performing a lumbar puncture (**choice C**), or CT scan (**choice E**). Although there is a theoretical risk of interfering with culture results by giving antibiotics before performing lumbar puncture, the potentially rapid progression of meningitis dictates that antibiotics not be delayed.

Calling Child Protective Services (**choice A**) and social work (**choice B**) are incorrect for two reasons. First, as emphasized above, initiating antibiotic therapy is the first priority. Second, failure to have money to pay for antibiotics is not a form of child neglect. Similarly, insurance for prescription medications is not vital at this time, as this child will be admitted for at least several days of observation and intravenous antibiotics.

37. **The correct answer is B.** This is somewhat of an ethical and a procedural question. It is up to the physician to assess difficult situations such as this and provide the best information to the patient or patient's family. Then, in general, physicians let the family decide the best course of action based on the provided information. This is why telling the parents that you have the final say (**choice A**) is incorrect. It is possible in extreme circumstances of medical futility to declare this as such, and withdraw care despite the patient's/parents' wishes. It is usually wise to obtain a consultation from the hospital's ethics committee prior to making such a decision.

Trying to involve the relatives in the decision (**choice C**) is often appropriate, but it should be an open discussion and you should not pit the family members against each other.

Telling the parents that this situation is medically futile and that they are simply prolonging their own suffering and wasting money at this point (**choice D**) and withdrawing life support despite the parents' wishes (**choice E**) are clearly insensitive and inappropriate.

38. **The correct answer is A.** The child in this vignette has the classical anticholinergic toxidrome. Signs and symptoms of anticholinergic ingestion include: hyperthermia, dry mouth, flushed skin, dilated pupils, delirium, and urinary retention. Antihistamines, tricyclic antidepressants, and scopolamine ingestions can lead to this syndrome.

The cholinergic toxidrome (**choice B**) includes diarrhea, diaphoresis, urination, miosis, muscle fasciculations, bradycardia, salivation, and emesis.

The narcotic toxidrome (**choice C**) includes miosis, bradycardia, hypotension, hyperventilation, and coma.

Salicylate ingestion (**choice D**) often presents with nausea, vomiting, and hyperventilation. It is a gastric irritant and directly stimulates the respiratory center of the brain.

The sympathomimetic toxidrome (**choice E**) includes mydriasis, tachycardia, hypertension, hyperthermia, and seizures.

39. **The correct answer is E.** A hand x-ray will allow an assessment of bone age, which will confirm the most likely diagnosis in this case: constitutional delay of growth and development. Constitutional delay occurs when, for unknown reasons, a child's pubertal development and consequently their growth spurt is delayed past the usual chronological age when this occurs. Final adult height, though, is always what would be predicted based on the parent's height. In other words, acquisition of their adult height simply occurs later than their peers. Bone age, or the degree of skeletal maturity, actually correlates much better with the onset of puberty than chronological age. Hence, if this child's bone age is delayed, given a normal growth velocity for his bone age and lack of any other signs of disease on examination, the parents and the child can be reassured that he will eventually obtain a full, normal, adult height. The delay in bone age is actually detectable long before puberty, around age 3.

Monthly testosterone injections (**choice A**) will speed up the child's progression through puberty, which may be socially desirable, but should not be undertaken without first confirming the diagnosis with a bone age and discussing the options with the parents.

Magnetic resonance imaging (**choice B**) is not necessary in the face of a normal growth velocity and no other signs of illness.

Growth hormone deficiency (**choice C**) will produce short stature, but is not compatible with the normal growth velocity.

A serum cortisol (**choice D**) may be abnormal in pituitary disease, but again, there is no evidence on history or examination to suggest this.

40. **The correct answer is B.** It is important to recognize that this infant is hemodynamically unstable despite her normal blood pressure and to intervene aggressively. An infant will maintain a normal blood pressure despite being in shock until they are literally at death's door. All bilious emesis in infants must be thoroughly evaluated to exclude midgut volvulus. The story here is classic enough that further radiographic imaging is probably not warranted and may cost valuable time. The consequences of delay here are catastrophic. If the volvulus is not corrected before the bowel dies, the baby will be left with short-gut syndrome and will be TPN-dependent for life with all the complications that entails, including, ultimately, liver cirrhosis and transplant. If the baby is felt to be stable enough to evaluate more thoroughly, an upper GI with small bowel follow-through will demonstrate the abnormal position of the ligament of Treitz, confirming malrotation and indicating laparotomy.

Neither admitting her for intravenous rehydration and evaluating for bacterial gastroenteritis (**choice A**) nor beginning oral rehydration and giving her close followup (**choice C**) is sufficient to correct this potentially catastrophic problem.

An abdominal CT without contrast (**choice D**) may not be adequate to demonstrate the lesion.

Abdominal ultrasound (**choice E**) will be difficult to interpret with the excess bowel gas from the obstruction and is not the imaging modality of choice.

41. **The correct answer is B.** This child most likely has idiopathic thrombocytopenic purpura, given his age and history. The most concerning differential diagnosis is, of course, a new leukemia. It is extremely rare for acute lymphoblastic leukemia, the most common type in childhood, to present solely with an isolated thrombocytopenia. Usually, there will be other cell lines that are clearly involved. This child's hemoglobin and hematocrit are normal for his age and the leukocyte count is normal with no blasts seen. Hence, a presumptive diagnosis of ITP can be made. An appropriate therapy would be IVIG.

A bone marrow biopsy (**choice A**) is not necessary at this point, unless he fails to respond to therapy. The platelet count is so low in this case though that treatment should be undertaken.

At this low platelet count there is a much higher risk of intracranial hemorrhage, and this child should be excluded from sports until the platelet count returns to normal. However, given the absence of any neurologic signs of hemorrhage on examination, no imaging of the head is indicated yet (**choice C**). An MRI would not be the appropriate choice in any case, as recent blood is more easily detected on a CT scan. This child's ultimate prognosis is excellent, with chronic ITP being extremely rare in children.

Transfuse 2 units of platelets and recheck the platelet count (**choice D**) is inappropriate at this time because if he has ITP, the platelets will be destroyed very quickly. It is sometimes used in situations when life-threatening bleeding is occurring.

42. **The correct answer is D.** Developmental dysplasia of the hip is critical to detect in the newborn period because if treatment is undertaken then the outcome is likely to be good, while if treatment is delayed past 4 to 6 months the outcome is likely to be a lifetime of painful disability. Many different screening protocols have been investigated, including ultrasound or radiographic screening, examinations by nurses, orthopedists, or pediatricians, or combinations of all of the above. The most useful and cost-effective measure is clinical screening by pediatricians. The diagnosis remains a clinical one and even if an ultrasound is normal, given the examination above, treatment must be undertaken. It can be stopped later if the examination returns to normal and no other evidence of hip dysplasia exists. A Pavlik harness is a relatively benign intervention until the diagnosis can be confirmed and may well avert a disaster.

By 4 months there will be significant dysplasia of the acetabulum, and so intervention is necessary before this point, and following the examination until then is indefensible (**choice A**).

Ultrasound (**choice B**) is useful in the evaluation of neonatal hips once a problem is detected, but they still give a significant number of false negatives. The diagnosis remains a clinical one, and even if an ultrasound is normal, given the examination above, treatment must be undertaken. It can be stopped later if the examination returns to normal and no other evidence of hip dysplasia exists. A Pavlik harness is a relatively benign intervention until the diagnosis can be confirmed and may well avert a disaster.

Plain radiographs (**choice C**) are difficult to interpret at this age, as the femoral head has not ossified, so these will likely not be useful until the child is at least 4 months old. By 4 months there will be significant dysplasia of the acetabulum, and so intervention is necessary before this point, and following the exam until then is indefensible. Incidentally, while social work may be useful in this case to ensure that the home environment is a stable one, the initial information available indicates a financially and socially supportive home. The identity of the father, while useful information, is at this point the least of the child's worries.

Rechecking the hip later (**choice E**) without any intervention is not appropriate given the examination findings. Also note that the breech delivery is a strong risk factor for hip dislocation.

43. **The correct answer is D.** Disk batteries require emergent removal because there is a risk for esophageal corrosion in the first 4 hours after ingestion. Sharp objects, such as open safety pins, also need to be removed emergently. Any child with a foreign body ingestion who is symptomatic (i.e., stridor, respiratory distress, drooling, pain) also requires endoscopic evaluation.

Admission to the hospital for observation (**choice A**) is not appropriate in this situation because time is a critical factor after the ingestion of a disk battery in order to prevent corrosive injury to the esophagus.

Discharging the patient home, either to followup with their pediatrician (**choice B**) or a gastroenterologist (**choice C**), is also not appropriate in this vignette.

Scheduling the patient for a followup chest x-ray in 24 hours (**choice E**) would be appropriate in this case if the child had ingested a coin rather than a disk battery. The child in this vignette is asymptomatic and the foreign body is located in the distal esophagus. If this were a coin, a followup x-ray in 24 hours may show movement of the coin into the stomach; this would then require careful followup on the parents' part to ensure that the foreign body passes into the stool.

44. **The correct answer is C.** Children at the age of 3 cannot yet fully comprehend the concepts of death and terminal illness. The primary concern of this population of sick children is their imminent physical comfort and fear of the unknown.

Telling her that her concerns can only be addressed in the presence of her parents (**choice A**) is also not supportive or sensitive to the patient's substantial fears.

Stating that nothing bad will befall the patient if she is well behaved (**choice B**) is also inappropriate and incorrect. First and foremost, it is a dishonest response insofar as the patient will eventually die from her leukemia regardless of her behavior. Secondly, it will instill a new fear within the patient and a perception that when her course of illness deteriorates, it is a consequence of her bad behavior.

Telling the patient she will die soon (**choice D**) is completely inappropriate and would likely be very anxiety-provoking to a patient who does not yet have a full comprehension of the concept of death.

Avoiding the patient's question altogether (**choice E**) is not a sensitive or appropriate response to any patient's concerns regardless of the age of the patient. Although the patient's question is a difficult and painful one to answer, she does deserve the respect of a sensitive and empathic response.

45. **The correct answer is E.** This newborn most likely has trisomy 21, or Down syndrome. This syndrome has an increasing prevalence based on maternal age. The prevalence for a 20-year-old woman is 0.69 per 1000 live births and increases to 39 per 1000 live births for a 45-year-old woman. The diagnosis of Down syndrome can be made clinically and verified by chromosomal analysis. The majority of neonates with Down syndrome are hypotonic and hyperextensible. Their fontanels are enlarged and close late. They typically have epicanthal folds, upslanting palpebral fissures, a short nasal bridge, a downturned mouth, and an enlarged tongue. About 40 to 50% of patients with Down syndrome have congenital heart disease; a perimembranous ventricular septal defect is the most common type of congenital heart disease and the murmur of the child in this vignette is consistent with this anomaly. Single palmar creases are common in the general population, but are found in high frequency among patients with Down syndrome.

Beckwith-Wiedemann syndrome (**choice A**) is diagnosed by the presence of three or more of the following: macrosomia, hemihyperplasia, macroglossia, abdominal wall defect, embryonal tumor, adrenocortical cytomegaly, ear anomalies, visceromegaly, renal anomalies, and neonatal hypoglycemia. The baby in this vignette has macroglossia, but does not have any other findings of Beckwith-Wiedemann syndrome.

Infants with congenital hypothyroidism (**choice B**) have macroglossia, hypotonia, and enlarged fontanelles. However, they also characteristically have dry, coarse skin, constipation, umbilical hernia, and a hoarse cry, which are not found in the infant in this vignette.

Trisomy 13 (**choice C**) is characterized by orofacial clefts, microphthalmia/anophthalmia, and polydactyly of the limbs.

Trisomy 18 (**choice D**), or Edwards syndrome, is characterized by prenatal growth deficiency, clenched hands with overlapping fingers, prominent occiput, and short sternum.

46. **The correct answer is C.** The infant in this vignette shows characteristic clinical features of fetal alcohol syndrome. Children with fetal alcohol syndrome often require a team approach to management because they often have significant behavioral and cognitive defects. Organic brain damage is a possibility in children with fetal alcohol syndrome and needs to be considered in children with microcephaly. A head circumference more than 2 to 3 standard deviations below the mean is a significant indicator of poor brain growth and should be further evaluated.

Intake of folic acid during pregnancy (**choice A**) is significant in children born with evidence of neural tube defects. The child in this vignette does not have any evidence of a neural tube defect.

Questioning a mother about her seizure history (**choice B**) may elicit use of phenytoin during pregnancy. Fetal hydantoin syndrome is characterized by intrauterine growth retardation and bleeding disorders in the neonatal period due to vitamin K deficiency. There are no classic lip findings associated with this disorder as described in this patient.

Cocaine use during pregnancy (**choice D**) can also result in intrauterine growth retardation and microcephaly, but does not have the classic facial findings described in this infant.

Isotretinoin (**choice E**) is used to treat severe acne and is a known teratogen. Its use is contraindicated during pregnancy because there is about a 20% risk of damage to the fetus; defects associated with its use include CNS, ear, and cardiovascular anomalies.

47. **The correct answer is E.** The most telling information in this vignette is the odor of mint on the toddler's breath. It is consistent with the ingestion of oil of wintergreen (methyl salicylate), which is a highly concentrated form of salicylate (1 cc equals 1.4 grams of salicylate). Therefore it can be quite toxic. Salicylates are also gastric irritants, which leads to vomiting shortly after a toxic ingestion.

Acetaminophen (**choice A**) ingestion can be associated with vomiting, diaphoresis, and fatigue in the first 24 hours after ingestion; however, it is not associated with any classic odor.

Ethylene glycol (**choice B**) ingestion is characterized in the early stages (1-12 hours) by nausea, vomiting, and drowsiness. It then progresses to cardiac arrhythmias. There is no classic odor associated with this ingestion either.

Iron (**choice C**) ingestion is characterized by abdominal pain, nausea, vomiting, and diarrhea about 6 to 12 hours after a large ingestion. This does not truly fit the history of the toddler in this vignette.

Methanol (**choice D**) ingestion is characterized by drowsiness, inebriation, nausea, and vomiting. It is a common ingredient in industrial solvents. There is no classic scent after ingestion.

48. **The correct answer is E.** This patient most likely has Kawasaki disease, which is associated with an elevation of the acute phase reactants, including platelets. Platelet counts may be initially normal, but by day 5 of illness, many patients will have thrombocytosis. This thrombocytosis contributes to the risk for myocardial infarction in these patients due to their predisposition to coronary artery aneurysms.

    Patients with Kawasaki disease will have sterile pyuria as part of their illness due to the inflammation of the urethral meatus. Mild proteinuria may be present but hematuria does not typically occur (**choice A**).

    Neutropenia (**choice B**) is not seen in Kawasaki disease. Commonly, these patients will have a normal to high white blood cell count during the course of their disease.

    Antinuclear antibody (**choice C**) and rheumatoid factor (**choice D**) are not found in patients with Kawasaki disease.

49. **The correct answer is D.** Toddlers are known to put things into their mouths, and a foreign body aspiration should be strongly considered in any young child with onset of cough without fever. Because of the anatomy of the bronchi, the foreign bodies are more likely to lodge on the right than on the left. The examination is usually significant for wheezing on the side with the foreign body because of airway hyperreactivity. Inspiratory/expiratory chest films in a child who will cooperate are helpful and will show hyperinflation of the affected side during expiration. The child in this vignette is too young to cooperate; therefore, a lateral decubitus film of the affected side will show inappropriate hyperinflation of that side.

    Cough-variant asthma (**choice A**) should be considered in any child with a persistent cough without fever, especially worse at night or after exercise. The examination typically shows wheezing bilaterally, not just on one side, and anteroposterior chest x-ray may reveal bilateral hyperinflation.

    Croup (**choice B**) should be considered in any child who has a cough accompanied by stridor, indicative of an upper airway process. The classic x-ray finding in a child with croup is the "steeple-sign" on lateral neck film, representing upper airway narrowing.

    Epiglottitis (**choice C**) is not a common finding in the pediatric population anymore due to the success of the *Haemophilus influenza type B* vaccine. Children with epiglottitis classicly are toxic appearing, in significant respiratory distress, and drooling with their heads tilted outward. The classic x-ray finding in epiglottitis is the "thumb sign" on lateral neck film, representing the swollen, enlarged epiglottis.

    Vascular webs (**choice E**) should also be considered in a child with stridor. Vascular anomalies in the upper airway affecting the trachea can cause compression and stridor on both inspiration and expiration. They are not typically seen on x-rays.

50. **The correct answer is A.** Albuterol is a beta-2-agonist and is believed to have some benefit in the management of respiratory syncytial virus. It is thought to relieve some of the small airway edema, which results in the increased airway resistance in this disease process.

    RSV is a viral illness; therefore, ampicillin (**choice B**), an antibiotic, is not indicated in this case. The baby is currently afebrile and there is no indication of bacterial superinfection given in the vignette.

    Dexamethasone (**choice C**) is a glucocorticoid that is often used in the management of croup. Studies have failed to show any benefit in the duration of symptoms, length of stay, and oxygen requirement when steroids are used in RSV bronchiolitis.

    Nebulized normal saline solution (**choice D**) is not indicated in the management of RSV bronchiolitis. It can act as an airway irritant and worsen the patient's respiratory status.

    Ribavirin (**choice E**) is an antiviral medication, that inhibits the replication of DNA and RNA viruses. It is indicated for use in severe RSV infection in children with underlying disorders, i.e., prematurity, bronchopulmonary dysplasia, and congenital heart disease. The child in this vignette has uncomplicated RSV bronchiolitis, and there is no indication to begin ribavirin therapy in this case.

Pediatrics: Test Four

1. A 22-year-old woman gave birth to a baby boy 6 days earlier. This first pregnancy was uneventful and the newborn was well until the previous night when he started developing crops of tiny blisters on the scalp. Some of them have become pussy and crusted. The baby also seems to have become very irritable during the past 24 hours. You arrange for them to come to the office immediately and on visual inspection of the baby's skin you note that there are discrete and confluent translucent and turbid vesicles on the parietal and occipital scalp of the baby boy. Some of the lesions are covered with a hemorrhagic crust. The fontanelles are bulging and the newborn is irritable and cries throughout the examination. You decide to initiate treatment immediately while waiting for laboratory study results. The study that should be performed in the office to help you establish a preliminary diagnosis is

   (A) a KOH examination of scrapings from the base of a lesion
   (B) a scotch tape test of scrapings from the base of a lesion
   (C) a Tzanck smear of scrapings from the base of a lesion
   (D) Wood light examination of the skin
   (E) Wood light examination of the urine

2. A mother brings her 2½-month-old son to see you because she noticed he had a swollen left scrotum. She reports that he seems fine without any symptoms and his birth history was normal. He was full-term with a birth weight of 8 pounds. There was no significant jaundice or other problems. On physical examination you confirm there is a left scrotal mass that does not reduce. It does transilluminate. The right scrotal area is normal. There is no bulge in either inguinal area. The most appropriate next step in management is to

   (A) observe
   (B) prepare him for immediate surgery
   (C) refer him for elective surgery in the next several weeks
   (D) refer him for genetic consultation
   (E) send him for a testicular scan

3. A 6-year-old girl is brought to the office with a large, swollen, and tender right axillary node. History reveals that a week or two ago she received multiple scratches from her playful kitten. She says, "my armpit really hurts, especially when I'm bored or trying to go to sleep at night." There is no drainage, but slight erythema, some induration, and definite tenderness in the right axillary region. The most appropriate next step in management is to

   (A) aspirate the node for Gram stain and culture
   (B) biopsy the node and send for pathology assessment
   (C) obtain a chest x-ray
   (D) place a PPD
   (E) treat with trimethoprim-sulfamethoxazole

4. A mother brings her child for an office visit because of a particularly annoying cough that he has had for several weeks. He seems to have "chains of coughs" where he will cough "again and again." Mostly, the cough continues on and off throughout the day, but he has no coughing at night. He has been able to attend school on most days, but sometimes the coughing is particularly bad after the long, busy weekends, causing him to miss Monday mornings at school. He has no past medical history for asthma or allergies. Family history for allergic diseases is negative. Over-the-counter cough medications have offered no relief to his cough. His appetite has been fine and he has no visible change in weight. Physical examination is normal except for some minimal erythema of the posterior pharynx. The most appropriate next step in management is

   (A) allergy testing
   (B) a chest x-ray
   (C) over-the-counter cough medication
   (D) counseling
   (E) placement of a PPD

5. A pregnant mother brings her 8-year-old daughter to the office because of a rash that the child had just 2 days ago, but that seems to have resolved by today. She would have canceled the appointment but a friend told her that there are certain childhood infectious diseases that may hurt the baby and she is anxious to learn if this was one of them. She tells you that the rash had started with no special prodrome around the hairline and on the face 5 days ago and then suddenly spread as if before their eyes over the next day or day and a half. It was fleeting, she tells you, and now it is already the second day that the rash is gone. You ask the girl if she has any pain or discomfort and she says that her feet hurt a little, but it seems to be getting better, too. On examination, the girl appears to be in no acute distress and her vital signs are within normal limits. Her skin is slightly desquamating on the hairline and on the trunk, but there are no active inflammatory lesions to be seen. You palpate her lymph nodes to conclude that she has bilateral enlarged posterior occipitocervical lymph nodes. Exposure to the cause of this illness is deleterious to the mother's unborn baby during the

   (A) first trimester of pregnancy
   (B) second trimester of pregnancy
   (C) third trimester of pregnancy
   (D) the entire pregnancy
   (E) the neonatal period

6. While you are busily working in the morning clinic the advice nurse turns to you for guidance. A mother is calling to say that her child has been exposed to tuberculosis as the grandmother was just diagnosed with cavitary tuberculosis. You should tell her that the incubation period for infection with tuberculosis to development of a positive tuberculin skin test is

   (A) 1 to 6 months
   (B) 2 to 4 weeks
   (C) 2 to 12 weeks
   (D) 10 to 21 days
   (E) 10 to 90 days

7. A 15-month-old toddler is rushed to the emergency department 30 minutes after she grabbed the handle of a pot on the stove spilling it down the front of her body and into her loosely fitting diaper, resulting in scalding burns over parts of her pubic and perineal area. The infant is wildly crying, afebrile, and has a blood pressure of 70 mm Hg systolic and pulse of 130/min. The skin burn areas consist of reddened second-degree burns with some blistering patches in the lower abdomen, perineum, and pubic areas of the body. The burn surface area is believed to be 3 to 5%. The most appropriate next step in management is to

   (A) admit the child to the hospital
   (B) contact the child protective services
   (C) order a complete blood count, serum glucose, electrolytes, BUN, and creatinine
   (D) recommend topical 1% silver sulfadiazine cream
   (E) recommend topical 1% silver sulfadiazine cream and prophylactic oral antibiotics

8. A 15-year-old diabetic boy returns for his annual check-up. He was diagnosed with insulin-dependent diabetes mellitus (IDDM) 2 years ago and has been in fairly good control. Recently he has been having glycosuria and high blood glucose measurements during the morning and afternoon. His mother is very involved with his diabetic management and assures you that he is compliant with testing his daily glucose levels. There has not been a major change in his diet or exercise. He has a history of allergic rhinitis, but has not taken any medications for this. His temperature is 36.7 C (98.1 F). He has slightly boggy turbinates, and his post pharynx has erythema without exudate. There is no lymphadenopathy. Chest and abdomen are normal. Sexual maturity rating is 3. You conclude that the most likely reason for poor glycemic control is

(A) end of the honeymoon period
(B) occult infection
(C) puberty
(D) renal disease
(E) Somogyi effect

9. An African American boy is brought to your office as he is recovering from an illness. He was prescribed sulfisoxazole for chronic otitis earlier in the week by another doctor. He felt somewhat better but now has a new symptom of weakness. His physical examination is normal except for pallor. Laboratory studies show a normal leukocyte and platelet count. Hemoglobin is 9.4 g/dL, reticulocyte count is 4%. The peripheral smear shows Heinz bodies, some nucleated red cells, a few spherocytes, and some "bite" or blister cells. Bilirubin is 5.1 mg/dL, with a direct bilirubin of 1.3 mg/dL. The direct Coombs is negative. Hemoglobin electrophoresis is normal. The best diagnostic test to perform to establish the diagnosis is

(A) bone marrow examination
(B) a G6PD assay
(C) indirect Coombs test
(D) a Monospot test
(E) pyruvate kinase levels

10. One Friday evening at the local emergency department, 14 adolescents aged 17 to 19 are seen for symptoms of abdominal pain, vomiting, diarrhea, and some had low-grade fever. The hospital epidemiologist is called in to question the teens and is able to identify 11 other persons who were ill with similar symptoms but did not seek medical help. All had attended the high school graduation reception earlier that day. Further investigation reveals that 33 others who did not become ill had attended the same post-graduation party. Chicken salad and crème-filled pastries are implicated in this outbreak of *Staphylococcus aureus* food poisoning. The best estimate of the attack rate of staphylococcal poisoning for those who attended the party is

(A) 25.0
(B) 25.0%
(C) 43.1
(D) 43.1%
(E) 75.8%

11. A 5-year-old boy has had increasing abdominal pain over the past 24 hours. He has no vomiting, diarrhea, or other symptoms of illness except for mild decrease in appetite. On physical examination he appears ill and is in mild distress. Temperature is 38.3 C (102.0 F), pulse is 112/min, and respirations are 45/min. Abdominal examination reveals mild tenderness and guarding in the right upper quadrant area. The next best step in management is to obtain

(A) an abdominal ultrasound
(B) a chest x-ray
(C) a CBC and blood culture
(D) serum amylase and lipase
(E) a urine culture

12. A 4-year-old child is brought to the office for a followup for ear pain. You saw her 4 days ago for a low-grade fever and earache, diagnosed an acute otitis media, and prescribed amoxicillin 40 to 60 mg/kg/day. Her mother reports that she still seems to have a slight fever and continues to complain of earache. She appears "no better, no worse." Your examination is essentially the same as it was the few days before. The most appropriate next step in management is to

    (A) change to a broad-spectrum antibiotic
    (B) continue amoxicillin for 4 more days and re-evaluate
    (C) obtain a CBC and blood culture
    (D) perform myringotomy
    (E) prescribe an antihistamine/decongestant medication

13. A 19-year-old woman, upset by a breakup with her boyfriend, is found unconscious in her dorm room. The floor is littered with bottles of cola and one empty bottle of rum. In the emergency department she is unarousable. Her temperature is normal, blood pressure is 80/55 mm Hg, and respirations are 15/min. Neurologic examination reveals that her pupils are equal, slightly dilated. The remainder of the examination is normal. Laboratory studies show a blood alcohol level of 100 mg/dL and blood glucose of 85 mg/dL. As you order further tests, you consider the best test to explain her unconscious state will be

    (A) an ammonia level
    (B) a CBC
    (C) electrolytes and repeat blood glucose
    (D) further drug testing
    (E) a head CT

14. A 12-year-old boy returns home after being away for 3 weeks at sleep-away summer camp. He participated in all sorts of activities, including hiking, swimming, archery, and tennis. The morning after his return he tells his mother about an earache that he had for the last few days of camp. She brings him to your office for examination. His past medical history is unremarkable. His right ear appears slightly swollen, erythematous, and there is definite, foul-smelling, purulent discharge in the canal. The most appropriate next step in management is to

    (A) administer amoxicillin
    (B) culture the ear discharge
    (C) give hydrocortisone otic drops
    (D) order a CT scan
    (E) prescribe polymyxin B/neomycin/hydrocortisone otic drops

15. A 3-year-old girl is brought to the emergency department by her mother who barely speaks English. They are refugees from a poor and war-torn country recently given asylum. They just transferred from a facility in another state after having spent 3 months there upon immigration to the United States. You manage to learn from the mother that the girl had suddenly become sick 7 days earlier with worsening fever, malaise, and upper respiratory symptoms. Her eyes have been red for a few days and she cries when exposed to bright light. The mother shows you her skin rash and signals that it started 2 days ago on the forehead and behind the ears and is now spreading downward to involve the trunk and extremities. You inquire about immunizations but the mother starts crying and says, "No, none, war." You examine the child to find that she is in moderate distress with a fever of 38.5 C (101.3 F), a pulse of 120/min, and respirations of 24/min. She is at the fifth percentile for height and weight and appears dehydrated. The conjunctivas are injected and the girl is photophobic. Her face, neck, trunk, and proximal extremities are covered with dull red macules and papules that coalesce to form irregular concentric patterns on the extremities and a more confluent pattern on the trunk. There is some brownish discoloration and fine scaling only behind the ears. In addition to obtaining blood for serologic studies the finding that would most likely aid you in confirming the diagnosis is

    (A) Forscheimer sign
    (B) Herald patch
    (C) Koplik spots
    (D) strawberry tongue
    (E) vesicular enanthem

16. You are at a conference for primary care physicians in Hawaii and are about to go put on your swimsuit when you hear that a pharmaceutical representative is specifically requesting your presence at his lecture that is scheduled to begin in 5 minutes. You know this man pretty well, as he has been to your office many times over the past few years and knows that you have a thriving practice. You reluctantly agree to attend the lecture. He begins the talk discussing erythromycin, which you know is most appropriate for

(A) chemoprophylaxis for close contacts to someone with *Bordetella pertussis*
(B) prophylaxis for a human bite
(C) *Salmonella* gastroenteritis in a toddler
(D) secondarily infected tinea corporis
(E) sinusitis in a 5-year-old

17. You are called to the labor and delivery floor to examine a newborn who is noted to have a meningomyelocele. You are concerned about other findings that are frequently associated with this condition. At this time the most appropriate study to order to evaluate this newborn for coexisting conditions is

(A) a chest x-ray and echocardiogram
(B) a CT scan of the head
(C) an ophthalmologic examination performed by an ophthalmologist
(D) a renal scan
(E) sonography of the hips

18. A mother calls the answering service one night because her 12-month-old is "ill". She was not feeling well earlier in the day and has become increasingly ill. On and off she will play and eat, but then she has episodes where she stops and cries out in pain. The mother thinks she is experiencing abdominal pains. This morning her daughter had one stool that was softer than usual and then she vomited one or two times. Her last stool was soft with some mucus mixed with blood. The infant still breast-feeds and also eats table foods. It is peak season for rotavirus. An older sibling had diarrhea a few days ago, but so far no one else has been ill with vomiting or diarrhea. At this time the best advice to give this mother is to

(A) continue to breast-feed, but give additional clear liquids
(B) let the infant eat and drink as she wants but call the office for followup in the morning
(C) stop the breast-feeding and only give clear liquids
(D) take her daughter's temperature and give a trial dose of liquid acetaminophen
(E) take her daughter to the emergency department

19. A 15-year-old girl comes to the clinic for a well physical examination. She has not had an annual checkup for 3 years. She denies any significant past illnesses and takes no medications. Menarche was at age 12 years. Review of systems is negative and she has no complaints. She is a good student with a GPA of 3.5 and is very active in sports year round for about 1 hour each day. Physical examination is unremarkable except for the suggestion of mild pallor. As the results of a complete blood count and cholesterol come back, you are surprised to see that the hemoglobin is 10 mg/dL and the red cells are microcytic and hypochromic. As you discuss the results with the patient you explain that the most likely cause of her anemia is low iron due to

(A) excessive milk drinking
(B) inadequate dietary intake of iron
(C) increased need for iron due to pubertal growth
(D) menstrual blood loss each month
(E) microscopic blood loss in her urine due to sports

20. A very concerned mother brings her 6-month-old boy to the office because he sometimes appears "cross-eyed". Past medical history reveals he was a full-term, 8-pound baby at birth with normal growth and development. Immunizations are up-to-date. Physical examination reveals strabismus that was not detected on previous well examinations. A white reflex of the right eye is seen. The next best step in management is to obtain

(A) a CT scan of the head
(B) a neurology consult
(C) an ophthalmology consult
(D) a renal scan
(E) TORCH titers

21. A 4-month-old infant is brought to the emergency department because of a swelling on his head. The mother explains that she came home from work and noticed a reddened area on the scalp. She explains that the baby-sitter told her that the infant fell off an upholstered armchair. The infant has been fussy and irritable, wanting to feed continuously. On examination there is a large diffuse erythematous swelling over the left occipitoparietal area of the head. There are no other abnormalities. An x-ray of the head reveals three to four nondepressed linear fractures over the left occiput. The next best management of this is to order

(A) aPTT, PT, and platelet count
(B) calcium and phosphate
(C) a CBC and platelet count
(D) a child protective service consultation
(E) a skeletal survey

22. A 7-year-old boy is brought to the clinic for a well checkup. His mother is concerned about some "pimples" on his cheeks and wonders whether he is too young to be having acne. Otherwise review of systems is negative. When asked about family history, she thinks there is a strong family history of acne. There is no family history of heart disease or high blood pressure. Her brother has a type of seizure disorder. The boy's physical examination is essentially normal except for clusters of red papules on the center of his cheeks, malar area, and a few on his chin. You also note hypopigmented macules on his back. The boy reports he never noticed them before and his mother was unsure if they have been there for a while or not. You are able to see them even better with the help of a Wood lamp. Having considered possible diagnoses, you now decide the best management would include

(A) benzoyl peroxide to facial papules, clotrimazole cream to hypopigmented spots
(B) benzoyl peroxide to facial papules, no therapy for the hypopigmented spots
(C) genetic counseling
(D) serum testosterone
(E) topical steroid cream to the face papules and hypopigmented spots

23. An African American girl is brought to the office for her 3-year-old checkup. She has been healthy and growing just fine. If anything, the parents have noticed she seems to have put on a little weight with a noticeably full abdomen. Her temperature is 37.0 C (98.6 F). Physical examination reveals a firm, nontender, well-demarcated abdominal mass and mild hepatomegaly. The remainder of the examination is otherwise normal. An ultrasound reveals a mass with extension into the inferior vena cava. A complete blood count is normal. The diagnostic study result that would most likely confirm the most probable diagnosis is

(A) an abnormal bone scan
(B) an abnormal brain scan
(C) elevated urinary vanillylmandelic acid
(D) a gene deletion of 11p13
(E) an N-*myc* gene

24. A 4-year-old boy is brought to the office for a preoperative examination before a scheduled herniorrhaphy. His mother says that he has been tired over the past week or so, but attributes this to his anxiety about the surgery. On examination you note multiple anterior cervical nodes and feel the tip of his spleen. His leukocyte count is $3000/mm^3$, hemoglobin is 9.0 mg/dL, and platelet count is $70,000/\ mm^3$. The next best step in management is to

(A) begin a sepsis workup
(B) evaluate his bone marrow
(C) order a Monospot test
(D) perform a lumbar puncture
(E) send blood for type and cross-match

25. A 12-month-old boy is brought to the office for a well-child examination. He is doing well at home and the mother has no complaints. His vital signs and physical examination are within normal limits. After reviewing his immunization history, you inform the mother that the child should receive the combined measles, mumps, and rubella (MMR) vaccine as well as the varicella vaccine at this visit. She explains that she is concerned because of a recent television news story linking the MMR to autism. The most appropriate response to her concern is:

(A) "It may be safer to give the MMR as separate injections on separate days, as the association between the MMR and autism has been shown only when the three components of MMR are given together."
(B) "Postponing the MMR until after his third birthday is one way of decreasing the risk of MMR-associated autism."
(C) "Since the delivery of multiple vaccines simultaneously increases the chance of a serious side effect of one or more of the vaccines, we can give them as separate injections on separate days."
(D) "While there is a theoretical risk of neurological disease as a result of the use of live vaccines, neither the MMR nor the varicella vaccine is a live virus, and so concern is unwarranted."
(E) "While there may be widespread concern about an epidemiologic link between vaccines and autism, no studies have convincingly shown such an association."

26. During a routine 4-month-old infant well visit a mother wonders how she will know if her child has hypertension. There is a strong family history on both sides for cardiovascular disease. You explain to her that routine blood pressure measurements are typically taken starting at the age of

(A) 6 months
(B) 1 year
(C) 3 years
(D) 5 years
(E) 10 years

27. A 12-month-old infant is brought to the office for an initial assessment. The family just moved from a neighboring state. The parents are concerned that the infant's speech is not as developed as his older brother was at the same age. Their son has no words and very poor vocalization. On examination you observe that he is microcephalic and when you plot him on the growth curve his height and weight are less than the fifth percentile. The most appropriate next step in management is to

(A) determine bone age
(B) get a CT scan of the head
(C) obtain a genetic consult
(D) send blood for T_4 and TSH levels
(E) send TORCH titers

28. You are called to the newborn nursery to see a full-term infant who is vomiting at 24 hours of age. The baby was born to a 40-year-old mother who has no significant past medical history. The initial physical examination at 4 hours of age revealed findings of mild hypotonia, small, low-set ears, and Brushfield spots. Taking these findings into consideration, the best initial test to order is

(A) an abdominal x-ray
(B) an echocardiogram and electrocardiogram
(C) electrolytes, BUN, and creatinine
(D) an MRI of the head
(E) serum T_4 and TSH levels

29. A 12-year-old girl is brought to the office for a rash. She went to school yesterday but the teacher noticed her rash and said the girl could not return to class until a doctor checked her and said that she is not contagious. She says that she does not feel ill. She recalls that she may have had a runny nose a few days ago and her stomach hurts a bit, but she is due to have her period soon. The rash began 2 days ago in the creases under her arms, around her neck, and in the groin area. Her past medical history is unremarkable. Just 2½ weeks ago she had a well visit and received her second MMR. Physical examination reveals a fine maculopapular rash over most of her body that blanches with pressure. Hyperpigmented areas are noted in the creases of her arms. The most appropriate next step in management is to

(A) order a CBC and blood culture
(B) order a CBC, erythrocyte sedimentation rate, and ANA
(C) provide reassurance
(D) send a rubella titer
(E) send a throat culture

30. A 10-year-old child is brought to the clinic complaining of a "bad sore throat". He has tender anterior cervical lymph nodes, palatal petechiae, and a temperature of 38.3 C (101 F). His rapid strep test is positive for *Streptococcus pyogenes*. The most appropriate advice to give the mother is:

(A) All ill siblings should have rapid strep tests.
(B) All siblings sick or well should have rapid strep tests.
(C) All siblings who are over 3 years of age and have a sore throat should have rapid strep tests.
(D) The boy may return to school after he has been afebrile for 24 hours.
(E) The boy may return to school after 3 days of antibiotics.

31. While you are about to leave for the emergency department around midnight, a close friend and neighbor asks you for medical advice regarding his 4-year-old son. As he is a close friend and neighbor, you gladly offer advice and do not charge him any professional fees. The boy does not get better and the father decides to sue you. The most likely outcome would be that the courts

(A) would hold you liable
(B) would not admit the case
(C) would not hold you liable because the advice was requested and not volunteered by you
(D) would not hold you liable because the father of the patient is a close friend
(E) would not hold you liable because you did not take any fees

32. A 9-year-old girl is brought to your office by her parents with fever and a rash of two days duration. She was healthy until a week ago, when she had a flu-like viral illness with sore throat and conjunctivitis. Five days later she started breaking out with a very itchy skin rash on the face and trunk. She has been getting new breakouts of the rash daily and the itch is disrupting her sleep. Otherwise, she does not have any significant past medical history and the only medication her parents gave her was over-the-counter cold syrup that helped a little with the fever and discomfort. The parents tell you that they have two other children at home, ages 5 and 11, who do not appear to be ill at this time. You examine the girl to find that she is in mild acute distress with a fever of 38.0 C (100.4 F) and pulse of 100/min. She is at the appropriate height and weight for her age. On her oral mucosa there is a vesicular enanthem, mainly on the palate. On the face and trunk there are 30 to 40 vesicles, fresh and umbilicated pustules, and crusted papules, most on a faint erythematous base. Many of the lesions are excoriated. At this time the medication that is absolutely contraindicated in this child is

(A) acetaminophen
(B) amoxicillin
(C) ampicillin
(D) aspirin
(E) cephalexin

33. A 12-year-old boy is brought to the office by his mother because of a 5-day history of a skin rash that seems to be getting worse every day. She tells you that the boy had a slight fever and runny nose last week that resolved without treatment. The mother is very concerned that this could be the same illness her husband had 3 weeks ago, and he is still at home being treated for pneumonia that developed as a complication. She is very concerned that her boy could also have some grave complication and she would like to prevent it if possible. She has also heard that this illness may come back many years later and she inquires if this is true. The boy is in no acute distress and has a total of 3 to 4 vesicles and about a dozen umbilicated pustules and crusted papules on his face and upper trunk. He has no complaints and is tolerating the rash well. At this time the most correct statement about his condition is:

(A) It is impossible that the father and son have the same disease because the boy has a childhood viral exanthem that does not affect adults.

(B) Such mild cases of the illness in children usually resolve uneventfully but he may develop herpes zoster later in life.

(C) Such mild cases of the illness in children usually resolve uneventfully without further appearing in any form because of lifelong immunity.

(D) The child will most certainly develop pneumonia as a complication because his father has developed it.

(E) The father and the child should be physically separated from each other until their diseases resolve because they could keep on reinfecting each other.

34. A 15-year-old girl is brought to the office by her mother for a skin rash that appeared 3 weeks earlier. It has not been bothering her but is rather unsightly and does not seem to be getting any better. It started with a large, red, scaly patch on her right arm, and approximately 10 days later spread to involve the entire trunk, upper arms, and thighs. The girl is otherwise healthy and has no complaints. She is in high school, has good grades, and is on the cheerleading team, but her gym teacher suspended her since the rash began because it would get very red and "juicy" every time she engaged in vigorous physical activity. You find the girl to be in no acute distress. She is well developed, well nourished, and appears overall in good health save for the skin lesions. The largest patch located on the right upper arm is 3 cm in diameter, oval, with an erythematous and scaly border. Many salmon-colored, oval and round discrete macules and papules are fairly evenly distributed over the trunk and proximal extremities. Their surface is finely crinkled and some have a collarette-type scale. You notice that all of the lesions are distributed so that the long axis runs parallel to the lines of cleavage. The mother insists her daughter receive specific treatment for the disease because it is compromising her extracurricular sports activities. At this time the most correct statement about his condition is:

(A) Daily long, soaking baths in hot water will hasten the recovery.

(B) Long-acting oral antihistamines will shorten the course of her disease.

(C) There is no specific treatment for her disease, but ultraviolet B light in erythema exposures may shorten the duration.

(D) A 7-day course of oral penicillin is indicated to shorten the duration of her disease.

(E) A single dose of oral fluconazole 150 mg is the preferred method of treatment.

35. On a sunny and warm September day a 45-year-old mother brings her 3-week-old firstborn boy to the office because of a rash that developed over the past 2 or 3 days and seems to be getting worse. She fears the child has "caught a cold" with the unusually high temperatures we were having over the past 2 weeks because he has been very cranky, doesn't sleep well, and has long episodes of crying during the feeding times. She meticulously cleans and sterilizes all the baby's bottles and pacifiers, bathes him only for a short few minutes every other night and has kept him nice and warm, but to no avail. You remember that the pregnancy and delivery went well, and that the newborn boy scored 9 and 10 on the 1-minute and 5-minute Apgar scores, respectively. When you ask to examine him, the mother starts unwrapping the crying baby and you note 2 blankets, a cap, mittens, and 2 pairs of long-sleeved overalls. As soon as she undresses the boy he stops crying and falls asleep. On the cheeks, trunk, and extremities the baby's skin is covered with myriad discrete, erythematous papules, vesicles, and papulovesicles. The anatomic location of the underlying pathologic process in this otherwise healthy neonate is most likely the

(A) apocrine ducts
(B) eccrine ducts
(C) hair follicle infundibulum
(D) sebaceous ducts
(E) subcutaneous fat

36. After returning from a camping trip, a 16-year-old boy has diarrhea, increased flatus, and abdominal pain. Physical examination is unremarkable. Enzyme-linked immunosorbent assay testing of the stool establishes the diagnosis of *Giardia lamblia*. You provide treatment with metronidazole for 5 days. In addition, you feel it is best to give the following advice:

(A) *Giardia* may be acquired from freshwater streams and food that is washed in that water, but it is not spread by fecal-oral route.
(B) Household contacts may be examined for *Giardia*, but if they are asymptomatic they are usually not treated.
(C) It is a self-limited disease and pregnant women should not be treated.
(D) Trimethoprim-sulfamethoxazole is indicated as a preventive measure when traveling in infested areas.
(E) When camping, *Giardia* infection can be prevented by drinking only water that is chlorinated or boiled.

37. A 16-year-old boy comes to the office complaining of a rash for 2 weeks. Upon examination of his skin you see scaly hypopigmented and hyperpigmented macules located over both shoulders, the sides of his neck, and a few macules even on his lower face. A Wood lamp examination shows a yellow or brownish fluorescence. Hyphae and spores are seen on the KOH wet prep. The most appropriate therapy for this rash is

(A) calcipotriene ointment
(B) discontinuation of all medications
(C) low-potency topical corticosteroids
(D) selenium sulfide shampoo
(E) topical trichloroacetic acid (TCA)

38. You get a call from the father of a 12-year-old girl. He tells you that he is out of town on a business trip and was just informed by the family taking care of his daughter at home that she has been diagnosed with mumps. He wants to know when it is "safe" for her to go to school. You advise him that according to the recommended policy she may return to school

(A) 1 week after the parotid gland swelling began
(B) 2 weeks after the parotid gland swelling began
(C) 6 days after the parotid gland swelling began
(D) 9 days after the parotid gland swelling began
(E) when she is fever free and feeling better

39. A 7-month-old boy is brought to the clinic by his mother because of a 2-day history of a cough. He developed a "runny nose" about 1-week ago, which she attributed to the upper respiratory illness that her teenage son had several weeks before that. The baby then developed a cough, which she describes as "rough" and "coming in fits". He has, on occasion turned red in the face while coughing, but has never become cyanotic. You notice in his chart that the last time the child was in the clinic for a routine visit was at 1-month of age, and when questioned the mother reports that he has not been seen by any other health care provider because of difficulties in the home. However, he has been completely well until this recent illness. His temperature is 37.0 C (98.6 F), pulse is 100/min, respirations are 33/min, and blood pressure is 100/60 mm Hg. His lung fields are clear, heart sounds are normal, and abdomen is unremarkable. He is in no respiratory distress, and a chest x-ray appears normal. He has a single paroxysm of coughing in your office that lasts approximately 1 minute. There is no color change associated with this episode. The most appropriate next step in management of this patient is to

(A) begin antibiotic therapy with amoxicillin for 7 to 10 days for presumptive bacterial pneumonia
(B) begin therapy with amantadine for presumptive influenza A infection
(C) obtain a nasopharyngeal culture for *Bordetella pertussis* and empiric therapy with erythromycin
(D) provide reassurance and reevaluate in 2 to 3 days
(E) repeat the chest x-ray in 1-week

40. A 3-year-old boy was walking around the family's living room when his parents noticed that he seemed to be "gagging and choking." He never had any real trouble breathing but they decided to bring him to the emergency department because after he stopped gagging, they gave him some ice cream (his favorite food) and they were alarmed when he spit it up immediately. The boy is now running around the examining room and looks very comfortable. He is otherwise healthy. Vital signs are: temperature 37.1 C (98.7 F), blood pressure 108/60 mm Hg, pulse 120/min, respirations 18/min, and oxygen saturation 96% on room air. His lungs sound clear to auscultation. The most appropriate next step in management is to

(A) admit the patient to the hospital for observation as a precaution
(B) give the patient something to eat, and if he swallows it without difficulty that will rule out any serious abnormality
(C) obtain a chest x-ray and if that is normal, reassure the parents that anything that made the patient gag has undoubtedly cleared
(D) obtain chest and neck x-rays, but regardless of their findings consult the otolaryngology team because of your high suspicion of an esophageal foreign body
(E) reassure his parents that because he seems comfortable in the emergency department and never developed respiratory distress that he should be clear to go home with them

41. During an annual physical examination an apparently healthy 16-year-old girl inquires about the freckles she first noticed on her face as a child. She complains that they have been increasing in number over the years and even started appearing on her hands. She is afraid that they make her look unattractive and would like to get rid of them. When you ask her about sun exposure and sun protection measures she admits to being an avid hiker but not a very consistent sunscreen user. On inspection, you note that she has blonde hair and blue eyes. Multiple small brown macules are present on the sun-exposed areas of her face, neck, shoulders, and dorsal hands. They are all homogeneous in color and 2 to 3 mm in diameter with smooth, well-demarcated borders. Otherwise, her skin examination is unremarkable. Concerning these macules, you should recommend

(A) complete avoidance of sun exposure because that will result in the freckles fading away
(B) daily use of a broad spectrum ultraviolet A and ultraviolet B sunscreen with an SPF of at least 15, along with wide-brimmed hats, long sleeves, and trousers if prolonged sun exposure is anticipated
(C) regular use of self-tanning preparations that will even out her skin color to make the freckles less noticeable as well as protect her during prolonged sun exposure
(D) that she really doesn't need to do anything because the freckles will eventually go away on their own
(E) ultraviolet A treatment to "harden" the skin before repeated prolonged sun exposure

Items 42-44

A previously healthy 16-year-old boy is brought to the clinic after "blacking out" a couple of times. These "blackouts" occurred on two separate occasions while practicing football alone in his backyard. He is the captain of his school team and the county tournament begins in 2 days. He denies any previous episodes, any visual disturbance, funny smells or tastes, numbness or tingling, or limb weakness. He has no breathing difficulties. His blood pressure is 100/60 mm Hg lying down and 100/65 mm Hg while standing, pulse is 65/min lying down and 67/min standing, and respirations are 16/min. There is no clubbing and all pulses are present and equal. He has an active precordium and there is a mid to late systolic murmur (grade 3/6) that increases when he stands. His neurological and funduscopic examinations are normal. His asks if he can play in the upcoming tournament.

42. The most appropriate response is:

(A) "Let me contact the football coach to see if there were any witnessed episodes, but you may continue playing for the moment."
(B) "Next time you play football be sure to have somebody with you to witness any further episodes."
(C) "Next time you play, stop if you notice any funny sensations, such as funny smells or visual disturbances."
(D) "No more strenuous exercise is allowed pending further evaluation."
(E) "You will not be allowed to participate in any contact sports, but low-impact sports such as swimming or track are fine from now on."

43. The boy's mother would like to know specifically what type of evaluation is going to be required for her son. You should explain that the best diagnostic study for this condition is an

(A) echocardiogram
(B) electrocardiogram
(C) electroencephalogram
(D) exercise stress test with supervision
(E) MRI of the brain

44. Two days later, you attend the first football game of the county high school tournament. You see that one of the players takes a hit to his helmet and you evaluate him on the sideline. He was disorientated for about 4 minutes after the hit, but he had no loss of consciousness. The remainder of the physical examination is normal. You are reminded that this player had similar symptoms after a hit 3 weeks earlier but he had been asymptomatic since that time. The most appropriate next step in management is to

(A) observe him on the sideline and then tell him he can return to play after he has been asymptomatic for 1 month

(B) observe him on the sideline and then tell him he can return to play after he has been asymptomatic for 1 week

(C) observe him on the sideline and then tell him he can return to play after he has been asymptomatic for 20 minutes

(D) transport him to the hospital and then tell him he can return to play after he has been asymptomatic for 1 month

(E) transport him to the hospital and tell him that he cannot play for the remainder of the season

45. You are working in the clinic and many children are brought in throughout the afternoon for well-child examinations. As part of the assessment of each child you need to document any evidence of developmental delay. The situation that would require documentation of developmental delay is

(A) an 18-month-old boy who pulls up to standing position and walks unaided

(B) a 5-month-old boy who utters no intelligible words to his parents

(C) a 5-year-old girl who is unable to copy a drawing of a square

(D) a 4-month-old girl who locates a sound by looking

(E) a 6-month-old boy is who unable to scribble with a crayon on paper

46. A 28-year-old second-year pathology resident that delivered a healthy, full-term baby boy 5 days earlier calls you at your office because of a rash her son developed the previous day that covers practically his entire body. The baby is otherwise doing well. The pregnancy was uneventful and lasted a full 42 weeks. He was 20 inches long and weighed 3950 g at birth. His Apgar scores were 9 and 9 at 1 and 5 minutes, respectively, and he has successfully started breast-feeding at home. He sleeps 2½ hours between feedings and does not seem to be in any distress. The mother tells you that he is covered with hundreds of pinpoint pustules with an erythematous halo. They are present everywhere: on the scalp, face, trunk, and extremities. Only the palms and soles are spared for now. She thinks that some of the lesions have already disappeared, but new ones have erupted, too. You stop by after work to check on the baby and you then confirm that the 5-day-old baby boy has over 100 discrete 1 to 2 mm pustules on an erythematous base, and also some erythematous papules interspersed. The palms and soles are indeed unaffected. He is sleeping peacefully and does not appear to be bothered by this rash at all. You reassure the mother that all will be well and describe this common condition to her. You should explain to her that the most likely histopathologic finding in this disorder is

(A) accumulation of eosinophils around the pilosebaceous follicle just below the dermoepidermal junction

(B) accumulation of mucin in the hair follicles with a lymphoid perifollicular infiltrate

(C) hyperkeratotic plugs in pilosebaceous orifice

(D) noninflammatory subepidermal blisters

(E) spongiotic vesicles in the epidermis

47. An 8-year-old girl is brought to the office by her parents for a skin lesion that appeared on her cheek about 2 months ago. They say it started as a pimple and grew very rapidly over several days to the size of a small pea. It has since bled several times rather profusely and they are scared that this will happen again. The girl is very irritated by it and constantly picks at it. Finally, when her teacher called you because of a bleeding episode in school, they made the appointment to see you. The child is otherwise healthy and has no medical problems. She does well in school and spends a lot of spare time playing outdoors with her neighborhood friends. You find the girl to be a talkative, pleasant 8-year-old in good overall health. On her right cheek there is a 0.5-mm reddish-brown, moderately firm, pedunculated nodule covered by crust-scale. The most appropriate therapeutic approach to this skin disorder is

(A) methods of physical destruction
(B) Mohs micrographic surgery
(C) no treatment is indicated at this time
(D) topical antibiotic ointments
(E) topical corticosteroid ointments

48. A 30-year-old woman gives birth to a full-term, 19-inch baby boy of 3200 grams after an unremarkable third pregnancy. The boy receives Apgar scores of 9 and 10 at 1 and 5 minutes, respectively, and only when he is cleaned and dried off you notice that on the right upper arm there are several confluent erythematous macules and papules that have a nodular component on palpation. They cover a total area of 10 cm^2. You reassure the mother that this is most likely a congenital hemangioma and that nothing needs to be done at the present time except regular followup to assess growth of the lesion and appropriate blood work. When the mother returns for the boy's 1- and 3-month followup visits, your records show that the lesion is progressively enlarging and now covers a total area of 30 cm^2. It is an ill-defined, dull red, mottled plaque with a bluish hue and a firm, multinodular deeper component on the right upper arm. The most appropriate laboratory analysis to detect a possibly fatal complication that can develop as a result of this lesion is

(A) differential white count
(B) erythrocyte sedimentation rate
(C) liver function tests
(D) platelet count
(E) urine analysis

49. A 28-year-old African American woman has just delivered a healthy baby girl at full term after an uneventful pregnancy. The baby weighs 3.5 kg and is 47 cm long. Her Apgar scores are 9 and 10 at 1 and 5 minutes, respectively. On close examination you notice that there are clusters of superficial vesicles and pustules under the chin and on the forehead. A few are present on the lower back and shins also. Some of them have ruptured during the first bathing only to leave a collarette of fine white scale surrounding a 1-mm hyperpigmented brown macule. The mother is concerned about these lesions. The most appropriate next step in management is to

(A) begin phototherapy
(B) prescribe oral antibiotic therapy
(C) prescribe topical antibiotic cream
(D) provide reassurance that no treatment is necessary
(E) provide topical corticosteroid cream

50. A 3-year-old girl is brought to your office by her parents because of a skin eruption that developed while she was visiting her grandparents at the shore. They tell you the child was healthy when she left 2 weeks ago, and everything was fine until 10 days later when the lesions started appearing. The grandparents noted that the child had multiple mosquito bites on her arms and legs but did not treat them. They got alarmed when she developed blisters at the sites of the insect bites, and by the time her parents arrived to pick her up, many of these had ruptured to leave weepy, crusted areas that the girl persistently scratches. They also noticed she had become weak and had been febrile for the past 2 days. On physical examination you find the child to be in mild distress with a temperature of 37.8 C (100 F), pulse of 100/min, and respirations of 22/min. Her height and weight are appropriate for her age. On the skin of the trunk and extremities there are multiple moist, weepy, denuded circular areas with yellowish, purulent crusting, peripheral scale, and small bullae adjacent to them. Bullae on an erythematous base are seen interspersed between the circular patches. There are also many excoriations. In addition to an oral medication, the most appropriate topical medication is

(A) azelaic acid
(B) fluocinonide
(C) hydroquinone
(D) ketoconazole
(E) mupirocin

Pediatrics Test Four: **Answers and Explanations**

ANSWER KEY

1. C
2. A
3. E
4. D
5. A
6. C
7. A
8. C
9. B
10. D
11. B
12. A
13. D
14. E
15. C
16. A
17. B
18. E
19. B
20. C
21. D
22. C
23. D
24. B
25. E
26. C
27. E
28. A
29. E
30. A
31. A
32. D
33. B
34. C
35. B
36. B
37. D
38. D
39. C
40. D
41. B
42. D
43. A
44. B
45. C
46. A
47. A
48. D
49. D
50. E

1. **The correct answer is C.** This patient has neonatal herpes, and performing a Tzanck smear will help visualize multinucleated giant cells with intranuclear inclusions found in scrapings from the base of a blister. Frequently, an apparently previously well newborn will become ill on the fourth to eighth day of life and develop vesicular lesions on the skin or buccal mucosa. The lesions may be erythematous depressed patches or vesicles with an erythematous halo that become pustules within 24 hours and continue to become crusted or ulcerate over the next few days. Purpura, petechiae, erosions, and large blisters may also develop. The scalp and face are most commonly affected as they are in prolonged contact with the cervical area from which the infection is transmitted during childbirth. At times, conjunctivitis and keratoconjunctivitis may be seen as the presenting sign. This is subsequently followed by lethargy, anorexia, fever, hepatitis, pneumonia, coagulopathy, and central nervous system involvement with irritability, bulging fontanelles, seizures, paralysis, opisthotonus, or coma in the most severe cases. If untreated, neonatal herpes will end fatally in 90% of cases. Early treatment, therefore, within 24 hours of onset preferably, should be initiated if there is suspicion of neonatal herpes. The diagnosis may be aided by a Tzanck smear, viral cultures, or biopsy of the cutaneous lesions.

   A KOH examination (**choice A**) is performed when skin infection with a yeast or dermatophyte is suspected. This simple test helps visualize spores, hyphae, and pseudohyphae present in scrapings of skin taken from the suspicious lesion. It is easily performed in the office setting and does not require more than 10 to 20 minutes to complete (although it may take longer to examine some specimens if the fungal elements are scarce).

   A scotch tape test (**choice B**) is performed in search of ova and parasites in the stool of a patient. It is best done in the morning before the patient has defecated and wiped or washed the perianal area. A strip of scotch tape is applied to the anus and perianal skin and firmly pressed. Subsequent microscopic examination commonly yields evidence of ova or parasites in infestations such as pinworm and hookworm.

   Wood light examination of the skin (**choice D**) would be indicated if the patient were suspected of having an infection of the skin, such as tinea versicolor or erythrasma. It is also useful in disorders of pigmentation to differentiate between epidermally and dermally located pigment (epidermal pigment or lack thereof is enhanced by Wood light, whereas dermal pigment remains the same color).

   Wood light examination of the urine (**choice E**) is used in the diagnosis of porphyrias. A sample of freshly voided urine is stored for 2 hours to facilitate oxidation of uroporphyrins that subsequently fluoresce a coral red color when exposed to Wood light.

2. **The correct answer is A.** The most likely diagnosis is a hydrocele. It is usually present at birth, but may occur at a later age. Hydroceles are usually asymptomatic. If the swelling is in the inguinal or inguinoscrotal area it may be difficult to differentiate from a hernia. Observation and followup are the appropriate management. Most hydroceles will spontaneously resolve.

   This is not a case of testicular torsion, tumor, or incarcerated hernia that would need immediate surgery (**choice B**).

   Elective surgery is rarely needed in such cases. If a hernia is found in association with the hydrocele then surgery can be planned electively in the near future (**choice C**).

   Genetic consultation is not necessary (**choice D**). Hydroceles do not suggest genetic conditions.

   A testicular scan might only be indicated if the diagnosis was unclear (**choice E**).

3. **The correct answer is E.** This young girl has a history for cat scratch disease (CSD). Typically, the incubation period is 1 to 2 weeks following a cat (usually kitten) scratch. There may be appearance of a cutaneous papule and then regional lymphadenopathy follows. The gram-negative bacterium responsible for CSD is *Bartonella henselae*. Management is usually symptomatic, but in this case because of the pain and mother's distress you opt to treat with trimethoprim-sulfamethoxazole. Ciprofloxacin and rifampin are alternative choices of therapy.

   Sometimes with CSD the affected nodes suppurate and aspiration is necessary. In this vignette aspiration is not necessary (**choice A**).

   Infrequently with CSD there is a solitary nodule or a systemic illness that could be confused with malignancy, and biopsy or node excision may be required (**choice B**). This child has the more classic presentation of CSD, however, with regional lymphadenopathy following a history for kitten scratch.

   A chest x-ray is not indicated (**choice C**).

   A PPD may be placed if the diagnosis is confusing, particularly if there is no history of kitten contact (**choice D**).

4. **The correct answer is D.** The data given in this case are suggestive of a psychogenic cough. There is no nighttime awakening and the Monday morning absences from school may even suggest school phobia. The cough has not been responsive to medications and the boy is otherwise well. Exploring the psychosocial factors in this case is important, as is seeking appropriate counseling.

   Referral to an allergist is not indicated at this time. There is no indication that this cough is caused by allergies (**choice A**).

   A chest x-ray is not indicated at this time (**choice B**). In this case there is enough information to suggest a psychophysiologic basis for symptoms, and one should seek to obtain further data about school, family, or life stressors. Performing studies to rule out organic disease would not be indicated first.

   Over-the-counter cough medication has been tried before without success, so would not likely be helpful (**choice C**). Cough medications with codeine also should not be prescribed.

   A PPD would be a good screening test, but not the best first step in this case (**choice E**). It is important to address underlying behavioral and psychogenic issues.

5. **The correct answer is A.** This child has rubella (German measles), one of the most benign of all diseases of childhood, except for possible infection of the fetus during pregnancy. A pregnant woman who contracts rubella in the first trimester of pregnancy has a high probability that intrauterine transmission will give rise to the congenital rubella syndrome. The portal of entry of the rubella virus is the respiratory mucosa, and the incubation period is 16 to 18 days. The exanthem begins around the hairline and face and spreads rapidly to involve the trunk and extremities within 24 hours. The rash is evanescent and generally disappears within 3 days. The clinical diagnosis in the 8-year-old girl is suggested by the maculopapular rash that begins on the face, progresses rapidly downward to the trunk and extremities, and subsides within a few days. Postoccipital and postauricular lymphadenopathy is characteristic, although not specific, for it may be seen, albeit not as consistently, with other infectious diseases such as measles, chickenpox, adenovirus infections, infectious mononucleosis, and others. A low-grade fever may or may not be present, and, with the lymphadenopathy, precedes the rash by a day or 2. In older children and adults, arthritis may affect approximately 30% of females and 5% of males. It usually involves the small joints of the hands and feet, knees, elbows, shoulders, and spine. It may last up to 2 weeks and be associated with an elevated erythrocyte sedimentation rate and false-positive latex fixation test that generally reverts to normal within 18 months. Other rare complications include thrombocytopenic purpura and encephalitis. Present prophylactic recommendations include vaccination of all children with the live attenuated vaccine alone or in combination with mumps and measles (MMR) at age 15 months, and revaccination at age 11 to 12 years. In addition, prenatal or antepartum screening for rubella infection should be routinely undertaken, but vaccination during pregnancy is not recommended because infection of the fetus with the live attenuated virus is a possibility.

   Congenital rubella occurs following maternal rubella infection during the first 20 weeks of pregnancy. Therefore, the second trimester of pregnancy (**choice B**), third trimester of pregnancy (**choice C**), the entire pregnancy (**choice D**), and the neonatal period (**choice E**) are incorrect. The earlier in pregnancy the infection develops, the greater the risk for the fetus.

6. **The correct answer is C.** The silent incubation period for infection with tuberculosis to development of a positive tuberculin skin test is 2 to 12 weeks.

   One to 6 months is not the incubation period for tuberculosis (**choice A**).

   Two to 4 weeks is the approximate incubation period for mumps, not tuberculosis (**choice B**).

   Ten to 21 days is the incubation period for varicella, not tuberculosis (**choice D**).

   Ten to 90 days is the approximate incubation time for primary syphilis, not tuberculosis (**choice E**).

7. **The correct answer is A.** Generally, if the burn is less than 10% burn surface area for an infant (or less than 15% for a child) and there is no third degree or full thickness burn, then outpatient management with followup is appropriate. If critical body areas are involved, however, including the face, hands, and perineum, or if potentially dangerous types of burn such as electrical or those with other life-threatening injury potential, then inpatient management is recommended.

   Child protective services should be notified when burns appear to have resulted from abusive injury. One needs to consider whether the burn pattern fits the history of what occurred and if there was delay in seeking medical care. In this case the scalding injury fit the described accident (**choice B**). Scalding is the most common type of burn during the first 3 years of life. Usually a child pulls a cup of coffee or cocoa from the counter or a pot down from the stove.

CBC, serum glucose, electrolytes, BUN, and creatinine are obtained with more life-threatening burns or those with greater than 10% body surface area (**choice C**).

Cleaning the wound with water and applying 1% topical silver sulfadiazine cream may be used in the management of partial thickness burns; however, the best answer is to admit this patient to the hospital (**choice D**).

Sometimes, in addition to topical silver sulfadiazine cream, prophylactic antibiotics may be used for severe burns. The most appropriate first step, however, would be to admit the child to the hospital (**choice E**).

8. **The correct answer is C.** Glycemic control is difficult to achieve during adolescence. In boys, the peak height velocity occurs usually between 14 and 15 years of age at SMR of 3 or 4. This boy is surely undergoing physical as well as hormonal and psychologic changes. As he reaches these mid-teenage years, blood glucose control may deteriorate and insulin requirements change.

   The diabetic "honeymoon period" usually begins within a few weeks after the diabetes is diagnosed and initial insulin therapy begins. The duration of the honeymoon may be weeks to months. This boy was diagnosed two years ago, however, so this is not the correct answer (**choice A**).

   This boy has a red throat but no other signs or symptoms that would indicate he has some underlying infection (**choice B**).

   Renal disease would be unlikely to present within the first 2 years after the diagnosis of diabetes (**choice D**). Diabetic nephropathy would usually not cause clinical problems for several years after diagnosis.

   Somogyi effect (**choice E**) refers to a rebound hyperglycemia following an episode of hypoglycemia. As one attempts to achieve better diabetic control with increasing doses of insulin, Somogyi phenomenon can occur in response to very low blood sugars. Hypoglycemia would go unrecognized, especially in the middle of the night, and then there would be rebound hyperglycemia in the morning. This patient has problems with high blood glucose throughout the day and the control problems are more likely related to puberty.

9. **The correct answer is B.** This boy has evidence of a hemolytic process with significant anemia, reticulocytosis, and hyperbilirubinemia. Together with a history of sulfamethoxazole therapy, this boy most likely has an illness caused by glucose-6-phosphate dehydrogenase (G6PD). G6PD deficiency is the most common hereditary enzyme disorder. It is an important cause of neonatal jaundice and also causes life-threatening hemolytic crisis in childhood. Illnesses and exposure to certain drugs such as antimalarials, sulfas, and nitrofurantoins cause hemolysis among G6PD deficiency patients. The frequency and severity is influenced by genetic factors. It is common in Mediterranean, African, and some East Asian populations. A G6PD assay needs to be determined after the hemolytic episode is over, because at times of increased reticulocytosis the level of enzyme in the red cells will be higher than usual.

   A bone marrow examination would only help establish that there is a hemolytic process going on with evidence of increased erythropoietic activity (**choice A**).

   Just as the direct Coombs test was negative, an indirect Coombs would also be negative in this case of G6PD. It would not be a helpful test. The indirect Coombs tests for the presence of anti-RBC antibodies in the serum. It would be positive in immunohemolytic anemias (**choice C**).

   A Monospot test would not be indicated (choice D). Infectious mononucleosis can cause thrombocytopenia and, more rarely, hemolytic anemia. There are really no symptoms or physical signs to suggest that this is mononucleosis (e.g., hepatosplenomegaly, lymphadenopathy, and thrombocytopenia).

   Pyruvate kinase deficiency is a very rare disease and usually occurs in individuals of northern European descent. Peripheral smear in these patients may show echinocytes or spiculated red blood cells. Although pyruvate kinase deficiency may also result in severe hemolytic anemic episodes triggered by infections, G6PD deficiency would be much more common a diagnosis and is particularly suggested by this patient's history of being African American and taking sulfa medication (choice E).

10. **The correct answer is D.** The attack rate of staphylococcal poisoning refers to the incidence rate expressed as a percent. It is obtained by dividing the total number of persons who became sick by the total number of persons who could have become sick, or those who attended the party. Thus, it is 14 + 11 divided by 14 + 11 + 33 = 25/58 = 43.1%.

The answer of 25.0 is incorrect, as this is the number of ill cases, not the attack rate (**choice A**).

The answer of 25.0% is also incorrect, but has been expressed as a percent (**choice B**).

The answer 43.1 needs to be expressed as a percent (**choice C**).

The answer of 75.8%, or the ratio of cases to noncases, is not the correct answer (**choice E**).

11. **The correct answer is B.** With lower lobe pneumonia, children commonly refer pain to the upper abdomen. In this case, pneumonia is suggested because of the fever, tachypnea, and abdominal pain. A chest x-ray should be obtained first.

An ultrasound may be helpful in identifying certain abdominal diseases such as cholecystitis, but would not be the best to order in this vignette (**choice A**).

If a diagnosis of pneumonia is made either clinically or by x-ray, a CBC and blood culture may not be necessary. It is not the next best step (**choice C**).

Serum amylase and lipase might be obtained, especially if one suspects pancreatitis and gallbladder disease. These conditions are uncommon in childhood. Although they may both display right upper quadrant tenderness on examination, the acute onset of illness and tachypnea would make these diagnoses less likely (**choice D**).

Five-year-old children may not localize abdominal pains very well, but the physical examination reveals upper quadrant tenderness, which would not really support a diagnosis of urinary tract infection. This child is old enough that other symptoms such as urinary frequency and dysuria might be present. If all other tests were normal, a urine culture might be obtained, but it is not the first or best choice answer (**choice E**).

12. **The correct answer is A.** After 3 to 4 days of antibiotics, the child with otitis should be better either in symptoms or upon ear examination, if indeed the causative organisms are sensitive to treatment. That the child still has low-grade fever and earache suggests that a change in antibiotics is needed. Amoxicillin-clavulanate would be a good choice. If on the other hand she is clinically much worse, then a full reevaluation is needed to be sure another underlying diagnosis (such as meningitis or sepsis) was not missed.

If she is really unchanged and still has fever and earache, then continuing the antibiotic for a full week course is not the best answer (**choice B**).

A CBC and blood culture would not be helpful because she is no worse and this vignette does not provide additional symptoms of concern to warrant further workup (**choice C**).

Although from a purist point of view it might be of interest to identify the causative organism, it would not be practical to perform myringotomies on children who did not get better in 2 to 3 days after initiation of antibiotics (**choice D**). A myringotomy would be an appropriate procedure to perform if the child was less than 6 weeks old, had an underlying immune disorder, or if the otitis persisted after 2 or more courses of different antibiotics.

Research has not consistently shown that antihistamine/decongestant combinations are efficacious in the treatment of otitis media and this is not the best answer (**choice E**).

13. **The correct answer is D.** The blood level of 100 mg/dL would not entirely explain this girl's unconscious state. Instead, it would correlate with less severe symptoms including impaired speech and behavior and drowsiness. Although it is true that more toxic levels (200 mg/dL) would lead to unconsciousness, hypoglycemia, and respiratory failure, because the blood alcohol level in this case is lower one must look for additional drug ingestion. Alcohol may potentiate the sedative effects of other drugs, notably narcotics or antidepressants. Screening needs to be done for other likely drugs.

An ammonia level would be unlikely to be useful in this case. Ammonia levels may be mildly elevated in cases such as this but these mild elevations are not of significance (**choice A**).

A CBC would not be helpful in the management of this case. There is nothing to suggest significant trauma or underlying problem of anemia. It is not the next best step (**choice B**).

Severe alcohol poisoning can result in metabolic acidosis and, importantly, in hypoglycemia. Starting an IV with D5W or D10W can be an important first step in management. With an initial normal blood glucose (85 mg/dL), hypoglycemia or accompanying acidosis is not the cause of her condition (**choice C**).

This girl's physical examination is normal and there is no evidence of injury or focal neurologic signs to suggest a significant fall or intracranial bleed (**choice E**).

14. **The correct answer is E.** This is a case of external otitis that should be initially treated with topical antibiotics. An additional first step in management is to gently remove the debris in the canal and use ear wicks to get the antibiotic drops effectively in the canal. Antibiotics should be chosen for their coverage against the most frequent pathogens, *Pseudomonas aeruginosa* and *Staphylococcus aureus.*

Oral antibiotics would not be the best initial management of otitis externa (**choice A**).

Cultures would be necessary only in cases resistant to therapy or in immunocompromised hosts (**choice B**).

Steroid drops may be effective in decreasing the inflammation, but should be used in combination with antibiotics (**choice C**).

Postauricular swelling, erythema, and edema might suggest mastoiditis or osteomyelitis of the temporal bone. These symptoms are not present in this vignette and these conditions are very rare in association with otitis. This case would not warrant a CT scan (**choice D**).

15. **The correct answer is C.** This girl has a typical case of measles (morbilli, rubeola), an infectious disease caused by the Morbillivirus and transmitted through respiratory droplets. It is not as common as it used to be because of obligatory immunization of children worldwide. After an incubation period of approximately 10 days, the prodromal symptoms of fever, malaise, and upper respiratory catarrh begin acutely. The conjunctivae are injected and there may be photophobia. From the second day, Koplik spots are usually present on the buccal mucous membrane opposite the premolar teeth. They appear as bluish-white spots with bright red areolae. Fever, catarrh, and cough increase for 3 to 5 days. The exanthem typically develops on or around the fourth day on the forehead and behind the ears, and then spreads "like a shower" to the face, trunk, and limbs. At first it is macular, and then dull red papules form with a tendency to coalesce into irregular concentric patterns or become more diffusely confluent. From the sixth to the twentieth day the rash starts fading, leaving behind brownish discoloration and fine scaling. In very severe forms it may become hemorrhagic. Complications are more common in young children, the malnourished, and the chronically ill. Bronchopneumonia, enteritis, and otitis have decreased in incidence with the advent of efficacious antibiotics. The most serious complication, encephalitis, develops in 1 out of 200 affected children. Specific antibodies become detectable 3 to 4 days after the rash appears, and maximum titers are reached 2 to 4 weeks later. Viral antigen can be detected by immunofluorescence in cell smears from the nasopharynx early in the course of the illness. Treatment consists of bedrest, symptomatic therapy, and antibiotics to control secondary bacterial complications. Passive protection is possible using normal human immunoglobulin given within 5 days of exposure, which prevents or attenuates the infection in contacts, and should be used only for children at special risk. Active immunization with the live attenuated vaccine (MMR, measles-mumps-rubella) has reduced the incidence of measles infection but may be followed by a mild illness and rash in the 3 weeks following immunization.

Forscheimer sign (**choice A**) is an enanthem observed in up to 20% of patients during the prodromal period or first day of the rash in rubella (German measles). Petechiae or reddish pinpoint or larger spots on the soft palate constitute this sign.

The herald patch (**choice B**) is the prototypical skin lesion of Pityriasis rosea, a benign self-limiting disease of unknown etiology. It frequently begins with a single herald or mother patch that is usually larger than succeeding lesions and may persist alone for a week or 2 before the other lesions appear. The incidence is highest between the ages of 15 to 40, and the disease is most prevalent in the spring and autumn. Women are more frequently affected.

Strawberry tongue (**choice D**) is seen with scarlet fever, a bacterial infection caused by beta-hemolytic streptococcus group A, most frequently seen in school-age children. A denuded, red tongue with prominent edematous papillae is characteristic.

A vesicular enanthem (**choice E**) may be seen in a variety of viral infections, most commonly but not limited to varicella, primary herpetic gingivostomatitis, and hand-foot-and-mouth disease. It is useful to remember that vesicular lesions in the mouth accompany vesicular lesions of the skin. If the skin rash is not vesicular, chances are that the enanthem won't be either.

16. **The correct answer is A.** Erythromycin is recommended for all household and other close contacts of a patient with *Bordetella pertussis* (whooping cough) to prevent secondary transmission.

Prophylactic antibiotics are sometimes used in human bites, especially those caused by closed-fist injuries. Coverage is needed for staphylococcus, streptococcus, and Eikenella corrodens organisms. Amoxicillin-clavulanate would be a good choice, but not erythromycin (**choice B**).

Not all cases of *Salmonella* must be treated. When therapy is indicated, amoxicillin, trimethoprim-sulfamethoxazole, and third-generation cephalosporins are all good choices, not erythromycin (**choice C**).

Secondarily infected tinea should be handled as impetigo with antibiotics such as amoxicillin-clavulanate or dicloxacillin, not erythromycin (**choice D**).

Amoxicillin may still be the drug of choice for sinusitis. Amoxicillin-clavulanate and third-generation cephalosporins may be used, but erythromycin is not the most ideal pharmacotherapy (**choice E**).

17. **The correct answer is B.** Meningomyeloceles are commonly associated with hydrocephalus and Arnold-Chiari malformation. A CT scan is indicated.

There is not a high association of meningomyeloceles with congenital heart disease (**choice A**).

There is not an increased incidence of cataracts or eye diseases with meningomyeloceles (**choice C**).

Polycystic kidneys or other renal anomalies are not commonly associated with meningomyeloceles (**choice D**).

Developmental dysplasia of the hip is not commonly associated with meningomyeloceles (**choice E**). Many times developmental dysplasia of the hip can be detected on physical examination. When the diagnosis is unclear a sonogram may be obtained.

18. **The correct answer is E**. The signs and symptoms in this 12-month-old infant should suggest the diagnosis of intussusception. Even during the peak season for rotavirus, all possible diagnoses must be considered for children presenting with vomiting and diarrhea. One cannot assume that it is just another case of gastroenteritis. The on-and-off nature of the abdominal distress and the passage of a bloody mucus stool (a possible currant jelly stool) must alert one to the possibility of intussusception. This infant must be evaluated right away in the ER, not simply wait to be seen in the morning. For most cases of intussusception the cause is not known; however, adenovirus or rotavirus infections may be predisposing factors.

Recommendations about feeding should not be given until the infant is evaluated (**choice A**).

This infant should be further evaluated for possible surgical diagnosis right away (**choice B**). The passage of a currant jelly-like stool is a late finding in intussusception.

In episodes of gastroenteritis, breast-feeding may be continued; however, this infant needs to be seen in the emergency department to rule out other etiologies for the vomiting and abdominal pains (**choice C**).

With intussusception there may be low-grade fever, but giving Tylenol elixir may only mask the symptoms and further delay the appropriate treatment (**choice D**).

19. **The correct answer is B**. Inadequate dietary intake of iron is the most important cause of iron deficiency among adolescents.

Excessive milk drinking can decrease the absorption of iron and is a contributing factor in iron deficiency for infants, but it is unlikely to be a cause of iron deficiency among teens. Most teenagers lack sufficient calcium intake and do not usually get enough milk products in their diet (**choice A**).

There is an increased need for iron during puberty, however this girl is 3 years past menarche so nearly all of her pubertal growth is complete. It is not the most important factor in iron deficiency among adolescents (**choice C**).

Heavy menstrual periods may account for iron loss, but nothing in this vignette suggests that the girl has prolonged or more frequent menses (**choice D**).

The prevalence of iron deficiency anemia may be higher in athletic adolescents, but iron deficiency is more likely to be the result of increased calorie requirement and inadequate dietary intake of iron. Proteinuria and microscopic hematuria have been reported in long-distance runners, but this would not likely cause significant iron deficiency anemia (**choice E**).

20. **The correct answer is C**. This infant with a new onset of strabismus must be seen by the ophthalmologist right away. He may have retinoblastoma. The differential diagnosis for a white pupillary reflex (leukocoria) includes other eye conditions such as a cataract. The ophthalmologist is the best consultant to help distinguish retinoblastoma from other disorders.

A CT scan is not the next best step (**choice A**). In a case of retinoblastoma, however, it may reveal intraocular calcifications.

This infant has strabismus but no other neurologic symptoms, such as increased intracranial pressure or cranial nerve palsies, to support a referral to neurology (**choice B**).

A renal scan is not necessary in this infant with eye problems. Retinoblastoma does not metastasize to the kidney (**choice D**).

TORCH (toxoplasmosis, other agents, rubella, cytomegalovirus, and herpes) titers would not be the best initial step in workup. The intrauterine infections, including toxoplasmosis, rubella, cytomegalovirus, and herpes, may all be associated with congenital cataracts (**choice E**).

21. **The correct answer is D**. There is enough information to suggest possible child abuse and child protective services need to be involved. This injury is unlikely to be caused by such a fall.

    Activated partial thromboplastin time (aPTT), prothrombin time (PT), and platelet count (**choice A**) are all screening tests to investigate for possible bleeding disorders such as hemophilia. They may be important tests to perform, especially if there is other evidence of bruising or bleeding, however, this is not the next best step in management. The swelling without early bruising suggests child abuse.

    Calcium and phosphate levels (**choice B**) are unlikely to be helpful in this case. There is no mention that the skull x-ray revealed osteoporosis or other underlying bone abnormalities.

    CBC and platelet count (**choice C**) would not be the first steps in management of this case.

    A skeletal survey (**choice E**) may be useful in children less than 3 years of age in the workup for child abuse, especially if other injuries are suspected. It is not, however, the next best step.

22. **The correct answer is C.** There is enough information in this case to suggest that this boy may have tuberous sclerosis, and genetic counseling is needed. Tuberous sclerosis is an autosomal dominant neurocutaneous disorder associated with hypopigmented oval macules with irregular borders ("ash-leaf spots") and adenoma sebaceum. The hypopigmented macules may light up and appear as a bright violet color under a Wood lamp. Adenoma sebaceum lesions may be confused with acne. They consist of pink to red facial papules that frequently occur in early childhood years before puberty. They represent angiofibromas and occur typically on the cheek, chin, and malar areas of the face. Tuberous sclerosis is associated with mental retardation, seizures, and tumors of the brain, heart, and kidney. A family history for seizures is given in this vignette. Seizures are the most common presenting complaint of tuberous sclerosis.

    The described facial papules are unlikely to be acne (**choice A**). They are not comedones or pustular lesions and they are not present at the typical regions for acne (such as in the nasolabial folds and on the shoulders and back). The occurrence of acne after the first few months of life and before 8 years of age is rare. The clinical description of the hypopigmented spots is not sufficient to suggest a fungal infection.

    Benzoyl peroxide is an effective topical agent for acne, however, the facial papules are not acne (**choice B**).

    A serum testosterone would not be useful (**choice D**). Androgens are important in the pathogenesis of acne, but serum free and total testosterone levels are frequently normal.

    Topical steroid cream or ointment is not indicated for these papules and macules (**choice E**). There is no history to suggest these skin lesions may be caused by other disorders, such as atopic dermatitis.

23. **The correct answer is D.** The most common presentation of Wilms tumor is an asymptomatic abdominal mass. The mean age for presentation is 3 years. Wilms tumor is known to be associated with the chromosome deletion involving 11p13. It may invade the inferior vena cava in more advanced cases.

    Wilms tumor is unlikely to metastasize to the bones and therefore it would be rare to have an abnormal bone scan (**choice A**). Wilms tumor may more frequently metastasize to the lungs.

    Wilms tumor is unlikely to metastasize to the brain and therefore it would be rare to have an abnormal brain scan (**choice B**).

    Urinary vanillylmandelic acid is commonly elevated in children with neuroblastoma, not Wilms tumor (**choice C**).

    The N-*myc* gene is associated with neuroblastoma, not Wilms tumor (**choice E**). Children with neuroblastoma might present with an abdominal mass, but they typically have symptoms of fever, weight loss, and irritability. Anemia is frequently present. Neuroblastoma metastasizes to the bone.

24. **The correct answer is B.** This 4-year-old boy most certainly has acute lymphoblastic leukemia (ALL). The bone marrow will surely show a number of blast cells. This boy has lymphadenopathy, probably splenomegaly, anemia, neutropenia, and thrombocytopenia. Some children with *all* also present with signs and symptoms

of fever, anorexia, bone pain, bleeding, ecchymoses, and hepatomegaly.

Sometimes a sepsis workup is indicated in the child with *all*, but unless the child is critically ill, the bone marrow evaluation is performed first (**choice A**).

A Monospot will not be helpful (**choice C**). Infectious mononucleosis may frequently be asymptomatic. Decreased platelet count and neutropenia may be seen, but there is usually lymphocytosis with atypical lymphocytes.

A lumbar puncture is performed as part of the workup of *all* because there may be occult CNS involvement at the time of diagnosis (**choice D**). The bone marrow evaluation is performed first, however, to establish the diagnosis.

Herniorrhaphy needs to be postponed and preoperative tests canceled. A preoperative type and cross-match (**choice E**) of blood for surgery, therefore, is not indicated.

25. **The correct answer is E.** Despite large-scale publicity of small, uncontrolled studies that purport to demonstrate a link between vaccines and autism, this association has been consistently disproved in subsequent larger trials. There is no evidence linking MMR (or any other vaccine) with autism or any other developmental disorder.

The delivery of multiple antigens together as components of combination vaccines has been an enormous boon to pediatricians, parents, and patients. The currently licensed combination vaccines (including MMR) must demonstrate that co-administration of the components provides sufficient immunogenicity without increasing the incidence of side effects (**choice A**).

As mentioned above, there is no epidemiologically established link between MMR and autism. Other than some special clinical circumstances (such as immunodeficiency), there is no reason to postpone the administration of MMR beyond the recommended time period of 12 to 15 months of age (**choice B**).

The current vaccine schedule calls for the delivery of multiple vaccines at a single visit. To date, studies have not demonstrated a decrease in efficacy or an increase of side effects when delivering the recommended combinations of injections at separate sites on the same day (**choice C**). Thus, the administration of MMR and the varicella vaccine on the same day should pose no increased risk to this child.

Both MMR and varicella vaccine are live-attenuated viral vaccines that rely on induction of T-cell immunity for protection from disease. There is no indication that either this class of vaccine or any other predisposes recipients to developmental disorders (**choice D**).

26. **The correct answer is C.** Blood pressure measurements are screened during well child visits beginning at 3 years of age. Determinations of blood pressure may be necessary before this time if a child has an underlying pediatric condition such as known kidney disease.

Routine blood pressures are not taken at 6 months of age (**choice A**).

Blood pressures are not routinely taken at the 1-year checkup (**choice B**).

Blood pressure measurements should be taken at the 3-year-old well visit and annually thereafter (**choice D**).

Blood pressures are taken routinely after age 3 years (**choice E**). Their determination should also be considered part of a full cardiac examination.

27. **The correct answer is E.** Titers for the more common viral intrauterine infections (TORCH stands for toxoplasmosis, other agents, rubella, cytomegalovirus, and herpes) would be a good first step in the workup for a small infant with language delay. All of these infections may lead to intrauterine growth retardation, and affected children will continue to grow on the low percentiles of the growth chart. Rubella and cytomegalovirus may cause sensorineural hearing losses and result in mental retardation. These problems may first be noticed as speech delay.

A bone age is unlikely to be helpful (**choice A**). This infant does not have global developmental delay or findings of endocrinopathy.

A CT of the head is unlikely to reveal the underlying etiology (**choice B**). Many intrauterine infections or genetic disorders associated with mental retardation may have abnormalities including intracerebral calcifications. This test is nonspecific, especially with the absence of any neurologic signs on physical examination.

A genetic consultation is unlikely to be helpful because no specific anomalies are present (**choice C**). Some genetic syndromes are associated with small size and microcephaly, but usually additional birth defects or anomalies are present.

Thyroid disease is unlikely to present with less than fifth percentile height and weight, microcephaly, and speech delay (**choice D**). Infants with hypothyroidism may be asymptomatic or present with intellectual retardation, growth delay, and delay in suture closure. They would not have microcephaly.

28. **The correct answer is A.** The infant has physical examination findings that suggest trisomy 21 or Down syndrome. Children with Down syndrome have an increased risk for congenital heart disease, duodenal atresia, pelvic dysplasia, and hypothyroidism. Duodenal atresia usually presents with progressive vomiting during the first day of life. An abdominal x-ray reveals the classic "double bubble" with distention of the stomach and proximal duodenum. There is absence of air distal to the obstruction.

    Echocardiogram and EKG may be obtained in infants with Down syndrome suspected to have congenital heart disease. Generally a murmur, cyanosis, or signs of cardiac failure may suggest a heart defect. Vomiting would be a late or unusual symptom for underlying heart disease (**choice B**).

    Electrolytes, BUN, and creatinine may be ordered if an underlying renal disorder is suspected. There does not appear to be a strong consistent association of Down syndrome with renal malformations. In a newborn with Down syndrome, gastrointestinal anomalies need to be considered first (**choice C**).

    No consistent data suggest any association of CNS anomalies with Down syndrome, so an MRI (**choice D**) of the head is not indicated.

    There is an increased incidence of hypothyroidism among children with Down syndrome. Vomiting is usually not a symptom of thyroid disease, however, therefore, serum T_4 and TSH levels (**choice E**) are not indicated at this time.

29. **The correct answer is E.** This girl most likely has scarlet fever. A fine maculopapular or papular rash that blanches with pressure and begins in the groin, neck area, and axilla should be considered group A streptococcal infection until proven otherwise. A throat culture should be obtained. Although the details of an HEENT examination were not given in this vignette, she most likely has some degree of pharyngitis. Some children with scarlet fever may not complain of sore throat.

    A CBC and blood cultures are unnecessary if the throat culture is positive for strep. Blood cultures should be obtained in cases in which a child is suspected to have sepsis. This girl appears well (**choice A**).

    There is not enough information to suggest that this girl has a diagnosis of systemic lupus erythematosus or other collagen vascular disease, so a complete blood count, an ESR, and ANA are not needed (**choice B**).

    Reassurance that it is nothing serious is not a correct answer (**choice C**). If this rash were related to the earlier administration of MMR, then reassurance should be given. A rash and mild illness following MMR should occur within 5 to 12 days, however, not 2½ weeks later. If a mild viral illness with a rash is considered, it is fine to follow her over time. A throat culture needs to be done, however, to ensure she does not have strep.

    A rubella titer is unnecessary as she just had her second immunization (**choice D**).

30. **The correct answer is A.** All siblings who are ill should probably have rapid strep tests. Classic strep throat affects children ages 3 years and older. Children frequently have fever, vomiting, and sore throat. Children younger than 3 years of age may have a streptococcal illness presenting with low-grade fever and nasopharyngitis. If any sibling at home is sick he should be examined, cultured, and treated if positive.

    It is not advisable to perform rapid strep tests on siblings who are completely well or asymptomatic (**choice B**).

    Although it is true that siblings over 3 years of age should have rapid strep tests if they have pharyngitis or sore throat, one cannot ignore siblings who are 3 years or less (**choice C**). If they are sick with low-grade fever, nasopharyngitis, and cervical adenopathy, they too should be tested for strep.

    It is sensible for the child to stay home until he has been afebrile for 24 hours. In the case of strep throat, however, he must receive at least 24 hours of antibiotics before returning to school (**choice D**).

    The boy does not have to wait for 3 days of antibiotics before returning to school (**choice E**).

31. **The correct answer is A.** The physician would be liable. Although the service was rendered free, by offering to advise/treat, the physician had established a physician/patient relationship that is binding. The courts would not entertain the defendant's contention that no professional charges were sought for the advice given to the plaintiff, nor would it be swayed by his plea that he proffered the advice to save the plaintiff inconvenience as it was past midnight. The moral is that gratuitous service is liable for a lawsuit, because once you offer advice, no matter how well meaning, you have entered

into a physician/patient relationship. Another aspect of service relates to treatment of professional colleagues, wherein as a matter of "professional courtesy" the physician may elect not to charge or charge a minimal amount. In these instances, the care must be of the same standard as would be given to other patients who paid in full, notwithstanding the financial arrangement agreed to by the two parties. In these cases, it is important that there should be no constraints on time or resources. Shortcuts to render care should not be used, as it would be in direct conflict with the standard of care that would have been normally used. It is also important for physicians to try to refrain from treating family members, as there may be a tendency to overlook aspects of history, allow emotion to cloud judgment, or conduct perfunctory examinations. They should be advised to have unrelated family physicians take care of their health-care needs. From the explanation above, it is obvious that **choices B, C, D, and E** are incorrect.

32. **The correct answer is D.** This little girl has varicella (chickenpox), a primary infection with the varicella zoster virus. Administration of aspirin to children with varicella is highly associated with Reye syndrome, and aspirin is absolutely contraindicated. In temperate regions 90% of cases occur in children less than 10 years of age, whereas in the tropics it affects mostly teenagers. The incubation period is 10 to 21 days. Transmission is by direct contact with the lesions and by respiratory route, with initial viral replication in the nasopharynx and conjunctiva. There is an initial viremia between days 4 to 6 seeding the liver, spleen, lungs, and other organs. At days 11 to 20, a secondary viremia occurs that culminates with seeding of the epidermis and formation of the characteristic skin rash. Individuals are infectious for at least 4 days before and 5 days after the skin lesions appear. Slight fever, headache, and malaise are usually present. The skin lesions are typically "teardrop" vesicles on an erythematous base that start as faint erythematous macules 24 hours earlier. Successive fresh crops of vesicles appear for a few days, mainly on the face, trunk, and oral mucosa. The vesicles quickly progress to pustules, umbilicate, and then crust over. Usually there is no scarring, unless very large lesions develop or they become secondarily infected with *Staphylococcus aureus* or Streptococcus organisms (which happens commonly). Rare complications are pneumonia, osteomyelitis, cerebellar ataxia and encephalitis, asymptomatic myocarditis and hepatitis, symptomatic thrombocytopenia and purpura fulminans. Reye syndrome, a syndrome of hepatitis and acute encephalopathy, is associated with the use of aspirin to treat symptoms of varicella. Aspirin is absolutely contraindicated in patients with varicella, and any child with varicella and severe vomiting or lethargy should be referred immediately to exclude Reye syndrome.

Acetaminophen (**choice A**) is a cyclooxygenase inhibitor that works well for the treatment of fever and noninflammatory pain. It is safe to use, has few side effects, and does not interact with other medications in a significant way. The only persons who should avoid taking acetaminophen are those with chronic liver problems in whom hepatic toxicity may be a concern.

Amoxicillin (**choice B**) and ampicillin (**choice C**) are penicillin-type antibiotics that may be given to children with varicella if need be. Considering that this is a viral disease, antibiotics are generally not indicated, but if there is severe superinfection of the skin lesions, you may have to resort to oral antibiotics.

Cephalexin (**choice E**) is a first-generation cephalosporin that arrests bacterial growth by inhibiting bacterial cell wall synthesis. It has bactericidal activity against rapidly growing organisms. Cephalexin is used for the treatment of bacterial skin infections and as prophylaxis in minor procedures. It is not contraindicated in a child with varicella.

33. **The correct answer is B.** The father and son have chickenpox (varicella), an infection caused by the varicella zoster virus. The father is described as having a complication, pneumonia, whereas the boy has a very mild case with no systemic symptoms and few skin lesions. Varicella may affect persons of any age group, 90% of cases occur in children less than 10 years of age in temperate climates, whereas in the tropics it affects mostly teenagers. The incubation period is 10 to 21 days. Transmission is by direct contact with the lesions and by respiratory route, with initial viral replication in the nasopharynx and conjunctiva. There is an initial viremia between days 4 to 6 seeding the liver, spleen, lungs, and other organs. At days 11 to 20, a secondary viremia occurs that culminates with seeding of the epidermis and formation of the characteristic skin rash. Individuals are infectious for at least 4 days before and 5 days after the skin lesions appear. Slight fever, headache, and malaise are usually present. The severity of the disease is age-dependent, with adults having more severe disease and a greater risk of visceral disease. The skin lesions are typically "teardrop" vesicles on an erythematous base that start as faint erythematous macules 24 hours earlier. Successive fresh crops of vesicles appear for a few days, mainly on the face, trunk, and oral mucosa. The vesicles quickly progress to pustules, umbilicate, and then crust over. Usually there is no scarring, unless very

large lesions develop or they become secondarily infected. Pneumonia is uncommon in normal children but is seen in 1 in 400 adults with varicella. Rare complications are osteomyelitis, cerebellar ataxia and encephalitis, asymptomatic myocarditis and hepatitis, symptomatic thrombocytopenia and purpura fulminans. Reye syndrome, a syndrome of hepatitis and acute encephalopathy, is associated with the use of aspirin to treat symptoms of varicella.

Following natural infection or immunization, the varicella zoster virus remains latent in the sensory dorsal root ganglion cells. The virus begins to replicate at some later time, traveling down the sensory root to the skin, and manifesting as herpes zoster. The incidence of zoster increases with age. For white persons more than 80 years of age the lifetime risk of developing zoster is 10 to 30%. Herpes zoster clinically occurs unilaterally within the distribution of a cranial or spinal sensory nerve, often with some overflow into the dermatomes above and below. It is frequently preceded by several days of pain that may persist long after the skin lesions have resolved (postzosteric neuralgia). Apart from immunosuppression and age, the factors involved in reactivation are unknown.

Even though varicella occurs most commonly in children less than 10 years old, it may affect persons of any age group. Therefore, it is not impossible that the father and son have the same disease (**choice A**). Chickenpox is often more severe in older people, especially adults, and complications are much more frequent than in childhood disease. Even the skin lesions tend to be more numerous as the age of the primarily infected patient increases. Pneumonia is the most common complication in adults with an incidence of 1 in 400 cases.

Although the boy has a very mild case of varicella (**choice C**) he will still carry the latent virus in his sensory root ganglion and, later in life, have the propensity to develop herpes zoster caused by unrelated immune suppression or advancing age. Infection with the varicella zoster virus does not recur in the form of varicella, but may recur in the form of herpes zoster.

Varicella in immunocompetent children usually follows a benign course and complications are infrequent. Pneumonia is seen as a complication in 1 out of 400 adults with varicella, but rarely affects children. Also, that the father has pneumonia as a complication of varicella does not in any way indicate that the same complication will develop in the son (**choice D**).

There is no need to have the father and the child physically separated from each other until their diseases resolve (**choice E**) because they have already been infected with the same varicella zoster virus that will progress to latency once the acute illness is overcome, so they cannot reinfect each other. In addition, chickenpox is followed by immunity, so even if the virus starts replicating later in life, it will take the form of herpes zoster and not varicella.

34. **The correct answer is C.** This girl has pityriasis rosea, a mild inflammatory exanthem of unknown etiology most frequently seen between the ages of 15 to 40, more often in women. The disease is most prevalent in the spring and autumn. It frequently begins with a single herald or mother patch that is usually larger than succeeding lesions and may persist alone for a week or 2 before the other lesions appear. The individual patches are oval or circinate, covered with finely wrinkled, dry skin, or, when it desquamates, with a collarette of scale. By that time, involution of the herald patch has begun, and the salmon-colored macular and papular discrete and coalescing lesions start fading away after a total of 3 to 8 weeks. The fully developed eruption has a striking appearance because of orientation of the longer axis of the oval macules and papules along the lines of skin cleavage, creating the well-known "Christmas tree" pattern on the back, especially. The eruption usually affects the trunk and proximal extremities and spares sun-exposed surfaces. Sometimes the lesions are purpuric and sometimes papular (more commonly seen in children under age 5 and African American children). Moderate pruritus may be present, and there may be mild constitutional symptoms before the outbreak. Relapses and recurrences are common, especially with strenuous physical activity or exposure to heat or irritation of the skin, such as rubbing with a rough towel after bathing. Treatment is symptomatic, but it is questionable whether it can shorten the natural duration of the illness. Ultraviolet B in erythema-dose exposures can be used to hasten involution after the acute inflammatory stage has passed. Topical steroids and oral antihistamines provide symptomatic relief to patients who experience pruritus, but do not affect the duration. For severe, generalized forms, a short course of oral steroids may be given. Simple emollients will alleviate the dryness and scaling.

Daily long, soaking baths in hot water (**choice A**) will only make the disease worse and may prolong the course by interfering with the natural resolution of the skin lesions. It is well known that pityriasis rosea renders the person's skin supersensitive to stimuli such as heat and friction. We commonly recommend that patients take short lukewarm showers as opposed to hot baths, and to gently dab their skin dry, as opposed to rubbing it with a rough towel.

Long-acting oral antihistamines (**choice B**) will not shorten the course of her disease but may alleviate any associated pruritus (which this patient does not have). Sometimes the lesions are itchy as they emerge, and oral antihistamines or topical steroids help in controlling this symptom. Neither one will affect the duration of the illness, though.

Pityriasis rosea is of unknown etiology, and systemic antibiotics offer no improvement. Thus, a 7-day course of oral penicillin is not indicated (**choice D**).

A single dose of oral fluconazole 150 mg (**choice E**) is used in the treatment of vaginal candidiasis. It is an antifungal antibiotic with no effect on pityriasis rosea.

35. **The correct answer is B.** This baby has miliaria rubra ("prickly heat") precipitated by continuous overheating and inability to eliminate sweat because of immaturity of the eccrine sweat glands in the skin. Differentiation of the epidermal appendages is frequently incomplete at birth. As a result, a high incidence of sweat retention may be seen in the newborn. Miliaria, a common skin disorder of the newborn period caused by sweat retention, is characterized by a vesicular eruption with subsequent maceration and obstruction of the eccrine ducts located in the epidermis (the acrosyringium). Keratinous plugging of the eccrine ducts and elimination of sweat into the adjacent epidermis and dermis below the level of obstruction leads to formation of the clinical lesions. Virtually all infants would develop miliaria under appropriate conditions. There are two forms of miliaria: *1*) miliaria crystallina, consisting of clear, superficial vesicles without an inflammatory component, and *2*) miliaria rubra, with small, discrete, erythematous papules, vesicles, and papulovesicles. The incidence of miliaria is greatest in the first few weeks of life owing to the immaturity of the sweat gland system, favoring closure of pores and sweat retention. Therapy is directed toward avoidance of excessive heat and humidity. Light clothing, frequent cool baths, and air conditioning all help in alleviating the skin disorder.

Apocrine miliaria is a similar condition based on occlusion of the apocrine ducts (**choice A**) in the epidermis, but in these cases, the erythematous papules and papulopustules that are present are confined to apocrine areas of the body (axillae, breasts, and groin).

The sebaceous duct (**choice D**) enters hair follicles near the infundibulum of the hair follicle (**choice C**) so they form a unified pilosebaceous unit. Occlusion of the pilosebaceous apparatus from retention of keratin and sebaceous material yields tiny, 1 to 2 mm, pearly white or yellow papules (milia), particularly on the cheeks, nose, chin, and forehead of the neonate.

The subcutaneous fat (**choice E**) is located deep beneath the epidermis and the dermis. Any pathologic changes affecting the subcutaneous fat would clinically manifest as either nodules or plaques, and not vesicles or papulovesicles.

36. **The correct answer is B.** Household contacts may be examined for *Giardia*, but if asymptomatic they are usually not treated. However, one may treat asymptomatic carriers to prevent household transmission from young children to their pregnant mothers or family members with immunodeficiency disorders.

It is true that *Giardia* may be found in freshwater mountain streams; however, it is also true that it is frequently spread by fecal-oral route. In fact, preschool epidemics may occur and children attending day care centers may be at especially high risk (**choice A**).

If a pregnant woman is infected and needs to be treated, paromomycin (a nonabsorbable aminoglycoside) can be used as an alternative to metronidazole (**choice C**).

Antimicrobials such as trimethoprim-sulfamethoxazole and doxycycline may be given to decrease the incidence of travelers' diarrhea, but would not be helpful against *Giardia* (**choice D**).

Boiled water is a good preventive measure, but concentrations of chlorine used to disinfect drinking water do not effectively prevent *Giardia* (**choice E**).

37. **The correct answer is D.** Selenium sulfide shampoo is the first line treatment for tinea versicolor. The hyphae and spores seen on the KOH wet prep are sometimes thought to look like "spaghetti and meatballs".

A skin rash is one of the most common side effects of medications. However, this case illustrates the typical findings of tinea versicolor, not a drug eruption (**choice A**). Drug eruptions can vary according to the medication and the host. Maculopapular, morbilliform, urticarial, erythema multiform, erythema nodosum, exfoliative, and acneform rashes are common forms of skin rashes that may result from reaction to drugs or medications.

Calcipotriene ointment is a good choice of treatment for psoriasis, not for tinea versicolor (**choice B**).

A topical steroid cream may be useful as an adjunctive therapy, but is not the best choice treatment for this case (**choice C**).

TCA is used to treat condyloma acuminata and is therefore not the appropriate therapy (**choice E**).

38. **The correct choice is D.** Nine days after the appearance of parotitis is the acceptable time for a child with mumps to return to school so that transmission will be prevented.

Returning to school 1 week after parotid swelling (**choice A**) is incorrect. One week of exclusion from school is appropriate for rubella. Policy states that children with rubella may return to school 7 days after the rash begins.

Returning to school 2 weeks after parotid swelling (**choice B**) is incorrect.

Returning to school 6 days after parotid swelling (**choice C**) is incorrect. Six days of exclusion from school is appropriate for measles. Policy states that children with measles may return to school 6 days after the rash begins.

When the girl is fever free and feeling better (**choice E**) it seems reasonable to think that she may return to school, but this is incorrect. Mumps virus is spread by the respiratory route, and if this girl returns too early to school she will transmit the infection to others.

39. **The correct answer is C.** This patient exhibits the classic signs of pertussis, a respiratory illness caused by the gram-negative rod *Bordetella pertussis*. Following an incubation period of 6 to 20 days, the syndrome begins with upper respiratory symptoms (catarrhal phase), which progress to fits of coughing (including the characteristic "whoop" in some cases) in the paroxysmal phase. The symptoms slowly resolve in the convalescent phase, which can last for weeks. Potential complications of pertussis include pneumonia, apnea (especially in young children), and seizures. There is a safe and effective vaccine against pertussis, and many cases are seen in unimmunized or incompletely immunized patients (such as the one in this question). Culture of nasopharyngeal secretions for pertussis has its greatest yield in the late catarrhal or early paroxysmal phases, but even in the absence of culture conformation, if there is a clinical scenario consistent with pertussis, antimicrobial therapy with a macrolide antibiotic such as erythromycin is indicated. Therapy often does little to lessen the impact of the disease, but does decrease spread to others. Prophylaxis of susceptible close contacts of known cases is also of importance in limiting spread.

Although this child clearly has a respiratory illness, a clear lung examination and a negative chest x-ray make the diagnosis of bacterial pneumonia unlikely. Thus, therapy with amoxicillin (**choice A**) is not indicated at this time.

Amantadine, an antiviral compound with activity against influenza A, is approved for use in children (though not those under one year of age) at high risk of complication of influenza infection. Its use is not indicated in this case (**choice B**), as there is not a confirmed infection with influenza A, and the patient is clinically stable.

While this patient appears stable and would likely improve at home with simple observation (**choice D**), his course is compatible with a diagnosis of pertussis, and he thus requires antibiotic therapy as described above.

There is no role for serial chest radiography (**choice E**) in this case. While x-ray findings of pneumonia can lag clinical clues by days to weeks, the absence of fever or rales on examination make this diagnosis unlikely.

40. **The correct answer is D.** Esophageal foreign bodies can be a life-threatening emergency. Children, particularly at the age of 2, due to their curiosity and tendency to place items in their mouth, are at high risk of both airway and esophageal foreign bodies. In the esophagus, these objects can lodge anywhere but usually will be found at one of two narrow areas: the upper esophageal or lower esophageal sphincter. Esophageal foreign bodies can produce esophageal obstruction that manifests as gagging, choking, difficulty swallowing secretions, or difficulty with intake of solids or liquids. The assessment of patients for esophageal foreign bodies is based on the triad of history, physical exam, and radiographic findings. Of these, history is the most sensitive factor. History includes either a witness who saw the patient placing something in their mouth or simply a history of prolonged coughing, gagging, or choking. Physical examination findings include difficulty controlling secretions (swallowing their own saliva) but generally do not include respiratory abnormalities. Finally, radiographic imaging can detect radiopaque foreign bodies. Commonly, esophageal foreign bodies are coins, and these flat objects will be seen on chest x-ray, oriented in the coronal plane posterior to the tracheal air column; this corresponds to the position of the esophagus. The standard treatment for esophageal foreign bodies is removal through rigid esophagoscopy performed under general anesthesia. Ideally, this is performed when it is safe for the patient to undergo a procedure. Local edema can progress to complete obstruction and potential esophageal perforation, but removal of esophageal foreign bodies is not as urgent as for airway foreign bodies.

Admitting the patient to the hospital for observation as a precaution (**choice A**) is incorrect because patients with a suspected esophageal foreign body should be evaluated by an otolaryngologist in the emergency department.

Giving the patient something to eat, and believing that if he swallows it without difficulty that will most likely rule out any serious abnormality (**choice B**) is not correct because any patient who may undergo general anesthesia in the near future should be on NPO status with IV fluids.

Obtaining a chest x-ray, and, if that is normal, reassuring the parents that anything that made the patient gag has most likely cleared (**choice D**) is incorrect. The patient's history is convincing for esophageal foreign body aspiration and should be evaluated by an otolaryngologist.

Reassuring his parents that because the boy seems comfortable in the emergency department and never developed respiratory distress so he should be clear to go home with them (**choice E**) is not correct because history is the most sensitive factor in assessment of patients for esophageal foreign bodies, and since the history suggests aspiration, he requires further evaluation.

41. **The correct answer is B.** Freckles are small (<0.5 cm) brown macules that occur in profusion on the sun-exposed skin of the face, neck, shoulders, and backs of hands. They become prominent during the summer when exposed to sunlight and subside, sometimes completely, during the winter when there is no exposure. Blondes and redheads with blue eyes and of Celtic origin (skin types I and II) are especially susceptible. They usually appear around age 5. The best way to encourage their fading and prevent future appearance to a certain degree is to practice photoprotection on a regular basis during the summer months with the use of protective clothing and sunscreens. Clothing constructed of tightly woven sun-protective fabrics, irrespective of color, affords substantial protection. Wide-brimmed hats, long sleeves, and trousers all reduce direct exposure. Sunscreens are of two major types: chemical and physical. Chemical sunscreens are chromophores that absorb energy in the ultraviolet B and/or ultraviolet A regions, thereby diminishing photon absorption by the skin. Sunscreens are rated for their photoprotective effect by their *sun protective factor* (SPF). The SPF is simply a ratio of the time required to produce sunburn erythema with and without sunscreen application. SPF ratings of 15 or higher provide effective protection against UV-B and, to a lesser extent, UV-A.

Although complete avoidance of sun exposure would eventually result in the disappearance of freckles (**choice A**) this is very impractical and would be an unacceptable lifestyle for a healthy person of any age.

Self-tanning lotions (**choice C**) are becoming an increasingly popular alternative method of acquiring a socially desirable tanned appearance without the dangers of ultraviolet light exposure. Since they act through chemical oxidation of the skin's corneal layer, they cause an equal degree of darkening throughout the treated area. Thus, the freckles would get darker too and still stand out from the surrounding skin. Also, they do not provide sun protection to a significant degree and regular sunscreen application is recommended.

It is true that in most cases freckles do tend to disappear as a person gets older (**choice D**) but waiting several decades for that to happen will certainly be an unacceptable alternative for this young lady who expressed the desire to improve her current appearance.

In this era of increased awareness of the carcinogenic potential of ultraviolet light, the so-called "hardening" regimens (**choice E**) earlier used to induce tolerance to naturally occurring sunlight by ultraviolet A treatments are all but obsolete.

42. **The correct answer is D.** This patient has a history and physical signs supporting the diagnosis of hypertrophic cardiomyopathy. Since this is the most common cause of sudden death during participation in sports for children, the patient is absolutely forbidden from all strenuous exercise pending further evaluation. Worrisome symptoms include exertional syncope, as in this case, chest pain, and palpations.

"Let me contact the football coach to see if there were any witnessed episodes, but he may continue playing for the moment" (**choice A**), and "Next time you play football be sure to have somebody with you to witness any further episodes" (**choice B**) are inappropriate, as they allow the patient to return to strenuous exercise that may be dangerous. Obtaining a witnessed account can be extremely useful for assessments of syncope (e.g., when evaluating for seizure disorders), but the probable suddenness in symptoms and signs are more indicative of a cardiac disorder. In addition, there were no presumptive symptoms of visual, olfactory, or gustatory aura.

"Next time you play, stop if you notice any funny sensations, such as funny smells or visual disturbances" (**choice C**) is also inappropriate, as it allows the patient to return to strenuous exercise and presumes it is a possible seizure disorder as the cause. If a seizure disorder were suspected you would advise the patient not to go to large open spaces alone, not to swim alone, keep the restroom unlocked when in use (in case of a seizure in the restroom), and, if they drive, inform the motor vehicle authority. A seizure is not a contraindication for sports.

"You will not be allowed to participate in any contact sports, but low-impact sports such as swimming or track are fine from now on" (**choice E**) is incorrect since in this case any strenuous exercise is forbidden, including low- or non-impact sports. This type of action may be implemented if the patient has had two or more concussions.

43. **The correct answer is A.** The diagnosis of hypertrophic cardiomyopathy is most easily confirmed with an echocardiogram, which can evaluate the thickness of the ventricular wall.

An electrocardiogram (**choice B**) will not be the best test to diagnose hypertrophic cardiomyopathy, but suspicion might be aroused when looking at the size of the S and the R waves in the lateral leads (V1 and V6). A rare familial syndrome involving prolongation of the QT interval could increase the athlete's risk of sudden death.

An electroencephalogram (**choice C**) is a useful test when evaluating for seizure disorder, which is not the most likely cause of the patient's syncope.

An exercise stress test, even with supervision (**choice D**), is dangerous because it requires that the patient reach a maximal heart rate while exercising for a reliable interpretation. This may exacerbate syncope in this patient.

An MRI of the brain (**choice E**) is an excellent method to delineate soft tissue, especially when ruling out organic causes for syncope (e.g., tumor that may cause seizure disorder, etc.). For this patient, who has a diagnosis of probable cardiac cause, an MRI would not be very useful. Radiologically, there are no studies on the effectivity of MRI scans when evaluating ventricular hypertrophy.

44. **The correct answer is B.** This player/patient had a mild concussion (defined as a significant blow to the head that may result in unconsciousness). Most authorities would allow return of a player to competition after the athlete has been asymptomatic for 15 to 20 minutes. After a second concussion, even a mild one, the patient may return to competition after 1 to 2 weeks if asymptomatic for 1 week.

Observing him on the sideline and then telling him he can return to play once asymptomatic for 1 month (**choice A**) is correct if there had been a more severe concussion (with concussion symptoms lasting more than 30 minutes).

Observing him on the sideline, and then telling him he can return to play once asymptomatic for 20 minutes (**choice C**) would be correct if this were the patient's first concussion.

Hospital evaluation is not needed for the initial assessment of mild concussion, even if it is recurrent. Most authorities recommend transportation to a hospital for any loss of consciousness, and for further evaluation if the episode lasted longer than 5 minutes. None of these took place in this situation and therefore transporting him to the hospital and then telling him he can return to play when asymptomatic for 1 month (**choice D**), and transporting him to the hospital and telling him that he cannot play for the remainder of the season (**choice E**) are incorrect.

45. **The correct answer is C.** By the age of 5 years a child should be able to copy a circle, a square, a cross, and the capital letters V, T, H, O, X, L, Y, U, C, and A as part of the motor (visual) developmental milestone. Thus, a 5-year-old girl who is unable to copy a drawing of a square exhibits developmental delay and should be documented for review.

An 18-month-old boy (**choice A**) should be able to walk unaided with his feet slightly apart.

A 5-month-old boy who utters no intelligible words to his parents (**choice B**) would not exhibit developmental delay unless he is 18 months old, by which time he should be able to voice 6 to 20 recognizable words and echo the last word spoken to him.

The communication milestone of a 6-month-old child includes being able to turn to their parent's voice (even if across the room), babble using single and repetitive syllables, and locate a sound by looking (**choice D**).

The 6-month-old boy should be able to use his whole hand (palmer grasp) to obtain objects, reach with two hands for objects up to one foot away, and transfer objects from one hand to the other. One would not expect them to scribble with a crayon (**choice E**) at this age, and so he is not developmentally delayed.

46. **The correct answer is A.** This baby boy has the typical clinical picture of erythema toxicum neonatorum (toxic erythema of the newborn), an asymptomatic, idiopathic, benign, self-limiting skin eruption of the neonatal period. The eruption may first appear as a blotchy erythema that evolves into firm pink papules or pustules on an erythematous base. The erythematous macules may be confluent into patches several centimeters in diameter and stand out sharply from normal skin. Erythema toxicum neonatorum usually appears during the first 3 to 4 days of life, but may start as late as the 14th day. It may wax and wane for 2 weeks and then resolve completely. Individual lesions last from several hours to 2 weeks. Various reports quote the incidence rate to be anywhere from 5 to 71% of all newborns. It is somewhat less frequent in premature infants. The histopathologic appearance is rather characteristic, with typical accumulation of eosinophils around the pilosebaceous follicles just below the basement membrane zone (dermoepidermal junction). Perifollicular or intraepidermal accumulation of eosinophils is seen when pustules are biopsied. Peripheral eosinophilia may be seen in a fraction of these patients. Because it is a benign, self-limited disorder, only reassurance of the parents is needed. In cases of doubt, rapid confirmation of the diagnosis may be done by preparing a cytologic smear of the pustule, and staining with Giemsa or Wright stain reveals clusters of eosinophils in the absence of other inflammatory cells.

Accumulation of mucin in the hair follicle with a lymphoid perifollicular infiltrate (**choice B**) is seen in follicular mucinosis, a condition sometimes encountered in children in the form of pink, scaly patches devoid of hair on the trunk and extremities. Identical lesions, albeit with eosinophils sprinkled among perifollicular lymphocytes, is seen as a manifestation of cutaneous T-cell lymphoma (mycosis fungoides).

Hyperkeratotic plugs in pilosebaceous orifices (**choice C**) are seen in keratosis pilaris, a condition frequently associated with atopic dermatitis that clinically presents as firm, keratotic follicular papules on the extensor arms and legs of children or young adults.

Noninflammatory subepidermal blisters (**choice D**) are seen in epidermolysis bullosa, a genodermatosis with many subtypes ranging from benign to lethal with nuances in between. These children lack certain components of the basement membrane zone that results in formation of spontaneous or trauma-induced blistering of the skin, sometimes evident at birth. The blisters can be 1 mm to several cm in diameter and are typically located on sites of friction or trauma.

Spongiotic vesicles in the epidermis (**choice E**) are seen in many eczematous dermatitides of the skin, such as atopic dermatitis, nummular dermatitis, and allergic contact dermatitis. All of these diseases clinically manifest with scaly red patches and plaques studded with clear vesicles that often weep a serous fluid and often crust. It is unusual for any type of eczema to present in a child less than 2 months of age.

47. **The correct answer is A.** This child has the typical clinical presentation of pyogenic granuloma, a common vascular lesion most often seen in children and young adults. Pyogenic granulomas develop rapidly and are solitary most of the time. Although they may appear on any skin or mucocutaneous surface, they most commonly develop in areas subject to trauma, such as the hands, forearm, face, and oral mucosa. They are bright red to reddish-brown, soft or moderately firm, usually at least slightly pedunculated nodules. The size varies from pinpoint to 2 cm in diameter, and they bleed easily and sometimes profusely, even with the slightest trauma. Although it was once believed, as the name pyogenic granuloma implies, that it was a consequence of infection (Staphylococcal), current opinion is that it is a true benign neoplasm or reactive vascular process, possibly associated with trauma. It is not contagious or infectious in nature. Pyogenic granulomas are usually easily diagnosed clinically because of their very characteristic clinical presentation. Histopathologically, a vascular, hemangioma-like proliferation of blood vessels is embedded in a loose stroma. There is an epidermal collarette at the periphery and it may be covered by scale or scale-crust over a flattened epidermis. Treatment is with physical methods of destruction, such as curettage and electrodesiccation of the base, liquid nitrogen, or pulse-dye laser surgery. Pyogenic granulomas often recur after treatment because of persistence of the proliferating blood vessels deeper in dermis. In those cases, repeating the destructive process or using CO_2 laser or classic surgical excision may be curative.

Mohs micrographic surgery (**choice B**) is used in the surgical treatment of malignant neoplasms of the skin that are not amenable to classic surgical methods because of recurrence within a scar, location in high-risk areas (planes of embryonal fusion), malignancies that have clinically poorly defined borders (e.g., morpheaform basal cell carcinoma), or when tissue sparing is a great concern. It is not used in the treatment of benign lesions such as pyogenic granuloma.

It is incorrect that no treatment is indicated at this time (**choice C**) because this is a proliferating lesion that has already bled on multiple occasions and is located in areas of high risk for trauma that may lead to unwanted complications.

Topical antibiotic ointments (**choice D**) will not cause resolution of pyogenic granuloma by themselves. They may be used to prevent secondary infection once the lesion has been removed by other methods.

Topical corticosteroid ointments (**choice E**) are not indicated in the management of pyogenic granuloma, a benign neoplasm that may easily be complicated by superinfection. They have no effect on the course of the disease.

48. **The correct answer is D.** This patient has a congenital cavernous hemangioma. The most serious complication of such a lesion is the Kasabach-Merritt syndrome, a variant of disseminated intravascular coagulopathy in which thrombocytopenia is caused by sequestration of platelets in giant cavernous hemangiomas, most commonly of the kaposiform endothelioma type. Most hemangiomas associated with Kasabach-Merritt syndrome are exceedingly large, but it has developed in patients with lesions as small as 5 to 6 cm in diameter, as well as in patients with visceral hemangiomas, disseminated neonatal hemangiomatosis, and the Klippel-Trenaunay syndrome. During the first few weeks of life thrombocytopenia as low as 2000 to 4000/mm^3, anemia, decreased fibrinogen levels, increased prothrombin time, and decreased partial thromboplastin time may be detected. Thus, children with rapidly expanding hemangiomas, with or without other visible signs of coagulopathy, should be checked for platelet entrapment and thrombocytopenia. The danger of Kasabach-Merritt syndrome is in acute hemorrhage and compression of vital structures by the rapidly enlarging hemangioma. Thirty percent of infants with this syndrome die from complications of bleeding, respiratory distress, infection, or malignant transformation. Thus, infants with large hemangiomas and thrombocytopenia should be promptly treated.

A differential white count (**choice A**) would be appropriate if an infectious or myeloproliferative disorder was suspected, but not in the case of enlarging cavernous hemangiomas.

Erythrocyte sedimentation rate (**choice B**) is a nonspecific indicator of certain chronic inflammatory processes, such as juvenile rheumatoid arthritis, lupus erythematosus, dermatomyositis, and many other diseases, but is not elevated in the case of a congenital hemangioma in which platelet entrapment is occurring.

Liver function tests (**choice C**) are performed to exclude certain congenital infections or metabolic diseases. They are not indicated in the workup of a congenital hemangioma.

Urine analysis (**choice E**) with additional special tests is performed when infections (e.g., pyelonephritis) or inflammatory disorders (e.g., nephrotic syndrome) of the genitourinary tract are suspected. In addition, some metabolic diseases (e.g., the porphyrias) and endocrinologic disorders (congenital adrenal hyperplasia) may be diagnosed through specific analysis of the urine. There would be no specific change in this laboratory assessment with a congenital cavernous hemangioma.

49. **The correct answer is D.** This baby girl has transient neonatal pustular melanosis, a benign, self-limiting disorder of unknown etiology that affects up to 4% of newborns. Lesions are usually present at birth in the form of superficial vesicles and pustules that rupture easily during the first bathing and leave a collarette of fine, white scales around a pinhead-sized hyperpigmented brown macule. These usually fade in 3 weeks to 3 months. Clusters of lesions usually appear under the chin and on the forehead, lower back, and shins. Less frequently they involve the cheeks, trunk, and extremities, and only rarely do frank bullae appear on the palms and soles. The content of the vesicles and pustules is sterile, and smears of the lesional fluid stained with a Wright stain reveal mostly neutrophils (in contrast to erythema toxicum neonatorum, in which eosinophils abound) and cellular debris. Histopathologically, intracorneal or subcorneal pustules and focal hyperpigmentation of the basal layer are seen. Transient neonatal pustular melanosis has no known systemic associations and requires no treatment. The vesicles and pustules disappear within 24 to 48 hours, leaving hyperpigmented macules that resolve spontaneously over the ensuing weeks or months.

Phototherapy (**choice A**) is used in the treatment of neonatal hyperbilirubinemia. It has no indication for use in transient neonatal pustular melanosis, which is a self-limiting, spontaneously resolving disorder.

Neither oral (**choice B**) nor topical (**choice C**) antibiotics are indicated in the treatment of transient neonatal pustular melanosis because the disorder is not a bacterial infection, nor do the lesions have a tendency to become secondarily infected.

Topical corticosteroid cream (**choice E**) would not be indicated because the lesions resolve spontaneously, and the fragile skin of a newborn baby would be extremely susceptible to side effects of topical corticosteroids and systemic absorption.

50. **The correct answer is E.** This child has bullous impetigo, a skin infection frequently seen in children that is most commonly caused by phage type 71 coagulase-positive *Staphylococcus aureus.* The neonatal type is highly contagious and a serious threat to nurseries. Children with bullous impetigo may have a history of insect bites at the sites of onset of lesions. Crowding, poor hygiene, neglected wounds, and minor trauma contribute to the spread of this infectious disease. Secondary infection of preexisting skin lesions, such as insect bites, abrasions, herpes simplex, or eczema, is common. The bullous variant starts with fragile bullae that rupture to leave a circinate, weepy, or crusted lesion that at this stage is called impetigo circinata. Initially, constitutional symptoms are absent, but with time or with extensive lesions, malaise and fever or a subnormal temperature may be present. The diagnosis is easily confirmed by doing a Gram stain and culture of the base of the erosions. Treatment is necessary for resolution, and with bullous lesions an oral semisynthetic penicillin or cephalosporin is recommended. Topical therapy should be done simultaneously with either mupirocin ointment or bacitracin ointment. For localized, non-bullous varieties, topical therapy may be sufficient. Mupirocin is highly effective in skin infections caused by *Staphylococcus aureus,* and resistance has not been an issue.

    Azelaic acid (**choice A**) is a topical medication that inhibits melanogenesis by way of competitive inhibition of the enzyme tyrosinase. It is commonly used to treat pigmentary disorders of the skin, such as melasma or postinflammatory hyperpigmentation. It has no antibacterial effect and would not be useful in treating impetigo.

    Fluocinonide (**choice B**) is a topical corticosteroid preparation of medium potency frequently used for inflammatory conditions of the skin, such as contact dermatitis or lichen simplex chronicus. It has immunosuppressive activity, causes vasoconstriction, and decreases fibroblast activity. It has no antibacterial properties, and may in fact help the infection to spread more rapidly. It is not used in the treatment of bacterial infections of the skin.

    Hydroquinone (**choice C**) is used for its bleaching properties in the treatment of hyperpigmentation of the skin, such as in melasma or postinflammatory hyperpigmentation secondary to acne. It blocks melanin synthesis in a reversible fashion. Long-term use has been associated with secondary ochronosis, a skin disease in which yellow-brown pigment is deposited in the dermis permanently. Two percent hydroquinone is available in many over-the-counter skin care products that advertise bleaching (lightening) properties, and is also available as a 4% preparation by prescription.

    Ketoconazole (**choice D**) is an antifungal available in systemic and topical formulations and commonly used in the treatment of yeast and dermatophyte infections of the skin. It blocks ergosterol synthesis, thus preventing normal wall formation of the microorganisms. It is not approved for use in children under age 2.

Psychiatry: **Test One**

1. A 32-year-old woman with recurrent, moderate major depressive disorder comes to the office for a routine followup appointment. She has been stably maintained on paroxetine 40 mg qd since her last depressive episode approximately 6 months ago. She had her first depressive episode at the age of 16 and has had five depressive episodes since then. She has never made a suicide attempt, but she has lost employment and relationships secondary to her depressive illness. She tells you that she currently feels well and that she does not have any neurovegetative complaints, such as sleep or appetite disturbances. She adamantly denies any suicidal intent, ideation, or plan. She inquires today as to whether she should still take her antidepressant medication and of the risks of discontinuation. The most appropriate response to her question is:

   (A) "Given your history of recurrent depression, you would incur a significant risk of relapse if the antidepressant medication were discontinued or decreased."

   (B) "There is no evidence to suggest that you would benefit from additional antidepressant treatment given the remission, and you may stop paroxetine immediately."

   (C) "You can stop taking paroxetine on a scheduled basis and may have a prescription for an as-needed dose of paroxetine when feeling depressed."

   (D) "You have passed the 6-month threshold for the need of full doses of antidepressant, and the paroxetine dose may be cut in half without incurring any risk of recurrence."

   (E) "You should have another antidepressant medication added at this time to maintain remission of the depression."

2. You are called to assess a 56-year-old homeless African American man with a past history of alcohol dependence and gastritis who wants to leave the hospital against medical advice. The patient was admitted to the medical floor 13 days ago with a bleeding gastric ulcer and aspiration pneumonia. He is medically stable for discharge, but the patient's medical team (including yourself) and social work services have been pursuing placement for the patient in a residence with outpatient alcohol treatment. The patient now states that he does not wish for such treatment. He tells you that he is not depressed and does not feel suicidal. There is no evidence that the patient is hallucinating, and he does not appear paranoid. He tells you that he enjoys his present lifestyle and does not feel that he is hurting anyone by living in the manner that he does. Mini-mental status examination score is 30/30. The patient, when asked, states that he would never have left against medical advice when he was medically ill, but because it has been explained to him that the acute phase of his illness is over, he feels that it would be appropriate for him to leave, given that he does not want to live in the suggested residence or pursue alcohol treatment. He does, however, agree to medical followup as an outpatient. The most appropriate next step in management is to

   (A) allow the patient to be discharged only on the condition that he is escorted to an inpatient alcohol detoxification facility

   (B) allow the patient to sign out of the hospital against medical advice and give him a referral for an outpatient alcohol program

   (C) have a psychiatrist state that the patient must allow the hospital to make his health care and placement decisions

   (D) sedate, physically restrain, and then reassess the patient

   (E) seek guardianship over the patient because of his poor judgment

3. A 13-year-old girl with no past medical history comes to the clinic with her mother for a routine annual examination. The patient has always been a good student and athlete. The patient's mother states that her grades have deteriorated significantly in the last 4 months and that she refuses to do her schoolwork. She does not want to go to see her friends and has stopped going to her after-school activities. The patient, in private, denies that she is sexually active or using illicit drugs or alcohol, and a urine hCG and drug screen are both negative. The patient, who is normally very bright and talkative, is unusually short-tempered and curt during your interaction today. She angrily denies any suicidal intent, ideation, or plan, perceptual disturbances, or paranoia. Physical examination is unremarkable, and there are no indications of physical or sexual abuse. The most appropriate next step in management is to

(A) explain to the patient and her mother that these symptoms are part of a normal adolescent maturing process
(B) prescribe a low dose of olanzapine for what may be a first-break psychotic illness
(C) prescribe a trial dose of methylphenidate for the patient's inattention to her schoolwork
(D) refer her to an adolescent psychiatrist for possible antidepressant medication and verbal or group therapy
(E) send her for an electroencephalogram for suspected seizure disorder

4. A 20-year-old woman has new onset panic disorder with recurrent panic attacks consisting of chest pain, palpitations, shortness of breath, a fear of dying or "going crazy," and distal paresthesias. She was started on paroxetine 30 mg a day at her last visit 9 days ago and is here for a followup visit. The patient presently complains of "being anxious all the time," having feelings of internal restlessness, and poor sleep. She tells you that she actually feels more anxious since starting paroxetine and would like to consider a change in medication. The most appropriate next step in management is to

(A) augment the paroxetine the patient is receiving with haloperidol 2 mg twice a day
(B) augment the paroxetine the patient is receiving with phenelzine
(C) increase the dosage of paroxetine to 40 mg a day and reassure the patient that these side effects are "treatment emergent"
(D) recommend that the patient's starting dosage of paroxetine be lowered to 5 to 10 mg a day
(E) suggest that the patient change medications immediately to sertraline 200 mg a day

5. A 25-year-old Caucasian woman with bipolar disorder comes to the clinic for a followup appointment. She was discharged from the hospital 10 days ago after a manic episode that was successfully treated on the psychiatric ward with carbamazepine 400 mg bid. The patient is noted to have a completely normal mental status examination, with no evidence of racing thoughts, euphoria, irritability, or depressive symptoms. She gives no indication that she is having any problems understanding the manner in which she is supposed to take carbamazepine and insists that she is taking it as directed. However, the patient's blood level of carbamazepine today is 2 μg/mL (4-12 μg/mL therapeutic dosing range). It was 8 μg/mL upon discharge from the hospital. The patient is taking no other medications. The most appropriate next step in the management is to

   (A) add haloperidol to the patient's medication regimen to increase the level of cognitive organization and carbamazepine compliance
   (B) ask the patient if she would rather take her entire dosage of carbamazepine at bedtime to increase compliance
   (C) educate the patient about the dangers of her medication noncompliance
   (D) titrate the dosage of carbamazepine to therapeutic blood levels
   (E) rehospitalize the patient because of her impaired judgment and limited insight

6. A 30-year-old woman is brought to the emergency department by her husband after being found lethargic and confused. The patient has no known medical history and does not drink or use illicit drugs. According to the patient's husband, the patient recently got a prescription for a "medicine for anxiety that she takes only when she needs to." She has been under a great deal of stress lately and has been taking more and more of the pills. They do not remember the name of the medication and could not find the bottle. However, they are sure that the medication is not a stimulant. Urinary toxicology and routine laboratory studies are pending. The patient's vital signs are mildly depressed, and respirations are stable. After ensuring stable airway, breathing, and circulation, the most appropriate next step in management is

   (A) diuresis with intravenous furosemide
   (B) electroconvulsive therapy for precipitous depression
   (C) flumazenil to reverse benzodiazepine toxicity
   (D) methylphenidate to increase level of awareness and ability of the patient to cooperate with history taking
   (E) transcranial magnetic stimulation

7. A 42-year-old man who is status-post partial colectomy comes to the clinic for pain management. He is a highly functioning English professor and has recently returned to work on a part-time basis. The patient presents to you today because he is having difficulty weaning from the opiates that he received postoperatively. He admits that he has been having different physicians prescribe him narcotic analgesics because he cannot bear the symptoms of opiate withdrawal such as diarrhea, piloerection, nausea, and sweating. His postoperative pain is not as prominent a problem for him as the symptoms of narcotic withdrawal. He tells you that he does not want methadone or other opiate agonist maintenance therapy but "needs something" for this problem. The most appropriate option for this patient with respect to treating his opiate withdrawal symptoms is

   (A) clonidine
   (B) disulfiram
   (C) flumazenil
   (D) haloperidol
   (E) methylphenidate

8. You are seeing a 6-year-old boy who is brought to the clinic by his parents because of "behavioral problems." Since the birth of a younger sister 2 months ago, the patient has started to act in an immature manner that is inconsistent with his usually well-behaved and relaxed demeanor. He has started sucking his thumb and throwing temper tantrums in public. The parents have been attempting to ignore the patient's behavior and have not punished him for anything he has done. Physical examination and medical review of systems are normal. In the examination room alone with his parents and you, the patient is noted to be well behaved. Appropriate management to improve the patient's behavior is to

   (A) have the patient help his parents with some of the care of the baby
   (B) have the patient start antidepressant therapy that may be tapered when the baby gets older
   (C) have the patient undergo deep breathing and relaxation exercises on a regular basis
   (D) prescribe methylphenidate for the patient's impulsivity and immature outbursts
   (E) recommend that the parents use light spankings when the patient misbehaves

9. A 56-year-old woman is admitted to the hospital for evaluation of nausea without emesis and diffuse abdominal pain that she has had for 6 months. She has had a negative workup thus far that has included complete blood count, chemistries, liver function tests, amylase, lipase, esophagoscopy, colonoscopy, and contrast CT scan. You are called to see her because she is "completely dissatisfied" with her present nurse, and she demands that she be allowed to hand pick whomever will be assigned to work with her. Her specific complaint is that she is not given sufficient narcotic pain medication to manage her abdominal pain and that, whereas some nurses are prompt to call the doctor on call to assess her, other nurses seem indifferent to her needs. The patient's nurses have disagreement among themselves over the severity of the patient's actual symptoms and the appropriate way to interact with her. The patient has no symptoms consistent with psychosis and adamantly denies any suicidal intent, ideation, or plan. The most appropriate management is to

   (A) assemble the present nursing staff together to address the patient's defenses, including splitting of nursing staff assigned to work with the patient
   (B) attempt to transfer the patient to a psychiatric inpatient ward for somatization disorder
   (C) call for a surgical consultation because of escalating pain in the presence of narcotic treatment for her pain
   (D) comply with her wishes and allow her to interview nurses that will tend to her care
   (E) reprimand the patient's present nurse for not calling earlier regarding the patient's pain

10. A 35-year-old African American woman comes to the office because of anxiety for the past 3 weeks. She has also experienced brief periods of palpitations and diaphoresis while at work. She denies a history of syncopal episodes, chest pain, or shortness of breath, drug abuse, past medical history, or recent traumatic events in her personal life. The patient has added that she has started to work longer hours as an accountant during a busy tax season and that she has started to smoke one to two cigarettes per day and often drinks 4 to 5 cups of coffee while at work. Physical examination and laboratory studies, including complete blood count, chemistries, and thyroid function tests, are all normal. The most appropriate next step in management is to

(A) order a CT scan of the patient's head
(B) order a 24-hour Holter monitor for the patient
(C) prescribe a 14-mg nicotine patch for the patient
(D) prescribe a low dosage of sertraline to treat the patient's panic attacks
(E) recommend that the patient decrease her caffeine intake

11. A 45-year-old man is admitted to the cardiac telemetry floor because of electrocardiogram changes that occurred during a 2-day binge on crack cocaine. On admission, the patient has no signs of confusion, is fully oriented, and, aside from appropriate concerns regarding his condition, he has no complaints of recent depression or anxiety. On the patient's second hospital day, an electrocardiogram is normal, and the patient is ruled out for a myocardial infarction by cardiac enzymes. When you go to discharge him, he tells you that he "feels very depressed and tired." He adds that it feels "like I can barely move." He denies suicidal ideation, feelings of guilt, paranoia, or perceptual disturbances. His vital signs are stable. The most appropriate next step in management is to

(A) administer haloperidol to treat the psychiatric and physiologic symptoms of cocaine withdrawal
(B) observe his symptoms as the cocaine withdrawal resolves
(C) perform neuropsychological testing to assess the presence of bipolar disorder
(D) prepare him to receive electroconvulsive therapy
(E) start insight-oriented psychotherapy

12. A 21-year-old college junior comes to the student health center complaining of "extreme sadness." For the past couple of weeks he has been depressed, sleeping 12 hours per day, and has had "no appetite." He denies that he feels any suicidal intent, ideation, or plan. These symptoms began when his girlfriend of 2 years terminated their relationship and started dating one of their classmates. At the end of the interview, he calmly states that he feels frustrated to the extent that he feels like stabbing both his ex-girlfriend and her new boyfriend with a knife that he bought that day at a sporting goods store. At this time you should

(A) call the patient's parents regarding the situation
(B) maintain the confidentiality of the session while at the same time documenting what the patient said during the session
(C) medicate the patient immediately for agitation and reassess him after the medication has taken effect
(D) protect and warn the patient's ex-girlfriend and her new boyfriend
(E) treat the patient's depression with medication or referral for electroconvulsive therapy

13. A 56-year-old woman with a history of bipolar I disorder that has been stably maintained on lithium carbonate comes to the office because of a mild intention tremor. She is very satisfied with lithium as her mood stabilizer and does not want to switch to a different medication or reduce the dose of lithium because her most recent hospitalization occurred when she and her past physician attempted to reduce her lithium dosage. Her blood pressure is 110/80 mm Hg, and pulse is 65/min. Her lithium level is in the middle of the therapeutic range, and complete blood count, thyroid-stimulating hormone, and chemistries are all normal. The most appropriate next step in management is to

(A) begin a trial of benztropine while honoring the patient's wish that the lithium dose be maintained
(B) begin a trial of propanolol for the patient's tremor while honoring the patient's wish that the lithium dose be maintained
(C) insist that the patient discontinue lithium treatment
(D) refer her for biofeedback to control the tremor
(E) tell her as empathetically as possible that nothing can be done to reverse this side effect of lithium

14. A 54-year-old African American woman with schizophrenia comes to the emergency department complaining of a 12-day history of a productive cough, fever, and chills. She is escorted by a case manager from the residence where she lives. The patient is compliant with all treatments and residence guidelines. She has no present psychiatric complaints, such as depression, auditory hallucinations, or paranoia. She takes clozapine and docusate. She is fully oriented and answers all questions appropriately. Her temperature is 39.1 C (102.4 F), blood pressure is 120/80 mm Hg, pulse is 105/min, and respirations are 20/min. A chest x-ray shows lower lobe pneumonia. The most appropriate next step in management is to

(A) administer a loading dose of phenytoin for seizure prophylaxis in the context of clozapine treatment and febrile illness
(B) obtain a complete blood count with differential
(C) obtain a serum chemistry to determine potassium level
(D) prescribe oral antibiotics and advise her to follow up as an outpatient
(E) send sputum for acid-fast bacilli and begin therapy for tuberculosis

15. A 14-year-old Haitian boy is referred to the clinic for evaluation of a potential psychotic illness. He is a well-groomed and well-related boy. He has many friends at school, is on the varsity baseball team, and maintains a B average in his schoolwork. The patient admits that he senses "spirits around me always" and that he recognizes these spirits as his deceased ancestors from Africa. The patient denies any auditory, visual, or tactile hallucinations. The patient's parents and maternal grandmother also believe in the presence of these spirits but insist that they will do whatever is in the patient's best interest and will follow your suggestions. He denies any history of drug or alcohol use. The patient denies any report of depression or anxiety and adamantly denies suicidal intent, ideation, or plan. The most appropriate intervention at this time is to

(A) admit the patient to an adolescent psychiatry unit for observation and organic workup for psychosis
(B) give the patient a prescription for low-dose haloperidol and follow the patient weekly as an outpatient
(C) look into foster care options for the patient
(D) order weekly urine drug screen monitoring for the patient for 2 months
(E) reassure the patient and his family that he has no obvious psychiatric illness

16. A 68-year-old Caucasian woman with hypertension and gout is brought to the office by her daughter because of mental status changes. The patient makes polite conversation and denies problems, but her daughter reports that she has abruptly stopped working as an accountant because she "just wasn't interested" anymore. She also has stopped attending church functions and cooking for the family. She specifically denies a depressed mood, anhedonia, poor appetite, or problems sleeping. She is reportedly becoming more forgetful and less "outgoing." She has had recent dosage change in the metoprolol that she has taken for several years. Her temperature is 37.0 C (98.6 F), blood pressure is 115/70 mm Hg, pulse is 70/min, and respirations are 20/min. She does not appear depressed. Her physical examination is normal, except for a slight systolic murmur and an ataxic gait. She scores 25/30 on the mental status examination. She has severe difficulty drawing, naming a pen or a table, and recalling objects. You suspect dementia of the vascular and/or Alzheimer type and send for a B_{12}, folate, TSH, and RPR, all of which are negative. You start her on tetrahydroaminoacridine. She returns for her 3-week followup visit in a wheelchair. Her daughter explains that the patient has had increasing difficulty walking and has a wide-based "wobbly" gait. She also has had frank confusion and new onset urinary incontinence. She does not answer your questions. Her examination is unchanged from the previous visit except for an even more ataxic gait. Complete blood count and electrolytes are normal. At this time you should discontinue the tetrahydroaminoacridine and order

(A) a CT of the head and urinalysis
(B) an echocardiogram and liver function tests
(C) an electrocardiogram and liver function tests
(D) an electroencephalogram and liver function tests
(E) a radiograph of the pelvis and urinalysis

17. A 37-year-old man has a history of recurrent major depression. He was hospitalized 4 years ago after a serious overdose and has failed previous antidepressant trials of amitriptyline and nefazodone. He has been unable to achieve remission since his hospitalization despite faithful compliance to his treatment plan. He was finally stabilized on fluoxetine over the last 3 months with near total therapeutic response. His functioning at work and home has improved significantly, and he has not had any suicidal ideation whatsoever after being on the fluoxetine for 4 weeks. He has no major medical problems or allergies and is not taking any other medications. He comes to your office today grateful for his remarkable improvement regarding his depression but complains of sexual dysfunction with decreased sexual desire and delayed ejaculation. There is no difficulty achieving or maintaining an erection. He asks for your help. The most appropriate next step in management is to

(A) add bupropion
(B) add sildenafil
(C) stop the fluoxetine and give him a trial off medications
(D) stop the fluoxetine and switch to bupropion
(E) stop the fluoxetine and switch to nortriptyline

18. A 31-year-old man with bipolar illness comes to the urgent care clinic because he is concerned that he broke his ankle while running on an uneven road. He has taken ibuprofen, aspirin, acetaminophen, and codeine over the last 2 days for pain with good results. He reports that his mood has been stabilized with lithium, with only one hospitalization since starting the medicine 10 years ago. He had several admissions before taking lithium. He denies increased thirst, nausea, diarrhea, and has no tremor or ataxia. You examine the leg and read the radiograph and decide to send the patient home with rest and an air cast, to be followed with his regular physician. At this point it is important to advise the patient to stop taking

(A) acetaminophen, aspirin, codeine, and ibuprofen because all may increase his lithium level
(B) acetaminophen because it may increase his lithium level
(C) aspirin because it may increase his lithium level
(D) codeine because it may increase his lithium level
(E) ibuprofen because it may increase his lithium level

19. A 38-year-old woman with schizoaffective disorder, diet-controlled diabetes, and cervical stenosis with neuropathic pain is brought to the emergency department after "passing out" at home. She has a long psychiatric history, including several episodes of delusions that she is being chased by devils, two suicide attempts while depressed and psychotic, and a history of cocaine and benzodiazepine use. She denies any current depressive or psychotic symptoms. Her medicines include haloperidol, amitriptyline, and trazodone. She denies taking any illicit drugs, but all of her medicines have been increased recently. During the physical examination particular attention should be given to

(A) ataxia, signifying an acute reaction to haloperidol
(B) coarse tremor, signifying amitriptyline toxicity
(C) orthostatic hypotension from taking medications with α-adrenergic antagonism
(D) pupillary dilation or nystagmus from illicit drug intoxication
(E) retinal examination for signs of long-standing diabetes

20. A mother brings her 5-year-old son to the clinic for the first time. She has recently moved here from a rural area where they only had one doctor to cover all the needs of the residents of the community. She is now trying to find a physician to take care of her son, who has been diagnosed with attention deficit hyperactivity disorder. He has been treated with pemoline in the past year and needs a refill of the prescription now. You explain to her that it would be safer and reasonable to try to change the child to another medication. She is initially upset but finally agrees to a change and to blood tests on the child because of reported possible side effects of pemoline. At this time you should order

(A) a complete blood count
(B) liver function tests
(C) a platelet count
(D) a serum creatinine
(E) thyroid function tests

21. A 32-year-old new patient comes to the office complaining of nausea, fatigue, and abdominal pain. She has been hospitalized approximately six times in the past few years for both similar and different conditions. She tells you about a lump in her throat that caused difficulty swallowing that was so "debilitating" that she was admitted to the hospital, but the workup was negative. She had a miscarriage when she was 27 and was hospitalized for evaluation, which was also unremarkable. She also cannot tolerate high-fiber foods because of heartburn and bloating, and over the past couple of years she has had frequent migraine headaches and blurred vision and has seen several neurologists. These workups were also negative. She is extremely concerned about her "negative workups" because she really feels sick and believes that the "right tests" were never ordered. She hands you five large bundles of paper that she tells you are her medical records from the past. You flip through them and notice that she has had two colonoscopies, an upper endoscopy, a small bowel series, a hysteroscopy, two laparoscopies, and a CT scan and MRI of the head. The most appropriate management at this time is to

(A) do as the patient requests and run a series of tests
(B) explain to her that she will be fine within a day or two because it is probably something transitory and that no further evaluation is indicated
(C) perform a complete physical examination and explain that tests are not necessary now, but schedule regular followup visits every few weeks
(D) run a series of tests because, even though her workup is negative, one should be on the safe side
(E) tell the patient that her condition is based on stress and refer her to a psychiatrist

22. A 73-year-old woman is brought to the office for the assessment of behavioral changes. She lives with her daughter, who tells you that the patient has become gradually more confused in the past 3 years. She forgets to do things like lock the door or pick up mail. She often puts on two different shoes, misplaces things, and accuses her daughter of stealing her clothes or other items that she has misplaced. She has refused to see a doctor for years, but because she has not been sleeping well her daughter convinced her to see a doctor for insomnia. The patient has been generally healthy over the years and has suffered no major illnesses. She responds to your questions with short answers and explains that her daughter is exaggerating. You decide to do a test to determine who is telling the truth. The most appropriate test at this time to detect cognitive deficits is the

(A) Mini-mental status examination
(B) Minnesota Multiphasic Personality Inventory-2
(C) thematic apperception test
(D) Wechsler Adult Intelligence Scale
(E) Wisconsin card-sorting test

23. A 35-year-old woman with bipolar disorder type I has been taking lithium for a few years. She has managed to stay out of the hospital and keep her job as an accountant. She has been married for 3 years and has talked to you in the past about pros and cons of having a child given her history. She comes to see you now because she thinks that she is pregnant. A urine hCG is positive. She is concerned about the effects of lithium on the fetus. You should tell her that

(A) lithium causes fetal neural tube defects when taken during pregnancy
(B) lithium causes some congenital heart anomalies that are incompatible with fetal survival
(C) lithium is completely safe to take in pregnancy as long as the lithium level is within normal range
(D) lithium sometimes causes pigmentary retinopathy in the fetus
(E) she should have an abortion because lithium is toxic to the fetus

24. A 24-year-old graduate student is rushed to the emergency department after he was found unconscious in his apartment. His roommates report that he has used heroin in the past, but they thought he had been clean for the past 2 years after completing a rehabilitation program. He has pinpoint pupils and shallow breathing. Physical examination shows multiple needle scars. At this time you should administer

(A) buprenorphine
(B) clonidine
(C) methadone
(D) naloxone
(E) naltrexone

25. You are covering in the office for your colleague who is on a vacation when you receive a call from the mother of one of his patients. She is very concerned that her child has developed "some nerve disease" because he has a twitch in the eye and the side of his mouth. She swears that her son has never had these problems before. You ask her to wait on the phone while you check his medical records. It seems that the child was diagnosed with attention deficit hyperactivity disorder recently and was started on a stimulant. You conclude that the child seems to have developed tics. The most appropriate intervention at this time is to

(A) confront the mother that her inadequate parenting caused stress to her child resulting in tics
(B) explain that this is a side effect of his medication that will go away on its own
(C) tell the mother that child has new onset tics and needs further exploration by a neurologist
(D) tell the mother to bring the child in so that you can examine him and suggest further treatment
(E) tell the mother you will call her pharmacy for an antipsychotic agent to counteract the tics

26. A 68-year-old man comes to the office for a followup visit after being discharged from the hospital following a myocardial infarction. He is a widower and lives alone in his house. He tells you that he is doing "pretty well" and reports no complaints, except for decreased sleep, which he feels is normal for his age. He seems a little bit depressed. When you start inquiring about the symptoms, you find that he may have some mild form of depression, which you explain is very common after a myocardial infarction. You also remember reading that depression significantly increases the risk of death in patients with cardiovascular disease, independent of other risk factors for cardiovascular disease. Therefore, you talk to him about the possibility to starting medication. The medication that has been proven to decrease mortality in this population is

(A) alprazolam
(B) bupropion
(C) nortriptyline
(D) paroxetine
(E) pimozide

27. A 6-year-old boy is brought to the clinic because of behavioral problems. The patient's mother tells you that her son has a normal activity level at home, but there is a complaint of "hyperactivity," inattention, and aggressiveness with his stepbrother and stepsister when the patient goes to his father's house for weekend visits. The mother wants you to prescribe a medication for the patient to "calm him down for his visits to his father's house." He has had recurrent ear infections and eustachian tube placement but has no past psychiatric history. The most appropriate next step in management is to

(A) obtain information from the patient's teacher with regard to level of activity, behavior, and attention to academic performance
(B) order a CT scan of the patient's head
(C) order an electroencephalogram
(D) prescribe fluoxetine
(E) prescribe methylphenidate

28. While working in the clinic, you see a 10-year-old boy whom you feel has a diagnosis of attention deficit hyperactivity disorder. The patient's presenting problems include not paying attention in class, constant fidgeting, not waiting his turn, and impulsive behaviors in school and at home. You decide to start the patient on methylphenidate. At each visit you should

    (A) determine complete blood count
    (B) determine fasting blood glucose level
    (C) do audiology testing
    (D) measure height and weight
    (E) send a urinalysis

29. A 67-year-old woman with hypertension, which is well controlled on her current regimen of antihypertensives, comes to the clinic for a health maintenance examination. Her husband of 30 years died 1 month ago. She tells you that she feels sad but is regaining her appetite and sleeping well, and she adds that she is happy to be alive to enjoy her grandchildren. However, she sometimes hears her husband's voice calling her. Complete examination, including neurologic and Mini-Mental Status Examination (30/30), is unremarkable. She is concerned about her current psychologic condition. The most appropriate next step in management is to

    (A) prescribe risperidone for auditory hallucinations
    (B) reassure the patient that hearing her husband's voice calling her may be a part of normal grieving
    (C) recommend an MRI of the patient's head
    (D) recommend a psychiatric inpatient hospital stay
    (E) recommend that the patient receive donepezil to help her level of orientation

30. A 42-year-old man comes to the office for a periodic health maintenance examination. He is generally healthy and has no known medical or psychiatric history. He does, however, admit to a 20 pack-year history of smoking. He would like to quit and is wondering if there are any recommendations or medications that may help him. He explains that he recently attempted to quit "cold turkey" but experienced dysphoric mood, insomnia, irritability, and a weight gain, so he started smoking again. Physical examination and laboratory studies are all unremarkable. Appropriate management at this time is to

    (A) prescribe bupropion
    (B) prescribe haloperidol
    (C) recommend an increase in his caffeine intake
    (D) recommend an increase in his caloric intake
    (E) recommend the temporary use of alternate forms of tobacco intake, such as chewing tobacco

31. An 11-year-old boy is brought to the clinic by his foster mother because she is "having difficulty controlling him." The boy constantly starts fights with other children and steals money from them. Additionally, the patient has a history of multiple arrests for shoplifting and vandalism. There are no abnormalities on physical examination. On mental status examination, the patient is found to be very well behaved and charming but does admit to the behaviors described by his foster mother. As an adult, the patient has a higher likelihood of developing

    (A) antisocial personality disorder
    (B) autistic disorder
    (C) pica
    (D) rumination disorder
    (E) schizophrenia, chronic paranoid type

32. A 43-year-old man with no known past medical history or psychiatric history comes to the emergency department because of a 3-month history of fulminant episodes of heart palpitations, shortness of breath, feelings of "claustrophobia," and distal paresthesias. He appears calm on examination but states that earlier in the morning, he had "an attack." His blood pressure is 150/100 mm Hg and pulse is 105/min. He is diaphoretic and has dilated pupils. Urinary toxicology is positive for cocaine. The most appropriate next step in management is to

    (A) give him a prescription for lorazepam and a followup appointment with his internist
    (B) give him a prescription for paroxetine and a followup appointment with a walk-in psychiatric clinic
    (C) provide agonist therapy for cocaine dependence
    (D) recommend cognitive behavioral therapy for relaxation training
    (E) refer him for cocaine dependence treatment

33. A 37-year-old man comes to the clinic complaining of repeated, intrusive thoughts that his hands are dirty. He has begun compulsively washing his hands to the point that anytime he touches a surface, such as a table or a doorknob, he needs to wash. He explains that he does not want to take medication for this condition because of side effects that he experienced from previous trials of psychiatric medications. He has read about "something called exposure and response prevention treatment" and would like to try it. Exposure and response prevention therapy for this patient may involve

    (A) free association of thoughts
    (B) having the patient touch a dirty surface and not wash his hands
    (C) induction into a hypnotic state
    (D) interpretation of unconscious drives
    (E) keeping a diary of when he feels the need to wash his hands

34. A 45-year-old woman is brought to the emergency department by her family because she is "in a manic state." The patient has not slept for several days, has flight of ideas, has maxed out five credit cards, and believes that she is indestructible. She has always been extremely reluctant to seek treatment and has never had consistent outpatient followup in the past. She has had two distinct depressive episodes, with consistent sadness, tearfulness, and passive suicidal ideation, and two other manic episodes in the last 6 months. In addition to hospitalization, the most appropriate pharmacotherapy for this patient is

    (A) amitriptyline
    (B) lithium
    (C) propanolol
    (D) theophylline
    (E) valproic acid

35. A 36-year-old woman with borderline personality disorder comes to the clinic requesting to see a new physician because she is "sick of medications and wants to start fresh with someone new." The patient's history reveals the hallmark symptoms of borderline personality disorder, including chronic emptiness, chronic suicidality, fear of perceived loss, extreme emotionality, and multiple suicide attempts. Her record confirms that she has not made any appreciable improvement despite multiple trials of medications and psychiatric hospitalizations. A therapeutic modality with proven efficacy for this patient's condition is

    (A) aromatherapy
    (B) biofeedback
    (C) dialectical behavior therapy
    (D) flooding
    (E) hypnotherapy

36. A 45-year-old man returns to the clinic 3 weeks after beginning therapy with paroxetine 20 mg for minimal to moderate major depression. He has no previous psychiatric history before this past month, when he began to experience a consistently depressed mood, poor sleep, decreased appetite, and loss of interest in many of his leisure activities. Now, when asked how he feels, he says, "I'll have one good day and one bad day. But I have been eating and sleeping better." However, he remains frustrated that his depression is not "fixed" and wonders if he should discontinue his medication. The most appropriate management is to

(A) agree that he is not responding to paroxetine and discontinue it
(B) ask the patient if he would like to change antidepressant medication after a brief "washout period"
(C) augment the patient's current medication with haloperidol
(D) augment the patient's current medication with thyroid hormone
(E) reassure the patient that the optimal effect of the paroxetine may have yet to be reached

37. A 31-year-old man is admitted to the hospital for an acute manic episode. He is intrusive and threatening and requires intramuscular haloperidol injections every 4 hours to control his agitation. After a week in the hospital, his agitation is under control, and he only has symptoms of hypomania. He has a history of three prior hospitalizations for mania. At a team meeting, the patient's medication regimen of oral haloperidol and lithium carbonate is discussed. If the patient were to be maintained on haloperidol, his bipolar illness would place him at an increased risk for

(A) agranulocytosis
(B) Cushing syndrome
(C) dementia, Alzheimer type
(D) hypophosphatemia
(E) tardive dyskinesia

38. A 33-year-old Hispanic woman who works as an accountant for a large corporation comes to the office for a periodic health maintenance examination. She has an "anxious personality" but says that over the past year she has been unable to stop worrying about reality-based concerns such as her job security, finances, and the health of her parents. She has been experiencing difficulty concentrating, tension headaches, and fatigue from "the constant stress I'm under." She does not drink alcohol, smoke, use illicit drugs, or ingest caffeine. Physical examination and review of systems are all within normal limits. Appropriate management for her symptoms is

(A) buspirone
(B) electroconvulsive therapy
(C) flooding
(D) haloperidol
(E) propanolol

39. A 64-year-old woman with a 25-year history of bipolar disorder, rapid cycling type, comes to the clinic for a followup visit. She has not had a hospitalization in over 3 years and is currently on a regimen of valproic acid and thyroid hormone. She has no manic or depressive symptoms at this time. Laboratory studies show no abnormalities, and her valproic acid level and thyroid-stimulating hormone levels are normal. As part of this patient's therapeutic drug monitoring, you should include assessment for

(A) breast cancer
(B) drug-induced parkinsonism
(C) osteoporosis
(D) pulmonary embolism
(E) tardive dyskinesia

40. A 45-year-old African American woman comes to the office for a followup visit. You have been seeing her since an inpatient hospitalization for her first episode of depression 9 months ago. She had psychotic features to her depressive illness at the time, including auditory hallucinations instructing her to kill herself. The patient has been in full symptomatic remission for the past 7 months on haloperidol and venlafaxine. Today, she asks if she can have her medication regimen changed and wonders if she should still be taking any medication at all. Appropriate management at this time is to

(A) explain that she can safely be taken off of haloperidol and venlafaxine if she undergoes electroconvulsive therapy once a month
(B) explain that she should continue with both medications for at least 5 years
(C) halve the dosage of both medications following today's appointment
(D) recommend that she continue the medications but that she can take them every other day
(E) slowly taper her off the haloperidol

41. A 4-year-old boy is brought to the clinic by his parents because his preschool teacher is concerned that he may be "autistic." On examination, the patient displays little interest in you, the nurse working with you, or his parents. During the assessment, he picks up a toy truck and spins the back wheels with his fingers for minutes at a time. Physical examination and laboratory studies, including chemistries, complete blood count, and toxicologies, are all within normal limits. To make the diagnosis of autism in this patient, you need to document

(A) a comorbid elimination disorder
(B) impairments in communication
(C) an IQ of less than 70
(D) sleep-wake cycle dysregulation
(E) vocal or motor tics

42. A 44-year-old HIV-positive man who is dependent on heroin is brought to the emergency department from the clinic with paranoid delusions that his landlord is attempting to poison him by sending poisonous gas through the ventilation system. The patient is not agitated, expresses no suicidal or homicidal ideation, and denies depressive complaint. His clinic chart notes that this is the first time he is experiencing delusions. Physical examination is unremarkable. A biochemical profile, toxicology studies, complete blood count, lumbar puncture, and head CT with contrast are all unremarkable. The patient is admitted to the psychiatric floor with a diagnosis of psychotic disorder not otherwise specified versus psychosis secondary to HIV infection. An appropriate treatment regimen for this patient is

(A) amitriptyline 200 mg at bedtime
(B) diazepam 10 mg 4 times a day
(C) haloperidol 10 mg 3 times a day
(D) methylphenidate 5 mg once daily
(E) olanzapine 5 mg at bedtime

43. A 55-year-old African American woman with diet-controlled hypertension comes to the office because she is feeling depressed following the death of her sister. She has had difficulty sleeping, a poor appetite, and feelings of guilt. She no longer enjoys running and playing the piano, which were her two favorite hobbies. She would like to try an antidepressant medication but, as she says, "not one that will affect my blood pressure." The antidepressant medication that would most likely result in an increase in blood pressure in this patient is

(A) amitriptyline
(B) bupropion
(C) fluoxetine
(D) sertraline
(E) venlafaxine

44. While working in an emergency department you are called to assess a 32-year-old woman who has had a sudden increase in blood pressure. She explains that she recently started taking medication for "social phobia" but has forgotten the name of the pills. She was having a glass of wine after work with a group of friends when she had the sudden onset of a headache, "the sweats," and blurry vision. The medication that most likely caused this clinical presentation is

(A) bupropion
(B) fluoxetine
(C) lorazepam
(D) phenelzine
(E) sertraline

45. You are called to the GI/liver floor to assess a 48-year-old man with hepatitis C cirrhosis and bipolar disorder. The patient has a clear sensorium and is fully oriented. However, he has symptoms of a depressive episode with tearfulness, crying, poor sleep, and hopelessness. He has a history of unipolar, manic, and depressive episodes that occur on average twice a year. He has never been compliant with psychiatric outpatient care and is currently not taking any medications for his psychiatric condition. The most appropriate pharmacotherapy for this patient is

(A) carbamazepine
(B) haloperidol
(C) lithium
(D) nefazodone
(E) olanzapine

46. A 54-year-old woman with migraine headaches and bipolar disorder comes to the clinic for a followup appointment. Although she does not feel depressed at this time, she is frequently tired, frequently feels cold, and has gained 30 pounds in the last 6 months. She tries to exercise and eat a healthy diet and promises that she is compliant with her lithium therapy. Her blood pressure is 110/80 mm Hg, and pulse is 65/min. On physical examination you note that she is more hirsute than on previous evaluations but is otherwise normal. The next appropriate step in this patient's management is to

(A) prescribe an antidepressant
(B) prescribe a psychostimulant
(C) recommend phototherapy
(D) send her for genetic testing for Huntington disease
(E) send thyroid function tests

47. A 22-year-old college student is brought to the emergency department following a rape that occurred while she was walking home from her classes this evening. She is visibly shaken and is crying throughout the whole interview and physical examination. You ask the patient if she would like some sort of counseling or therapy for herself, and she tells you that she would very much appreciate that. At this time the most appropriate mode of therapy for this patient is

(A) Amytal interview
(B) dialectical behavior therapy
(C) hypnotherapy
(D) psychoanalysis
(E) supportive psychotherapy

48. A 34-year-old woman comes to the office because of a depressed mood, fatigue, loss of interest in activities, excessive somnolence, and weight gain. These symptoms occur every winter and then gradually resolve during the springtime. She is much less productive during the winter, and would like treatment because she has already begun to feel "slowed down." She does not want to use antidepressant medication but would consider dietary supplements or "alternative treatments" to help her with her depression. Given her request, the most appropriate recommendation for her condition is

(A) biofeedback
(B) kava lactones
(C) phototherapy
(D) vitamin B_{12}
(E) vitamin E

49. A 26-year-old man with borderline personality disorder comes to the office for a followup visit. He recently had a brief psychotic episode and was started on risperidone. He tells you that he has this intense feeling that he is "jumping out" of his skin. He is unable to sit still and constantly feels the need to stretch his legs. His mother has noticed that he paces around the house. He promises that he has been compliant with his medication. He denies any psychotic symptoms. After a short conversation, you determine that this is a side effect of the medication. You observe that even during the interview the patient is unable to sit still for more than 2 minutes. The most appropriate next step in management is to

(A) admit him to the hospital for further treatment
(B) discontinue the risperidone
(C) recommend no change because the side effect will eventually subside
(D) start propranolol
(E) switch to a different antipsychotic agent

50. A 45-year-old man with a history of depression and anxiety comes to the office because of irritability, feelings of sadness, and a lack of desire to "do anything." His relationship with his wife has been very poor lately, and their "intimate life" is nonexistent. He has taken sertraline in the past and is willing to go back on medication, but he insists on something that will not cause impotence. In the past he had problems with libido and erection. He has heard from other patients that attend the same group therapy that there are other types of medications available without these side effects, and he is willing to give them a try. Given this patient's concerns, you should prescribe

(A) bupropion
(B) maprotiline
(C) paroxetine
(D) trazodone
(E) venlafaxine

Psychiatry Test One: **Answers and Explanations**

ANSWER KEY

1. A
2. B
3. D
4. D
5. D
6. C
7. A
8. A
9. A
10. E
11. B
12. D
13. B
14. B
15. E
16. A
17. A
18. E
19. C
20. B
21. C
22. A
23. B
24. D
25. D
26. D
27. A
28. D
29. B
30. A
31. A
32. E
33. B
34. E
35. C
36. E
37. E
38. A
39. C
40. E
41. B
42. E
43. E
44. D
45. C
46. E
47. E
48. C
49. D
50. A

1. **The correct answer is A.** The patient's history of over three depressive episodes places her at high risk for recurrent depressions as opposed to a patient with a single index episode of depression. The standard of care for recurrent depression is the continuation of the dosage or dosages of antidepressant medicine that facilitated remission.

   Discontinuation of medicine without presuming a risk of recurrence (**choice B**) is incorrect. There seems to be significant evidence that patients with recurrent depressions benefit from maintenance therapy to prevent recurrence of depressive illness.

   Taking paroxetine on an as-needed basis (**choice C**) has no support from clinical evidence. Antidepressant efficacy is most commonly achieved after at least 2 weeks of consistent administration. Paroxetine has never been shown to be an effective treatment for depression when used on a prn basis.

   Decreasing the dosage of paroxetine (**choice D**) is inappropriate management because there is no evidence to support a 6-month threshold after which a patient with recurrent depression can have a decreased dosage of antidepressant without incurring a risk of recurrence.

   The addition of another antidepressant (**choice E**) is incorrect and excessive. The patient has achieved remission on her present regimen of medication. The addition of another antidepressant in a well patient has not been supported by the clinical literature.

2. **The correct answer is B.** It is often frustrating to observe the self-destructive alcoholic patient, and a natural inclination of health care professionals and social workers may be to attempt to impose treatment and placement on such individuals. However, the patient in question clearly demonstrates competence and self-determination over his life circumstances, even taking into consideration how contrary to his own benefit his decisions may seem to his medical and social work team.

   Allowing the patient to be discharged only on the condition that he is escorted to an inpatient alcohol detoxification facility (**choice A**) is incorrect. The patient has demonstrated competence and does not require detoxification from alcohol because he has been medically hospitalized for almost 2 weeks.

   Having a psychiatrist to state that the patient must allow the hospital to make his health care and placement decisions (**choice C**) is incorrect for two reasons. The first is the competence of the patient. The second is that a psychiatric consultant does not have the jurisdiction to assign the hospital power to make decisions on behalf of the patient. Only through a legal hearing can someone appointed by the hospital be given those powers.

   Physical and chemical restraint (**choice D**) is incorrect and is a serious violation of the civil liberties of a mentally competent patient.

   Seeking guardianship (**choice E**) is incorrect because the patient has demonstrated competence. He does not represent an imminent danger to himself or others, and his acute medical issues have been resolved.

3. **The correct answer is D.** The patient is manifesting signs of adolescent depression. Adolescents, as opposed to adults, may have signs of depression that include irritability and academic difficulties rather than overt sleep or appetite changes. The patient in question is a formerly high-achieving student, and there is no reason why she should not be able to reattain her former level of functioning if her depression is adequately treated.

   The patient's symptoms are not a part of normal adolescence (**choice A**). The patient's presenting problems should therefore not be attributed to normal maturation, and intervention for this patient should be sought.

   The use of methylphenidate (**choice B**) to aid in the patient's attention to schoolwork is not appropriate at this time. The diagnosis of attention deficit hyperactivity disorder is not appropriate for this patient. The patient's declining school performance is more a reflection of deterioration in performance secondary to depressive illness. The patient's high premorbid school performance is also indicative of not having an innate attentional problem.

   The patient does not show symptoms of a psychosis. Therefore, no antipsychotic medication, such as olanzapine (**choice C**), should be given to the patient.

   There is nothing episodic or intermittent in the patient's presentation to indicate an epileptic illness as the etiology of her deterioration in function. Therefore, an electroencephalogram (**choice E**) is incorrect.

4. **The correct answer is D.** Selective serotonin reuptake inhibitors (SSRIs), such as paroxetine, fluoxetine, and sertraline, are considered to be the first-line treatment for panic disorder. However, patients with panic disorder (and other anxiety disorders) may experience some treatment-emergent anxiety with SSRIs that can be avoided if the medication is started at low doses and titrated slowly. The patient's starting dosage of paroxetine was much too high for a patient with panic disor-

der and likely caused or contributed to the patient's worsened anxiety. A lower starting dosage and slow titration may alleviate the patient's panic disorder without making the patient feel more anxious.

There is no known evidence to support the use of haloperidol (**choice A**) in panic disorder.

Potentially dangerous interactions, such as serotonin syndrome, occur with the simultaneous use of SSRIs and monoamine oxidase inhibitors such as phenelzine (**choice B**), tranylcypromine, and isocarboxazid.

An immediate increase in the second week of treatment to 40 mg a day of paroxetine (**choice C**) would likely only exacerbate the patient's present condition.

Switching the patient to sertraline 200 mg a day (**choice E**) is incorrect. A 200-mg daily dose of sertraline is too high and would likely cause treatment-emergent anxiety in this patient. A switch to a lower dosage of sertraline, such as 25 mg or 50 mg daily, could be an appropriate choice.

5. **The correct answer is D.** Carbamazepine is a medication that can induce its own metabolism. Patients may therefore have a need for dosage increase to maintain a therapeutic blood level of carbamazepine. The patient's presentation for this outpatient appointment gives no indication that she is at all confused or noncompliant with respects to her outpatient regimen.

   The patient gives no indication that she is psychotic or disorganized in her process of thought. Therefore, the addition of haloperidol (**choice A**) is not indicated or recommended.

   Giving the patient her entire dose of carbamazepine at bedtime (**choice B**) is incorrect. The elimination half-life of carbamazepine is approximately 8 to 12 hours, necessitating at least bid dosing of this medication.

   The patient indicates that she understands her medication regimen and is taking her medication as directed. There are no observable signs on mental status exam to indicate a lack of reliability (**choice C**) on the part of the patient.

   The patient does not display impaired judgment or insight on mental status exam. Her low blood level of carbamazepine is likely caused by the pharmacokinetics of the medication. There is no indication to rehospitalize this patient (**choice E**).

6. **The correct answer is C.** The patient presents with symptoms and clinical signs consistent with the over-ingestion of benzodiazepines. Benzodiazepines are generally considered safe if taken alone in overdose. The patient's presentation of confusion and decreased level of awareness in the context of relatively stable medical presentation while on a flexibly dosed regimen of a medicine for anxiety is suggestive of benzodiazepine intoxication. These signs can be quickly reversed with the administration of flumazenil. Keep in mind that flumazenil can cause seizures in patients who have taken stimulants or tricyclics in addition to benzodiazepines.

   The patient's presentation is much more suggestive of an intoxication than a precipitous depression (**choice B**). Nothing gleaned from the patient's history is suggestive of a major depressive disorder.

   There is no indication to diurese (**choice A**) a patient with benzodiazepine toxicity. Patients with over-ingestion of anxiolytics will more likely have decreases in blood pressure that could be exacerbated by active diuresis.

   The administration of methylphenidate (**choice D**) does not address the underlying cause of the patient's lethargy and obtundation. There is no evidence of clinical benefit that would occur from giving methylphenidate to a benzodiazepine-intoxicated patient.

   Transcranial magnetic stimulation (**choice E**) is an experimental treatment that is under investigation for indications similar to those of electroconvulsive therapy. It is not indicated or well studied for the over-ingestion of benzodiazepines.

7. **The correct answer is A.** Clonidine, which is an α_2-agonist, can be used alone or in conjunction with opiate agonists such as methadone in the treatment of the autonomic symptoms of opiate withdrawal. It is worth noting, however, that craving for opiates may not be appreciably ameliorated with clonidine.

   Disulfiram (**choice B**) is an inhibitor of aldehyde dehydrogenase that may be effective as aversive therapy for patients who are dependent on alcohol. It has no role in the treatment of opiate withdrawal.

   Flumazenil (**choice C**) is a benzodiazepine antagonist used to treat intoxication or over-ingestion of benzodiazepines. It has no known role in the treatment of opiate withdrawal.

   Haloperidol (**choice D**) is an antipsychotic medication that has no indication in the treatment of opiate withdrawal.

Methylphenidate (**choice E**) is a psychostimulant used primarily in the treatment of attention deficit hyperactivity disorder. It has no role in the treatment of opiate withdrawal.

8. **The correct answer is A.** The patient's behavior is indicative of regression in response to a decreased amount of attention caused by the demands on the parents after having a second child. Having the patient help his parents with some chores relating to the care of the infant would help the patient adjust to having a new younger sibling and give the patient a sense of being paid attention to.

    The patient does not appear to have a syndrome depressive disorder for which an antidepressant (**choice B**) is indicated. Other interventions, such as having the patient help his parents with some of the care of the baby, are preferable to committing the patient to medication therapy.

    Relaxation and deep breathing exercises (**choice C**) are indicated primarily for adult patients with anxiety-spectrum disorders. The patient in question, a child acting immature for his chronologic age, would not likely benefit from this mode of therapy.

    The patient does not manifest symptoms that indicate attention deficit hyperactivity disorder (especially notable is the calm manner the patient demonstrated in the doctor's office). Therefore, a trial of methylphenidate (**choice D**) is not indicated.

    Spanking the patient (**choice E**) would likely result in worse behavior from the patient. The patient clearly craves attention from his parents. Although seemingly an aversive stimulus, a spanking would positively reinforce his need for attention from his parents.

9. **The correct answer is A.** This patient shows traits of a cluster B (dramatic type) personality disorder. Frequently, these patients use techniques such as splitting of hospital staff to obtain attention, preferential treatment, and, in this patient's case, an increase in her narcotic pain medication. This patient has obviously succeeded in being able to create a divided opinion among nurses in terms of what constitutes appropriate responses to her complaints. In doing so, the patient is able to convince at least some of the nurses assigned to her care to recommend to other nurses and doctors that she needs as much narcotic pain medication as she is demanding. The most appropriate way to handle such patients is a team approach where the opinions of nursing staff are addressed with a consensus arrived on how to handle the patient's repetitive complaints and demands.

    Somatization disorder (**choice B**) is a psychiatric disorder that involves somatic complaints from multiple organ systems and is a diagnosis of exclusion after workup has proved to be negative. It is not usually treated as a psychiatric inpatient treatment unless a concomitant component of depression or psychosis exists, which makes the patient a risk for potential self-harm.

    The patient has no indication of a surgical abdomen because of a 6-month history of the same abdominal complaint. Additionally, there is no indication from the battery of tests conducted that a lesion requiring imminent surgical attention is needed. Therefore, surgical consultation (**choice C**) is not necessary at this moment.

    Allowing the patient to pick her nursing staff (**choice D**) is incorrect. Allowing the patient to choose her own nursing staff would serve as reward for the patient's manipulative behavior and would reinforce the patient's existing belief that she will automatically get what she wants by making aggressive demands.

    Reprimanding the patient's nurse (**choice E**) is not an appropriate intervention. It would be especially harmful in this instance because of the potential that staff would be further divided on the issue of patient management and because it would strengthen the patient's perception that staff is split among nurses who genuinely care for her and nurses who are indifferent to her needs.

10. **The correct answer is E.** The patient's presentation is highly suggestive of intoxication on caffeine. The patient describes palpitations and diaphoresis exclusively at work where she is known to ingest larger quantities of caffeine than she would normally given the seasonal increase in demands of her employment.

    A CT scan of the head (**choice A**) is also not indicated given that there is nothing in the patient's clinical presentation to suggest a neurologic lesion.

    A 24-hour Holter monitoring (**choice B**) would be premature given that the patient experiences palpitations only at work (e.g., situationally) and that she has no history of syncope or past cardiac history.

    A 14-mg nicotine patch (**choice C**) is inappropriate because the patient does not smoke an equivalent to 14 mg nicotine per day (a basic filtered cigarette contains 1 mg nicotine). Additionally, over-ingestion of caffeine appears to be a more likely etiology for the patient's presentation than the one to two cigarettes that she smokes daily.

    Prescribing a low dosage of sertraline to treat the panic attacks (**choice D**) would be premature for this patient.

She does not give a history of overt panic attacks, and she not impaired by her presenting problem. A decrease in caffeine intake is a more reasonable choice before committing the patient to medication.

11. **The correct answer is B.** The patient is in obvious cocaine withdrawal following his cocaine binge preceding hospitalization. The patient, before having cocaine withdrawal, gave no history of recent symptoms of depression or mania. The patient's intense dysphoria will most likely be self-limited and improve coincidentally with resolution of his withdrawal from cocaine.

Treating the patient's cocaine withdrawal with haloperidol (**choice A**) is incorrect. At present, there are no known pharmacologic agents that have demonstrated consistent improvement in the symptoms of cocaine withdrawal. Although cocaine withdrawal is an intensely unpleasant experience, it does not carry the same dangers as withdrawal from alcohol, benzodiazepines, or barbiturates.

The patient's rapid shift in mood may incline some physicians to believe that he has a bipolar-spectrum disorder. However, the history is more clearly indicative of withdrawal from cocaine, and neuropsychological testing (**choice C**) while the patient is craving cocaine and in active withdrawal would not yield an accurate baseline of the patient's range of psychopathology.

Given that the patient most likely has a self-limited depression and is not catatonic, delirious, suicidal, or psychotic, electroconvulsive therapy (**choice D**) for this patient would be extremely premature.

The practice of insight-oriented psychotherapy (**choice E**) requires participation from the patient and a frustration tolerance that would be in excess of what someone in cocaine withdrawal could provide.

12. **The correct answer is D.** First and foremost, the physician in this case is legally obligated to protect any potential victims from imminent harm, even in the event of a breach of patient confidentiality. The landmark case in this matter is Tarasoff versus the Board of Regents of the University of California. A long-standing shortcoming of this obligation is that "to protect and warn" potential victims is not firmly defined by statute.

The patient in this case is a legal adult. There is no obligation of the physician in this case to call his parents (**choice A**). Additionally, merely calling the patient's parents would likely not qualify as protecting and warning the potential victims of this patient.

Maintain the confidentiality of the session while at the same time documenting what the patient said during the session (**choice B**) is incorrect because doctor-patient confidentiality must be breached to protect potential victims of a patient.

The patient in this case does not appear agitated, and his desire to harm his ex-girlfriend and her new boyfriend would not likely change in the event of a prn dose of anti-agitation medicine. Therefore, medicating the patient immediately for agitation and reassess the patient after the medication has taken effect (**choice C**) is incorrect.

Treating the patient's depression with medication or referral for electroconvulsive therapy (**choice E**) may be viable at a later time, especially if the patient is admitted to an inpatient psychiatric ward. However, the most exigent legal matter for this physician is the protection of potential victims of the patient.

13. **The correct answer is B.** A β-blocker such as propanolol can be used as effective treatment to control this patient's tremor, especially given the fact that dosage reduction (another viable option to decrease or eliminate lithium-induced tremor) is not desired by the patient.

Benztropine (**choice A**) is an anticholinergic medication used to treat extrapyramidal side effects of neuroleptic medication. It has no use in the treatment of lithium-induced tremor.

The patient may continue with lithium treatment given that tremor is usually a benign and treatable side effect of lithium. Therefore, insisting that the patient discontinue lithium treatment (**choice C**) is incorrect.

Biofeedback (**choice D**) is not considered to be a first-line option in the treatment of lithium-induced tremor. There is, however, literature supporting biofeedback in many other conditions, such as chronic pain.

Telling the patient as empathetically as possible that nothing can be done to reverse this side effect of lithium (**choice E**) is incorrect because of the aforementioned options available to patients who develop tremor while on lithium.

14. **The correct answer is B.** The patient is on clozapine therapy, which carries a potentially fatal risk of agranulocytosis. Complete blood count is usually obtained weekly to bi-monthly depending on the length of time a patient has been taking clozapine. From the patient's history, it is noted that she was away for 3 weeks and may not have had complete blood count monitoring.

A dosage-dependent risk of seizures does exist for patients taking clozapine. However, there is no clinical data to support seizure prophylaxis (**choice A**) for patients taking clozapine in the context of a fever.

Metabolic abnormalities in this context have been reported with clozapine treatment; however, abnormalities pertaining to potassium (**choice C**) are not as common, nor are they as potentially life threatening as agranulocytosis.

Because of the risk of agranulocytosis with clozapine treatment, the patient should not be discharged from the emergency department with advise to followup as an outpatient (**choice D**) before having a complete blood count performed.

Given the patient's history of schizophrenia and institutionalized living, she is at higher risk for tuberculosis. However, the patient's most exigent and potentially life-threatening matter presently is agranulocytosis in the context of an infection. Evaluating and treating for tuberculosis (**choice E**) may be appropriate but is secondary to ensuring that the patient has an adequate granulocyte count.

15. **The correct answer is E.** The patient's beliefs are consistent with his cultural background and are supported by the patient's parents and grandmother. The patient does not show any other psychiatric symptoms, and his functioning academically and socially is excellent.

The patient does not have a psychotic illness and is functioning optimally academically and socially. He does not warrant an inpatient psychiatric hospitalization (**choice A**) or further laboratory workup at this time.

Haloperidol (**choice B**) is often used as a treatment for patients with delusional disorder. A delusion is defined as a fixed, false belief that is not accepted as true by a person's culture. Because the patient's belief in spirits is accepted by his parents and grandmother, it does not represent a delusional belief, and there is no indication for antipsychotic treatment.

There is no indication that he is being abused or neglected by his parents. A referral for foster care (**choice C**) is absolutely inappropriate for this patient.

Weekly drug screening (**choice D**) for this patient is not necessary. There is no indication that the patient is using any illicit drugs habitually, and the patient demonstrates excellent academic and social functioning. There is no indication to regularly screen this patient for illicit drugs.

16. **The correct answer is A.** This patient has an acute mental status change, and delirium is the main concern. The number one cause of delirium in this age group is a urinary tract infection, and this patient has incontinence, so the urinalysis is ordered. Medications are often a cause of delirium, which is why the tetrahydroaminoacridine was discontinued. Tacrine can cause confusion but does not explain the incontinence or gait problems. A CT scan of the head is also part of the mental status workup. This patient has the symptoms of normal pressure hydrocephalus. The classic triad is unsteady gait, incontinence, and confusion. It is a potentially treatable dementia. A CT scan would show enlarged ventricles, and the treatment is a lumbar puncture to decrease the pressure.

An echocardiogram (**choice B**) would be indicated if the patient had evidence of embolic events. Tacrine can elevate liver function tests and this should be followed, but the patient has signs of normal pressure hydrocephalus.

An electrocardiogram (**choice C**) is indicated if the patient has signs of arrhythmia (episodic lightheadedness or syncope). Again, this patient has the classic triad of normal pressure hydrocephalus.

An electroencephalogram (**choice D**) would be indicated if the patient had obvious signs of seizure (motor movements, tongue lacerations). This test is a good idea in a confused incontinent patient if there is reason to suspect seizures (history of head trauma, medicines that lower the seizure threshold) or if the workup for more likely causes has been negative.

A radiograph (**choice E**) is indicated to rule out hip fracture if the patient had recently fallen or has had an abnormal lower extremity neurologic exam.

17. **The correct answer is A.** The patient has SSRI-induced sexual dysfunction, a common side effect. Given that he has had such serious depression in the past and failed trials of two other classes of antidepressants, it would be advantageous to keep him on the fluoxetine if at all possible. Antidotes for SSRI-induced sexual dysfunction are not well studied, but the addition of bupropion to the existing effective therapy has the best evidence.

The patient does not have erectile dysfunction, so sildenafil (**choice B**) is not an appropriate choice.

With the patient's serious history of depression with a suicide attempt and only 3 months of remission, stopping the antidepressant medication completely (**choice C**) would not be prudent.

Switching to bupropion (**choice D**) is a reasonable choice because it has the lowest incidence of sexual dysfunction of the drugs mentioned. However, it would be risky to stop the fluoxetine because a therapeutic response has finally been obtained with it.

Switching to nortriptyline (**choice E**) would not be advisable as a next step because the patient has a history of a failed trial on another tricyclic antidepressant.

18. **The correct answer is E.** Ibuprofen and several other NSAIDs are thought to increase lithium levels by inhibition of renal prostaglandin synthesis. This is probably the most common interaction with lithium. Lithium has a low therapeutic index, and changes in renal clearance are likely to be clinically significant.

Acetaminophen (**choice B**), aspirin (**choice C**), and codeine (**choice D**) are metabolized by the liver and will not affect his lithium level (**choice A**).

19. **The correct answer is C.** The classic antipsychotics and antidepressants often cause orthostatic hypotension, and patients often complain about this and the anticholinergic symptoms of dry mouth and constipation. This patient is on three medicines that commonly cause hypotension by α-adrenergic blockade.

Ataxia (**choice A**) is associated with lithium toxicity. Dystonias are common acute reactions to haloperidol.

Coarse tremor (**choice B**) is associated with lithium toxicity. Arrhythmias are associated with tricyclic toxicity.

It is reasonable to consider illicit drug use (**choice D**), especially if the patient was having psychiatric symptoms, but this patient is experiencing a common side effect of psychiatric medicines.

Some of the newer antipsychotics, such as olanzapine, are known to cause diabetes and elevation of lipids. Haloperidol is not associated with diabetes (**choice E**). It would be reasonable to check this patient's glucose, but this patient is most likely experiencing a common side effect of increasing her psychiatric medicines.

20. **The correct answer is B.** Pemoline is sympathomimetic approved for the treatment of attention deficit hyperactivity disorder. Given the rate of reported cases of hepatic failure, which range from 4 to 17 times higher than expected in the general population, pemoline can be used only if informed consent of the risks and benefits has been obtained from the patient. Liver function tests should be ordered at this time.

It is not typically necessary to order a complete blood count (**choice A**) in patients taking pemoline. It is necessary to monitor in patients taking clozapine, an antipsychotic agent, because of its association with agranulocytosis.

Platelet count (**choice C**) is usually not affected with the use of pemoline. Aplastic anemia has been reported in some patients.

Serum creatinine (**choice D**) is usually not changed with the use of pemoline because it does not affect renal function. Elevated acid phosphatase can be seen in the adult male population because of potential prostate enlargement on pemoline.

Thyroid function tests (**choice E**) are not necessary because the thyroid is not affected by the use of pemoline.

21. **The correct answer is C.** This patient suffers from somatization disorder defined by multiple somatic symptoms in four different areas (CNS, genitourinary, gastrointestinal, and pain). The workup is usually negative, and patients undergo multiple admissions and interventions to satisfy their needs. The most appropriate treatment for this disorder is regularly scheduled visits with the primary care physician. This should limit increased need for visits elsewhere and decrease the cost of medical workup yet provide enough attention for the patient. Treatment with mental health counselors is sometimes a necessary part of management.

Doing what the patient requests (**choice A**) is not appropriate. It increases costs and confirms once again the patient's suspicion that something is really wrong.

Telling the patient that she will be fine (**choice B**), even though it may be true, sends a message that you are not willing to listen to her and understand her problems. It may only cause her to change physicians.

Running tests (**choice D**) just to be on the safe side, even though a review of documentation or a physical examination does not support it, is not a well-justified option. Clinical judgment needs to be used to proceed with diagnostic procedures.

Telling the patient that it is all because of stress (**choice E**) and referring her to a psychiatrist is not an appropriate choice. Even though the symptoms may be stress related, referring her to somebody else is avoiding dealing with her. Also, the patient may not want to see a psychiatrist because she feels convinced she has medical problems.

22. **The correct answer is A.** The Mini-mental status examination is a brief instrument designed to grossly assess cognitive functioning. It assesses orientation, memory, calculation, language, reading, writing, and visuospatial abilities. It is easy and therefore widely used in any clinical setting. In this case it would be the first appropriate test to use.

The Minnesota Multiphasic Personality Inventory-2 (**choice B**) is designed to provide an objective measure of abnormal behavior. It contains 10 scales with major psychopathology and three validity scales (lie, infrequency, and correction) that can be interpreted to detect the absence of pathology. It is used and interpreted by skilled mental health professionals.

The thematic apperception test (**choice C**) is a projective test used to reveal a patient's emotions, motivations, and core personality conflict. It is used by skilled mental health professionals for the purposes described. It is not helpful for detecting cognitive deficits in dementia.

The Wechsler Adult Intelligence Scale (**choice D**) is not appropriate in this case. It is used by skilled professionals to assess intelligence. It takes longer and is not primarily used by primary care physicians.

The Wisconsin card-sorting test (**choice E**) is a neuropsychologic test used to assess executive functions and abstract thinking. It is used by skilled professionals more frequently when a specific battery of tests needs to be done. It is usually not applied by primary care physicians.

23. **The correct answer is B.** Lithium may cause fetal harm when administered to pregnant women. Data suggest an increase in cardiac and other abnormalities, especially Ebstein anomaly, which happens in every 2,000 cases (which is 10 to 20 times higher than in the general population). Pregnant women who have been taking lithium should always be appraised for potential hazard to the fetus.

Fetal neural tube defects (**choice A**) are more often seen with the use of valproic acid in pregnancy.

"Lithium is completely safe" (**choice C**) is an incorrect statement as explained above.

Pigmentary retinopathy (**choice D**) is not caused by lithium. In adults it can be caused by thioridazine.

Abortion (**choice E**) may be considered only after a discussion and assessment of potential hazard to the fetus have been done. Whereas fetal anomalies may occur, they are not observed in all cases.

24. **The correct answer is D.** Naloxone is a short-acting opioid antagonist used intravenously to reverse respiratory depression caused by ingestion of large amounts of opioids. Depending on the half-life of the opioid, it can be used until the effects abate. The reversal is seen as an increase in blood pressure and respirations and reversal of constricted pupils.

Buprenorphine (**choice A**) is a partial μ-agonist analgesic that is effective in detoxification from opioids. It is available only parenterally and exhibits few respiratory depression effects. It can be used as a first step in detoxification. Because it is a partial agonist, it is not indicated in patients who already have signs of overdose on opioids.

Clonidine (**choice B**) is an α_2-adrenergic agonist that reduces the symptoms of opioid withdrawal by inhibiting noradrenergic activity. It is used in detoxification but not for initial treatment of overdose.

Methadone (**choice C**) is a long-acting synthetic opiate agonist used for detoxification, providing smoother withdrawal from opiates. It cannot be used in a patient with overdose because it suppresses respirations.

Naltrexone (**choice E**) is used in detoxification, significantly shortening the time of the complete process when combined with clonidine. It is a long-acting oral opioid antagonist that helps to maintain abstinence for up to several months.

25. **The correct answer is D.** Even though you suspect that the tics are related to the use of the stimulant, establishing a diagnosis over a phone on a child you have never seen before is bad practice. Therefore, it would be appropriate to see the child, which would also help with the mother's stress.

Confrontation about parenting skills (**choice A**) is completely inappropriate because it does not address the current problem and should not be done over the phone without knowing the family situation. This could only be counterproductive.

Tics may be present off and on (**choice B**), but you need to examine the patient first to establish the diagnosis.

Further exploration by a neurologist (**choice C**) may not be required after you examine the child and assess the severity of symptoms. Adjusting the dosage, leaving the dosage as is if the tic is mild, or adding benzodiazepine at times may help.

Adding antipsychotics (**choice E**) to the current regimen without ever seeing a patient is unacceptable. Dopaminergic antagonist may indeed help with involuntary movements, but the risks and benefits of such treatment should be seriously considered.

26. **The correct answer is D.** It has been well documented in clinical studies that SSRIs are helpful not only in treating depression but also in preventing further clotting by virtue of their effect on platelets. Therefore, the patient should be prescribed paroxetine at this time.

Alprazolam (**choice A**) is a short-acting benzodiazepine that has no effect on mortality rate in cardiovascular disease. It was initially thought that it had an antidepressant effect. It should not be used because of its strong addictive potential.

Bupropion (**choice B**) has dopaminergic and noradrenergic properties as an antidepressant but has not been proven to decrease mortality in this population of patients.

Nortriptyline (**choice C**) could treat depression but, given its potential cardiotoxicity, is not recommended.

Pimozide (**choice E**) is an antipsychotic not indicated here. It can also cause Q-T interval prolongation, leading to arrhythmias and death.

27. **The correct answer is A.** The patient displays hyperactive and inattentive behaviors that occur most prominently when visiting his father and his father's new family. The differential diagnosis includes attention deficit hyperactivity disorder (ADHD), adjustment disorder, depression, and separation anxiety disorder. It is indeed possible that the patient's mother is able to control the patient in the context of the home environment, whereas in other environments the patient displays out-of-control behavior, impulsivity, and hyperactivity, meeting the criteria for ADHD. However, the diagnosis of ADHD requires two settings in which these behaviors are evident. Further information from the patient's school is therefore necessary.

A CT of the patient's head (**choice B**) is also not indicated. Intermittent behavioral problems in a specific social context are not indicative of an anatomical lesion.

Intermittent behavioral problems in a specific social context are not indicative of an underlying seizure disorder, so EEG (**choice C**) is incorrect.

Nothing in the history indicates that the patient is syndromic and continually depressed. Fluoxetine (**choice D**) is therefore inappropriate.

Committing the patient to methylphenidate therapy (**choice E**) is inappropriate and premature given the details missing from the patient's history. Of particular importance is the patient's school performance, which may be a better indicator of the patient's innate ability to attain to tasks than the intrinsically stressful environment of being in his remarried father's residence.

28. **The correct answer is D.** Methylphenidate is a psychostimulant in the family of compounds that includes amphetamines. Loss of appetite and subsequent failure to maintain a normal growth curve can occur in some patients. Weight and height should be taken at every monthly medication visit for these patients.

Hematologic and infectious complications are not commonly seen in patients taking methylphenidate. Therefore, monitoring his complete blood count (**choice A**) at every visit is not indicated.

Insulin resistance or hypoglycemia are not commonly seen and have not been attributed to methylphenidate therapy. Therefore, fasting glucose monitoring at every visit (**choice B**) is not indicated.

Audiologic complications (**choice C**) are not commonly seen in patients taking methylphenidate.

Urinalysis (**choice E**) does not need to be a part of routine monitoring for methylphenidate. It is of note, however, that methylphenidate should be avoided in patients with renal failure.

29. **The correct answer is B.** The patient does not show any signs of a pathologic bereavement. She is eating and sleeping well and does not appear to have a mood that is decompensating toward depression. Hearing a recently deceased loved one's voice is a common complaint following that person's death. In isolation from other symptoms, it is not an indication for imminent treatment.

The patient does not show evidence of a primary psychosis or psychotic depression. The hearing of her deceased husband's voice is likely a limited condition that does not require treatment with risperidone (**choice A**).

The patient presents with a condition of normal bereavement. There is nothing from the history given (medical or psychiatric) to warrant an MRI (**choice C**).

The patient does not show any suicidality, homicidality, or psychotic symptoms. There are no indications for inpatient psychiatric stay (**choice D**) for this seemingly well-adjusted and grieving woman.

The patient does not give evidence of a dementing illness. There is no indication to treat her with anti-Alzheimer medication such as donezipil (**choice E**).

30. **The correct answer is A.** Bupropion has been approved for the treatment of nicotine dependence. Alternate forms of treatment for this patient may include nicotine taper through patches or gums and behavioral therapy. Patients taking bupropion should not have a history of seizures or bulimia.

    Haloperidol (**choice B**) is not an appropriate treatment for smoking cessation. In fact, a dopamine-blocking agent such as haloperidol may increase a patient's desire to smoke. Several reports suggest that schizophrenic patients chronically taking haloperidol reported an improvement in concentration from smoking.

    Caffeine intake (**choice C**) is often a trigger for smoking behaviors and is therefore incorrect.

    Eating large meals and increasing caloric intake (**choice D**) is also a trigger for many smokers and would not be effective as a treatment for smoking cessation.

    The patient is addicted to nicotine. There is no benefit from changing the delivery system of the nicotine temporarily (**choice E**). If the patient were to begin chewing tobacco, he would likely either continue chewing tobacco or begin smoking again.

31. **The correct answer is A.** The patient is demonstrating behaviors consistent with conduct disorder, which is thought to be the pediatric antecedent to adult antisocial personality disorder. The pervading pattern among patients with conduct disorder is a disregard for the rights of others and an inability to conform to acceptable societal limits.

    The patient's social engagement and reciprocity indicate that he is not at an increased risk of developing an autistic disorder (**choice B**). Additionally, pervasive developmental disorders usually develop long before age 11.

    The patient has not demonstrated any signs that he is eating substances that would not qualify as food. Therefore, pica (**choice C**) is incorrect.

    Rumination disorder (**choice D**) is a disease that generally begins in childhood and involves the patient eating his or her own emesis. The patient manifests none of this.

    The patient demonstrates good social reciprocity and is described as engaging and charming. There is no evidence of any social maladaptation or psychotic symptoms. He is not at an increased risk of developing schizophrenia (**choice E**).

32. **The correct answer is E.** The patient's anxiety symptoms most likely stem from his cocaine use. Intoxication with cocaine can produce psychiatric symptoms that are indistinguishable from panic attacks. In this particular patient, cessation of cocaine use will likely be sufficient to stop the patient's panic attacks.

    The patient should not be given any type of prescription for a controlled substance in the emergency room setting. A prescription for lorazepam (**choice A**) with a followup appointment is inappropriate given the low probability that the patient would go to his appointment and the rewarding qualities of lorazepam.

    The patient's panic attacks are most likely precipitated by cocaine intoxication, so a prescription for paroxetine (**choice B**) for panic disorder is inappropriate.

    There is presently no established agonist therapy for cocaine dependence (**choice C**).

    The patient's panic attacks most likely occur in the context of cocaine intoxication. Relaxation training works optimally when the patient is trained to relax during circumstances that are similar to those that provoke anxiety. In the cocaine-intoxicated patient, the ability to effectively use relaxation techniques (**choice D**) is highly circumspect.

33. **The correct answer is B.** Exposure and response prevention treatment for obsessive-compulsive disorder involves exposure to an anxiety-provoking stimulus (in this case touching a dirty surface) and subsequent prevention of the compulsive response (washing hands). It is hoped that patients will gradually not feel compelled to perform their compulsive rituals in real-life situations after this sort of "practicing."

    Free association (**choice A**) is considered to be a central component of psychoanalysis. It is defined as a patient stating what is on his/her mind without censoring his/her thoughts. It is not compatible with the problem-focused method of exposure and response prevention.

    Induction into a hypnotic state (**choice C**) does not constitute exposure and response prevention. Exposure and response prevention is a cognitive-behavioral technique that requires a patient's conscious awareness and concentration.

    Interpretation of unconscious desires (**choice D**) is a central aspect of analytically oriented psychotherapy. It is not a component of exposure and response prevention.

Journal and diary entries (**choice E**) can be used in behavioral therapy to identify triggers or situations that are coupled with specific emotional states (anxiety, depression, etc.). There is, however, no active component to this exercise that is tantamount to exposure and response prevention.

34. **The correct answer is E.** The patient has symptoms suggestive of a bipolar I diagnosis. More specifically, the patient demonstrates the rapid cycling subtype of bipolar disorder, the criterion being four or more discrete mood episodes within one calendar year. Valproic acid is the best studied pharmacotherapy for rapid cycling bipolar disorder, with superiority over lithium demonstrated for this subtype.

    Amitriptyline (**choice A**) is a heterocyclic antidepressant that could further exacerbate the patient's manic presentation. It should not be a part of this patient's initial management.

    Lithium (**choice B**) is a mood stabilizer effective in bipolar disorder. However, the efficacy for lithium is significantly compromised if the patient's presentation includes mixed or dysphoric mania or rapid cycling bipolar disorder.

    Propanolol (**choice C**) is a β-blocker used occasionally for performance anxiety or social phobia. It has no indication in the treatment of bipolar disorder.

    Theophylline (**choice D**) is an anti-asthmatic medication that has no known psychiatric indications and is not appropriate for the treatment of this patient.

35. **The correct answer is C.** Dialectic behavioral therapy was developed by Marsha Linehan at the University of Washington specifically for the treatment of patients with borderline personality disorder and chronic suicidality. The techniques involved in this treatment include the use of confrontation, humor, and self-regulation and exploration of patient affect. Controlled studies of this therapeutic modality confirm its efficacy.

    Aromatherapy (**choice A**) has been used experientially for patients with such conditions as anxiety and adjustment-related stress. It is not, however, a well-studied modality for any mental health condition.

    Biofeedback (**choice B**) has been used to treat chronic pain and many medical conditions thought to have a psychosomatic component, such as hypertension and asthma. There is no evidence to suggest that it is an effective treatment for borderline personality disorder.

    Flooding (**choice D**) is a cognitive-behavioral technique with documented efficacy for patients with a history of specific anxiety-provoking situations (such as fear of contamination in obsessive-compulsive disorder or fear of riding elevators for agoraphobic patients). Given that this patient does not have a specific stimulus that is anxiety provoking, it is difficult to flood the patient situationally.

    Hypnotherapy (**choice E**) has no documented efficacy in the treatment of behavioral disturbances and chronic suicidality associated with borderline personality disorder.

36. **The correct answer is E.** The full effect of an antidepressant medication generally takes between 4 and 6 weeks to achieve. The patient shows improvement after only 3 weeks of treatment and will likely continue to improve on the same dosage of medication.

    Discontinuation of paroxetine (**choice A**) is not recommended because of the patient's steady improvement on the medication and likely continued improvement in the ensuing weeks.

    The patient's initial response to treatment indicates that he will continue to improve if his treatment is allowed to continue the 4 to 6 weeks needed to observe a response. Changing the patient's antidepressant regimen (**choice B**) at this point would be premature.

    Haloperidol (**choice C**) is not an effective agent for augmentation of antidepressant response in the unipolar, nonpsychotic depressed patient.

    Augmentation with thyroid hormone (**choice D**) would be indicated only if, after a sufficient amount of time for a full trial, the patient were only partially responsive to treatment. In this patient, augmentation with thyroid hormone or lithium would be premature.

37. **The correct answer is E.** Patients with mood disorders (manic or depressed) are at increased risk for developing tardive dyskinesia when placed on long-term neuroleptic treatment. This risk appears to exceed that of patients with psychotic illness without mood symptoms.

    Bipolar patients treated with haloperidol do not have an increased risk of agranulocytosis (**choice A**). Agranulocytosis is an uncommon complication of clozapine, an atypical antipsychotic, and mirtazapine, an antidepressant.

    Cushing syndrome (**choice B**) has not been shown to develop at a higher rate in either the bipolar population or the neuroleptic-treated population.

Treatment with haloperidol has not been shown to increase the risk of development of Alzheimer disease (**choice C**).

There is no documented evidence that bipolar patients with chronic neuroleptic treatment are at a higher risk of hypophosphatemia (**choice D**).

38. **The correct answer is A.** The patient has symptoms consistent with generalized anxiety disorder. Buspirone is a serotoninergic medication used specifically to treat generalized anxiety. Venlafaxine and a short course of benzodiazepines are also approved treatments for generalized anxiety disorder.

    Electroconvulsive therapy (**choice B**) is not indicated in the treatment of generalized anxiety disorder unless a severe depressive illness is a comorbid presenting feature.

    Flooding (**choice C**) is a technique that forces large amounts of an anxiety-provoking stimulus or situation onto a patient. For example, a patient who has a phobia of snakes may be placed in an enclosed space with live snakes. For generalized anxiety, there is a lack of specificity, and a flooded situation is difficult to simulate.

    Haloperidol (**choice D**) is an antipsychotic medication that is also used to treat acute agitation. It has no indication in the clinical treatment of generalized anxiety disorder.

    Propanolol (**choice E**) is a β-blocker that is used for patients with performance anxiety, frequently in the context of social phobia. The patient does not give a history consistent with performance anxiety, and propanolol would likely be of little benefit to this patient.

39. **The correct answer is C.** Thyroid supplementation is a well-documented treatment for bipolar disorder, especially for female patients with the rapid cycling subtype. Among the complications for patients taking thyroid supplementation is osteoporosis, especially if patients become hyperthyroid. Periodic assessment for osteoporosis is recommended in these patients.

    There is no known increased risk of breast cancer (**choice A**) in patients taking thyroid hormone or valproic acid. The patient should have breast cancer screening as part of her physical health maintenance but not necessarily as part of therapeutic drug monitoring.

    Tremor can develop as part of valproic acid therapy or in hyperthyroid conditions. However, actual parkinsonism (**choice B**) with bradykinesia, rigidity, and postural instability is not well documented for patients taking these medications.

    Pulmonary embolism (**choice D**) and peripheral coagulopathies do not typically develop with valproic acid treatment or with thyroid hormone treatment.

    Tardive dyskinesia (**choice E**) is a complication associated with older neuroleptic medications and not with thyroid supplementation or with valproic acid treatment. Therefore, tardive dyskinesia is incorrect.

40. **The correct answer is E.** The patient's stable presentation without psychotic or depressive features warrants that she should be tapered off of haloperidol. The present guidelines are such that after a 6-month well period for a patient with a history of single-episode psychotic depression, antipsychotic treatment may be discontinued. In this patient, the added risk of tardive dyskinesia with extended use also warrants discontinuation of haloperidol.

    The patient should not be taken off antidepressant medication in favor of maintenance electroconvulsive therapy (**choice A**). There is no data to support the antidepressant maintenance efficacy of an abrupt switch from maintenance medication to maintenance electroconvulsive therapy.

    The patient's stable presentation warrants a taper of antipsychotic medication (although a year's maintenance of the antidepressant is warranted). A 5-year history of haloperidol (**choice B**) treatment in a patient with a history of mood disorder also places the patient at a high risk for tardive dyskinesia.

    For maintenance of remission from depressive illness, patients should be given the dose of medication that produced remission. Halving the dosage of both the antidepressant and antipsychotic medications (**choice C**) for this patient is therefore not advised.

    There are no data to support the efficacy of the use of venlafaxine or haloperidol every other day (**choice D**) in the maintenance of remission from depression.

41. **The correct answer is B.** The diagnosis of autism requires criteria from three major categories of impairment: social interaction, communication, and repetitive stereotyped behaviors. Asperger disorder, a disorder with a slightly better prognosis than autism, requires only social interaction deficiencies and repetitive stereotyped behaviors.

    A comorbid elimination disorder (**choice A**), such as encopresis or enuresis, is also not a requirement of autistic disorder.

Although a high percentage of autistic children have IQs less than 70 and comorbid mental retardation, an IQ of less than 70 (**choice C**) is not a diagnostic requirement of autistic disorder.

Sleep-wake dysregulation (**choice D**) is also not a requirement for the diagnosis of autism. However, the repetitive and ritualized nature demanded by many autistic patients can result in odd circadian patterns.

Autistic children very often have vocal or motor tics (**choice E**) in their presentation, and a history of tics in a socially restricted child should alert the clinician to a potential autism-spectrum diagnosis. However, tics are not a diagnostic requirement of autism.

42. **The correct answer is E.** HIV infection, even in the absence of AIDS, can produce new onset psychotic symptoms in patients. Patients with HIV infection are exquisitely sensitive to the extrapyramidal effects of neuroleptic medications used to treat psychosis. Therefore, a low dose of an atypical antipsychotic that is less prone to cause extrapyramidal symptoms is the treatment of choice for this patient.

The patient does not show any depressive symptoms on examination, and the patient's psychotic presentation does not seem to be in the context of a psychotic depression. An antidepressant such as amitriptyline (**choice A**) is therefore not indicated.

The patient does not show any agitation or need for sedation. The use of diazepam (**choice B**) is therefore not indicated as a part of the treatment regimen at this time.

Haloperidol at doses approaching 30 mg/d (**choice C**) would likely cause unacceptable extrapyramidal effects in this patient. Additionally, risks for neuroleptic malignant syndrome would be high given the factor of using a high dose of medication in a haloperidol-naive patient.

Methylphenidate (**choice D**) is often used for appetite stimulation in the cachectic HIV and cancer populations. It is not indicated as a treatment for psychosis, and its dopamine activity may even exacerbate psychotic states.

43. **The correct answer is E.** Venlafaxine is an antidepressant medication that has comparable efficacy to selective serotonin reuptake inhibitors in mild to moderate depression and may have an even greater efficacy in more severe depressive disorders. However, doses in excess of 150 mg/d of venlafaxine are associated with systolic blood pressure increases.

Amitriptyline (**choice A**) is not associated with increases in blood pressure, and, as with many heterocyclic antidepressants, orthostatic hypotension may occur with the use of this medication.

Bupropion (**choice B**) is not typically associated with increases in blood pressure.

Fluoxetine (**choice C**) and sertraline (**choice D**) are selective serotonin reuptake inhibitors that are not associated with increases in blood pressure.

44. **The correct answer is D.** Monoamine oxidase inhibitors, such as phenelzine, tranylcypromine, and isocarboxazid, are effective antidepressant and anxiolytic medications. Tolerability of these medications can be limited by dietary restrictions to tyramine-containing foods placed on patients because of tyramine-induced (in this case from the glass of wine) hypertensive crisis.

Bupropion (**choice A**) is an antidepressant medication thought to act on the dopaminergic and noradrenergic systems. It is not associated with tyramine-induced hypertensive crisis. A specific danger of bupropion is seizures, especially in the bulimic population.

Fluoxetine (**choice B**) is a selective serotonin reuptake inhibitor that is not associated with tyramine-induced hypertensive crisis.

Lorazepam (**choice C**) is a benzodiazepine medication that is not associated with elevations in blood pressure.

Sertraline (**choice E**) is a selective serotonin reuptake inhibitor that is not associated with tyramine-induced crisis. It should be noted that a washout period for a switch to or from a monoamine oxidase inhibitor and a selective serotonin reuptake inhibitor is required.

45. **The correct answer is C.** Of the medications listed, only lithium has an exclusively renal metabolism and elimination. Renal failure, therefore, can be a complication of lithium treatment. However, it should be most safely tolerated by this patient with liver disease.

Carbamazepine (**choice A**) is an antiepileptic medication that can be used for the treatment of bipolar disorder. Elevation of liver enzymes, however, is a very common complication of carbamazepine treatment, with overt hepatitis occurring in some patients.

Haloperidol (**choice B**) is an antipsychotic medication with hepatic elimination. It can also inhibit the metabolism of other medications that the patient may be taking.

Nefazodone (**choice D**) is an antidepressant medication that has a new warning of potential hepatic failure and is an inhibitor of the cytochrome p450 system.

Olanzapine (**choice E**) is an antipsychotic medication with an exclusively hepatic metabolism. Cases of fulminant hepatic failure have occurred with olanzapine use.

46. **The correct answer is E.** The patient is evidencing clinical signs consistent with hypothyroidism, a common complication of treatment with lithium. Thyroid function tests should be checked at least yearly in patients on lithium therapy.

    The patient's presentation of hypothyroidism in the context of lithium treatment is reversible with proper adjustment of lithium or addition of thyroid hormone. An antidepressant (**choice A**) is not indicated for this patient.

    A psychostimulant (**choice B**) is not the treatment of choice for this patient given the reversible nature of her presentation with proper correction of thyroid status.

    Phototherapy (**choice C**) is a treatment specific for patients with seasonal affective disorder. There is nothing from the history that includes a distinct seasonal component to the patient's presentation.

    Huntington disease (**choice D**) is an autosomal dominant condition that has many psychiatric manifestations, including depression, psychosis, anxiety, and dementia. There is also an accompanying movement disorder that may precede or follow the psychiatric manifestations of illness. There is nothing from the patient's history consistent for this disorder.

47. **The correct answer is E.** Patients coming off a terribly traumatic event or the news of a serious illness are, at least initially, best counseled by supportive psychotherapy. Supportive psychotherapy involves using the patient's strengths to customize coping strategies that can help patients recover from stressful life circumstances.

    An Amytal interview (**choice A**) is used for patients who have a conversion disorder to observe a resolution of neurologic symptoms. It would be inappropriate to use such a technique in this patient.

    Dialectical behavior therapy (**choice B**) is a therapeutic modality specifically designed for borderline personality disorder patients that involves cognitive/behavioral techniques that examine their stereotypically extreme behaviors and perceptions. It would be inappropriate to use this in a patient immediately after a sexual assault.

    Hypnosis (**choice C**) can be used as a tool to help the patient arrive at conflicts outside of his/her conscious awareness. The patient in question has been abused and is likely to feel powerless and helpless. Hypnotizing this patient in the days ensuing a sexual assault will likely be of little value.

    Psychoanalysis (**choice D**) involves the use of transferential reactions, the uncovering of unconscious drives, and working through conflict that arises during treatment to gain an insight into neurotic patterns. This would be too much to demand of this patient at the present time.

48. **The correct answer is C.** The patient has seasonal affective disorder. Part of the pathogenesis of the disorder is thought to lie with disrupted circadian rhythms that can be artificially corrected with phototherapy.

    Biofeedback (**choice A**) can be efficacious in the treatment of some pain and anxiety-related syndromes. It does not have any proven efficacy in the treatment of seasonal affective disorder.

    Kava lactones (**choice B**) are a naturally occurring extract that can be useful as a treatment for some anxiety-related conditions. It does not have a proven efficacy for seasonal affective disorder.

    Vitamin B_{12} (**choice D**) is important for the proper development of the nervous system, and B_{12} deficiency can cause neurologic symptoms, dementia, and depression. Vitamin B_{12} supplementation does not have a proven efficacy for seasonal affective disorder.

    Vitamin E (**choice E**) is a fat-soluble vitamin that is thought to have anti-inflammatory properties that may make it useful in the treatment of Alzheimer disease. It does not have a proven efficacy for seasonal affective disorder.

49. **The correct answer is D.** There are several ways of treating akathisia. One is by adding low doses of propranolol to the current treatment. This is the first choice because this patient has otherwise responded to therapy. Lowering the dose or adding benzodiazepines or anticholinergics are other options.

    Admission to hospital (**choice A**) would be indicated in a severe case of akathisia where major changes in medication are required and where the risk of exacerbation of symptoms is great. This is not the case with this patient.

Discontinuing risperidone (**choice B**) in a patient who has had a recent psychotic episode is not appropriate management of the problem.

Recommending no change (**choice C**) is not appropriate because akathisia does not subside over time. The patient is complaining about it, and if nothing is done, it may negatively affect the patient's compliance.

Switching to a different antipsychotic (**choice E**) can be considered only if other options are exhausted but not as an initial step.

50. **The correct answer is A.** Bupropion is a relatively pure norepinephrine reuptake inhibitor with some dopamine reuptake blocking activity. Its advantages include no significant effects on cardiac conduction, low switch to mania potential, few anticholinergic side effects, no weight gain, and no sexual side effects. It is also used effectively in treatment of smoking cessation.

    Maprotiline (**choice B**) is an antidepressant of an older generation, belonging to tetracyclics. It is rarely used because of side effects, which are similar to the ones of tricyclics (sedation, orthostatic hypotension, lower seizure threshold, anticholinergic effects, etc.).

    Paroxetine (**choice C**) is a selective serotonin reuptake inhibitor that causes sexual side effects, such as decreased libido, anorgasmia, and impotence.

    Trazodone (**choice D**) is a highly specific serotonin reuptake blocker and serotonin 5HT-2 antagonist. It can be arrhythmogenic and cause sedation and orthostatic hypotension. It can cause priapism. Because of these properties, it is currently used as a sleeping agent rather than as an antidepressant.

    Venlafaxine (**choice E**) is a serotonin-norepinephrine reuptake inhibitor. It has no significant interaction with adrenergic, muscarinic, histaminergic, or serotonergic receptors. It can cause anorgasmia and abnormal ejaculation as well as impotence, but its most common side effects are related to increased blood pressure, gastrointestinal symptoms, somnolence, dizziness, nervousness, and dry mouth.

Psychiatry: **Test Two**

1. A 38-year-old woman comes to the office because of upper respiratory symptoms. After a taking a brief history and physical examination, you provide the appropriate treatment for this condition. You notice in her chart that on the last visit you noted something about possible mild depressive symptoms. You mention it to her and begin a discussion about depression. She admits that she has been feeling depressed and has recently started taking St. John's wort. She has not noticed much improvement but admits that she is not quite clear what to expect. She asks you to prescribe a low dosage of an antidepressant, such as fluoxetine. She wants to take the St. John's wort and fluoxetine, but she only wants a low dosage of the prescription so that she does not become dependent on it. At this time you should

    (A) agree with the combination of the two medications and prescribe fluoxetine
    (B) explain that the combination of the two medications could have dangerous results
    (C) explain that studies show that St. John's wort has no antidepressant properties
    (D) tell her not to take ibuprofen and St. John's wort because the combination could cause renal failure
    (E) tell her St. John's wort is unsafe to use and that she should discontinue it

2. A 38-year-old woman with schizoaffective disorder comes to the office because of weight gain. She has been taking olanzapine for a few months and is very concerned about the 10 lb that she has gained since starting the medication. She has a family history of cardiovascular disease and diabetes mellitus. You discuss the possibility of switching her to ziprasidone because it is not usually associated with weight gain. She is willing to try it after you discuss risks and benefits. Before starting her on the new medication you should order

    (A) a complete blood count with differential
    (B) an electrocardiogram
    (C) an electroencephalogram
    (D) a prolactin level
    (E) a thyroid panel

3. A 42-year-old woman with depressive disorder with atypical features has recently been switched to a new antidepressant. During a weekend trip with her boyfriend to visit his Italian family, she was cautious not to drink red wine and eat any of the hams or sausages they serve. However, over the weekend she comes to the emergency department complaining of flushing, restlessness, tremors, headache, and sweating. Her blood pressure is 185/115 mm Hg, and a tremor and myoclonic jerks are observed. She tells you that she is on a monoamine oxidase inhibitor. When asked about her diet she swears that she stuck to it and is unable to understand the reason for this crisis. On further questioning, her boyfriend adds that they went to a Thai restaurant with his cousins. You realize that this is most likely a case of tyramine-induced hypertensive crisis. The most appropriate next step in managing this patient is to

   (A) admit her to hospital for treatment
   (B) discontinue the monoamine oxidase inhibitor, send her home with a few benzodiazepine pills, and advise her to see her psychiatrist as soon as possible
   (C) keep her unmedicated in the emergency department and observe her for several hours in a dark, quiet room
   (D) send her home with antihypertensive medication
   (E) send her home with no medication because the effect will subside on its own

4. A 78-year-old woman with diabetes mellitus is brought to the emergency department from her nursing home because of a change in behavior. According to the accompanying records she has been disoriented and hallucinating for the past 3 days. She does not seem to recognize the staff and has been complaining that it has been raining in her room. According to the documentation, 2 weeks ago she was started on low doses of amitriptyline for chronic pain. She is uncooperative during questioning and examination and appears agitated. Her skin is warm and flushed, and mucous membranes are dry. She is mildly tachycardic, and her temperature is 38.8 C (101.8 F). Laboratory studies show no significant abnormalities. The most appropriate next step in management is to

   (A) administer haloperidol intramuscularly
   (B) administer physostigmine intravenously
   (C) admit her to the intensive care unit
   (D) discontinue amitriptyline and send her back to the nursing home
   (E) provide safety for the patient and others in the emergency department

5. While in the hospital checking on a patient of yours who delivered a healthy baby 24 hours earlier, you are approached by a colleague who is examining a patient on the same floor. During the course of the conversation, he seems distracted and irritable, at one point launching into a diatribe about the inefficiency of the administration of the hospital. At the end of the conversation, he thanks you for listening and confesses that he has been under a great deal of stress lately. "But I've put myself on benzodiazepines and that keeps me sane," he concludes. At this point, the best response to your colleague is:

   (A) "As you know, I am required to report you to the State Medical Board."
   (B) "Have you thought about going for counseling? I have someone very good to recommend."
   (C) "How long have you felt like this?"
   (D) "I agree. This hospital never has been very efficient."
   (E) "Is there anything I can do to help?"
   (F) "Sometimes this whole profession gets the better of me, too."
   (G) "Well, I hope that you feel better soon."
   (H) "Why don't you make an appointment to see me for a physical exam? We can check and make sure that you are holding up OK."
   (I) "You need to take some time off. Let's talk about how to arrange coverage for your patients."
   (J) "You really should not be prescribing for yourself. If you need benzodiazapines, I'd be happy to prescribe them for you."

6. A 36-year-old woman with depression comes to the office because of a 4-day history of fever and chills that started while she was on a business trip. She has also been feeling “spaced out,” dizzy, and shaky and has been having difficulty sleeping. She has been taking sertraline for the past 3 months but admits that she forgot to take it on her recent trip. She is not sure if her depression is getting worse or if she just caught “the flu” on her trip. Either way, she did not continue with the medication upon her return. Physical examination is unremarkable. The most appropriate management at this time is to

    (A) advise her to stop taking sertraline because her symptoms are most likely an adverse reaction
    (B) consider sending her to a neurologist because of the symptoms described
    (C) tell her to restart sertraline to counteract the discontinuation syndrome
    (D) tell her that you would like to increase the dosage of sertraline because these symptoms are most likely signs of worsening depression
    (E) treat the “flu” with symptomatic therapy and stop sertraline

7. A 27-year-old bank teller was held up at gunpoint during a bank robbery several months ago. She comes to the clinic now because she “needs help with some problems.” She believes that she is depressed because she has been having flashbacks of the incident and nightmares. She is unable to concentrate at work because memories of the event continuously come to her mind. She has quit her job and is unable to go into any banks. When she walks down the street she feels as if she is constantly monitoring for signs of danger. Given the functional impairment related to her symptoms, the most appropriate management at this time is to

    (A) begin insight-oriented psychotherapy
    (B) prescribe alprazolam
    (C) prescribe sertraline
    (D) refer her for electroconvulsive shock therapy
    (E) suggest that she should go back to work because that is the only way to overcome the fear

8. A 25-year-old woman comes to the office because she gets extremely irritable, moody, and tearful a week or so before her menstrual period. She has crying spells and often has an increase in appetite with cravings for chocolate and sweets during this time. This has caused problems at work because she has difficulty controlling her temper with the customers. Her boyfriend has noticed that they fight much more on those days, so he tries to stay away from her during that “time of the month.” She has seen television commercials about premenstrual dysphoric disorder and has tried to follow some of the dietary recommendations she read about in magazines. This has helped her a bit, but the mood swings remain. She is willing to try anything that would help. Before starting her on pharmacologic treatment you should

    (A) assess whether she has regular ovulatory cycles
    (B) discuss the possibility of couples therapy for her and her boyfriend
    (C) obtain a thyroid panel
    (D) recommend increased salt consumption
    (E) recommend increased vitamin C consumption

9. A 10-year-old boy is brought to the clinic for evaluation. He comes with his parents who provide teachers’ reports that say that in the past couple of months the boy has been restless and fidgety. He repeatedly coughs as if he is trying to clear the throat. He has recently become disruptive in class, making loud, barking noises and screams that he would try to modulate and incorporate into a word. While the parents are explaining these issues, the boy blinks and touches his knee with one hand repeatedly. He has been doing well academically and is a very fastidious boy. There is no one else in the family with these symptoms. You should

    (A) explain that the boy needs psychotherapy to resolve conflict that caused this condition
    (B) explain that there is some evidence that this disease is inherited through sex chromosomes
    (C) inquire about a family history of obsessive-compulsive disorder or attention deficit hyperactivity disorder
    (D) tell the family that there are some specific tests that can confirm the diagnosis
    (E) tell the family that unfortunately this disorder usually leads to early dementia

10. A 26-year-old man is brought to the emergency department by ambulance after calling 911 and telling the operator that he is suicidal and plans to throw himself in front of a bus. He called for help because he was afraid that he might do "something stupid." He tells you that he is very depressed and wishes to die. He feels worthless and extremely fatigued, and, to "top it all off," he has been having unpleasant dreams. He denies any previous psychiatric history but admits to occasional use of street drugs. These depressive symptoms came on abruptly after a 4-day binge of crack cocaine. His vital signs are stable, and a complete physical examination is normal. The most appropriate next step in management is to

(A) admit him to the hospital for observation
(B) order an electrocardiogram
(C) order urine toxicology
(D) prescribe an antidepressant and send him home with a followup appointment in the clinic the following day
(E) proceed with involuntary commitment to the hospital

11. A 32-year-old woman with schizophrenia, paranoid type has been maintained on risperidone for 1 year. She is now complaining of two missed menstrual periods, before which she had one or two short and irregular periods. She knows she is not pregnant because she has not been in a relationship in the past year, nor did she have any sexual encounters. She denies having had any similar problems in the past. She recalls that this can be a side effect of the medication but reports that it concerns her because she fears that she will develop an "imbalance" that will be difficult to treat. The most appropriate next step in management is to

(A) add an anticholinergic to counteract the effects
(B) lower the dosage of risperidone
(C) obtain a prolactin level
(D) order an abdominal ultrasound
(E) start bromocriptine along with current medication

12. A 27-year-old stockbroker comes to the clinic complaining of easy distractibility at work, difficulty concentrating, and increased fidgeting. He has had these problems since early childhood but was able to compensate for them with a good memory. He admits to a past history of cocaine abuse, explaining that cocaine had a "calming effect" for him, whereas the friends he used cocaine with became more excited and expansive in their demeanor. At this time he would like medication to improve his attention and optimize his performance but does not want any medication with addiction or abuse potential. A medication that may be useful for this patient is

(A) bupropion
(B) fluoxetine
(C) haloperidol
(D) olanzapine
(E) risperidone

13. A 19-year-old student comes to the health center complaining of "depression." He just completed his final exams yesterday morning and had been sleeping for 18 hours before coming to see you. He was using "some pills" that he got from a friend to stay up for "marathon studying sessions." For the past day, he has been feeling "depressed" and "exhausted" in spite of his good performance on his exams and the full day of rest. He feels like crying and cannot seem to get enough to eat. The patient denies any suicidal intent, ideation, or plan, and there are no perceptual disturbances or paranoia. The most appropriate next step in management is to

(A) administer a one-time dose of flumazenil
(B) prescribe a clonidine taper for 1 week
(C) prescribe a methadone taper for 1 week
(D) prescribe methylphenidate
(E) provide supportive treatment and monitor the patient as an outpatient for 2 to 3 days

14. A 22-year-old woman comes to the office stating, "You've got to do something about my hideous skin." She tells you that she is so embarrassed of what she perceives as "obvious defects" on her face that she is unable to go out and socialize on most nights and that she cannot feel comfortable in settings with other single people. On examination, you notice that the patient has flawless skin and is actually very attractive. She has gone to five other doctors, and none of them have been able to provide any "help" to her. This patient is most likely suffering from

(A) body dysmorphic disorder
(B) conversion disorder
(C) hypochondriasis
(D) major depressive disorder with psychotic features
(E) somatization disorder

15. A 17-year-old Japanese boy with no past psychiatric history comes to the clinic complaining of feelings of sadness and impaired memory. His mother adds that his personality has changed a bit lately, too. You notice that he is jaundiced and has a resting tremor. On mental status examination, the patient has speech difficulties and difficulty maintaining attention. The most appropriate next step in management is to

(A) advise him to have phototherapy
(B) measure blood ceruloplasmin levels
(C) prescribe an antidepressant for major depression
(D) prescribe an antipsychotic for impending psychosis
(E) recommend electroconvulsive therapy

16. A 31-year-old previously healthy man comes to the emergency department because of a 3-hour sustained, painful penile erection that occurred spontaneously without any sexual stimulation. He denies any illicit drug use but does acknowledge that he has been taking a friend's prescription sleeping medication for the past 2 to 3 days. The medication most likely to have caused his condition is

(A) alprazolam
(B) chloral hydrate
(C) diphenhydramine
(D) trazodone
(E) zolpidem

17. A 24-year-old actress with bulimia nervosa comes to the office because of a depressed mood, anhedonia, low energy, and concentration difficulties. There is no suicidal intent, ideation, or plan, and she does not have any hallucinations or paranoid ideation. She is not currently taking any medications but would like you to prescribe "something for her depression." Over the years, she has had improvement in her binging and purging behaviors, but her work in the entertainment industry has compelled her to continue vomiting at least twice a week. In considering antidepressant agents for this patient, you recall that she would be at an increased risk for seizures with

(A) bupropion
(B) citalopram
(C) fluoxetine
(D) paroxetine
(E) sertraline

18. A previously healthy 21-year-old woman is brought to the clinic by her mother because of the acute onset of abnormal involuntary movements. She has choreoathetoid movements of her trunk that occur at rest and with movement. They do not occur while the patient is asleep. The mother tells you that these movements occurred suddenly one day after the patient found out that her husband was having an affair, and she shows you results from genetic, infectious, and metabolic testing as well as neuroimaging that other specialists have performed, all of which are normal. An intervention that may be helpful in the diagnosis of this patient's disorder is

(A) an Amytal interview
(B) an edrophonium challenge
(C) a phenobarbital challenge
(D) phototherapy
(E) 24-hour electroencephalogram monitoring

19. A 45-year-old African American man with diabetes mellitus, obesity, and hypertension comes to the office because of fatigue and daytime sleepiness. He is somnolent throughout his workday in spite of getting at least 8 hours of sleep per night. His wife complains of his constant loud snoring throughout the night and often worries that he has abruptly stopped breathing while he is sleeping. He denies hypnagogic or hypnopompic hallucinations or sleep attacks. The most appropriate management of his condition is to

(A) begin a trial of acupuncture
(B) begin therapy with continuous positive airway pressure
(C) prescribe desipramine
(D) prescribe dextroamphetamine sulfate
(E) prescribe haloperidol

20. An HIV-positive 44-year-old man comes to the clinic because of depression, anxiety, and sleep difficulties. He was diagnosed with HIV 8 years ago and has a history of multiple hospitalizations for pneumonia. Currently, he is only taking cisapride for gastroesophageal reflux disease while he decides whether he wants to have a more extensive treatment regimen for his HIV infection. However, he would like antidepressant or anxiolytic treatment before beginning HIV treatment. A potentially fatal cardiac interaction could occur if this patient were prescribed

(A) gabapentin
(B) lithium
(C) nefazodone
(D) risperidone
(E) thyroid hormone

21. A 10-year-old previously healthy boy is brought to the clinic by his mother because of "delusions." The mother explains that for the last 10 days her son has started to believe that an unspecific government agency is tapping the family's phone and has video cameras throughout the family's house. He has an older brother who is currently in a psychiatric hospital for the same paranoid beliefs. The patient's older brother, age 17, has had these beliefs for approximately the last 2 months and has, according to the mother, been "telling my younger son about what he calls 'the hidden truth.' " On mental status examination, the patient is fully alert and calm, with normal speech. He has no mood complaints or perceptual disturbances, is not psychomotor agitated, and has no difficulties in concentration. Serum chemistries, complete blood count, and neuroimaging are all normal. The most likely diagnosis is

(A) bipolar disorder, most recent episode manic
(B) major depressive disorder with psychotic features
(C) schizophrenia, disorganized type
(D) schizophreniform disorder
(E) shared psychotic disorder

22. A healthy 7-year-old girl is brought to the office for an evaluation of attention deficit hyperactivity disorder. The patient was referred by her teacher who, in a letter to you, describes the patient as "very bright and sociable" but also as inattentive during class, unable to finish assignments on time, lacking in attention to details, and easily distracted. The patient's parents also notice a pattern of inattention that is evident in their daughter when they attempt to help her with homework. In your office, she is noted to be very polite and appears happy. She does not display any disruptive or impulsive behaviors. Physical examination is normal. The parent's are concerned about the teacher's letter and want you to do whatever necessary to help with her problem. The most appropriate management for this patient is to

(A) evaluate her for mental retardation
(B) prescribe methylphenidate
(C) treat her for major depressive disorder
(D) refer her for sleep study evaluation
(E) report the patient's parents for seeking a prescription for a controlled substance

23. You are called to assess a 35-year-old woman because of "management problems." She was admitted to the hospital 2 days ago because of "generalized malaise of unknown origin." Some of the staff taking care of her describe her as manipulative and unreasonable, whereas others demand that you reprimand the staff members who are not "taking good enough care of this poor woman." On interview, the patient states that there is a wide and unpredictable gamut of care given to her. Whereas she gives small gifts to some staff members for excellent caregiving, the patient refuses to cooperate and screams when approached by other staff members. The defense mechanism that the patient is most clearly demonstrating is

(A) blocking
(B) projection
(C) reaction formation
(D) splitting
(E) sublimation

24. A 72-year-old woman with a history of chronic schizophrenia comes to the clinic for a routine followup visit. She reports that she has been feeling increasingly sedated for the past several months after her daily dose of haloperidol was increased to 10 mg. She denies any current mood or psychotic symptoms and is not suicidal or homicidal. She has been able to live independently in the community for many years and has not been hospitalized in over 15 years. She is not manifesting any extrapyramidal symptoms, and her physical examination and routine chemistries, thyroid function tests, and complete blood count are normal. At this time the most appropriate next step in management is to

(A) add lithium to her treatment regimen
(B) begin a supervised decrease in her haloperidol dose
(C) discontinue the haloperidol and switch her to maintenance electroconvulsive therapy
(D) prescribe an antidepressant
(E) prescribe a psychostimulant

25. You are seeing a 24-year-old woman with borderline personality disorder in the clinic for a followup appointment because her regular physician is on vacation. The patient has recently been discharged from an inpatient unit following a suicide attempt by cutting her wrists. During the course of the interview, the patient asks if you are married. The most appropriate next step in management is to

(A) ask the patient why she is asking you this
(B) discontinue the assessment
(C) ignore the question and continue with your assessment
(D) reprimand the patient
(E) tell the patient that you will tell her at the end of the assessment if she cooperates with the rest of the interview

26. A 35-year-old man with depression comes to the office for a followup visit for chronic back pain caused by a disk rupture and motor vehicle accident many years ago. His pain is usually controlled with ibuprofen, moderate exercise, and good sleep hygiene. Rarely he takes diazepam for muscle strain spasms. He has developed symptoms of neuropathic pain in the last 6 months, and you started him on a low dosage of amitriptyline at bedtime. He has also continued taking fluoxetine because of his history of five previous depressive episodes. He has responded well to the antidepressant medication but has developed sexual side effects, which responded nicely to the addition of bupropion. This patient is at greatest risk for

(A) amitriptyline toxicity with electrocardiogram changes
(B) diminished efficacy of bupropion with the return of sexual side effects
(C) diminished efficacy of fluoxetine with the return of depressive symptoms
(D) sedation and CNS depression from increased diazepam levels
(E) severe pain with increased metabolism of ibuprofen

27. You are seeing a 35-year-old woman in the clinic who has been previously diagnosed with psychotic disorder not otherwise specified. She has been receiving disability payments since she was in her early twenties and has always been socially isolated; she has never been able to work in any type of employment for more than 3 days at a time. During your assessment she acknowledges that she "hears voices sometimes" and often feels like people are following her. Currently, she cannot take public transportation because of a fear of people being able to read her thoughts. She denies any prominent mood symptoms such as depression, euphoria, racing of thoughts, or grandiosity. There are also no neurovegetative signs of depression or mania on mental status examination. From review of the patient's medical record, you see that she has had, in addition to her history of chronic delusions and hallucinations, discrete episodes of depressed mood, weight loss, guilty ruminations and delusions, and psychomotor retardation. This patient is most likely suffering from

    (A) autistic disorder
    (B) bipolar disorder with psychotic features
    (C) major depressive disorder with psychotic features
    (D) schizoaffective disorder, depressed type
    (E) schizophreniform disorder

Items 28–29

28. A 29-year-old woman with schizophrenia comes to the office with her husband because of a "strange feeling of tight muscles" in her neck. She says that she recently started taking chlorpromazine and "it's not working yet." Her husband is sitting quietly in the corner with his head down, nodding his head in agreement. Her temperature is 37.0 C (98.6 F). Physical examination shows that her neck is twisted to the right. The next best step is to

    (A) administer benztropine intramuscularly
    (B) administer bromocriptine intravenously
    (C) advise her that she would benefit from massage therapy
    (D) reassure her that this is normal and that no treatment is necessary
    (E) refer her to a neurologist

29. The appropriate management is undertaken, but she returns 3 months later with her husband who says that she is more socially withdrawn than ever and that she usually sits staring out the window for hours each day. You note that she has a flat affect. You discuss alternative therapy with the couple and decide that clozapine may be the solution. You tell them that she will need to come back to the office every week. They want to know the reason for this "great inconvenience." You explain that close monitoring is required because there is a slight risk of a disorder that is characterized by

    (A) dysfunction of the thyroid gland
    (B) life-threatening elevations in prolactin levels
    (C) life-threatening hypertensive crises
    (D) a great reduction in the number of white blood cells
    (E) reduced glucose levels

30. A 2-year-old boy is brought to the emergency department by his single mother and her boyfriend. The mother had noticed that the child was crying in his sleep when she returned from a social outing at 3 AM. In the morning, he was somnolent and emotionally distant. The boy had been in the care of her 17-year-old brother, who also lives in the household. Before this event, the child had been healthy and only had some trouble with potty training, according to the mother. On entering the examination room the mother's first words are "Will you take him away from me?" The child is lying on the examination table in a fetal position with a fixed gaze. His temperature is 96.7 C (98.0 F), and his pulse is 120/min. You notice that he is small for his age and poorly nourished. Centered on his buttocks are large flaccid bullae filled with serohemorrhagic fluid. They extend over the boy's gluteal regions and involve the posterior scrotum as well. In view of the clinical setting and physical examination, the most appropriate next step in the evaluation of this child is

    (A) a chest x-ray
    (B) a complete blood count with differential
    (C) an oral glucose tolerance test
    (D) a rectal swab
    (E) a skeletal survey

31. A 15-year-old boy with no significant past medical or psychiatric history is brought to the clinic for a routine visit. You remember him as a friendly, high-achieving student; however, the mother states that he has had a deterioration of school performance and activities over the last several months. He recently quit the cross country team and was caught smoking cigarettes and suspended from school. Physical examination and laboratory studies, including toxicology, are all within normal limits. The patient is noted to be much less friendly than usual with you during the appointment. When asked about what is bothering him, he curtly replies, "nothing." The most appropriate next step in management is to

    (A) prescribe a mood stabilizer
    (B) prescribe a psychostimulant
    (C) question him about neurovegetative symptoms of depression
    (D) reassure the patient's mother that he is going through normal "issues" associated with adolescence
    (E) send him for neuropsychologic testing, including IQ testing

32. You are called to the medical floor to evaluate a 20-year-old man for "change in mental status." He has severe mental retardation and was recently admitted to the hospital for a urinary tract infection. The patient has a history of serious injury from beating his head against walls. He has been intermittently agitated and assaultive to staff during his hospitalization. For agitation, he has received a total of 10 mg of lorazepam over the last 24 hours. When you arrive, the nurse tells you that he is now masturbating in his room in the presence of staff and laughing uncontrollably. The patient's one-to-one observer states that this is the first time he has ever acted in this manner. The patient's vital signs, chemistries, and complete blood count are all within normal limits. The most appropriate next step in management is to

    (A) administer benztropine 2 mg intramuscularly immediately
    (B) administer lorazepam 2 mg intramuscularly immediately and repeat in 1 hour if not effective
    (C) discontinue the lorazepam
    (D) switch from lorazepam to diazepam for agitation
    (E) write a behavioral contract for this patient to reinforce more controlled expressions of frustration

33. A 41-year-old man has a history of cocaine dependence and cocaine-induced depressive disorder. He has multiple arrests for cocaine possession and petty theft. He has never followed consistently with outpatient care upon discharge from his multiple psychiatric hospitalizations. The patient is also noted to have had a history of at least five suicide attempts by overdose and by hanging. He comes to the emergency department today in withdrawal after a 3-day cocaine binge. He states that he is extremely depressed and that he wants to kill himself. The most predictive risk factor for this patient making another suicide attempt is

    (A) cocaine abuse
    (B) criminal record
    (C) male gender
    (D) poor treatment compliance
    (E) previous suicide attempts

34. You are called to assess a patient for capacity. The patient is a 72-year-old man with no past psychiatric history who has Stage III congestive heart failure. The patient was admitted to the medical intensive care unit of your hospital hypoxic and in respiratory distress. You were originally called to assess the patient's capacity for accepting intubation and intensive measures when the patient presented to the emergency department. At that time, the patient was hypoxic, disoriented, and agitated. He could not communicate anything to you verbally, and you found that he did not have the capacity to decide on heroic measures in his care. The patient was intubated and transferred to the medical intensive care unit. The patient has been extubated and extensively diuresed and is now communicative and oriented. He has communicated that he would like all heroic measures, including intubation, to be done in the future and would like a written statement to that effect in his medical record. The patient's medical team is consulting you on the appropriateness of this request given his previous delirium. On mental status examination, the patient is fully oriented, conversant, and able to pay full attention to you during the interview. He tells you that he wants all measures to be done in the future to save his life. He indicates that he realizes the extensive and irreversible nature of his cardiac illness but would like to stay alive as long as possible. The patient denies depressive or psychotic symptoms. The appropriate recommendation to give to his primary team is to

(A) encourage the patient to accept the irreversible nature of his illness and to reconsider his wishes
(B) explain to the patient the binding nature of your original capacity assessment
(C) honor the patient's wishes for self-determination of his future care
(D) offer the patient antidepressant therapy
(E) seek legal counsel to over-ride the patient's wishes given the severity of his illness

35. A 35-year-old woman with no past psychiatric history comes to the clinic for the evaluation and treatment of panic attacks. Her first panic attack occurred 3 months ago while she was trapped in an elevator for an hour. She now experiences chest pain, palpitations, feelings of derealization, and shortness of breath every time she has to get on an elevator. She is an attorney, and her office is on the 35th floor, which makes avoidance of elevators all but impossible. She does not want to take any psychiatric medications and has heard about cognitive-behavioral therapy for treatment of situation-specific panic attacks. The most appropriate cognitive-behavioral approach to this patient's presenting problem is

(A) an Amytal interview
(B) free association
(C) graded exposure to elevator riding
(D) hypnosis
(E) interpretation of transference reactions

36. A 5-year-old African American boy with no past medical or psychiatric history is brought to the clinic by his parents because for the last 3 months the patient "doesn't speak at all in front of anyone except us." He has had a thorough audiologic and cognitive workup that was negative. The parents report that their son's speech is not lacking in vocabulary and is not mispronounced at all. On examination, the patient communicates with you by nodding and smiling appropriately. He refuses to speak to you. Physical examination and laboratory studies are normal. The parents play an audiotape for you in which the patient's speech is normal and age appropriate. Appropriate management of the patient is

(A) antipsychotic therapy
(B) behavioral therapy, including positive reinforcement for the patient when he speaks
(C) psychodynamically oriented psychotherapy
(D) schedule of punishment if the patient fails to speak
(E) sleep deprivation therapy

37. A 4-year-old boy is brought to the clinic for evaluation of "bizarre behavior." His foster mother says, "he just doesn't act appropriately." He cries uncontrollably when he leaves his preschool and frequently jumps into the arms of a social worker he does not know or an acquaintance of his foster mother's whom he meets for the first time. The foster mother also adds that the patient often behaves indifferently to or unaware of the other foster children in her house with whom the patient has lived for several months. He was given up for adoption by a 16-year-old mother who had normal prenatal care and no substance abuse or past medical history. The patient is up to date with immunizations and has been a physically healthy child with age-appropriate intellect and normal scores on cognitive testing. He has been in at least ten different foster homes since he was born. There has never been any evidence of physical abuse or sexual abuse necessitating a change in foster placement. There are no abnormalities on physical examination. The patient's presentation is most likely attributable to

(A) an autistic disorder
(B) frequent changes in environment
(C) mental retardation
(D) an occult infection
(E) prodromal socialization defects of schizophrenia

38. A 31-year-old woman comes to the office for a routine health maintenance examination. She has no physical complaints but says that every time she has to give a presentation for work, "I feel like I'm going to faint, and I have palpitations and sweats, and it's like the environment fades in and out in front of my eyes." Public speaking is the only situation that provokes such a response in her. She asks if there is something that she could be prescribed to help with this or if she should "do anything." She has no significant past medical history except for acne vulgaris. At this time the most appropriate management is to

(A) begin biofeedback therapy
(B) prescribe a low dosage of haloperidol for her to take every day
(C) prescribe a low dosage of propanolol for her to take before public speaking
(D) recommend an increase in caffeine intake before public speaking
(E) recommend sleep deprivation therapy

Items 39 and 40

Three months after witnessing her best friend being shot to death by another classmate in school, a 14-year-old girl is brought to the office by her parents because her teacher says that she seems to be having trouble concentrating. Ever since that "awful day" she has been very "sad" and withdrawn, often sitting on her bed and staring at the wall "for hours." She has frequent crying spells and refuses to play with friends or participate in her normal after-school activities. Her appetite has "dwindled down to nothing," and she feels very guilty that she survived the shooting. On further questioning, she reluctantly admits that she has constant thoughts of "joining her friend." She did not receive any counseling after the incident.

39. The most likely diagnosis is

(A) adjustment disorder
(B) brief psychotic disorder
(C) dysthymic disorder
(D) major depressive disorder
(E) normal grief

40. The most vital question to ask at this time is:

(A) "Are you hearing voices?"
(B) "Do you have any friends that you feel comfortable talking to at school?"
(C) "Do you wear a helmet when you ride your bicycle?"
(D) "Can you describe your typical weekly alcohol intake?"
(E) "Have you thought of the means by which you can 'join your friend'?"

41. A 6-year-old girl who is familiar to you from the last shift that you worked 2 days ago is brought to the emergency department because of diarrhea that has persisted despite the prescription of an antidiarrheal medication. The patient's mother looks very emotional and states that she "doesn't know what to do." The patient herself seems less concerned and scared than her mother. The mother requests that the patient be admitted to the hospital so that "some people can please take care of her." The mother says that she cannot take care of her daughter because of her daughter's "terrible illness" and that she feels "very scared." The patient's physical examination is remarkable for hyperactive bowel sounds and decreased skin turgor. Laboratory studies reveal small elevations in sodium, BUN, and creatinine. Stool from the patient's previous visit was negative for cultures, ova, and parasites. Today you send the patient's stool for toxicology. The pathologist calls you back to state that the patient's stool came back positive for laxatives. You confront the patient's mother with this information, and she admits that she has been putting laxatives in her daughter's food so that she would be admitted to the hospital so "someone would take care of us both." This patient's mother most likely

(A) has bipolar disorder
(B) has factitious disorder NOS
(C) has schizophrenia, chronic paranoid type
(D) has somatoform disorder NOS
(E) is malingering

42. A 14-year-old boy who has no past medical or psychiatric history comes to the office for a pre-participation sports examination. He is a straight A student and is a member of his school's basketball and hockey teams. He has no complaints today but says, "I think that I might be gay. I'm sexually attracted to other boys my age, and I'm really not aroused at all by girls. At first it was a little awkward, but I think I'm OK with it now. I have a cousin who is gay, and he's really helped me out." The patient denies a depressed mood, suicidal ideation, or sleep and appetite disturbances. This patient most likely has

(A) adjustment disorder with depressed mood
(B) gender identity disorder
(C) no diagnosis on Axis I
(D) paraphilia NOS
(E) sexual disorder NOS

43. A 41-year-old man comes to the clinic with his wife because of "temper problems." He says, "it seems like the slightest thing can tick me off, and it's embarrassing." As an example, the patient states that when he found some trash in his car left by his wife, he suddenly yelled and screamed and then knocked over an entire table of tools in his garage. His wife gives a similar history of the patient: "just completely going ballistic and losing his cool over a little thing and then calming down later and apologizing for getting so upset." There are no depressive symptoms, no history of assaultive behavior toward anyone, and no criminal history. At baseline, the patient is described as "the sweetest man I'll ever know" by his wife. He has no past medical or psychiatric history. He has been married to the same woman for 12 years, works as an executive for a large building supply company, and is active in community affairs and in his church. At this time the most appropriate management is

(A) anger management classes
(B) dialectical behavioral therapy
(C) electroconvulsive therapy
(D) maintenance antipsychotic therapy
(E) maintenance benzodiazepine therapy

44. A 40-year-old man with treatment refractory schizophrenia, undifferentiated type since his early twenties comes to the clinic for a scheduled followup appointment. He has been on multiple neuroleptic medications and has a history of neuroleptic malignant syndrome that was attributed to treatment with haloperidol. The patient has also had failed trials of risperidone and olanzapine. He has no past substance abuse or past medical history. On mental status examination, he is poorly related, with probable thought blocking, restricted affect, and poverty of thought content. The most appropriate next step in management is

(A) a carefully monitored trial of clozapine
(B) permanent state hospitalization because of treatment refractoriness
(C) a rechallenge of haloperidol with lithium augmentation
(D) reintroduction of haloperidol, but only in intramuscular formulation and on an as-needed basis
(E) symptomatic observation on no medications because of the patient's history of neuroleptic malignant syndrome

45. A 49-year-old homeless man is brought to the emergency department. He has a history of depression and alcohol abuse and reports that he has not had alcohol for the past 36 hours. He is on no medications and has no allergies to any medications. On examination, he appears agitated and complains of feeling "shaky." His temperature is 37.0 C (98.6 F), blood pressure is 156/88 mm Hg, pulse is 105/min, and respirations are 27/min. His cardiac rhythm is regular, and his lungs are clear to auscultation bilaterally. A serum glucose is 105 mg/dL. The most appropriate intervention at this time is to administer

(A) gabapentin
(B) glucose
(C) lorazepam
(D) morphine
(E) phenytoin

46. A mother brings her son to see you at the request of the boy's teacher at school. The teacher noted over the past few weeks that the boy is having these brief, "weird episodes" with facial and whole body twitching, and she notes that he is frequently clearing his throat as if he has allergies. The teacher thinks that he might have epilepsy. He has a long history of attention deficit hyperactivity disorder, and the school is aware that he takes methylphenidate. At the beginning of this semester there was a parent-teacher meeting, and the boy's progress was reported to be fine. He gets Bs and Cs at school and otherwise seems to be doing fine. Physical examination is normal. You decide that the next best step is to

(A) discontinue the methylphenidate
(B) do a urine drug screen
(C) order an MRI of the head
(D) prescribe clonidine
(E) schedule an electroencephalogram

47. A 3-year-old boy is brought to the clinic because his parents are worried about his delayed language development. They also tell you that their son always appears to be "in his own little world." You are told that his previous doctor had diagnosed the child with autism, but they did not believe her. They are here for a second opinion. When observing the child, the finding that is most consistent with autism is

(A) ability to develop peer relationships
(B) ability for spontaneous play
(C) communication through gestures
(D) microcephaly
(E) stereotypical hand flapping

48. A 14-year-old girl is coming to see you for a checkup. She will soon be moving out of town to live with her mother because her parents are in the process of getting a divorce. Her dad will live in their present house, but she and her mother and younger sister will get an apartment in a nearby town. She will go to a new high school and visit her dad during the summers. As your patient is changing her clothes in the examination room, the mother wants some advice about what to expect regarding her daughter's reaction to their divorce and move. Wisely, you inform her that adolescents react differently than younger children or older adults and that there may be potential for significant depression. She should particularly be alerted to the most likely depressive symptoms of

(A) acting-out behavior
(B) increased separation anxiety
(C) open grieving and talking about their anger at the parents
(D) sleep disturbance
(E) temper tantrums

49. A 35-year-old Caucasian woman with a history of headaches comes to the clinic in December with joint pains. When pursuing her history you note that she also has intolerance to lots of different food types, stomach bloating, rectal pain with defecation, dysmenorrhea, chronic irregular periods, and difficulty swallowing. She denies feelings of depression or sleep disturbances over the past year, and when asked about hobbies she happily talks about her active interest in jazz music. She also denies substance abuse. She takes several vitamins and acetaminophen but no prescribed medications. Physical examination is normal. A complete blood count, erythrocyte sedimentation rate, and renal and liver panels are all normal. The most likely diagnosis is

(A) depression with melancholia
(B) Lyme disease
(C) somatization disorder
(D) systemic lupus erythematosus
(E) ulcerative colitis

50. A 34-year-old woman who works as a technician for a major company comes to the clinic complaining of fatigue, low energy, and a depressed mood. She states, "I have felt this way for most of my life." She feels depressed most of the time and denies any recent stressors or significant losses in her life. She tells you that she is doing well in her job and that recently she even received a promotion. She has no interests outside of her job, she has no happy thoughts, and her self-esteem is very low. She denies suicidal thoughts but states that she does not care if she dies. She has had no sleep disturbance, change in appetite, or difficulty concentrating. She is taking no medications and denies substance abuse. Physical examination is unremarkable. An electrocardiogram is normal. Laboratory studies show

Hemoglobin	12.6 g/dL
Hematocrit	36.5%
Platelet	354,000/mm^3
Sodium	136 mEq/L
Potassium	4 mEq/L
Chloride	102 mEq/L
Bicarbonate	21 mEq/L
Glucose	100 mg/dL
Blood urea nitrogen	12 mg/dL
Creatinine	0.6 mg/dL
Thyroid-stimulating hormone	0.9 mU/mL
Thyroxine	9 mg/dL

The most likely diagnosis is

(A) adjustment disorder with depressed mood
(B) bipolar disease
(C) cyclothymia
(D) dysthymic disorder
(E) hypothyroidism
(F) major depression

Psychiatry Test Two: **Answers and Explanations**

ANSWER KEY

1. B
2. B
3. A
4. E
5. I
6. C
7. C
8. A
9. C
10. A
11. B
12. A
13. E
14. A
15. B
16. D
17. A
18. A
19. B
20. C
21. E
22. B
23. D
24. B
25. A
26. A
27. D
28. A
29. D
30. E
31. C
32. C
33. E
34. C
35. C
36. B
37. B
38. C
39. D
40. E
41. B
42. C
43. A
44. A
45. C
46. D
47. E
48. A
49. C
50. D

1. **The correct answer is B.** St. John's wort presumably has minimal monoamine oxidase inhibitor activity. If it is combined with an SSRI, serotonin syndrome could develop. You should explain that this could have dangerous results.

The combination of the two (**choice A**) could be dangerous because of the serotonin syndrome. It is also unjustified because two agents with potential antidepressant effects should not be combined. Instead, patients should be given a trial of one agent at appropriate doses and for the appropriate length of time.

St. John's wort has been shown to have mild antidepressant properties equal to those of a low dose of tricyclics (**choice C**).

The combination of ibuprofen (**choice D**) and St. John's wort will not result in renal failure because St. John's wort is not metabolized through the kidney.

St. John's wort appears to be fairly safe to use (**choice E**) even though there are no data available in overdose scenarios.

2. **The correct answer is B.** Ziprasidone belongs to the group of atypical antipsychotics indicated in the treatment of schizophrenia. However, in premarketing trials, ziprasidone caused prolongation of the Q-T interval and should not be used in patients with cardiac problems unless there is no alternative medication. EKGs should be done frequently. A baseline EKG, although not required, is suggested.

Complete blood count and differential (**choice A**) are not necessary because in clinical trials and in practice ziprasidone does not seem to significantly affect blood count.

Electroencephalogram (**choice C**) is not necessary because there is no evidence of increased seizure activity in patients without a history of seizures.

Prolactin level (**choice D**) is not required because ziprasidone does not affect the tuberoinfundibular system and does not increase prolactin like some other antipsychotics do.

Thyroid panel (**choice E**) is not affected by the use of ziprasidone. Thus, it would not be necessary to order that.

3. **The correct answer is A.** This patient is having a hypertensive crisis that is a result of tyramine-monoamine oxidase inhibitor interaction. She has developed serious symptoms that require inpatient treatment and monitoring because the risk of organ damage secondary to significantly elevated blood pressure is great. She should be given intravenous phentolamine or infusions of nitroprusside or intravenous β-blockers and should be placed in a dark, quiet room with continuous monitoring of vital signs and EKG. Cooling blankets and adequate rehydration should be provided.

Discontinuing the monoamine oxidase inhibitor and ordering benzodiazepine (**choice B**) is an option in milder cases. Discharging this patient is inappropriate.

Keeping the patient for observation in the emergency room unmedicated (**choice C**) would be an option in a milder case of hypertension but not in the presence of these blood pressure levels.

Sending the patient home with antihypertensive medication (**choice D**) in this case is inappropriate given the present clinical picture and the risk of serious consequences.

Sending the patient home unmedicated (**choice E**) is inappropriate with this clinical picture. It is true that side effects tend to subside after 24 hours, but in this case the symptoms warrant further inpatient treatment.

4. **The correct answer is E.** The patient developed anticholinergic delirium, commonly seen in elderly patients, even those on low doses of medication with anticholinergic properties. Because the delirious patient is confused, agitated, and actively hallucinating, the first priority after establishing the diagnosis of delirium is to provide safety for the patient and others in the emergency department by placing physical restraints and one-on-one observation until further measures are taken. Chemical restraints include the use of benzodiazepines. In the elderly population, however, benzodiazepines can produce paradoxical reaction.

Haloperidol (**choice A**) is contraindicated in anticholinergic delirium because of possible potentiation of anticholinergic and other side effects.

Administering physostigmine (**choice B**) is a choice of treatment for severe delirium; however, it requires close monitoring because of serious toxic side effects. Thus, it should not be the first next step but could be considered an option after you provide safety for the patient and others in the emergency department.

Admission to the ICU (**choice C**) can be considered after the initial measure of providing safety has been taken.

Discontinuing medication and returning the patient to the nursing home (**choice D**) is not an appropriate choice of management in this case scenario. This patient needs to be treated for delirium before being sent back to the nursing home.

5. **The correct answer is I.** Whether suffering from stress or a substance abuse problem, your colleague is likely to make serious medical mistakes as he cares for his patients. At the very least he is distracted and not able to give them his full attention. For this reason, he must be removed from patient contact, and the issue is best addressed directly in an empathetic and helpful manner.

   He has done nothing that can be acted upon by the State Medical Board (**choice A**), although as events progress this option remains open. At any rate, this is a harsh and non-empathetic reply to a colleague who has just expressed some vulnerability.

   Counseling (**choice B**) is a great option to pursue after the patients have been protected. For the physician to continue in his present state while he seeks counseling continues to place patients at risk.

   Discussion as to how long he has felt this way (**choice C**), commiserating about the hospital staff (**choice D**), confessing that the profession is hard (**choice F**), or wishing him well (**choice G**) miss the essential issue that he may be putting patients at risk and requires intervention.

   Although the concern for a colleague's health is admirable (**choices E and H**), it is his mental, not physical, health we need to be most concerned about. Concern for his health is good, but it does not address the main issue here, which is patient safety.

   Physicians should not prescribe for themselves, but neither should they prescribe for each other (**choice J**) as a casual act of friendship. Prescribe only for those people who are your patients and about whom you have exercised due care and consideration. Drugs do not solve the problem here. He must stop patient contact until he can deal with patients as a steady, competent practitioner of medicine.

6. **The correct answer is C.** The symptoms described are typical of discontinuation syndrome seen when a few doses of antidepressant are missed. Discontinuation events are usually mild and short lived. Symptoms occur more frequently with shorter acting SSRIs, such as paroxetine and sertraline, rather than longer acting fluoxetine. Somatic symptoms include flu-like symptoms, sensory disturbances, sleep disturbances, gastrointestinal symptoms, etc. Psychological symptoms include crying spells, irritability, and agitation. This patient should be told to restart sertraline to counteract her discontinuation syndrome.

   Stopping sertraline (**choice A**) is not appropriate because the patient had been responding well and had no initial complaints about side effects.

   Sending the patient to a neurologist (**choice B**) is inappropriate because her physical exam seems normal and because the symptoms are related purely to the discontinuation of her medication. If the symptoms continue after the treatment has been resumed, one should consider further exploration.

   Increasing sertraline aggressively (**choice D**) can cause more side effects, and it does not seem that there are enough data to support the worsening theory.

   Symptomatic therapy for flu (**choice E**) is recommended if needed, but there is no reason to discontinue sertraline. On the contrary, symptoms will subside once the sertraline treatment is resumed.

7. **The correct answer is C.** The patient has symptoms of post-traumatic stress disorder (PTSD) that seriously interfere with her everyday functioning. Sertraline is one of the antidepressants approved for treatment of this disorder. Other antidepressants and anticonvulsants have also been effective in treatment of PTSD.

   Insight-oriented psychotherapy (**choice A**) is focused on getting insight into the underlying unconscious conflicts based on exploration of transference feelings evoked during the process. It is not suitable for the treatment of acute PTSD.

   Alprazolam (**choice B**) can be used in acute stress reaction for symptom relief but is not indicated as long-term treatment of PTSD because of its addictive potential.

   Electroconvulsive shock therapy treatment (**choice D**) is not indicated for PTSD. It is sometimes used for depression refractory to other treatment modalities.

   Going back to work (**choice E**) is basically taking a behavioral approach in exposing the patient to the fearful situation. This is usually used in other phobias under controlled and supervised conditions. In the context of current active symptoms of PTSD, this is not a good treatment choice.

8. **The correct answer is A.** To determine the presence of luteal phase symptoms, one needs to determine whether the patient has regular ovulatory cycles. To do this, the patient can chart her basal body temperature to document the rise in temperature just after ovulation.

   Couples therapy (**choice B**) is not indicated in this case. The cause of the problem, which is most likely hormonal, should be sought and managed appropriately.

   Thyroid panel check (**choice C**) is not necessary because there has been no consistent evidence that the premenstrual dysphoric disorder is associated with abnormal levels of these hormones.

Increased salt consumption (**choice D**) is counterproductive because it produces more fluid retention and worsening of symptoms. On the contrary, decreasing salt consumption is suggested.

Increased vitamin C consumption (**choice E**) has no effect on these symptoms. Nutritional supplements such as calcium, magnesium, and vitamins E and B6 might alleviate the symptoms, but this is controversial.

9. **The correct answer is C.** Tourette disorder belongs to the group of tic disorders with an onset before age 18. It is most common in boys. Multiple motor and vocal tics are present during the illness many times a day, every day for more than a year. Patients often do not have a tic-free period for more than 3 months. The disturbance is not caused by a general medical condition or effects of a substance. Coprolalia and echolalia occur later. Obsessive-compulsive disorder, tic disorders, and attention deficit disorder are more frequently encountered in the families of these patients.

Psychotherapy (**choice A**), even though it may be helpful in dealing with the stress of disease, is not the treatment of choice.

Inheritance through sex chromosomes (**choice B**) is not seen. In some families there is evidence of autosomal dominant mode of inheritance.

Specific tests (**choice D**) are not available for Tourette disorder. Nonspecific abnormalities in EEG and CT scans can be found occasionally.

Early dementia (**choice E**) is not a result of chronic Tourette disorder. Emotional rather than intellectual problems are seen in these patients.

10. **The correct answer is A.** This patient is having suicidal ideas with a plan and called for help. He reports symptoms of depression that may well be related to his binging on crack cocaine. He should be admitted for observation and reevaluated for suicidality and need for further inpatient treatment once some of the cocaine effects have decreased.

Obtaining an electrocardiogram (**choice B**) is not a routine procedure for crack addicts. He is not complaining of any somatic symptoms, his vital signs are stable, and a complete physical examination is normal, so the decision about an EKG is up to the physician assessment.

Urine toxicology (**choice C**) in a patient who admits to using crack is not necessary and increases the cost. Only if the patient is unwilling to admit what he has taken, or doesn't know, is urine toxicology justified.

Prescribing an antidepressant and sending him home (**choice D**) is inappropriate because of reported suicidality and the inability to follow this patient once the medication is prescribed.

Involuntary commitment to the hospital (**choice E**) is not justified. The patient asked for help and most likely will voluntarily stay for treatment. Involuntary commitment should be considered only if there is suspicion that the patient is suicidal and able to carry out his threat and refuses voluntary admission.

11. **The correct answer is B.** The first option would be to try and reduce the dosage of risperidone and provide more frequent followups to ensure that there are no signs of worsening of mental disorder. In most cases this intervention helps in regulating menstrual periods.

Adding an anticholinergic (**choice A**) is useless because it will not affect the prolactin level.

Obtaining a prolactin level (**choice C**) can be done, but it is known that amenorrhea does not directly correlate with the prolactin level. Prolactin levels that are not as high can still cause menstrual irregularities.

Ordering an abdominal ultrasound (**choice D**) is not justified in this case because it seems that the problems are related to the use of risperidone. There are no other symptoms that indicate any structural pathology, such as pain or irregular bleeding. Also, if pregnancy is suspected, a pregnancy test should be performed, not an ultrasound.

Starting bromocriptine (**choice E**) can also be an option, but after all the others are exhausted. Bromocriptine is used to stop lactation but can exacerbate symptoms of psychosis.

12. **The correct answer is A.** The patient most likely has attention deficit hyperactivity disorder (ADHD). An interesting phenomenon that is observed with ADHD patients is that they have "paradoxical" reactions when abusing illicit stimulants such as cocaine or amphetamines, being calmer after their use. Bupropion has been used with success in the adult ADHD population and is especially desirable when the use of psychostimulants, such as methylphenidate or dextroamphetamine, is undesired.

Before the widespread use of psychostimulants for the treatment of ADHD, antidepressants such as desipramine were used. Attention deficit is now conceptualized as a relative dopamine deficiency in the frontal lobes of the cerebral cortex. Serotonin-specific antidepressants such as fluoxetine (**choice B**) are not used with regularity to treat ADHD.

Haloperidol (**choice C**) has no indication for ADHD. Dopamine blockade by haloperidol may actually make attentional difficulties worse.

Olanzapine (**choice D**) has no indication for ADHD.

There is no evidence to support the use of risperidone (**choice E**) for ADHD.

13. **The correct answer is E.** The patient is manifesting signs of withdrawal from stimulants. There is no pharmacotherapy that has been consistently proven to be helpful in the management of stimulant withdrawal. Fortunately, no autonomic instability occurs in the context of stimulant withdrawal. Supportive treatment and monitoring the patient as an outpatient (given the lack of imminent danger to self or others) will likely result in resolution of the patient's dysphoric appearance and depressed mood.

    Flumazenil (**choice A**) is a benzodiazepine receptor blocker that is used in the treatment of benzodiazepine intoxication or overdose. It does not have an indication in the treatment of stimulant withdrawal.

    Clonidine (**choice B**) is used to manage the autonomic hyperarousal associated with opiate withdrawal. It would not be appropriate in the management of this patient.

    A methadone taper (**choice C**) can also be used to manage withdrawal from opiates. It would not be appropriate in the management of this patient.

    Methylphenidate (**choice D**) is a controlled substance; it is a prescription psychostimulant that is used for attention deficit hyperactivity disorder. The patient's abuse of psychostimulants in the absence of a perceived attention deficit hyperactivity disorder makes the use of methylphenidate for this patient highly undesirable.

14. **The correct answer is A.** Patients with body dysmorphic disorder have an inordinate preoccupation with imagined defects in their physical appearance. The patient has no actual dermatologic problems but cannot help but focus on what she understands to be horrible-appearing skin. Frequent visits to physicians is a common presentation for patients with body dysmorphic disorder.

    Conversion disorder (**choice B**) involves neurologic symptoms that are judged to be associated with psychological factors or stressors. It is not evident in this patient's presentation.

    Hypochondriasis (**choice C**) involves a belief or preoccupation that one has a serious disease despite medical reassurances. The patient does not have a belief that she is having an actual medical illness.

    The patient is not depressed, nor does the patient's preoccupation with her appearance constitute a psychotic phenomenon. Therefore, major depressive disorder with psychotic features (**choice D**) is incorrect.

    Somatization disorder (**choice E**) involves multiple somatic complaints without known medical etiology. It is not consistent with this patient's presentation.

15. **The correct answer is B.** The patient is presenting with the initial signs of Wilson disease, or hepatolenticular degeneration. It is an autosomal recessive disorder more common in people of Japanese descent that is characterized by copper deposition in the liver and the neurologic systems (particularly the basal ganglia). Initial workup of suspected Wilson disease should include measurement of blood ceruloplasmin and 24-hour urinary copper levels. Once the diagnosis is confirmed, chelation therapy can offer significant resolution of symptoms if Wilson disease is detected early enough.

    The patient's jaundice secondary to hepatic dysfunction would be best treated with chelating the excess unbound copper. Phototherapy (**choice A**) does not address the underlying pathophysiology of Wilson disease.

    Hepatic, neurologic, and psychiatric manifestations of Wilson disease are potentially reversible with chelation therapy. It is therefore imperative to make this diagnosis rather than gauge this patient's improvement with an antidepressant (**choice C**).

    The patient is not manifesting any psychotic symptoms on examination (although psychotic symptoms can occur in Wilson disease). There is no indication for an antipsychotic (**choice D**) at this time.

    Electroconvulsive therapy (**choice E**) does not address nor correct the aberrant copper deposition seen in Wilson disease.

16. **The correct answer is D.** Priapism, or sustained penile erection in the absence of sexual stimulation, is a painful adverse effect of trazodone. The exact mechanism of its occurrence is not known. Treatment for priapism may involve surgical drainage or epinephrine injection.

Alprazolam (**choice A**) is a benzodiazepine medication that is not associated with priapism. It has sedative-hypnotic and anxiolytic properties. Notably, because of its short half-life, addiction and withdrawal potential are high for alprazolam relative to most other benzodiazepines.

Chloral hydrate (**choice B**) is an older sleeping medication whose active metabolite is ethanol. It is not associated with priapism.

Diphenhydramine (**choice C**) is an antihistamine that is used for management of agitation and as a sedative-hypnotic. Priapism is not associated with diphenhydramine with the same frequency as with trazodone.

Zolpidem (**choice E**) is a medication used specifically for sleep induction and maintenance. It does not have anxiolytic properties that have been well characterized. It is not associated with priapism.

17. **The correct answer is A.** Bupropion is associated with a slightly increased risk of seizures in the general population. An especially high risk of seizures, however, is noted when actively bulimic patients are prescribed bupropion. Rapid metabolic changes associated with bulimia are believed to contribute to the increased risk of seizures when bulimic patients are prescribed bupropion.

Citalopram (**choice B**) is not associated with an increased seizure risk in patients with bulimia.

Fluoxetine (**choice C**) is the medication that probably has the most robust literature supporting its safe and effective use for the maintenance of remission for patients with eating disorders. It is not associated with an increased risk of seizures in bulimic patients.

Paroxetine (**choice D**) is a medication that is not associated with an increased risk for seizures in bulimic patients and is a preferred treatment for the maintenance of remission of anorexia and bulimia.

Sertraline (**choice E**) is not associated with an increased seizure risk in bulimic patients and has a record of safe and efficacious use in the maintenance of remission for patients with eating disorders.

18. **The correct answer is A.** The patient is presenting with a classic case of conversion disorder. She has had an acute stressor (disclosure of husband's affair) that has been translated to neurologic rather than psychiatric symptoms. For a large population of patients with conversion disorder, an interview after having received a dose of intravenous Amytal will reveal a rapid resolution of these neurologic symptoms and confirm the diagnosis of a conversion reaction.

Edrophonium challenge (**choice B**) is used to detect the presence of myasthenia gravis. It would not be useful diagnostically in this patient or in a patient for whom choreoathetoid movements rather than fatigue is the primary presentation.

A phenobarbital challenge (**choice C**) is useful for ascertaining the amount of barbiturate that is needed for prevention of withdrawal symptoms in a patient addicted to barbiturates or benzodiazepines. It is not indicated in this patient.

Phototherapy (**choice D**) is not useful diagnostically or therapeutically for a patient having a conversion reaction.

This patient does not have intermittent-episodic symptoms suggestive of seizures. Therefore, 24-hour electroencephalogram monitoring (**choice E**) would not be helpful.

19. **The correct answer is B.** The patient presents with a classic history of obstructive sleep apnea. Continuous positive airway pressure can be used to keep the patient's airway patent throughout the time the patient is asleep and prevent the frequent, brief awakenings that occur during the course of the patient's sleep cycle.

Acupuncture (**choice A**) has no proven efficacy for obstructive sleep apnea.

Desipramine (**choice C**) is a tricyclic antidepressant that has been used for enuresis and for pediatric sleeping disorders, such as night terrors. It is not indicated for obstructive sleep apnea.

Dextroamphetamine sulfate (**choice D**) is frequently used in the treatment of narcolepsy. The patient clearly does not have the history of recurrent, abrupt sleep attacks that characterize narcolepsy.

Haloperidol (**choice E**) has no proven efficacy for obstructive sleep apnea, and, given its propensity for long-term neurologic side effects, it should be avoided in the treatment of isolated sleep complaints.

20. **The correct answer is C.** Ventricular arrhythmia can occur with the coadministration of nefazodone and cisapride. Nefazodone is a potent inhibitor of the cytochrome p450 3A4 isoenzyme system that metabolizes cisapride.

Both gabapentin (**choice A**) and lithium (**choice B**) have an exclusively renal metabolism and could be safely administered to this patient if there is no demonstrable renal toxicity for this patient.

Risperidone (**choice D**) does not have the same potential for drug-drug interaction if coadministered with cisapride.

Thyroid hormone (**choice E**) does not have the same potential for drug-drug interaction if coadministered with cisapride.

21. **The correct answer is E.** The patient's history is classic for shared psychotic disorder (also known as folie a deux). The patient has adopted the same paranoid delusional belief system as his older, and presumably dominant, brother. Interestingly, there is evidence to suggest that for the nondominant member of a folie a deux, mere separation from the dominant member may result in resolution of symptoms.

The patient is clearly not manifesting symptoms suggestive of a manic episode, although delusions of a grandiose, expansive, or paranoid nature are possible presentations of a manic episode (**choice A**). His regular appearance and intact concentration and normal speech are not consistent with mania.

The patient is not manifesting any syndromal depressive symptoms to suggest that his paranoid delusions are occurring in the context of a psychotic depression (**choice B**).

Schizophrenia, disorganized type (**choice C**) requires at least a 6-month history of some psychotic symptomatology. It is not consistent with the patient's presentation and clinical history.

Schizophreniform disorder (**choice D**) requires more than 1 month but less than 6 months of psychotic symptoms. The patient's presentation does not meet the criteria for this disorder.

22. **The correct answer is B.** Attention deficit hyperactivity disorder is something of a misnomer insofar as patients meeting the criteria for this disorder must be either inattentive or hyperactive/impulsive. Boys more commonly present with more overt disruptive behavioral problems, whereas girls are usually more inattentive. This patient's teachers and parents give a strong history of an inattentive-only presentation that would nonetheless be responsive to treatment with methylphenidate.

The patient is in regular classes and is described as bright and sociable by her teacher, which makes the diagnosis of mental retardation unlikely. There is no indication to evaluate the patient for mental retardation (**choice A**) from this presentation.

The patient does not appear depressed (**choice C**) on examination, and disruptive behaviors that may serve as depressive correlates are missing from the patient's history.

There is no report of disrupted sleep from the patient's history, and there is no indication of possible ictal activity. There is no indication for a sleep study (**choice D**).

The patient's parents provide documentation from the patient's teacher who made this referral that their daughter has attentional problems. There is no indication for reporting the patient's parents (**choice E**).

23. **The correct answer is D.** Splitting is a common narcissistic defense that involves others as being viewed as "all good or all bad." Patients in the cluster B spectrum of personality disorders (narcissistic, histrionic, borderline, and antisocial) commonly exhibit this defense in medical settings.

Blocking (**choice A**) is a temporary stoppage of thinking on the part of the patient. It is not evidenced by this patient's clearly delineated complaints.

Projection (**choice B**) is the attribution of one's own desires and wishes onto another person caused by intolerability of these desires and wishes to the patient.

Reaction formation (**choice C**) is when a drive that is unacceptable to the patient is changed to its exact opposite behaviorally. An example may include advocacy of public decency in a sexual deviant.

Sublimation (**choice E**) is considered to be one of the most mature defenses. It involves the diversion of drives or energies that may be unacceptable to the patient and society into socially acceptable ones. An example may include aggressive tendencies within a patient who subsequently becomes a star football player.

24. **The correct answer is B.** Pharmacokinetic parameters change in all patients as a function of age. The patient likely feels sedated because of a decreased rate of elimination of haloperidol. It would be appropriate to adjust the patient's dosage accordingly.

The patient is not manifesting any mood symptoms during this clinic visit. The specific complaint is of sedation. Prescription of an antidepressant (**choice D**) or lithium (**choice A**) is not indicated and would likely produce treatment-emergent sedation that would further exacerbate the patient's complaint.

The use of electroconvulsive therapy as a maintenance treatment for schizophrenia (**choice C**) is not indicated. Maintenance electroconvulsive therapy can be used as a treatment for depression, especially when remission of depression is initially achieved by electroconvulsive therapy.

Prescription of a psychostimulant (**choice E**) is rarely if ever indicated in a patient with a history of psychosis. Psychostimulants work to stimulate the cortical dopamine system, and a potential adverse consequence of this is production of positive psychotic symptoms such as hallucinations and paranoia.

25. **The correct answer is A.** By delineating the reason why the patient is asking you this question, a further clarification of the patient's perceptions, priorities, and response to stress can be attained. Additionally, boundaries within your therapeutic relationship with the patient may be produced.

The mere inquiry for personal information is not an indication to completely discontinue (**choice B**) an evaluation of a patient. Opportunities for further dynamic and diagnostic information from the patient is actually possible when this issue arises.

The patient would likely become uncooperative and agitated if her question were totally ignored (**choice C**) by you.

The patient should not be reprimanded (**choice D**) for asking if you are married. Patients may not be aware of what the appropriate boundaries are in a therapeutic relationship, and it is the therapist's duty to define these boundaries.

Contingencies involving your divulging personal information to the patient in exchange for her cooperation (**choice E**) are likely to produce an enmeshed relationship with the patient.

26. **The correct answer is A.** Fluoxetine has a myriad of predicted drug-drug interactions because of its inhibition of the p450 enzymes. By far the most common and well-documented interaction is a 2- to 10-fold increase in tricyclic levels (amitriptyline). Tricyclics are cardiotoxic and can be fatal.

Fluoxetine may increase, not decrease (**choice B**), the efficacy of bupropion, but it is of questionable clinical significance.

Fluoxetine inhibits the metabolism of other drugs because it is a potent p450 inhibitor. Usually patients taking fluoxetine have an increase in efficacy of a different drug, not an increase in fluoxetine (**choice C**).

Fluoxetine may increase diazepam levels (**choice D**), and it is something to consider when giving a long-acting benzodiazepine to a patient with increased risk for CNS depression and difficulty with metabolism, i.e., an alcoholic patient may be predisposed to a buildup of diazepam, and it would be good to be aware of the possible interaction between fluoxetine and several benzodiazepines. Again, by far the most common and well-documented fluoxetine interaction is a 2- to 10-fold increase in tricyclic levels.

Fluoxetine and the other SSRIs do not interact with ibuprofen and will not increase the patient's pain because of the increased metabolism of ibuprofen (**choice E**). Ibuprofen is not metabolized by the p450 system.

27. **The correct answer is D.** This patient is most likely suffering from schizoaffective disorder, depressed type. Schizoaffective disorder is defined in DSM-IV as the occurrence of a manic, mixed, or depressive episode concurrent with the active symptoms of schizophrenia. Additionally, there must be at least a 2-week history of delusions or hallucinations in the absence of mood symptoms.

Autism (**choice A**) is characterized by childhood onset of impairment in social reciprocity, stereotyped behaviors and restricted interests, and language impairment. This is not consistent with the patient's history.

The patient does not have a history of manic, hypomanic, or mixed episodes. Additionally, the patient's history is more indicative of a chronic and disabling psychotic process rather than an episodic and intermittent history consistent with bipolar disorder (**choice B**).

The patient does not have psychotic symptoms that occur exclusively in the context of a depressive diathesis. She is chronically psychotic in the absence of mood symptoms. Therefore, major depressive disorder with psychotic features (**choice C**) is incorrect.

Schizophreniform disorder (**choice E**) is often a transitional diagnosis that involves more than 1 month but less than 6 months of active psychotic symptoms. The patient's chronic disability is inconsistent with this diagnosis.

28. **The correct answer is A.** This patient is having an acute dystonic reaction that is caused by the antidopaminergic properties of the high-potency antipsychotic agent. Dystonia is a spontaneous contraction of individual muscles and can range from an "annoying" sensation of muscle spasms to laryngospasm. Treatment includes the cessation or reduction of the dose of the causal agent and the administration of an anticholinergic agent, such as benztropine, or an antihistamine, such as diphenhydramine, both of which are usually given intramuscularly for immediate effect.

    Bromocriptine (**choice B**) is typically given with dantrolene to treat neuroleptic malignant syndrome, which is characterized by fever, muscle rigidity, mental status changes, autonomic instability, tremor, and elevated levels of creatine kinase.

    This patient is having an acute dystonic reaction that requires treatment with an anticholinergic agent, not massage therapy (**choice C**).

    An acute dystonic reaction is not "normal," and it requires therapy with an anticholinergic agent, so reassuring the patient that this is normal and does not require treatment (**choice D**) is incorrect.

    There is no reason to refer the patient to a neurologist (**choice E**) at this time. An acute dystonic reaction can usually be treated with an anticholinergic agent and does not require the "expertise" of a specialist.

29. **The correct answer is D.** Clozapine is an atypical antipsychotic agent that is useful in treating the negative symptoms of schizophrenia (anhedonia, apathy, amotivation, avolition, and emotional and social withdrawal). There is a 1 to 2% risk of agranulocytosis and a 3% risk of leukopenia. This idiosyncratic reaction is most common within the first 6 months of treatment. Patients are required to have regular monitoring of the white blood cell count with differential.

    Thyroid dysfunction (**choice A**) is a side effect of lithium. It is not typically associated with clozapine.

    Clozapine is not typically associated with elevated prolactin levels (**choice B**).

    Clozapine is more often associated with hypotension and tachycardia than with hypertension (**choice C**).

    Clozapine has been associated with hyperglycemia, not hypoglycemia (**choice E**).

30. **The correct answer is E.** The clinical setting and physical examination are consistent with child abuse. The next most appropriate step in the evaluation of this child is to perform a skeletal survey for old fractures that would support the diagnosis of child abuse. Of all the child abuse cases diagnosed by the medical community, 5 to 22% are a result of burn injury. Scalding is the most frequent form of burn abuse, with more than 80% resulting from tap water scalds. Other forms of burn abuse include open flame burns and hot object "branding." Infants and toddlers are most frequently the victims of burn abuse, with ages typically ranging from 22 to 40 months. Boys are more frequently the victims of scald abuse than girls. Long-term physical abuse, nutritional and psychological neglect, and at least one other prior health-related problem are usually seen. Failure to thrive and delay in acquiring language skills are common. Prematurely born children and those with disabilities or behavioral problems are at increased risk of being abused. These children are often very submissive and withdrawn. The buttocks and perineum are the most frequently involved sites and are uncommonly involved in accidental scalds. Buttock immersion into hot water is typically used as punishment for failure to toilet train, enuresis, excessive crying, or other "unacceptable" behavior. The feet and hands are also commonly involved. Forced immersion scalds are characterized by symmetric burns with a tidemark. They tend to be deeper than accidental burns. Doughnut-hole burns occur when the child's buttocks is forced against the bottom of the hot fluid container that is cooler than the liquid it contains, and thus a sparing zone is formed in the center of the burn area. A striped appearance results from immersion of the child whose extremities are held flexed, and sparing of the skin folds then occurs. Parents from all levels of society and educational backgrounds abuse children. Those who abuse were often abused themselves, have violent backgrounds, poor stress management skills, are more likely to be single parents, and have other unstable social factors. Scald abuse is used as a form of punishment often triggered by a stressful event, such as unsuccessful toilet training. Caregivers often delay seeking medical attention. Physicians have a legal and moral obligation to investigate possible child abuse, and all states require it to be reported to the authorities. The child should be hospitalized, and a team approach should be used for determination of the accurate diagnosis and treatment. A thorough physical examination (including a full skin examination) should be performed, and a skeletal survey done because in 20 to 30% of cases, concurrent or old injuries are found, and there is up to a 70% risk that the abuse will happen again. Physician awareness is the key to early identification and intervention in child abuse cases.

A chest x-ray (**choice A**) would be done as part of the skeletal survey to detect old rib fractures, but alone it is not the most appropriate next step in the diagnostic evaluation of an abused child.

A complete blood count with differential (**choice B**) would be done in the case of suspected infectious or inflammatory disease process, neither of which is the case here. Subsequent evaluation of this child's nutritional status may warrant that a complete blood count be performed to exclude anemia, but not as a first step in the management of this child.

An oral glucose tolerance test (**choice C**) is not indicated because there are no signs or symptoms pointing toward a possible hyper- or hypoglycemic state in this child, nor are there family history indications that the child is at risk for developing diabetes mellitus.

A rectal swab (**choice D**) would be done if an infectious cause were suspected, such as a bacterial infection or parasitic infestation. The presentation of this child is inconsistent with an infection or an infestation.

31. **The correct answer is C.** As opposed to adult patients with depression, teenagers with depression are more likely to present with disruptions in behavior and are more likely to not want to volunteer their depressive symptoms. This patient presents with a history that is very consistent with adolescent depression. A thorough history of neurovegetative symptoms of depression and potential for self-harm is part of a complete assessment of this patient.

The absence of any present or past history of manic symptoms makes the prescription of a mood stabilizer (**choice A**) unnecessary.

The patient's age and lack of a history of academic problems pertaining to the inability to concentrate make a diagnosis of attention deficit hyperactivity disorder unlikely in this patient. Therefore, a prescription for a psychostimulant (**choice B**) is unwarranted.

A marked deterioration in function is not a part of normal adolescence (**choice D**). This patient requires intervention to restore his premorbid function.

Neuropsychological testing and IQ testing (**choice E**) is not indicated in this patient. The patient's diagnosis of depression is rather straightforward, and there is no history from his past academic achievement to indicate a learning disorder.

32. **The correct answer is C.** The patient's stable medical condition and acute change in mental status in the context of high lorazepam dosing makes the presentation highly suggestive of disinhibition secondary to benzodiazepines. Mentally challenged patients, children, and elderly patients are particularly susceptible to this complication of benzodiazepine treatment. A nonbenzodiazepine medication, such as an antipsychotic or mood stabilizer, would likely be a better agent for control of agitation in this patient.

Benztropine (**choice A**) is used in psychiatry to control extrapyramidal symptoms of neuroleptics. It would be of no use in this situation.

Giving more lorazepam (**choice B**) would likely further disinhibit this patient.

Switching to diazepam from lorazepam (**choice D**) would not improve the patient's behavioral disinhibition. Diazepam is a longer acting benzodiazepine than lorazepam, and it has a substantial lipid accumulation. With repeated dosing, diazepam would most likely lead to even longer periods of disinhibition in this patient.

This patient's baseline mental deficiencies and disinhibited state would make his comprehension of a written behavioral contract (**choice E**) virtually impossible.

33. **The correct answer is E.** Previous suicide attempts are the most predictive risk factor for subsequent suicide attempts. This patient's attempts by overdose and by hanging make him a high risk for later completed suicide.

Substance abusers have a higher risk of completed suicide than the general population. However, substance use is not as high a predictor of subsequent suicide attempts as previous suicide attempts. Therefore, cocaine abuse (**choice A**) is not the most predictive risk factor for this patient making another suicide attempt.

A history of criminal activity (**choice B**), specifically in the context of antisocial personality disorder, is a risk factor for completed suicide. In fact, antisocial personality disorder patients complete suicide more than patients with any other personality disorder diagnosis, including borderline personality disorder. However, previous suicide attempts are more predictive than a criminal record for subsequent suicide risk.

Collectively, men are noted to have more completed suicides than women. However, women as a group are noted to make more suicide attempts. The reason for this is that men are more prone to use violent means, such as self-inflicted gunshots, in their attempts than women. Regardless, gender (**choice C**) is not as predictive of potential for suicide attempts as previous suicide attempts.

Poor treatment compliance (**choice D**) with outpatient treatment does not have as high a predictive value for subsequent suicide risk as previous suicide attempts.

34. **The correct answer is C.** Assessments of patient capacity are specific and limited to the issue that capacity has been called into question and for the time that the evaluation is done. Capacity for the same treatment issue can change, meaning that patients can be deemed not to have capacity initially (such as in the case of a delirium) with the possibility that capacity can be achieved later. This is the case for this patient.

It is not appropriate for you to sway the competent patient into making decisions that are against his wishes (**choice A**).

Capacity determinations can change in favor of patient self-determination, especially in cases of a delirium. It would be incorrect to tell him that your original capacity assessment was binding (**choice B**).

The patient does not have prominent mood symptoms, and his desire for as much medical care as possible in the future is demonstrative of future-oriented thinking rather than the hopelessness that characterizes depressive illness. He therefore should not be given antidepressant therapy (**choice D**).

Seeking legal services to over-ride a patient's wishes when the patient clearly demonstrates capacity (**choice E**) is unethical and illegal. It would be especially inappropriate in this case given that the patient wants as much care to be given to him as possible.

35. **The correct answer is C.** Graded exposure is an in vivo cognitive-behavioral technique that involves putting patients in anxiety-provoking situations of increasing intensity to the point that these situations can be handled calmly by the patient. It is more useful and pertinent in situation-specific anxiety than for more generalized types.

An Amytal interview (**choice A**) is a technique used to make the diagnosis of conversion disorders. Patients with conversion reactions typically present with a recent stressful life experience and the subsequent sudden development of neurologic symptoms. These symptoms can be rapidly dissipated when patients are administered Amytal.

Free association (**choice B**) and interpretation of transference reactions (**choice E**) are fundamental components of psychoanalytically oriented therapies. These techniques are used to uncover and explore drives and desires that are outside of the patient's conscious awareness. These techniques are not used in a cognitive-behavioral oriented therapy.

Hypnosis (**choice D**) is not considered a cognitive-behavioral technique. Cognitive and behavioral therapies emphasize immediate thoughts and behaviors that are (or are made to be) within the conscious awareness of the patient and accessible to alteration.

36. **The correct answer is B.** The patient has selective mutism, whereby patients will not speak in specific circumstances. The most established treatment for selective mutism is behavioral therapy, including positive reinforcement for patient verbalization. More controlled evidence for pharmacotherapy of selective mutism, including fluoxetine, is being sought.

Patients with selective mutism are not responding to internal stimuli and are not to be considered psychotic; therefore, antipsychotics (**choice A**) are not indicated.

Psychodynamically oriented psychotherapy (**choice C**) is a treatment that requires, at a minimum, a verbal patient. Conflicts and urges are explored in dynamically oriented relationships centered on interpretation of transference reactions.

The use of punishment for patients with selective mutism is neither a proven effective treatment nor a humane one. Patients with this disorder are not exhibiting behavior that is manipulative or correctable by punishment (**choice D**).

Sleep deprivation therapy (**choice E**) can be helpful in some forms of depression. It does not have a theoretical or practical basis in the treatment of selective mutism.

37. **The correct answer is B.** The patient's diagnosis is reactive attachment disorder. Lack of environmental consistency is thought to potentially adversely affect a child's ability to form stable attachments. This can be manifested in a child displaying overly expressive attachment behaviors to people the child barely knows or in inhibited social interactions with people the child should know more personally.

The patient's lack of social appropriateness may lead some clinicians to label this child as autistic (**choice A**). Additional criteria for autism include observed deficiencies in language and stereotyped behaviors that are clearly absent in this patient's presentation.

The patient's normal cognitive testing rules out a diagnosis of mental retardation (**choice C**).

The patient's normal physical examination and medical workup make a diagnosis of occult infection (**choice D**) highly unlikely. Additionally, the circumstantial nature of the changes in the patient's behavior suggest a more psychiatric than medical presentation.

The patient's presentation does not indicate a schizophrenia-spectrum illness (**choice E**). The detection of a psychotic illness in a patient so young is rare and difficult.

38. **The correct answer is C.** A low dose of a β-blocker such as propanolol can alleviate the autonomic symptoms of performance anxiety, such as palpitations and diaphoresis, and the panic-like symptoms that occur.

Biofeedback (**choice A**) is not a proven treatment for performance anxiety.

Haloperidol (**choice B**) is not an accepted treatment for performance anxiety, and the cognitive and extrapyramidal motor effects for this patient make this an especially undesirable treatment alternative.

Caffeine intake (**choice D**) in patients prone to anxiety (circumstantial or generalized) usually exacerbates anxiety.

Sleep deprivation (**choice E**) can be a treatment for depression. It is not a treatment for performance anxiety and would likely have an adverse effect on the patient's ability to concentrate.

39. **The correct answer is D.** This patient most likely has major depressive disorder. To meet the criteria for this disorder a patient must exhibit a 2-week history of a distinct change in mood or a loss of interest or pleasure, along with at least four of the following: decreased appetite and weight loss, difficulty sleeping, psychomotor retardation or agitation, fatigue, feelings of worthlessness or guilt, inability to concentrate, and suicidal ideation. The symptoms must cause functional impairment.

This patient's suicidal ideation and marked functional impairment make it incorrect to diagnose her with adjustment disorder (**choice A**). An adjustment disorder, which may develop in response to a stressor, is characterized by a depressed mood and other symptoms that are similar to but less severe than the symptoms of major depressive disorder. If a patient meets the criteria for a major depressive disorder (as stated in the explanation above), you cannot diagnose her with an adjustment disorder. Also, individuals with an adjustment disorder typically return to baseline functioning within 3 months.

A brief psychotic disorder (**choice B**) is characterized by delusions, hallucinations, disorganized speech, or grossly disorganized behavior lasting for more than a day but less than a month. This patient does not fit this description.

Dysthymic disorder (**choice C**) is characterized by a depressed mood for more than 2 years. This patient has been symptomatic for only 3 months.

Normal grief (**choice E**) is an expected reaction to the loss of a loved one. It is characterized by feelings of loss, sadness, and decreased enjoyment. Individuals with normal grief may experience frequent crying spells and possibly minor dysfunction. It typically lasts a few months but may last longer. Major depressive disorder is diagnosed when there is suicidal ideation and feelings of worthlessness and guilt.

40. **The correct answer is E.** Because she has already told you that she has suicidal ideation ("joining her friend"), it is very important to ask if she has "thought of the means by which" she can "join her friend" or if she has made any preparatory actions.

It may be important to ask the patient if she is hearing voices (**choice A**) to determine if her depression is associated with psychotic features; however, this will not change the immediate management. You have already found out that she "constantly" thinks about "joining her friend," so now you need to question her about a plan.

Although is important to find out if she has friends that she can confide in, asking her, "Do you have any friends that you feel comfortable talking to at school?" (**choice B**) is not vital at this time.

It is important to counsel patients to wear helmets when riding their bicycle (**choice C**); however, this is not the most vital question to ask a patient with suicidal ideation.

All adolescents should be asked to describe their use of alcohol and other drugs (**choice D**); however, this is not the most vital question to ask a patient with suicidal ideation.

41. **The correct answer is B.** This presentation is classic for factitious disorder by proxy (classified under factitious disorder not otherwise specified in DSM-IV): "the intentional production or feigning of physical or psychological

signs or symptoms in another person who is under the individual's care for the purpose of indirectly assuming the sick role."

A history of mania or depression is clearly lacking in this narrative to determine that the patient's mother has a diagnosis of bipolar disorder (**choice A**).

There is no history given in this narrative to indicate that the patient's mother is chronically psychotic. Chronic paranoid schizophrenia (**choice C**) is therefore incorrect.

Somatoform disorders (**choice D**) as classified in DSM-IV do not allow provisions for the production or complaint of symptoms in people other than the patient.

Malingering (**choice E**) requires an incentive such as financial gain or the absolution of some legal responsibility motivating the fabrication of symptoms in a patient. The patient's mother in this question overtly states that she wanted to indirectly assume the sick role using her daughter's illness.

42. **The correct answer is C.** The patient is describing what seems to be an acceptance of his sexual orientation, which happens to be homosexual. Homosexuality in and of itself is not classified on any of the DSM-IV axes as a mental illness.

The patient does not seem to be at the point of having a difficult adjustment to his sexual orientation. He does not act depressed, nor does he complain of a depressed mood. Adjustment disorder (**choice A**) with depressed mood is therefore incorrect.

A diagnosis of gender identity disorder (**choice B**) is made in patients who identify with the gender opposite their own and who act or dress in a manner that is stereotypically of the opposite gender. The patient's participation in sports and identification as a gay man rule out a diagnosis of gender identity disorder.

Homosexuality, in DSM-IV, is not classified as a paraphilia (**choice D**).

Homosexuality, in DSM-IV, is not classified as a sexual disorder (**choice E**), such as disorders of arousal or sexual interest.

43. **The correct answer is A.** The patient has a clear case of intermittent explosive disorder. The patient does not meet criteria for a borderline personality disorder or antisocial personality disorder, as evidenced by the lack of problems that are seen within the patient's life from his social history. Anger management classes alone may be useful as a treatment for this patient. If this treatment is insufficient, propanolol, a β-blocker, has some clinical evidence to support its use.

Dialectical behavioral therapy (**choice B**) is used for chronically suicidal patients with a diagnosis of borderline personality disorder. Its use for patients with other disorders is being examined, but it is not an indicated treatment for intermittent explosive disorder.

Electroconvulsive therapy (**choice C**) has no data supporting its use in intermittent explosive disorder.

This patient does not appear psychotic, nor is there any evidence to suggest that his periods of anger are psychotically driven. The risks of antipsychotic treatment (**choice D**) in this patient clearly outweigh any benefits.

Maintenance benzodiazepine treatment (**choice E**) in this patient is not indicated and could be detrimental in terms of abuse or dependency. For acute agitation, short-term benzodiazepine treatment may be beneficial.

44. **The correct answer is A.** Clozapine is an antipsychotic medication that has been shown to have a superior profile over conventional neuroleptic medications with respect to extrapyramidal symptoms and in treating the negative symptoms of schizophrenia (flat affect, poverty of thought content). Some patients known to be "treatment refractory" with other antipsychotic medications have been shown to improve or remit with clozapine.

If viable treatments such as clozapine maintenance are available to this patient, "indefinite" state hospitalization (**choice B**) is neither humane nor appropriate.

Coadministration of lithium with haloperidol (**choice C**) confers a greater risk for neuroleptic malignant syndrome in patients.

Rapid dose changes and repeated intramuscular injections of haloperidol (**choice D**) are thought to be significant risk factors for the development of neuroleptic malignant syndrome. For obvious reasons, this should not be the treatment strategy for a patient with a preexisting history of neuroleptic malignant syndrome.

The patient is clearly manifesting signs of psychotic illness, and viable pharmacologic treatments should be offered. Therefore, no treatment with only observation (**choice E**) is incorrect.

45. **The correct answer is C.** From the available information, this patient is experiencing alcohol withdrawal. The treatment of this disorder, and appropriate intervention to prevent the onset of delirium tremens, is the administration of a benzodiazepine such as lorazepam.

Gabapentin (**choice A**) is a gaba-ergic agent used in the treatment of seizures. It has no role in the management of alcohol withdrawal or in the prevention of delirium tremens.

Glucose (**choice B**) is not useful in the treatment of alcohol withdrawal or in the prevention of delirium tremens. It is also unlikely that this patient's anxiety will improve with glucose administration because the patient is not hypoglycemic.

Morphine (**choice D**) has no role in the management of alcohol withdrawal or in the prevention of delirium tremens.

Phenytoin (**choice E**) is a sodium channel antagonist used in the treatment of seizures. It has no role in the management of alcohol withdrawal or in the prevention of delirium tremens.

46. **The correct answer is D.** This boy's story is consistent with a diagnosis of Tourette syndrome. Tourette syndrome is characterized by motor and phonic tics. They are frequently facial tics or tics that involve the entire body. Many children with Tourette syndrome have comorbid diagnoses, namely attention deficit hyperactivity disorder or obsessive-compulsive disorder. Although some stimulant medications may exacerbate Tourette syndrome in some children, in most cases the tic disturbance disappears over time without discontinuing the medication. The proper course of therapy is to use a medication such as clonidine.

Stopping the methylphenidate is not the best next step (**choice A**).

There is not enough supportive information provided in this case to suggest the need to do urine drug screening (**choice B**). His behavior and academic performance at school seem to be otherwise fine.

Ordering an MRI of the head would not be indicated at this time (**choice C**).

Although the teacher is concerned about epilepsy, the history supports Tourette syndrome to be the likely explanation for the boy's symptoms (**choice E**). There is no history that the boy's episodes are prolonged with lapses, tonic-clonic in nature, or associated with staring spells or loss of consciousness or alertness. A sudden drop in his overall school performance or a change in his behavior might make one more suspect of a seizure disorder.

47. **The correct answer is E.** Restrictive and stereotyped patterns of behavior, such as hand flapping, are common in autistic children and best correlate with this condition from the choices given.

The diagnosis of autism requires impaired social interaction, such as failure to develop peer relationships. Therefore, ability to develop peer relationships (**choice A**) is incorrect.

A lack of varied, spontaneous play is common in autism. Therefore, ability for spontaneous play (**choice B**) is incorrect.

A child who is able to communicate through gestures is unlikely to be autistic (**choice C**). In fact, an autistic child has an absence of any type of communication and has a qualitative impairment of communication with delay in, or complete lack of, development of the spoken language.

Microcephaly (**choice D**) is uncommon in autism as opposed to macrocephaly, which is prevalent.

48. **The correct answer is A.** Significant acting-out behavior can be a common sign of depression. Adolescents may act out by turning to substance use, being sexually active or promiscuous, skipping school, or having problems with the law.

Sleep disturbance may be a reaction for younger children or older adults but is less common among adolescents (**choice B**).

Increased separation anxiety is typical of preschool children, not adolescents (**choice C**).

Open grieving and talking about their anger at the parents is an unlikely response for mid-adolescence (**choice D**).

Temper tantrums are more frequent among younger children when they are frustrated about situations and are a depressive reaction seen often during adolescence (**choice E**).

49. **The correct answer is C.** This patient describes four pain symptoms, two gastrointestinal symptoms, one sexual/reproductive symptom, and one pseudomonal symptom, all with no apparent cause. This meets the criteria for the diagnosis of somatization disorder.

Depressive disorder (**choice A**) is unlikely. It consists of one or more major depressive episodes, each of which lasts at least 2 weeks. The most prominent symptoms of major depressive disorder are depressed mood and loss of interest or pleasure. Patients also tend to have other symptoms, but these vary from person to person. Insomnia and weight loss often accompany major depression, but depressed patients may also gain weight and sleep excessively.

Lyme disease (**choice B**) is a tick-borne disease caused by *Borrelia burgdorferi*. It is reported mostly in the months of May to August. It typically manifests with erythema migrans (dermatologic), seventh cranial nerve palsy, peripheral neuropathy (neurologic), atrioventricular block, myocarditis (cardiologic), and oligoarticular arthritis. This patient's story would not fit in with a pattern of symptoms and signs consistent with Lyme disease.

Her story does not fit with the pattern of systemic lupus erythematosus (**choice D**), the symptoms of which manifest as fatigue, malaise, weight loss, arthritis or arthralgias, fever, photosensitivity, rashes and serositis, thrombocytopenia, hemolytic anemia, nephritis, vasculitis, and pneumonitis, to name a few.

Her dysphagia, dysmenorrhea, and normal erythrocyte sedimentation rate cannot be explained with a diagnosis of ulcerative colitis (**choice E**). Ulcerative colitis is an idiopathic and chronic inflammatory bowel disease affecting the rectum and colon. It often presents with bloody diarrhea and weight loss.

50. **The correct answer is D.** This patient most likely has dysthymic disorder, which is characterized by depressed mood for at least 2 years and at least two of the following: change in appetite, alteration in sleep, low energy, low self-esteem, poor concentration, or feelings of hopelessness. There must be no history of a mania or hypomanic episode, substance abuse, chronic psychotic disorder, or organic cause.

Adjustment disorder with depressed mood (**choice A**) is characterized by impaired social or occupational functioning or abnormal symptoms within 3 months of a stressor.

Bipolar disease (**choice B**) is characterized by major depression with periods of mania.

Cyclothymia (**choice C**) is dysthymia with periods of hypomania.

This patient does not have hypothyroidism (**choice E**) because she has normal levels of thyroid-stimulating hormone and thyroxine.

Major depression (**choice F**) can be similar to dysthymia. The lifelong history of a depressed mood not triggered by any particular depressing event, however, and the predominance of patient complaints as opposed to objective signs, indicate that major depression is not the diagnosis in this case.

Surgery: **Test One**

1. A 38-year-old woman with allergic rhinitis and recurrent sinusitis comes to the clinic for followup. Approximately 1 month ago she underwent bilateral endoscopic sinus surgery for chronic sinusitis refractory to prior medical treatment with oral corticosteroids and multiple courses of antibiotics. She reports that her symptoms of headache and facial pain and pressure are much improved since the surgery. She is currently on no medications other than a daily topical nasal steroid spray prescribed by her otolaryngologist. Her only complaint is intermittent clear "runny nose" on the left side, which she notices almost every day. In addition, she has noticed the rhinorrhea to be exacerbated by straining or bending forward. Her symptoms are most consistent with

   (A) a common side effect of topical nasal steroid sprays
   (B) a leakage of cerebrospinal fluid
   (C) a recurrence of her allergic rhinitis symptoms
   (D) a recurrent episode of acute sinuitis
   (E) a viral upper respiratory illness

2. A 5-year-old child is brought to the emergency department by his mother because of pain and a "deformity in his right elbow." The child was playing at home and was trying to climb a tree when he fell on an extended outstretched arm. The child lives far from a medical facility and it took the mother an hour to reach the emergency department in her car. When the child is examined, he is in severe distress from the pain. There is a right upper extremity deformity at the right elbow and severe tenderness. The radial pulse is absent but the neurological examination is normal. A radiograph shows an extension-type supracondylar fracture of the humerus. The most appropriate next step in the management is

   (A) arteriography
   (B) closed reduction and reexamination of vascular status
   (C) closed reduction, reexamination of the vascular status, and immediate percutaneous pinning by the orthopedic surgeon
   (D) closed reduction, reexamination of the vascular status, and immobilization with a plaster cast
   (E) immediate operative exploration of brachial artery

3. A 73-year-old man with a history of tobacco abuse, hypertension, prior stroke, and laryngeal cancer is brought by EMS to the emergency department after being found unresponsive at his home. It is estimated by family members that he lost consciousness approximately 1 hour earlier. He underwent a total laryngectomy 10 years prior with no subsequent evidence of recurrent cancer. His current medications include ramipril and a daily aspirin. On physical examination, the patient is nonresponsive to voice or painful stimuli and his respirations are shallow. Vital signs are: temperature 37.1 C (98.7 F), blood pressure 199/98 mm Hg, pulse 92/min, respirations of 12/min, and an O_2 saturation level of 86%. There are no apparent signs of trauma secondary to a fall. The pupils are small, but equal and reactive. The patient's tracheostoma is widely patent; breath sounds are distant, but present bilaterally without crackles. An arterial blood gas reveals pH 7.28, PaO_2 59, and $PaCO_2$ 45. The most appropriate next step in management is to

   (A) establish a secure airway by intubating the patient with a transoral endotracheal tube and begin mechanical ventilation
   (B) initiate immediate treatment with thrombolytic therapy
   (C) obtain a CT scan of the brain to rule out cerebrovascular accident
   (D) perform an emergent cricothyroidotomy to secure the patient's airway and begin mechanical ventilation
   (E) place an endotracheal tube in the patient's tracheostoma and begin mechanical ventilation

4. A 25-year-old man comes to the emergency department because of left ankle pain that began after falling during a basketball game 1 hour ago. He is ambulatory but appears to be have significant pain. He denies any previous injuries or knee problems. He has no previous medical problems. His temperature is 37.6 C (100.0 F), blood pressure is 130/70 mm Hg, pulse is 105/min, and respirations are 14/min. On examination of his left lower extremity, the patient has a swollen left ankle with no bruises. He has good dorsalis pedis and posterior tibialis pulses and good sensory-motor function in the left foot. There is tenderness over the medial and lateral malleolus as well as the lateral and proximal part of his tibia. A plain x-ray of the ankle shows a non-displaced transverse fibular fracture higher than the level of the mortise. The most appropriate next step in the management of this patient is to

   (A) administer intravenous antibiotics and pain medication
   (B) admit him to the hospital for open reduction and internal fixation
   (C) apply a posterior splint and have him followup with an orthopedist in 2 weeks after the swelling subsides
   (D) prepare him for emergent closed reduction in the emergency department and admit him to the hospital for open reduction and internal fixation
   (E) x-ray his left hip to rule out any concomitant fracture

Items 5-6

A 20-year-old college student drove rapidly down a surface street and ran a red light. He lost control while trying to avoid another car, and slammed into a wall. His girlfriend, who was a front seat passenger, was killed instantly. In the emergency department he is hypotensive and tachycardic. He has a pelvic fracture, possible ruptured spleen, and a laceration to the right forearm. You are informed that one of the earliest persons at the scene was a physician who had his practice nearby. The physician did not bother to help the victims. You learn that the relatives are outraged, and have decided to sue him.

5. This physician would most likely
   (A) be found guilty by the court
   (B) be found not guilty by the court
   (C) have his license suspended
   (D) lose his hospital privileges
   (E) lose his medical license

6. The patient is now under your care. One of your concerns is the incredible amount of anger expressed by the relatives. They seem to dislike you as well, because you are part of the profession. The most appropriate initial intervention is to
   (A) assess circulatory status and control hemorrhage
   (B) establish a patent airway
   (C) hand over the patient to another doctor
   (D) inform the hospital attorney to avoid a lawsuit against you
   (E) secure good venous access

7. A 58-year-old woman comes to the office because of a "red bump" in the scar on her nose where you had removed a skin cancer 3 years earlier. About 4 weeks before her office visit she noticed what looked like a pimple appear in the center of the scar. When it would not go away after 4 weeks, she got concerned that her cancer had reappeared and came to see you. You review the chart and note that 3 years ago she had a biopsy confirmed basal cell carcinoma in the proximal part of the left nasolabial crease. You excised it with a 3 mm margin, and the pathology report confirmed that there was no tumor at the margin in the sections examined. You have been seeing her semiannually since and this is the first sign of what you think is most probably recurrent basal cell carcinoma based on clinical appearance. There is a 3-mm pearly, pink, translucent papule with telangiectasis traversing the surface located at the lower edge of a linear scar in the left nasolabial crease. If a biopsy of the lesion confirms your suspicion that this is recurrent basal cell carcinoma, the most appropriate next step in managing this patient is
   (A) cryosurgery
   (B) reexcision with a 5-mm margin
   (C) referral for Mohs micrographic surgery
   (D) topical 5-fluorouracil twice daily for 4 to 6 weeks
   (E) topical imiquimod cream under occlusion three times a week for 8 to 10 weeks

8. A 22-year-old man comes to the emergency department with a cut sustained to his right hand when he was hit with a sharp object during a physical altercation with his neighbor 6 hours ago. The patient complains of pain in his right index finger. He reports being allergic to lidocaine. He tells you that his last tetanus shot was 6 years ago. His temperature is 37.6 C (100.0 F). There is a 1-cm transverse laceration to the palmar aspect of his right index finger at the level of the proximal interphalangeal joint. No active bleeding is noted. There is good capillary refill distally as well as good sensorimotor function of the index finger. The most appropriate next step in management is to

    (A) administer tetanus toxoid as well as tetanus immunoglobulin
    (B) admit him for intravenous antibiotics with loose wound closure due to the location of the laceration and the relatively delayed presentation
    (C) exclude a fracture of the index finger, irrigate, and then repair under local anesthesia using procaine
    (D) irrigate the wound and provide local anesthesia using bupivacaine
    (E) irrigate the wound and provide local anesthesia using bupivacaine with epinephrine

Items 9-10

A 52-year-old man comes to the emergency department because of the acute onset of "excruciating abdominal pain." He says that he has had "gnawing" epigastric pain that radiates to his back for the past several months, but he did not have time to see a doctor about it because his job as a major newspaper editor keeps him busy until "all hours of the night." Previous episodes of abdominal pain occur about 3 hours after a meal, are relieved by eating food, and wake him from sleep. However, this episode came on 20 minutes after dinner and was not relieved by food. He is very concerned because his father-in-law was recently diagnosed with colon cancer, and he has been worrying that he may be suffering from the same disease. The sudden onset of this severe pain is what made him come to the hospital tonight. His blood pressure is 120/80 mm Hg and his pulse is 80/min. Physical examination shows a rigid, board-like abdomen with generalized rebound tenderness and hypoactive bowel sounds. Rectal examination shows dark, guaiac-positive stool, but no gross blood.

9. The most appropriate next step in management is to

    (A) arrange for an immediate exploratory laparoscopy
    (B) obtain an abdominal CT scan
    (C) obtain upright chest and abdominal x-rays
    (D) reassure him that this is not colon cancer
    (E) schedule an immediate upper endoscopy

10. Before you are able to perform the most appropriate step in management from the previous question, the patient suddenly develops severe nausea, hematemesis, and loses consciousness. His blood pressure is 80/60 mm Hg and pulse is 120/min. Bright red blood per rectum is noted. The most likely explanation for his worsening symptoms is

    (A) colonic perforation due to diverticulitis
    (B) dissection of the aorta
    (C) erosion of the gastroduodenal artery
    (D) ruptured abdominal aortic aneurysm
    (E) ruptured esophageal varices

11. A 60-year-old man with diabetes and hypertension comes to the office for a routine 6-month followup visit for his blood pressure. He is currently taking lisinopril and metformin. On examination, you discover a 1.5-cm mobile and nontender nodule on the right lobe of a thyroid gland. There is no lymphadenopathy. On further questioning, you find that he has no history of radiation to the neck and no family history of cancer. He feels well and review of systems is negative. Thyroid stimulating hormone level is normal. The most appropriate next step in management is to

(A) determine T_4 and T_3 levels
(B) order CT scan of the neck
(C) perform a fine needle aspiration (FNA), with or without ultrasound guidance
(D) recommend followup in 6 months
(E) refer him for surgical resection
(F) send him for thyroid scintigraphy with concurrent suppression by antithyroid medication
(G) send studies for thyroid peroxidase antibodies (TPO, also known as microsomal antigen)

12. During your afternoon rounds, you are asked to evaluate a 91-year-old bedridden woman who has been in the hospital for 4 weeks for multiple problems, including pneumonia, congestive heart failure, and dehydration. While in the hospital her condition has slowly deteriorated. Due to severe lower extremity contractures, she is no longer able to get out of bed. The nurses have asked you to evaluate her back for a "sore" which they say is getting worse. The "sore" initially started as something the size of quarter, but during her hospitalization it has increased in size. It is mildly tender and sometimes drains a clear fluid. She has been afebrile for 48 hours, is currently not on any antibiotics, and is tolerating her meals adequately. On examination, there is an ulcer the size of your palm over the lumbar and sacral area of the patient's back. The edges of skin are clean and there is no active purulent drainage. The superficial areas appear to be clean without exudate. The center of the ulcer is deep and you can touch an area that feels like bone. There are no "hidden areas" or pockets of fluctuance appreciated. The most appropriate course of action in order to heal this patient's ulcer is to recommend the appropriate dressing changes and

(A) antibiotics with appropriate coverage for skin flora
(B) incision and drainage of the ulcer
(C) total parenteral nutrition
(D) turning of the patient from side to side every 2 hours
(E) x-rays of the spine to look for degenerative changes

13. A 16-month-old child is brought to the emergency department by her parents because she has been crying and refuses to walk since she fell the night before. The parents report that she recently began to walk and has been unsteady on her feet. Examination reveals an irritable child with restricted movement of her right lower extremity. A radiographic examination reveals a displaced spiral mid shaft fracture of the femur. An orthopedic surgeon was called for stabilization of the fracture. In addition to stabilization of the fracture, you should order

(A) a bone biopsy
(B) an MRI of the femur
(C) serum calcium and phosphorus levels
(D) a skeletal survey
(E) urine mucopolysaccharide screen

14. A 22-year-old college student comes to the clinic for a followup visit after a wrist injury. He is still complaining of wrist pain. Three weeks ago, while ice skating, he fell on an outstretched hand. At that time, he complained of some tenderness in the wrist and went to the nearest emergency department. Physical examination at that time did not reveal any abnormality except for the point tenderness over the anatomic snuffbox. No associated deformity or sensory or motor deficit was noted at that time. A posteroanterior view of the wrist, in addition to lateral oblique and ulnar deviated views of the wrist, did not reveal any bony fracture. Because of the specific tenderness at the anatomic snuffbox, a plaster cast was applied and he was sent home with analgesics. Now, 3 weeks later he comes to the clinic for a scheduled appointment. You take off the plaster cast. Physical examination does not reveal any abnormality except for the same point tenderness at the anatomic snuffbox of the right wrist. Radiographs of the arm, forearm, and the wrist, including posteroanterior ulnar deviated and lateral oblique views, do not reveal any abnormalities. The most appropriate next step in management is to

(A) order a bone scan
(B) order a bone scan and reapply the plaster cast, if the scan is positive
(C) order a bone scan and reapply the plaster cast, even if the bone scan is negative
(D) prescribe more analgesics
(E) refer him to a psychiatrist

15. A 48-year-old man with coronary artery disease, hypertension, and diabetes returns to the clinic complaining of tongue pain. You have seen him three times over the past 4 months for a similar complaint. The pain is at 7/10 currently, which is worse than the previous visit of 4/10. He smokes one pack of cigarettes a day and drinks four drinks per week. Initially when you saw him, it appeared that he had this rather large superficial ulcer in the central portion of his tongue dorsum. Today the area of the lesion is smaller, although it appears to extend somewhat deeper. You have treated him with nystatin solution with limited improvement in the pain, but now the pain seems to be getting worse in spite of the nystatin. The most appropriate next step in management is to

(A) switch to fluconazole solution for presumed *Candida* infection
(B) switch to miconazole solution for presumed *Candida* infection
(C) switch to lidocaine solution for pain control
(D) switch to oral narcotic tablets for pain control
(E) take a biopsy in an attempt to establish a diagnosis

16. You are taking care of a 35-year-old man who has been shot in the abdomen and head by a fellow gang member. You learn that he is the most important member of an elusive and notorious gang. You also learn that he has a living will. His family wants him to be disconnected from the life support systems. In this situation, you would advise the family that you would have to wait for

(A) a decision by the hospital attorney
(B) a decision by the hospital ethics committee
(C) a decision by the state
(D) a second opinion from your colleagues
(E) the results of the electroencephalograph

17. A 32-year-old Caucasian woman comes to the clinic for a followup appointment for right upper quadrant abdominal pain. At the last visit she told you the pain is dull in nature, nonradiating, and occasionally associated with nausea. There is no weight loss, fevers, chills, or change in bowel habits. Upon further questioning you learned that she has no significant prior medical history. Her surgical history includes an appendectomy at age 8, and removal of her tonsils and adenoids as a toddler. Her only medication is oral contraceptive pills. She has no known allergies and does not smoke or drink. On physical exam 2 weeks ago, her vital signs were stable and her weight was appropriate for her height. Sclera were anicteric and there was no palpable adenopathy. Her heart and lung examinations were normal. Abdominal examination was significant for normal bowel sounds with mild tenderness in the right upper quadrant. Murphy sign was negative and there were no peritoneal signs or costovertebral angle tenderness. Pelvic and rectal examinations were within normal limits. Suspecting cholelithiasis, you sent her for laboratory studies and an abdominal ultrasound. Now she tells you there has been no change in any of her symptoms. Her laboratory results are all within normal limits including liver function tests and urinalysis. There were no gallstones seen on ultrasound; however, a 5-cm mass was noted in the periphery of the right lobe of the liver. The radiologist at the imaging center then performed a CT scan, which showed the mass to be consistent with a hepatic adenoma. With regards to her imaging results, the most appropriate thing for you to tell her is

(A) it is okay to continue with her oral contraceptive pills
(B) she should have an intravenous pyelogram to look for renal stones
(C) she will need a liver transplant
(D) that you recommend she should discontinue the oral contraceptive pills
(E) the mass is most likely cancer and she will need immediate surgery
(F) there is nothing to worry about
(G) you will refer her to an oncologist for chemotherapy

18. An 18-year-old bicyclist is brought to the emergency department by ambulance after being involved in a collision with a motor vehicle. A history is elicited from paramedics who transferred the patient that a car traveling 10 mph struck the patient's bike and the cyclist was thrown into an irrigation ditch on the side of the road. She was wearing a helmet and on arrival in the emergency department is complaining of only left lower leg pain. The paramedics noted a small wound around her ankle and that her ankle appeared deformed. She states that she is fine and can recall the entire accident. She denies any chest or abdominal pain and says, "Other than my ankle, I'm fine." Her blood pressure is 110/80 mm Hg, pulse is 75/min, and respirations are 16/min. She is holding a deformed left ankle with gauze dressing over the lateral aspect. The bandage is removed and reveals a 5-cm open wound with grass and mud covering exposed bone fragments. The left foot is warm, has 2+ dorsalis pedis and posterior tibial pulse, and normal sensation. Radiographs of the ankle have been ordered. The most appropriate next step in managing this patient is to

(A) bandage the wound using sterile technique and send her to a local orthopedic surgeon's office

(B) have the patient admitted to the hospital trauma service

(C) inquire about the patient's tetanus status and begin intravenous antibiotics

(D) irrigate the patient's wound with hydrogen peroxide and tell her to return to the orthopedic clinic in 2 or 3 days

(E) splint the ankle and give the patient crutches and pain medicine, tell her to return in 1 week for emergency department followup

19. As you are making afternoon rounds in the hospital, you are informed that one of your patients has a fever of 38.2 C (100.8 F). The patient is a 71-year-old man who is postoperative day 6 from a right hemicolectomy for colon cancer. Upon questioning, the patient tells you that he feels well other than a small amount of pain at his incision site. He has been tolerating his regular diet for 24 hours without any nausea or vomiting. He has passed flatus, but has not had a bowel movement. He has been ambulatory since postoperative day 3. He denies any cough, chest pain, shortness of breath, or dysuria. His Foley catheter has been removed for 3 days now. Physical examination reveals clear lungs with good inspiratory effort and no crackles, normal heart sounds, and nondistended and soft abdomen. There is erythema and increased tenderness around the distal half of the incision site. A small amount of purulent drainage is seen near the erythematous portion of the wound. He has no calf tenderness or lower extremity swelling. The most appropriate next step in the management of this patient's fever is to

(A) apply a dressing to the incision site drainage

(B) begin antibiotic therapy

(C) open, drain, and pack the incision site

(D) order a chest x-ray

(E) schedule a lower extremity venous Doppler study

20. A 70-year-old man returns for followup 3 weeks after his annual physical examination. On the prior visit you noted that he was in good health with no recent hospitalizations. He had a right knee replacement secondary to osteoarthritis 11 years ago and his only medication is an occasional ibuprofen for shoulder pain. He is a former tobacco user with a 50 pack-year history of smoking. Physical examination was normal. Urinalysis in the office showed 9-10 RBCs but no other abnormalities. Because of the hematuria, you referred him for CT scan of the abdomen and pelvis along with cystoscopy. As per the notes from the urologist, his cystoscopy did not display any abnormalities. However, his CT scan revealed a 6-cm contrast-enhancing mass in the mid pole of the left kidney. Chest x-ray is normal. In the office today the patient denies any back pain, gross hematuria, weight loss, nausea, vomiting, change in bowel habits, or new neurological symptoms. The most appropriate next step in the management of this renal mass is to

(A) begin high-dose IL-2 immunotherapy
(B) perform a percutaneous core biopsy
(C) refer the patient for chemotherapy
(D) refer the patient for radiation therapy
(E) refer the patient for removal of the left kidney, including Gerota fascia
(F) refer the patient for removal of the left kidney, leaving Gerota fascia intact

21. A previously healthy 12-year-old boy is brought to the emergency department because of abdominal pain that began earlier that same day. He did not eat any breakfast or lunch and when he developed a fever this afternoon, the parents became worried. The boy tells you that his pain was initially around his belly button but now it hurts more on the right side. He prefers to lie still since any movement makes the pain worse. He is not hungry and vomited one time in the car. His temperature is 38.8 C (101.8 F), blood pressure is 108/61 mm Hg, pulse is 106/min, and respirations are 20/min. He is lying perfectly still on the stretcher. His oral mucosa is dry. His abdomen is not distended, but has hypoactive bowel sounds. There is discrete tenderness on the right side of his lower abdomen with guarding and rebound tenderness. There is also pain on the right side when you palpate the left lower quadrant. You are unable to percuss the abdomen as the boy begins to cry in pain. Rectal examination is normal. Laboratory studies show a leukocyte count of 14,500/μL with a differential of 94% segmented neutrophils and 11 bands. His urinalysis has 3 to 4 RBC and 2 to 3 WBC. The most appropriate next step in management is to

(A) admit the patient for hydration and antibiotics
(B) admit the patient for serial abdominal examinations
(C) order a CT scan
(D) prepare the patient for emergent appendectomy
(E) prepare the patient for emergent exploratory laparotomy

22. A 45-year-old slightly obese woman comes to the office complaining of right-sided crampy abdominal pain. The pain became severe after she ate lunch and radiates to the area underneath the right shoulder blade. She has suffered from many similar episodes in the past 6 months and the pain typically lasts for several hours and then slowly dissipates. She denies any vomiting, dysuria, hematuria, fevers, chills, or change in bowel habits. She has just started menopause. On physical examination in your office, she is comfortable and afebrile with normal vital signs. She has hypoactive bowel sounds without abdominal distention. There is mild tenderness in the right upper quadrant without rebound or guarding. There is no costovertebral angle tenderness. Pelvic and rectal examinations are normal. Urine dipstick in the office is negative for blood, white cells, or bilirubin. At this time, the most appropriate imaging study to confirm this patient's diagnosis is

(A) an abdominal ultrasound
(B) a HIDA scan
(C) an MRI of the abdomen
(D) a plain film abdominal x-ray
(E) a renal/bladder ultrasound

23. A 22-year-old man is rushed into the emergency department after he was involved in a shooting. He is complaining of abdominal pain and tells you that he heard one shot and when he looked down at his shirt, it was covered in blood. You and your staff quickly complete the appropriate surveillance of the patient along with the placement of two large-bore peripheral intravenous lines. His blood pressure is 112/81 mm Hg, pulse is 120/min, and respirations are 32/min with an oxygen saturation of 94% on room air. His head and neck have suffered no injury. His lungs are clear to auscultation. There is a bullet entry site in the left lower quadrant and an exit wound in the left lower back. Blood is extruding from the entry site. His abdomen is nondistended but tender. There is no blood from the urethral meatus and rectal examination reveals good sphincter tone without any evidence of gross blood. His extremities have good distal pulses bilaterally. As you go to take an x-ray of his chest and abdomen, his blood pressure drops to 72/50 mm Hg and his pulse increases to 134/min. At this time he becomes cold, diaphoretic, and weak. He is given 1 liter of normal saline intravenously and his blood pressure and pulse improve. However, the pressure quickly drops and the pulse increases again. The most appropriate next step in management is to

(A) begin cardiopulmonary resuscitation
(B) give him a blood transfusion
(C) immediately perform a CT scan of abdomen and pelvis to evaluate his injuries
(D) place a central line
(E) prepare him for an emergent exploratory laparotomy

24. A 35-year-old man comes to the emergency department complaining of a generalized, persistent headache for the past 3 days. He denies chest pain or shortness of breath. He also states that he has had episodes about twice a month of severe headache, perspiration, rapid heartbeat, and facial pallor. They usually have an abrupt onset and last for several minutes. His blood pressure is 188/112 mm Hg, pulse 90/min, and respirations 18/min. The blood pressure after 3 min of standing is 152/94 mm Hg with a pulse of 112/min. Funduscopic examination shows constricted blood vessels, but no hemorrhages. Heart and lung examinations are normal. Serum chemistries and CBC are normal. An electrocardiogram is also unremarkable. The most appropriate next step is to

(A) begin therapy with captopril and followup to clinic in 6 months
(B) begin therapy with diltiazem and followup to clinic in 6 months
(C) begin therapy with hydrochlorothiazide and followup to clinic in 6 months
(D) begin therapy with metoprolol and followup to clinic in 6 months
(E) obtain a 24-hour urine collection for catecholamines after acutely controlling blood pressure

25. A 56-year-old man comes to the urgent care clinic with the acute onset of back pain. His vital signs are stable. He has point tenderness over the spinous process of T11. Rectal examination shows normal tone, brown, guaiac-negative stool, and a large nodule. There is 3/5 strength on the left and 5/5 strength on the right to dorsiflexion of the great toes. An MRI of the spine shows multiple lesions consistent with metastatic disease in the spine, and a compression deformity of T11 with spinal cord impingement. The patient is felt to have metastatic prostate cancer. You remember reading that an MRI of the prostate can be done in patients for preoperative staging. It has a sensitivity of 38% for spread of disease beyond the capsule of the prostate, but a specificity of 97%. Based on this data, an MRI of the prostate

(A) can rule out prostate cancer in 97% of patients
(B) will be more likely than not to show extracapsular spread of disease in patients with prostate cancer
(C) will only pick up 38% of all prostate cancers
(D) will pick up 3% of all prostate cancers
(E) would be a poor screening test to pick up disease in this patient

26. A 55-year-old man comes to the clinic with postprandial epigastric pain related to fatty meals. An abdominal ultrasound is ordered to evaluate for cholelithiasis. The results of the ultrasound confirm your suspicion, but also comment on a 1.3-cm simple cyst in the upper pole of the left kidney. No other abnormalities are identified on the ultrasound. He returns to the clinic 2 weeks later. He denies any hematuria, dysuria, or history of upper or lower urinary tract infections. Apart from the above history he is otherwise healthy, but is a 45-pack-a-year smoker. His temperature is 37.0 C (98.6 F), blood pressure 122/70 mm Hg, pulse 77/min, and respirations 18/min. Lungs are clear, heart is regular, and his abdomen is benign. Laboratory studies reveal a leukocyte count of 7400/µL, creatinine of 1.0 mg/dL, blood urea nitrogen of 12 mg/dL, hematocrit 46%. The most appropriate management of his ultrasonic renal finding is to

(A) drain the cyst and send the fluid for cytopathologic analysis
(B) explain that no treatment or followup is necessary
(C) followup ultrasound in 6 months to assure stability
(D) order a CT scan of the abdomen to rule out retroperitoneal adenopathy
(E) refer him to a urologist to evaluate for partial nephrectomy of the upper pole of the left kidney

27. A 23-year-old man is admitted to the hospital for chemotherapy treatment of metastatic seminoma. He presented 3 weeks ago with a painless testicular mass and underwent orchiectomy, yielding a diagnosis of seminoma. A CT scan of the abdomen confirmed metastatic disease to the retroperitoneal lymph nodes. His temperature is 37.0 C (98.6 F). He is well appearing, heart is regular without murmurs, lungs are clear, and abdomen is benign. Some postsurgical changes are present on inspection of the genitals. Laboratory studies show a leukocyte count of 6500/µL, hematocrit 45%, platelets 359,000/µL, blood urea nitrogen 12 mg/dL, and creatinine 0.6 mg/dL. As you are just finishing his admission chemotherapy orders, he states that he has changed his mind with regard to therapy and says that he now "has found God" and feels that God alone will cure his disease. The most appropriate management at this time is to

(A) discharge the patient and wish him well
(B) discuss his religious beliefs and point out the benefits that the chemotherapy will offer him
(C) have the patient placed on a psychiatric hold and administer the chemotherapy anyway
(D) tell him that God is not going to help him, only chemotherapy will
(E) tell him that the chemotherapy would likely not provide much benefit, however you still think it is worth a try

Items 28-29

You are seeing a 69-year-old man 1 day after having a gastric tube placed. The patient has a long history of dementia secondary to Alzheimer disease and was admitted to the hospital for failure to thrive (FTT). A full evaluation revealed only severe dementia but no obvious cause for the FTT. A swallowing study was performed that indicated likely aspiration of all oral foods. After discussion with the family, a decision was made to place a gastric tube for the purposes of feeding. The surgery was uneventful, and the patient appears to be doing well during a routine postoperative check.

28. The most accurate statement about this surgical procedure is that it

(A) allows the patient to take oral as well as tube-based foods
(B) eliminates the risk of aspiration
(C) has no effect on the risk of aspiration
(D) will improve the patient's long-term mortality
(E) will improve the patient's near term morbidity

29. Later that evening you are called to see the patient after he is found severely obtunded. The patient is now 34 hours postoperative. He had been getting tube feedings for the past 5 hours and had minimal gastric residuals at the 2-hour check time. On arrival he is cyanotic with labored breathing. His pulse oximeter reads 85% on 100% nonrebreathing mask. On inspection of the patient's mouth and oropharynx, there are tube feedings visible. The most likely etiology of this patient's respiratory distress is

(A) inadvertent oral consumption and aspiration of tube feedings
(B) oropharyngeal obstruction and hypoventilation
(C) over-sedation
(D) regurgitation and aspiration of gastric-tube infused tube feedings
(E) residual anesthesia

30. A 42-year-old man comes to the emergency department complaining of right knee pain and an inability to bend the knee. He explains that he was in a snowmobile race an hour ago and landed awkwardly on his right leg after a jumping maneuver. Normally he tries to land with his knees flexed to absorb the shock, however, his leg was extended and he felt something "snap" in his right knee as his snowmobile landed on the ground. He denies hitting his head or any loss of consciousness. Inspection of the right knee reveals intact skin with a slight depression or sulcus at the level of the inferior patellar pole. Distally the strength is 5/5 in the extensor hallucis longus, the gastrocsoleus muscles, and the anterior tibialis. The pulses are 2+ for the popliteal, dorsalis pedis, and posterior tibialis arteries. Knee x-rays show a posterior-lateral tibia dislocation. A closed reduction of the right knee is completed in the emergency department without complication. After the reduction, the knee is examined while the patient is still sedated. Gross global ligamentous instability is noted. The most appropriate next step in management is to

(A) apply a knee immobilizer or other splint with the knee in 45 degrees of flexion; discharge to home with crutches and non-weight bearing of right leg; schedule orthopedic surgery followup within 1 week

(B) apply a knee immobilizer or other splint with the knee in full extension; admit overnight for observation; if neurovascular status remains stable then discharge to home with crutches and non-weight bearing of right leg; schedule orthopedic surgery followup within 1 week

(C) apply a knee immobilizer or other splint with the knee in full extension; discharge to home with crutches and non-weight bearing of right leg; schedule orthopedic surgery followup within 1 week

(D) apply a knee immobilizer or other splint with the knee in full extension; order a stat MRI of the right knee to determine which ligaments are disrupted; consult the orthopedic surgery service regarding preoperative planning

(E) order an emergent right lower extremity angiogram and contact the vascular surgery service and the operating room personnel regarding a possible arterial injury

31. An inebriated 50-year-old man is brought to the emergency department because of a cut on his hand. He was walking down the road in front of the hospital when he decided to test the strength of a piece of glass lying on the curb against his hand. He came out victorious and exclaimed, "Yippie! Yoo hoo!" according to a witness, who brought him in. He has a laceration across the dorsal aspect of his hand that he refuses to let you treat. In this case

(A) the patient has no right to refuse treatment because he is drunk

(B) the patient has the right to refuse treatment

(C) you will be disciplined by the American Medical Association if you fail to treat him

(D) you will be disciplined by the state medical board if you fail to treat him

(E) you will treat him under the tenet of beneficence

32. A 31-year-old construction worker was walking along a steel beam when he fell, straddling the beam. There was no loss of consciousness. He was brought to the emergency department complaining of pain to his testes and perineum. On physical examination, his vital signs are stable, his abdomen is soft, and his bladder is palpable almost halfway to the umbilicus. There is no evidence of flank or back ecchymosis. Genital examination reveals gross blood at the urethral meatus. There is a butterfly pattern of ecchymosis over the scrotum and perineum. His testicles are palpable and mildly tender. The prostate is normal in location, size, and consistency. He complains of the urge to urinate but only a few drops of fresh blood appear at the meatus. The next best step in management is to

(A) check hemoglobin/hematocrit and BUN/creatinine

(B) obtain a scrotal ultrasound

(C) order a retrograde urethrogram

(D) perform a cystogram

(E) place a Foley catheter per urethra

(F) schedule a CT scan of abdomen and pelvis

33. A 67-year-old African American man comes to the emergency department complaining of urinary hesitancy. He has been treated for benign prostatic hyperplasia (BPH) with tamsulosin for the past 2 months. The patient states that for the past 2 days his urinary stream has become progressively weaker until the day of presentation when all he can do is "dribble a few drops" of urine. He feels the constant urge to urinate and admits to episodes of incontinence when he was unable to get to the bathroom in time. He is not leaking any urine when he coughs or sneezes. He denies any dysuria, hematuria, fevers, chills, or previously similar episodes. Physical examination reveals an uncomfortable male with normal temperature and vital signs. Heart and lung examinations are within normal limits. His abdomen is soft with normal bowel sounds. In the lower abdomen there is a palpable mass, dull to percussion, extending from the suprapubic area superiorly to the level of the umbilicus. The mass is nontender, smooth, slightly mobile, and firm. Examination of the penis reveals no abnormalities, and his prostate is enlarged but smooth and firm. Significant laboratory data include a serum BUN of 43 mg/dL and a creatinine of 2.6 mg/dL (he had normal lab values at his yearly physical 2 months ago) Prostate specific antigen is 11.4 ng/dL. He is unable to provide a urine sample. The most appropriate next step in management is to

(A) begin workup for prostate cancer
(B) increase dose of tamsulosin
(C) order sedation medication
(D) place Foley catheter
(E) schedule renal/bladder ultrasound
(F) transfer to operating room for emergent transurethral resection of prostate (TURP)
(G) wait for patient to provide urine sample for analysis and culture

34. A 51-year-old woman with hypothyroidism comes to the clinic complaining of left-sided facial pain and swelling that began approximately 3 to 4 days ago and has become progressively more swollen and tender. She had a similar but less severe episode that resolved spontaneously 4 years earlier. She recently recovered from a flulike illness with gastrointestinal symptoms. Her only medication is thyroxine and she has no known drug allergies. She is a nonsmoker, drinks alcohol only occasionally, and has never used intravenous drugs. Vital signs are: temperature 37.7 C (99.7 F), blood pressure 158/90 mm Hg, pulse 92/min, and respirations 20/min. On physical examination there is an area of swelling and erythema of the patient's left face just beneath the left earlobe, extending 4 cm anteriorly, and to the level of the angle of the mandible inferiorly. On palpation, the affected area is very tender, but there is no obvious fluctuance or discrete nodule or mass. The ear examination is normal bilaterally and all cranial nerves are grossly intact, including the facial nerve on either side. There is no additional tenderness or palpable adenopathy or mass on the neck. Oral cavity examination is without mass or mucosal lesion, erythema, or exudate. Bimanual palpation of the left buccal area elicits tenderness, but no mass is palpated. There is no evidence of drainage from Stensens duct on the left. Her leukocyte count is $13,000/mm^3$. The patient's clinical picture is most consistent with

(A) a benign salivary gland neoplasm
(B) an episode of acute parotitis
(C) HIV infection
(D) mumps
(E) squamous cell carcinoma of the left parotid

35. A 34-year-old woman is brought to the emergency department after a low-speed motor vehicle crash in which she was in the passenger seat and was not wearing her seat belt. She denies loss of consciousness or amnesia for the event. During the crash, her head bent forward and she hit the dashboard of the car. She is quick to dismiss the crash except for the annoying fact that her "teeth do not seem to fit together" like they did before the crash. Her oral cavity exam is normal, except that her teeth seem to contact each other on the right side before the left side. However, there are no cuts in the lining of her mouth and no bleeding. X-rays of her cervical spine and clinical assessment of her spine are normal. The most appropriate next step in management is to

(A) obtain a complete series of mandible x-rays
(B) provide the name and phone number of a dentist for the patient to make an appointment and followup on her dental concerns
(C) reassure her that her dental malocclusion is common after car crashes and that it should resolve spontaneously within a month
(D) reexamine her oral cavity to make sure there are no fractures of her mandible

36. A 53-year-old man returns to the clinic for followup, as he is in the process of being evaluated and worked up for new onset fatigue. He was found to have anemia with associated guaiac-positive stools. He has recently undergone a colonoscopy with biopsy of a mass in the ascending colon. Today he has brought along his wife for the biopsy results. It is your responsibility to tell the patient and his wife that his biopsy is positive for adenocarcinoma of the colon, which invades through the muscularis mucosa. Along with this information, you should also tell the patient that

(A) he has one of the rarer types of colon cancer
(B) he needs his entire colon removed
(C) he should undergo removal of a portion of his colon
(D) the biopsy removed all the cancer
(E) the primary site for his cancer to spread is to the brain
(F) with surgery he will definitely need a colostomy

37. A 44-year-old man is rushed into the emergency department after an accident. The patient was riding his bicycle, without a helmet, when he was struck on the left side by a car moving at a high speed. Per eyewitnesses, the patient was thrown from his bike approximately 10 feet, where he landed on top of another car parked on the street. He had a short loss of consciousness. Upon arrival in the emergency department he is awake, answering questions, but clearly short of breath. His neck has already been stabilized by the paramedics on the scene. His airway is patent, there are no loose teeth, and his oropharynx is clear of any blood or gastric secretions. There are no breath sounds on the left side of the chest. His left thorax has multiple abrasions and ecchymoses. The right lung field is clear to auscultation. His pulse oximeter is reading 84% while he is receiving oxygen at 6 L/min via nasal cannula. You continue to ask him questions, which he answers. The patient tells you that he is having trouble breathing. The most appropriate next step in the management of this patient's acute shortness of breath is to

(A) ask him if he smokes tobacco
(B) change his nasal cannula oxygen to face mask oxygen
(C) check an arterial blood gas
(D) perform a CT scan of the chest
(E) place a left-sided chest tube
(F) request a PA and lateral chest x-ray

38. A 61-year-old woman comes to the office complaining of "spidery veins." Occasionally, she has a dull, achy feeling in her legs that usually occurs at the end of the day. Recently her shoes have begun to feel tight at the end of the day. She used to work as a bank teller, spending many hours on her feet each day. She denies any shortness of breath or difficulty walking up stairs. There is no history of deep venous thrombosis. On physical examination her legs are symmetric in size, without evidence of trauma or skin breakdown. On the inner aspect of her upper and lower thigh are dilated superficial veins. There are good dorsal pedalis pulses bilaterally, and motor and sensory examination is normal. The most accurate statement regarding her condition is:

(A) Compression stockings may provide relief
(B) Sclerotherapy is not a reasonable treatment option
(C) There is no association with deep venous insufficiency
(D) These veins will never bleed
(E) Walking will likely improve her symptoms

39. A 37-year-old otherwise healthy woman comes to the urgent care clinic because of a 3-month history of vague abdominal pain. She has had a decreased appetite but has noticed an increase in her abdominal girth to the point where she can no longer wear her usual pants. She denies prior similar episodes, fevers, chills, or use of street drugs. She has never been hospitalized. Physical examination shows an obvious fullness of the abdomen with an easily apparent fluid wave. There is tenderness in the right upper quadrant with hepatomegaly. Laboratory studies show a normal CBC and serum chemistries other than a decreased albumin level. Liver function tests are also within normal limits. You perform an ultrasound guided paracentesis. The ascitic fluid reveals >3 g protein per deciliter. The most likely diagnosis is

(A) acute cholecystitis
(B) alcoholic liver cirrhosis
(C) Budd-Chiari syndrome
(D) gallbladder cancer
(E) hepatitis C

40. A 71-year-old man who you have not seen in 2 years comes to the office complaining of abdominal pain that he describes as "chronic" over the last 6 months. It occurs intermittently and is worse after meals. His wife questions how it can be worse after meals since he "never eats." When questioned, he is unable to localize the site of pain but describes it as crampy in nature. He has had a recent unintended 10-lb weight loss and he denies night sweats, fevers, or prior similar episodes before this period. His bowel movements are well formed and without blood. He has hypertension and coronary artery disease and underwent left femoral-popliteal artery bypass surgery 3 years ago. His vital signs are: temperature 37.2 C (99.0 F), blood pressure 151/89 mm Hg, and pulse 76 beats/min. Oral mucosa is moist. There is a right carotid bruit. Heart and lung examinations are unremarkable. His abdomen is non-distended with normoactive bowel sounds. There are no peritoneal signs, pulsatile mass, or organomegaly. There are well-healed incisions and palpable distal pulses in the extremities. This patient most likely has

(A) celiac sprue
(B) Crohn disease
(C) gastroenteritis
(D) irritable bowel syndrome
(E) mesenteric ischemia

41. A 62-year-old man comes to the office complaining of "red urine." For the past 11 years you have been taking care of his diabetes and hypertension, but he has never mentioned any blood in his urine before. He tells you that there is no pain associated with the blood, it occurs about once a week and persists through the entire urinary stream. The first episode was about 6 weeks ago, but he did not seek treatment because the bleeding stopped on its own. However, it has now persisted on a weekly basis and he is concerned. He denies fevers, back or abdominal pain, weight loss, history of urinary tract infection, or renal stones. Physical examination reveals no changes since his health maintenance examination 8 months prior. Urinalysis shows 12 to 14 red blood cells, 0 to 1 white blood cells, negative nitrite, and negative leukocyte esterase. Urine culture shows no growth. Complete blood count and biochemical profile are normal. Prostate specific antigen (PSA) is 1.1 ng/mL. A cystoscopy reveals a raised papillary frond, 1 cm in size, over the trigone. It is consistent with transitional cell carcinoma of the bladder. The most appropriate next step in management is to

(A) begin intravenous chemotherapy
(B) biopsy of the lesion through the cystoscopy
(C) give him intravesical BCG
(D) give him intravesical thiotepa
(E) resect the lesion through the cystoscope
(F) schedule external beam radiation to the pelvis

42. A 45-year-old construction worker comes to the clinic complaining of severe pain in his buttock area that started approximately 2 months ago with some vague anal discomfort. He also noticed some bright red blood on the toilet tissue and a feeling of incomplete emptying with bowel movements. However, today the pain became excruciating, to the point where he is unable to sit down. His foreman referred him to the clinic when he arrived to work that morning. He tells you that he has always strained at bowel movements and he does a lot of heavy lifting at his job. He has no other medical problems and no significant surgical history. He denies use of tobacco, alcohol, or illicit street drugs. He has never had a sigmoidoscopy and denies weight loss, fevers, chills, or family history of colon cancer. Temperature and vital signs are normal. His abdomen is soft and nontender. On rectal examination there is a very tender, firm, smooth-walled mass extruding from the anus. The mass is dark in color. There are a number of small hemorrhoids around the anus. When you attempt to reduce the mass to perform a digital rectal examination, the patient jumps off the table in pain. The most appropriate next step in management is to

(A) aspirate the mass with a small-gauge needle
(B) incise and drain the mass
(C) order a barium enema
(D) perform a colonoscopy
(E) prescribe sitz baths and warm packs to mass

43. A 78-year-old nursing home resident with end-stage Alzheimer disease is transferred to your emergency department because the floor nurses state that he has been refusing his meals and vomiting for the last 36 hours. The nursing home also reports a 2-day history of no bowel movements. It is unclear if the patient has recently passed flatus and his mental status is such that you cannot rely on his answer. Upon questioning, he states that his belly hurts. He had an inguinal hernia repair 15 years ago, but has no other chronic conditions besides Alzheimer disease. He takes medications only for Alzheimer. Occasionally the home will give him acetaminophen for a headache or joint pain. His temperature and vital signs are normal. His abdomen is grossly distended and there are high-pitched hyperactive bowel sounds. The entire abdomen is tympanitic to percussion. There is tenderness diffusely with guarding in the left lower quadrant. Rectal examination shows an empty rectal vault without masses or tenderness. Complete blood count reveals a mild leukocytosis. BUN and creatinine are mildly elevated, consistent with prerenal azotemia. An obstructive series shows a dilated sigmoid colon that is displaced and crossing the midline. There is no free air or dilated loops of small bowel. The most appropriate next step in management is to

(A) admit him for serial abdominal examinations
(B) order an upper GI series with small bowel followthrough
(C) perform sigmoidoscopy
(D) repeat the obstructive series after nasogastric tube is placed
(E) schedule an exploratory laparotomy

44. A 72-year-old woman comes to the emergency department with complaints of rectal bleeding. Over the past 2 days, she has developed crampy abdominal pain, nausea, and then a few hours prior to arrival had dark red blood mixed with stool. She denies hematemesis or coffee ground emesis. She has coronary artery disease, diabetes mellitus, and atrial fibrillation, for which she takes insulin, digoxin, and enteric-coated aspirin. Her blood pressure is 99/72 mm Hg, pulse 122/min, and respirations are 22/min. Cardiac examination reveals tachycardia and an irregularly irregular rhythm. Her abdomen is diffusely tender and moderately distended. Bowel sounds are decreased. Rectal examination shows dark red blood mixed with stool. Laboratory studies show:

BUN	52 mg/dL
Creatinine	1.1 mg/dL
Hematocrit	32%
Platelets	220,000/mm^3
Lactate	2.2 mEq/L

A CT scan of the abdomen shows thickening, mild dilation, and hyperemia of small bowel loops in the mid jejunum. Moderate aortic calcification is present. The solid organs appear normal. After stabilizing the patient and sending blood for type and cross-match, the most appropriate next step is to

(A) admit her to the medical service, rehydrate with normal saline, and follow up with a CT scan in 1 week
(B) order an arteriogram
(C) perform colonoscopy
(D) perform endoscopic gastroduodenoscopy
(E) send her for a small bowel followthrough study

45. A 48-year-old woman comes to the clinic complaining of hand pain after she fell forward on the pavement 24 hours ago. On examination, the left hand is swollen at the dorsum and palm. There is also swelling of the little finger and ring finger along with significant ecchymosis and pinpoint tenderness over the fifth metacarpophalangeal joint. She is unable to extend her little finger either at the proximal or distal interphalangeal joints. When asked to make a fist she does so but with extreme difficulty. There is no paresthesia noted. She has no scaphoid tenderness. Her elbow has a full and pain-free range of motion and appears normal. X-rays of the hand confirm a fracture at the head of the fifth metacarpal. X-rays of the elbow are unremarkable. Scaphoid views of the hand are negative. Besides the fracture of the metacarpal, based on the findings, you are concerned about

(A) compartment syndrome
(B) distal avulsion fracture of the extensor digiti minimi tendon (or extensor communes tendon)
(C) fracture to the head of the radius
(D) scaphoid fracture
(E) nerve ligation

Items 46-47

46. A 70-year-old man comes to the clinic for a preoperative examination 2 weeks before a total hip replacement. He has a past medical history of an embolic stroke 9 years ago, hypertension, type 2 diabetes mellitus, and neuralgia of the left hand. His medications include aspirin, torsemide, lisinopril, metformin, and gabapentin. He tells you that his neurologist recently decreased the dosage of the aspirin to 81 mg once daily. He is a nonsmoker and does not drink alcohol. His temperature is 37.0 C (98.6 F), blood pressure is 150/80 mm Hg, pulse is 72/min, and respirations are 16/min. His heart and lung sounds are normal. The abdominal examination is benign. His weight is 200 lb. His latest chest x-ray and electrocardiogram are normal. The recommendation that would have the greatest benefit in the perioperative stage of the hip replacement is to

(A) continue the metformin and recheck his serum glucose a week before the operation
(B) discontinue the aspirin
(C) increase the dosage of the torsemide
(D) increase the dosages of torsemide and lisinopril
(E) reduce his weight

47. You instruct the patient accordingly and send him home. He is routinely admitted to the hospital the day before the hip operation. He is started on an insulin sliding scale by the anesthesiologist, hydrated appropriately through an intravenous line, and given lorazepam for anxiety. In the evening, he is also kept nil by mouth as of midnight. At this time, the management that would have the greatest benefit in the perioperative period is to

(A) allow him to have his regular midnight snack
(B) discontinue all of his remaining medications as part of the *nil per os* policy
(C) discontinue all of his medications as part of his *nil per os* status except the metformin
(D) maintain his *nil per os* status except for water to allow him to take all of his regular medications
(E) maintain his *nil per os* status except for water to allow him to take all of his regular medications except for metformin

48. You are called to evaluate a 48-year-old man on the gastroenterology floor who is "being difficult to the staff." The patient is a successful executive who oversees a company with 2000 employees. He constantly complains about the "service" that he is receiving at the hospital. He was admitted for a bowel resection and colostomy for recurrent Crohn disease for which he had been treated with steroid therapy in the past. On interview, he states repeatedly that, "the staff here just don't know how to take care of people." He complains that they are not attentive to his needs and that he feels neglected. Additionally, the patient has asked that his wife and two young children not be allowed to visit him because, "I can't let them lose respect for me because of the way I'm looking." After a brief pause, the patient angrily declares, "I want to be treated like I'm someone who contributes to society and not like a bum." The most appropriate management is to

(A) discuss option of having his medical care transferred to another venue given his dissatisfaction
(B) discuss the difficulties of adjusting to a disfiguring surgery
(C) explain how fortunate he is for having had a life-saving surgery
(D) explain how steroid therapy is making his mood and thought process irrational
(E) prescribe haloperidol for body dysmorphic disorder

49. A 91-year-old man comes to the clinic for a followup appointment. He has a history of chronic obstructive pulmonary disease (COPD) and hypertension. He feels well and denies fever, weight loss, or any other problems. A complete physical examination was performed during his last visit 1 month ago. At that time, you found a prostate nodule on digital rectal examination and referred him to a urologist. A transrectal biopsy of the prostate was performed 2 weeks ago and reveals a Gleason grade 7 carcinoma. The most appropriate next step in the management of this patient is to

(A) begin antitestosterone treatment
(B) order a bone scan
(C) recommend a nerve-sparing prostatectomy
(D) send him back to the urologist for a radical prostatectomy

50. A 49-year-old woman comes to the office because of abdominal pain. She had a laparoscopic cholecystectomy 3 weeks ago and had an uneventful postoperative course. One week ago, she started to have intermittent mid-epigastric and right upper quadrant pain. She describes the pain as being nearly identical to her pain prior to her surgery. She also reports nausea, but denies fever or vomiting. Her temperature is 37.0 C (98.6 F). Physical examination shows tenderness in the right upper quadrant and mid-abdomen. Bowel sounds are normal and there is no rebound tenderness. The most appropriate next step in management is to

(A) obtain liver function tests, including alanine aminotransferase (ALT) and aspartate aminotransferase (AST)
(B) order a CT scan of the abdomen and pelvis
(C) order an ultrasound of the abdomen
(D) reassure the patient that some abdominal pain following surgery is to be expected
(E) refer the patient back to the surgeon because of a possible biliary leak

Surgery Test One: Answers and Explanations

ANSWER KEY

1. B
2. C
3. E
4. B
5. B
6. B
7. C
8. C
9. C
10. C
11. C
12. D
13. D
14. C
15. E
16. C
17. D
18. C
19. C
20. E
21. D
22. A
23. E
24. E
25. E
26. B
27. B
28. E
29. D
30. E
31. B
32. C
33. D
34. B
35. A
36. C
37. E
38. A
39. C
40. E
41. E
42. B
43. C
44. B
45. B
46. B
47. E
48. B
49. B
50. C

1. **The correct answer is B.** Cerebrospinal fluid (CSF) leaks are a potential complication of endoscopic sinus surgery. The patient's symptoms of unilateral clear rhinorrhea exacerbated by a Valsalva maneuver are consistent with a CSF leak. In the traumatic setting, CSF mixed with blood is suspected when "targeting" occurs, i.e., when a drop of fluid onto a sheet appears to separate out into clear fluid and bloody components. Fluid suspicious for CSF can also be evaluated for the presence of beta-2-transferrin, a protein present in CSF.

   Clear rhinorrhea is not one of the common side effects of topical nasal steroid sprays (**choice A**), which include epistaxis and minor throat irritation.

   Clear rhinorrhea is a symptom of allergic rhinitis (**choice C**), but is usually bilateral and would not be exacerbated by straining.

   Finally, she does not exhibit other signs or symptoms of recurrent sinusitis (**choice D**), such as fever, headache, purulent rhinorrhea or facial pain and pressure, or a viral upper respiratory illness (**choice E**).

2. **The correct answer is C.** A fall on an outstretched extended arm in children results in supracondylar fractures of the humerus. High incidence of neurovascular injury is associated with this fracture. In these types of fractures, accurate assessment of median, radial, and ulnar nerves and the brachial artery is essential. Immediate reduction under general anesthesia using fluoroscopy, is necessary in most cases, to restore radial pulse and peripheral circulation. Once the fracture is reduced, the distal extremity should be checked for the adequacy of the radial pulse. Fractures with significant displacements and brachial artery compression are often unstable, and application of plaster cast is difficult in these patients. Hence, the fracture should be stabilized with percutaneous pinning to maintain bone stability while allowing extension at the elbow. If arterial circulation is not restored with bone reduction, immediate arteriography and brachial artery exploration with the repair are indicated. For an extended ischemia of the forearm, forearm compartment fasciotomy is also indicated.

   Immediate arteriography (**choice A**) is only indicated when pulse does not return after the fracture is reduced successfully.

   Closed reduction of the fracture and reexamination of the vascular status (**choice B**) may itself prove that further intervention is unnecessary. But, in patients with severe displacement of the fractured fragment associated with brachial artery compression, further displacement should be avoided by fixation.

   Application of a plaster cast (**choice D**) in these fractures is not practical and, hence, external pinning should be used for the immobilization.

   Immediate open exploration of the brachial artery (**choice E**) is not indicated unless the fracture is associated with a severe crush injury of soft tissues and ischemia is suspected.

3. **The correct answer is E.** Regardless of the cause of this patient's loss of consciousness, he now demonstrates respiratory distress, meeting the criteria for assistance with mechanical ventilation. His arterial blood gas reveals poor oxygenation and a respiratory acidosis. Establishing a secure airway takes precedence over subsequent steps in evaluation and treatment of his underlying problem. Poor mental status or loss of consciousness alone may prompt the need for airway protection in some patients due to loss of pharyngeal tone and ability to protect the airway. This would not be the case with this patient, however. The key to this question is to understand the anatomy in a patient who has undergone a total laryngectomy. After a total laryngectomy, the digestive and airway tracts are completely separated and the patient's trachea is sewn to the skin, creating a "stoma" or "tracheostoma" just above the sternal notch. There is no longer any airway above this point. Therefore, a standard transoral intubation (**choice A**) is incorrect as there is no connection between the mouth and airway in this patient.

   Thrombolytic therapy (**choice B**) may be appropriate for some patients with ischemic stroke, although the cause of this patient's loss of consciousness has not yet been determined. In any case, the patient's history of hypertension and current SBP of 199 would likely be more consistent with a possible hemorrhagic stroke.

   A CT scan of the brain (**choice C**) might be helpful in determination of the patient's underlying problem, but not before securing the patient's airway.

   A cricothyroidotomy (**choice D**) is a surgical procedure for obtaining an emergent airway in a patient that cannot otherwise be intubated by making an incision through the cricothyroid membrane between the cricoid and thyroid cartilages. In this patient, however, the airway is widely patent and mechanical ventilation can be initiated via an endotracheal tube placed in the patient's tracheostoma. Having undergone a previous laryngectomy, the cricoid and thyroid cartilages are no longer present.

4. **The correct answer is B.** Admission to the hospital for open reduction and internal fixation is the correct management of such an ankle fracture. This is actually classified as a Weber C ankle fracture, as the fracture line in the fibula lies above the mortise. A Weber B fracture would be at the level of the mortise. A Weber A fracture line would be lower than the mortise and is managed as an ankle sprain with a splint

   Intravenous antibiotics (**choice A**), along with irrigation of the wound with sterile saline solution, are only indicated if the fracture is open. This fracture in this case is not open.

   Posterior splint and orthopedics followup (**choice C**) is not appropriate for this Weber C fracture, as explained above.

   Emergent closed reduction in the emergency department (**choice D**) is not indicated since the ankle is neurovascularly intact. A loss of the dorsalis pedis or tibialis posterior pulse would be an indication to reduce the ankle fracture emergently.

   Typically, the proximal parts of the tibia and fibula should be filmed rather than the hip (**choice E**), as those are commonly fractured concomitantly with the ankle.

5. **The correct answer is B.** There is no legal obligation enforced by the courts on any individual to rescue a person in distress. And, in the case of a physician, the law does not obligate him to treat a person who is unknown to him. **Choices A, C, D, and E** are incorrect.

6. **The correct answer is B.** The first intervention is to establish a patent airway. This includes looking for signs of obstruction that may be caused by fractures of the middle third of the face, the mandible, the larynx or trachea, or even foreign bodies.

   Assessing circulatory status and controlling hemorrhage (**choice A**) and securing venous access (**choice E**) come after an airway is established.

   This patient is already under your care. You cannot transfer him to the care of another doctor (**choice C**) without just cause.

   Informing the hospital attorney to avoid a lawsuit against you (**choice D**) is inappropriate because you must treat the patient and there is no reason to believe that you are going to be sued.

7. **The correct answer is C.** This patient has recurrent basal cell carcinoma in an area that corresponds to the facial planes of embryonic fusion and where sparing of tissue is very important, all criteria to perform Mohs micrographic surgery with the goal of minimizing the possibility of having deep penetrating segments of the tumor missed by conventional surgery. In Mohs micrographic surgery, the excision is performed in layers and, during the surgery, frozen sections are prepared that allow viewing of 100% of the margins of excised tissue. This minimizes the possibility of having thin projections of the tumor missed when classic "bread loafing" of the specimen is performed for conventional histopathologic sectioning (which allows approximately 2 to 3% of effective margins of the excision to be viewed). If tumor is viewed close to or near the specially prepared margins, another layer of tissue is excised and frozen sections prepared in the same manner. This procedure is repeated until the margins are clear. Excision of basal cell carcinoma with Mohs micrographic surgery has a recurrence rate of about 1%, compared to 8 to 9% with conventional surgery. It is preferable for lesions that are recurrent, in a high-risk location, or large and ill defined, and where maximal tissue conservation is critical.

   Cryosurgery (**choice A**) is not a good choice for this anatomic location due to the lack of margin control and probability that it would cause excessive destruction of the surrounding facial tissue and leave a considerable scar. It is performed by inserting a thermocouple into the central part of the tumor down to subcutaneous tissue, after appropriate local anesthesia is administered, and the area is frozen with liquid nitrogen or other cryogens. The depth and length of freezing vary considerably among surgeons and are largely based on experience.

   A recurrent basal cell carcinoma in the nasolabial margin carries a high probability of deep extension along the planes of embryonic fusion. Conventional reexcision (**choice B**) carries a high risk of "missing" parts of the neoplastic tissue. In addition, excising with a bigger yet still arbitrary margin on the face, where conservation of tissue is so important, is not practical and makes reconstruction difficult.

   Topical 5-fluorouracil (**choice D**) is a chemotherapeutic agent that is used for topical treatment of the superficial type of basal cell carcinoma in certain circumstances when other, more aggressive, types of treatment are either not indicated due to the poor overall health of the patient and associated risk of surgery, or if the patient refuses other treatment modalities. It is applied twice daily for a period of 4 to 6 weeks, leading to ulceration of the tumor and inflammation of the surrounding skin. Superficial basal cell carcinoma appears as a scaly red patch with a filiform pearly border (with or without pigmented areas within it) most commonly on the trunk or proximal extremities.

Imiquimod cream (**choice E**) is an immune modulator that is FDA approved for the treatment of genital warts. There have been multiple publications of case reports where it was successfully used for the treatment of superficial basal cell carcinoma in patients in whom more aggressive surgical treatment was not an option. This is not conventional treatment for basal cell carcinoma.

8. **The correct answer is C.** A fracture needs to be excluded prior to repair since the mechanism involved blunt trauma to the finger. The other issue that needs to be addressed is the choice of local anesthetic agent in view of this patient's allergy to lidocaine. Procaine is an ester, unlike lidocaine, which is an amide. Procaine is an alternative in case of allergy to lidocaine. Some advocate the use of cardiac lidocaine or single-dose lidocaine vials. This is due to the fact that they are devoid of methyl paraban, which is thought to be the cause of the allergy to lidocaine and present in multiple-dose lidocaine vials.

   Based on the patient immunization history and the absence of gross contamination of the wound, the patient only needs a tetanus booster. Had the wound been grossly contaminated, then the immunoglobulin would have been needed (**choice A**).

   IV antibiotics (**choice B**) are not required unless the patient has an open fracture or the laceration is at the metacarpopharyngeal joint or secondary to a human bite.

   Bupivacaine (**choice D**) is not an acceptable alternative, as it is an ester, like lidocaine, and my have cross reactivity with it.

   Using epinephrine (**choice E**) is also unacceptable in the finger where it may cause ischemia because of the presence of end arteries.

9. **The correct answer is C.** This patient is most likely suffering from a perforated duodenal ulcer and has free air in the peritoneum. These patients often present with a history that is consistent with a duodenal ulcer (gnawing abdominal pain that is relieved by food, wakes them at night, and radiates to the back), and the acute onset of severe abdominal pain with a rigid abdomen and rebound tenderness. The most appropriate way to detect this is to look for free air under the diaphragm with upright x-rays.

   An immediate exploratory laparoscopy (**choice A**) is not appropriate because the diagnosis of a perforated ulcer should first be established by finding free air under the diaphragm on upright x-rays. At that time, a laparotomy will most likely be necessary to repair the perforation.

   A CT scan (**choice B**) may be necessary if the upright x-rays, which are performed first, fail to show a perforation.

   Even though the symptoms seem to be related to a perforated duodenal ulcer, it is inappropriate to reassure him that this is not colon cancer (**choice D**) before performing any diagnostic studies.

   An immediate upper endoscopy (**choice E**) is not the most appropriate management in this case of a suspected perforated ulcer.

10. **The correct answer is C.** This patient most likely has a duodenal ulcer that eroded into the gastroduodenal artery, causing tachycardia, hypotension, syncope, hematemesis, and bright red blood per rectum. The history that this patient gave before he lost consciousness was consistent with a duodenal ulcer, and the radiation to the back may indicate that he has a posterior-penetrating ulcer. A fiberoptic endoscope is a safe and effective way to obtain the diagnosis quickly.

    A colonic perforation due to diverticulitis (**choice A**) is unlikely because this patient initially presented with classic symptoms of a duodenal ulcer, not with signs of diverticulitis (left lower quadrant pain, nausea, vomiting, anorexia, change in bowel habits, and a low-grade fever).

    Aortic dissection (**choice B**) typically presents with severe chest pain. They often have severe aortic insufficiency, pulmonary edema, and diminished pulses. A chest x-ray may show a widened mediastinum. This presentation is inconsistent with the patient in this case.

    A ruptured abdominal aortic aneurysm (**choice D**) typically presents with abdominal or back pain, a pulsatile abdominal mass, and shock. Since the patient in this case had the classic symptoms of a duodenal ulcer, and did not have a pulsatile mass on examination, this diagnosis is unlikely.

    Ruptured esophageal varices (**choice E**) would most likely present with upper gastrointestinal bleeding and hypotension in a patient with a history of hepatitis, cirrhosis, alcohol abuse, or chronic liver disease. The diagnosis is typically established with an upper endoscopy. The patient in this case describes the classic symptoms of a duodenal ulcer, and does not appear to have any evidence of liver disease or portal hypertension (spider angiomata, palmar erythema, gynecomastia, caput medusa, ascites, or a palpable spleen).

11. **The correct answer is C.** Asymptomatic thyroid nodules are often found on clinical examination. Most nodules are benign; however, approximately 5% are malignant. Risk factors for thyroid cancer include age >60 or <30 and patients with a history of radiation. For a given nodule, males are also more likely to have malignancy. An FNA is often recommended as the first step in evaluation, and may also be the most cost effective. An FNA may have an overall accuracy of as high as 95% in good centers. Results of the FNA may be nondiagnostic, benign (macrofollicular), indeterminant (microfollicular), or malignant. As most nodules are benign and without evidence of metastatic disease, a CT scan is not helpful (**choice B**). Given the utility of FNA, either proceeding directly to surgery (**choice E**) for a possible benign lesion or followup alone (**choice D**) for a potential carcinoma are not acceptable. A TSH in an asymptomatic patient is usually sufficient as a first step. T_3 and T_4 (**choice A**) are likely to be of less yield than an FNA, as the patient clinically is euthyroid. A low TSH may be helpful, however, in suspecting a hyperfunctioning adenoma; a high TSH may be indicative of autoimmune (Hashimoto) thyroiditis.

Thyroid scintigraphy (**choice F**) is recommended by some as an initial step to evaluate a thyroid nodule. The uptake scan can determine whether a nodule is autonomously functioning; these "hot" nodules are more likely to be benign. However, only about 10% of palpable nodules are "hot". In addition, smaller nodules are more likely to be indeterminate. An ultrasound is often used by thyroid specialists to assist in localizing and aspirating the nodule. It may reveal additional nodules or microcalcifications that may increase the risk of malignancy. However, its routine use after a thyroid scintigraphy or uptake scan is not indicated. For example, if scintigraphy showed a "cold" nodule the next best step would be biopsy; while if the nodule was "hot", suppression with medication could be attempted. Medical treatment is not an acceptable initial step for a thyroid nodule.

TPO antibodies (**choice F**) maybe helpful in a hypothyroid patient but would not be helpful in evaluation of the nodule.

12. **The correct answer is D.** This patient has a sacral decubitus ulcer secondary to pressure. The constant lying on her back has generated a pressure ulcer, which has gotten worse. The ulcer is not infected and is described as containing "healthy" tissue. However, unless the insulting agent (pressure) is removed, the sore will never heal. That is why it is so important for bedridden patients to be turned appropriately. This will prevent pressure sores and skin breakdown all over the body. The best dressings will be of little help if the constant pressure is not removed.

Because the wound is not infected, antibiotics (**choice A**) do not play a role in treatment.

The ulcer is not infected, therefore, there is no tissue to incise and drain (**choice B**). If a pocket of purulence were present then yes, incision and drainage would be necessary to help with healing.

While it is true that this patient will require adequate nutrition to heal this wound, total parenteral nutrition (TPN) (**choice C**) is not the best way to approach the problem. TPN is not without its own costs and complications. This patient can tolerate per os feedings, and therefore supplementation with intravenous nutrition is inappropriate.

Taking x-rays of the patient's spine (**choice E**) is not likely to contribute any information that will help in the care of this patient's ulcer. Imaging should be utilized when its results will help in the diagnosis or treatment of a problem. Neither is true in this case.

13. **The correct answer is D.** Spiral fractures in children are usually due to a twist or torsional injury. Spiral fractures of the femur are rare in toddlers and small children. When a spiral fracture of a femur or a humerus is seen in children from a fall, child abuse should be suspected and investigated unless the history and clinical examination strongly correlate with the fracture. A skeletal survey is indicated to document injuries in various stages of healing in cases of suspected child abuse.

A bone biopsy is not indicated (**choice A**) unless a metabolic disease is suspected.

An MRI of the femur (**choice B**) is not indicated to diagnose and treat an acute fracture. MRI is mostly useful for the soft tissue lesions rather than bony injuries, especially in the evaluation of extremities trauma.

Serum calcium and phosphorus levels (**choice C**) are not useful in an acute fracture in an infant. Fractures due to metabolic bone diffuse (nutritional rickets) occur more commonly as transverse metaphysial fractures. These fractures are associated with chronic radiographic changes.

Urine mucopolysaccharide screen (**choice E**) is not indicated routinely in an isolated single fracture of a long bone in an infant. When connective tissue or generalized bony disorders are suspected with involvement of multiple bones and fractures at different stages, then one should investigate the possibility of a metabolic disorder.

14. **The correct answer is C.** Scaphoid fracture in young adults is common after a fall on an outstretched hand. Hyperextension injuries of the wrist can also cause lunate dislocation or disruption of scaphoid lunate relation. Ulnar deviated, posteroanterior view of the wrist bring the scaphoid into full profile. PA and lateral views demonstrate lunate displacement. Oblique radiographs demonstrate a nondisplaced scaphoid fracture. Despite the negative radiograph, scaphoid fracture should be suspected with specific point tenderness in the anatomical snuffbox. Patients should be treated with a plaster cast immobilization, including the thumb and elbow. After 3 weeks, when the plaster cast is taken off, if the anatomical snuffbox specific tenderness persists, a bone scan should be ordered if the radiographs are still negative. A bone scan will highlight the fracture site. In the presence of negative radiographs and bone scan the plaster cast should be reapplied for at least 6 weeks for immobilization to avoid any future complication like posttraumatic arthritis of the wrist. The cast may sometimes be used for up to 3 months.

    Bone scans alone (**choice A**) may or may not prove an old fracture. The plaster cast must be reapplied for a prolonged time when scaphoid fracture is suspected in a young adult to prevent further complications.

    Bone scan and application of the plaster cast only when scan is negative (**choice B**) is not appropriate therapy when there is a clinically strong suspicion of scaphoid fracture.

    Simple administration of analgesics (**choice D**) will only mask the symptoms and delay the diagnosis without proper workup.

    Referral to a psychiatrist (**choice E**) is not necessary when clinical examination points to specific tenderness.

15. **The correct answer is E.** Squamous cell carcinoma of the upper aerodigestive tract is consistently among the top 10 neoplasms in terms of frequency and mortality. Smoking is by far the most significant risk factor for this type of neoplasm, and alcohol intake multiplies the risk. Even in the absence of this patient's smoking and alcohol history, the persistence of the lesion merits closer evaluation and likely biopsy. In particular, the fact that this lesion had initial improvement but is now clinically progressing is an ominous sign.

    Candidal infections of the oral cavity are common, particularly in immunocompromised patients. Nearly all of these respond well to topical antifungals. This patient may have had an ulcerated lesion with a superimposed infection, but the failure of the patient to continue their improvement is worrisome and requires a more thorough evaluation. Therefore, continued treatment with antifungals (**choices A and B**) is incorrect.

    Analgesics are effective for symptomatic relief of pain. Control of symptoms should not be confused with identification of the etiology of pain. While topical lidocaine (**choice C**) or oral medications (**choice D**) may be short-term temporizing measures, they are complementary interventions that can occur with a biopsy and should not be considered an essential step in management.

16. **The correct answer is C.** A decision by the state has to be awaited. Despite that this patient has a living will, the state has a primary interest in preserving this patient's life to establish the nexus and modus operandi of his organization in the larger interests of society. The family has no right to have life support systems withdrawn, and even if they had a durable power of attorney on behalf of the patient, the court would decree that the life support systems should be continued for reasons stipulated earlier. It must be pointed out that living wills have a narrow range of application, and in most states they relate to guidelines for terminal conditions. Unfortunately, there is no universal agreement with regard to the definition of a terminal condition, as this varies from state to state. In addition, a living will may not be applicable to a persistent vegetative state. Living wills are usually limited to the right to refuse interventions that would only prolong the process of dying. A durable power of attorney for healthcare is more encompassing than a living will. The other form of advance directive is oral statements to family members, friends, and healthcare personnel; this is the commonest form of advance directive. If the oral testimonies are vague or nonchalant assertions or remarks, however, then they will not stand the scrutiny of the law. It is important to remember that some states do not accept oral testimonies as credible. Despite the limitations of a living will, patients should be encouraged to provide advance directives, and a copy of this should be kept in the patient's records. In fact, under the Patient Self-Determination Act of 1990, hospitals, nursing homes, HMOs, and hospices that participate in Medicare and Medicaid programs are duty-bound to provide information to patients about their right to dispense advance directives.

The hospital attorney (**choice A**) does not have the right to make a judgment one way or the other in this case.

The ethics committee (**choice B**) cannot be called upon to help make a decision in this case.

Opinions of colleagues (**choice D**) would not be an admissible argument in court.

Awaiting the results of an electroencephalograph (**choice E**) is not justified.

17. **The correct answer is D.** This patient most likely has a hepatic adenoma. These lesions are typically found in young woman and oral contraceptives are a risk factor. Therefore, an appropriate first step in the management of a small, minimally symptomatic hepatic adenoma would be to stop any oral contraceptives. These masses carry a 10% risk of malignant degeneration as well as a risk of spontaneous rupture. For these reasons, most hepatic adenomas will ultimately require resection or embolization.

It is not unreasonable to stop her oral contraceptives and monitor the lesion, as many small ones will regress. For this reason, it is not appropriate for her to continue with her birth control pills (**choice A**).

The patient's urinalysis, ultrasound, and CT scan all show no evidence of renal stones. Performing an intravenous pyelogram (IVP) is unnecessary and a waste of resources (**choice B**). Besides, her symptoms are not typical of renal colic, which tends to be sharp, intermittent, and radiating toward the groin.

Patients who need liver transplants have liver failure (**choice C**). This patient provides no indication of that. She has no constitutional symptoms, and all of her liver function tests are completely normal.

Currently, this mass is most likely not cancer. Telling the patient that she has cancer and will need some type of oncological treatment (**choices E and G**) is inappropriate and will provide her with unnecessary worry. At the same time, it would also be unjust to tell her that she has nothing to worry about (**choice F**). As previously stated, these masses can become cancer or they may spontaneously bleed or rupture, all things that the patient should be made aware of.

18. **The correct answer is C.** This patient has an open (bone is exposed through disrupted soft tissues) fracture. The initial management of open fractures in the emergency department is crucial to obtain satisfactory results. Open fractures are *surgical emergencies*. Prompt stabilization and meticulous debridements are the keys to operative management. For most open fractures, a broad-spectrum cephalosporin and an aminoglycoside are started in the emergency department and the patient's tetanus status should be obtained. The application of a sterile dressing with minimal wound exploration until the patient can be taken to the operating room is appropriate.

As noted previously, open fractures, especially contaminated fractures as in this case, need surgical debridement as soon as possible. Sending this patient out of the emergency room to an office setting (**choice A**) only delays appropriate treatment.

This patient likely will not require admission to a trauma service (**choice B**). She had no loss of consciousness and this was a rather low-energy injury. The patient's physical examination is very benign at this point, and consulting the trauma service to admit this patient will again only delay the appropriate initiation of antibiotics and eventual surgical debridement.

Open fractures require adequate irrigation and debridement. Irrigating with hydrogen peroxide is not considered an adequate irrigation and does not qualify as a debridement (**choice D**).

Splinting the patient (**choice E**) may be appropriate to stabilize the fracture, but sending her out of the emergency department without the aforementioned antibiotics, irrigation, and debridement in the operating room is not sufficient for open fractures.

19. **The correct answer is C.** This patient has a postoperative wound infection. As with all types of infected fluid collections, the primary treatment is drainage of the fluid. In this case, that means removing the outer layer of closing (usually staples), releasing the pus, irrigating the now open wound, and packing the wound. Antibiotic therapy should then be initiated. Once the infection has been removed, daily dressing changes will allow the wound to heal by second intention.

Covering the drainage with a dressing (**choice A**) will prevent the patient from leaking on himself; however, it does nothing to halt the progression of the wound infection. If left untreated, this wound infection may disrupt the integrity of the abdominal fascial closure.

Using antibiotics (**choice B**) without opening the wound is inappropriate and incomplete.

It is appropriate to be concerned that any patient suffering from a postoperative fever may have or be developing pneumonia. It would not be inappropriate to order a chest x-ray on this patient. However, he has no respiratory distress, his lung examination is normal, and he has an obvious source for his fever (the wound). Therefore, the chest x-ray should be ordered AFTER the wound is drained (**choice D**).

A lower extremity thrombus may also cause a fever in the postop patient, and this may be evaluated by venous Doppler (**choice E**). However, the clinical suspicion here is low. There is no extremity edema, palpable cord, or tenderness or respiratory difficulty. Therefore, this test should not be ordered prior to opening the patient's infected incision site.

20. **The correct answer is E.** This patient has a stage I left renal-cell carcinoma (RCC) and the only currently known curative treatment is radical nephrectomy. When removing the entire kidney for cancer, the specimen should include the kidney along with Gerota fascia and the surrounding perinephric fat. If Gerota fascia is left in situ (**choice F**), this is called simple nephrectomy. Simple nephrectomy is usually reserved for nonfunctioning kidneys and should not be utilized when removing a kidney that contains cancer. Therapeutic options other than nephrectomy are reserved for those patient's who either have metastatic disease or are poor surgical candidates. Classic symptoms of RCC include hematuria, abdominal pain, and a flank/abdominal mass. However, this triad is present in less than 30% of patients presenting with RCC. In fact, with the widespread use of ultrasound and CT, the majority of renal-cell carcinomas are now found incidentally in asymptomatic patients.

    Interleukin-2 therapy (**choice A**) is reserved for those patients with metastatic disease. It may be used with or without and before or after nephrectomy. It plays no role as a primary treatment modality in a patient with localized disease.

    Percutaneous needle biopsy (**choice B**) is unnecessary in diagnosing this patient. The fact that this mass is contrast-enhancing confirms its diagnosis. Performing a biopsy is not indicated and should be reserved for those patients with multiple lesions, metastatic disease, or solitary kidneys.

    As previous stated, chemotherapy and radiation therapy (**choices C and D**) do not play a role in the primary treatment of localized renal cancer.

21. **The correct answer is D.** This patient is suffering from an acute appendicitis. This occurs when the appendiceal lumen becomes obstructed. Obstruction leads to increased production of mucus and entrapment of bacteria that dilates the appendix. Wall tension increases and blood flow becomes compromised, leading to vessel thrombosis and necrosis of the appendiceal wall. This process starts with luminal obstruction and inflammation. The most useful tools in establishing the diagnosis are history and physical. Typically, patients complain of periumbilical pain (caused by appendiceal contraction or distention of the lumen). As the inflammation spreads to the parietal peritoneal surface, the pain becomes somatic, steady, and more severe. It is aggravated by motion or cough and usually located in the right lower quadrant. Anorexia is so frequent that the presence of hunger should raise suspicion about the diagnosis. Temperature elevation is present with a commensurate tachycardia and mild leukocytosis. Urine may contain a few white or red blood cells if the appendix lies close to the right ureter or bladder. The treatment is early operation and appendectomy. This may be performed through a small incision in the right lower quadrant. Performing a midline incision with total abdominal exploration (**choice E**) is unnecessary with the current clinical scenario. A large midline incision will cause a prolonged recovery time with poor cosmetic results.

    While the patient is clearly dehydrated and does require intravenous fluids (**choice A**), this should not delay his necessary trip to the operating room. Antibiotics are important and they should also be administered, but again, should not delay a trip to the operating room.

    Performing serial abdominal exams (**choice B**) is beneficial in patients where the diagnosis and imaging studies are in doubt. In this case, neither is true, and delaying therapy will only lead to appendiceal perforation and increased risk of sepsis and other complications.

    A CT scan (**choice C**) may be beneficial in young women and other patients with atypical symptoms, or when the diagnosis is in doubt. That is not true here, where the patient has a classic presentation of acute appendicitis. Because the clinical suspicion for appendicitis is so high, his appendectomy should not be delayed for a test that will not change your plan.

22. **The correct answer is A.** This patient has the classic symptoms of biliary colic, or symptomatic cholelithiasis. This occurs when gallstones are formed and they pass into the common bile duct. It is estimated that almost 1 million new cases of cholelithiasis develop each year in the United States. There are three types of gallstones: cholesterol, pigment, and mixed cholesterol/pigment stones. Cholesterol stones are the most common stones in the U.S. These stones form because

of multiple factors, including *1)* bile supersaturation with cholesterol, *2)* nucleation of cholesterol monohydrate with subsequent crystal retention and stone growth, and *3)* abnormal gallbladder motor function with delayed emptying and stasis. Visualization of the gallbladder is done during routine sonography of the abdomen. It is very accurate in identification of gallstones. The test is rapid, not limited during pregnancy, and may detect very small stones. It is the test of choice for the initial screening of patients suspected of having gallstone disease.

The HIDA scan (**choice B**) is usually the test of choice for acute cholecystitis, but it is usually performed after an ultrasound. This is a nuclear study using radiopharmaceuticals with labeled, intravenously administered iminodiacetic acid. This material is rapidly extracted from the blood and excreted into the biliary tree. When the material cannot pass into the gallbladder, as occurs when a stone obstructs the cystic duct, this is pathognomonic for acute cholecystitis. In biliary colic (which this patient has) the pain does not persist. However, in acute cholecystitis, the pain persists and progression of inflammation causes gallbladder distention leading to inflammation of the parietal peritoneum. Many patients with acute cholecystitis experience anorexia, nausea, or vomiting.

MRI (**choice C**) plays no role in the evaluation of suspected gallstones. It is expensive and time consuming. There are many other cheaper and easier tests to utilize.

Plain abdominal x-ray (**choice D**) has a relatively low yield in the diagnostic evaluation of gallstones in the U.S. Only 10 to 15% of cholesterol and mixed stones contain sufficient calcium to be radiopaque. However, up to 50% of pigmented stones are radiopaque, although these form mostly outside this country.

While renal colic is in the differential diagnosis of this patient, it is unlikely. Besides, ordering only a renal/bladder ultrasound (**choice E**) is a poor imaging study for someone suspected of having renal stones (KUB, CT scan, IVP are better). This would not allow you to obtain the information you need to make an appropriate diagnosis.

23. **The correct answer is E.** This patient has received a penetrating injury to his abdominal cavity. He has become hemodynamically unstable in the trauma room and requires immediate exploration to evaluate his injuries and control bleeding. Based on physical examination, with visualization of his through-and-through gunshot wound, the abdominal wall fascia has been violated, making it highly probable that he has suffered injury to a hollow viscus organ, other organ, or vascular structure. In view of his physical examination and shock, an emergent laparotomy is the necessary form of treatment. If the penetrating injury is low velocity and the patient does not show any signs of shock, then the wound may be explored locally to evaluate for fascial disruption. If the fascia is not disrupted, then further workup with CT scan, serial examination, etc. may be considered. If during local wound exploration it is determined that the fascia was disrupted, then the patient requires exploratory laparotomy. Any patient with positive physical examination findings, shock, or evisceration requires immediate laparotomy.

This patient does not need CPR (**choice A**). He is suffering from shock secondary to acute blood loss. CPR is not necessary as long as he is able to maintain a blood pressure and pulse. With volume replacement, he is able to do this. However, if exploration is delayed then CPR may become necessary.

Due to his acute blood loss, the patient may require a blood transfusion (**choice B**). However, transfusion is futile unless the source of bleeding is discovered. Therefore, laparotomy should not be delayed for blood transfusion. This can be done in the operating room.

CT scan (**choice C**) will delay this patient's trip to the operating room. In a patient who is hemodynamically stable with questionable injuries, a CT scan may help with evaluation of injuries. This patient's survival requires quick control of his bleeding. CT scan will only help in the diagnosis and not the treatment of these injuries.

The patient already has two large peripheral intravenous lines placed. Taking the time to place a central line (**choice D**) will delay his laparotomy. The large peripheral IVs are placed as part of the early resuscitation and are frequently placed en route to the hospital. If they do not provide enough intravenous access, then a central line may be placed in the operating room.

24. **The correct answer is E.** This patient is presenting with classic symptoms of a pheochromocytoma. They typically present with paroxysmal spells (the 5 Ps); pressure (sudden increase in blood pressure), perspiration, pallor, palpitations, and pain (headache or chest pain). Orthostatic hypotension, as this patient has, is also a symptom, as is retinopathy. Pheochromocytomas are endocrine neoplasms that overproduce catecholamines such as epinephrine, norepinephrine, vanillylmandelic acid, and metanephrines. These can be picked up in a 24-hour urine collection. Predisposing factors are

familial forms, multiple endocrine neoplasia types II A and B, neurofibromatosis, and Lindau von Hippel syndrome.

Captopril (**choice A**), diltiazem (**choice B**), hydrochlorothiazide (**choice C**), and metoprolol (**choice D**) are all therapies for hypertension; however, the choices do not address multiple issues. Any young patient presenting with hypertension (particularly with his ancillary symptoms) needs an adequate evaluation for secondary causes. And, any patient presenting to the emergency department with newly diagnosed hypertension should also be seen more quickly than 6 months.

25. **The correct answer is E.** The easiest way to think about specificity is that it is used to rule in the presence of a certain entity (in this case, the presence of extracapsular spread of prostate cancer). Sensitivity, on the other hand, is used to rule out a certain entity. The most important aspect of a good screening test is a very high sensitivity, which this does not have, therefore making it a poor screening test.

Saying prostate cancer can be ruled out in 97% of patients (**choice A**) is suggesting that this test has a sensitivity of 97%, and this choice is similar to asking if this test has a high sensitivity, which it does not.

In this case the sensitivity is very low and the specificity is very high for extracapsular spread of disease *only*. Thus, MRI of the prostate should be able to rule in extracapsular spread if you see it, but you would not feel comfortable ruling it out if you do not see it (i.e., extracapsular spread of disease may very well be present even if the MRI does not show it!), therefore, saying that an MRI of the prostate will more likely than not show extracapsular spread of disease in patients with prostate cancer (**choice B**) is incorrect.

Saying that an MRI of the prostate will only pick up 38% of all prostate cancers (**choice C**) is incorrect because the test is not used to look at prostate cancer, but only extracapsular spread of cancer.

Saying that an MRI of the prostate will pick up 3% of all prostate cancers (**choice D**) is simply incorrect.

26. **The correct answer is B.** The Bosniak criteria exist for the classification of cystic lesions of the kidney. It is likely not important to memorize these unless you are either a urologist or radiologist. However, they are as follows. Type 1 is a simple cyst, as this patient has. It has no clinical significance and does not require any clinical followup whatsoever. These are very common in people over the age of 50. Bosniak class 2 lesions may have thin septations or calcifications in the wall. Ultrasound followup of these is not unreasonable (**choice C**), but often not necessary. Class 3 lesions have thick septae, and class 4 lesions have solid components. Class 4 lesions and usually class 3 lesions should be surgically removed (**choice E**). CT scan of the abdomen (**choice D**) would be performed prior to nephrectomy of stage 3 and 4 lesions.

Cyst drainage (**choice A**) is generally not performed for any renal lesions.

27. **The correct answer is B.** It is often difficult for the physician to understand and deal with the diverse religious beliefs encountered in the vast array of our patients. It is important not to dismiss these and at the same time rationally discuss what the medical alternatives have to offer. It is also important to remember that apart from certain psychiatric patients, you cannot force people to undergo treatments that they do not want. Discharging the patient without discussing all of the options with him (**choice A**) is inappropriate.

The patient is not overtly psychotic and is not demonstrating any evidence of psychiatric imbalance. These may very well be his true beliefs, and thus placing him on a psychiatric hold (**choice C**) is not an appropriate answer. If after discussing these issues with him, you find evidence of mental imbalance, then further psychiatric evaluation would be necessary.

Clearly, an abrupt response such as, tell him that "God is not going to help him, only chemotherapy will" (**choice D**) is inappropriate.

Telling the patient that chemotherapy is not likely helpful (**choice E**) in a patient with metastatic seminoma is not medically correct. This is one of the most treatable and potentially curable malignancies.

28. **The correct answer is E.** This procedure will most likely improve the patient's near term morbidity. The larger issue of providing tube feeding for severely demented patients is currently a topic under much debate. In addition to this patient's dementia, he has objective evidence that he aspirates when taking oral food. Patients such as this are one of the most common groups of patients given gastric or jejunal feeding tubes. Because this patient's primary problem is upper esophageal dysmotility and/or poor airway reflexes, a feeding tube placed in the stomach will only be of benefit if the patient does not regurgitate. If food travels retrograde through the lower esophageal sphincter and makes it to the mouth, the patient will be at

the same risk of aspiration. However regurgitation is less frequent when food is given via a gastric tube, therefore this patient's short-term prognosis is improved.

Although some patients get gastric tubes to augment nutritional intake, most, like this patient, do because of the inability to take oral food. Therefore it will not harm the patient to take oral as well as tube-based foods (**choice A**).

Based on the above discussion, feeding via the gastric tube does not eliminate the risk of aspiration (**choice B**). Once particulate matter makes it into the oropharynx, aspiration will likely occur.

Also, as discussed above, since food is not being given orally, the only way in which a patient can aspirate with a gastric tube is to have regurgitation. Therefore, this mode of feeding does reduce the risk of aspiration, making the statement that it will have no effect on the risk of aspiration incorrect (**choice C**).

Because nutrition is such a fundamental component of long-term prognosis, this patient will only worsen with time since gastric feedings are no substitute for intake of a variety of foodstuffs. Therefore, long-term mortality continues to be unaltered with tube feedings (**choice D**).

29. **The correct answer is D.** This patient's respiratory distress is most likely due to regurgitation and aspiration of gastric-tube infused tube feedings. As discussed previously, a gastric tube does not eliminate the risk of aspiration. Because this patient's primary problem is upper esophageal dysmotility and/or poor airway reflexes, a feeding tube placed in the stomach will only be of benefit if the patient does not regurgitate. If food travels retrograde through the lower esophageal sphincter and makes it to the mouth, the patient will be at the same risk of aspiration.

Although this patient is demented, inadvertent oral consumption and aspiration of tube feedings (**choice A**) is unlikely given that the tube feedings are not dispensed in a manner that patients can consume orally.

There is no evidence that this patient had previous upper airway difficulty. Therefore, oropharyngeal obstruction and hypoventilation (**choice B**) are unlikely.

Even if the patient had obstructed, it would not explain his ongoing hypoxia and respiratory distress. Although frequently invoked to explain altered mental status in elderly demented patients, there is no evidence that this patient was a victim of oversedation (**choice C**).

The time elapsed since the operation (34+ hours) makes residual hypnosis or sedation from general anesthesia (**choice E**) very unlikely. Again, even if this was a cause of initial apnea or hypoventilation, it does not explain the patient's continued hypoxia on 100% oxygen.

30. **The correct answer is E.** This otherwise healthy patient sustained a posterior-lateral dislocation of his knee. Knee dislocations require a significant amount of energy to occur. Keep in mind that the position of the knee on x-ray is usually much different than at the time of injury. This simply means that the degree of dislocation or displacement of the leg was initially much greater. Then, as the deforming forces declined, the tissues returned to a more anatomic position, albeit in this case one of dislocation. This is true too of fractures, especially pelvic fractures. The neurovascular structures at risk of injury in this patient include the popliteal artery and the tibial and peroneal nerves. This patient has an intact clinical neurovascular examination. However, the common type of arterial injury in this scenario is an intimal tear. The clinical vascular examination, including pulse checks and ankle brachial index (ABI), are often normal. Complications from intimal tears develop hours to days later. Essentially, this patient has an arterial injury until proven otherwise by angiography.

Splinting in 45 degrees of flexion (**choice A**) only risks redislocation of this globally unstable knee.

Observation (**choice B**) would be a good idea, but only after an angiogram rules out a vascular injury. Once the neurovascular status is determined to be intact, planning for knee ligament reconstruction can begin.

Splinting the leg (**choice C**) is essential and would be done before transport to the angiography suite; however, discharging to home risks missing a vascular injury.

MRI (**choice D**) would be helpful in the preoperative planning for the orthopedic surgery service. However, a possible vascular injury takes priority over ligamentous disruptions, making an angiogram the most appropriate next step.

31. **The correct answer is B.** The patient has a right to refuse treatment. The right to refuse treatment stems from the common law, tenets of democracy, and the constitution of the United States. This constitutes the fourth doctrine of ethics, namely, justice.

1. Under the doctrine of common law, any adult person who is of sound mind has the right to decide what can be done with his own body, and a physician who administers treatment without the express consent

of the individual is liable for damages, as he has violated the patient's rights by committing battery.

2. Under the democratic system of the United States, the fundamental right to decide one's personal choices rests with the individual. The right to refuse treatment has been implemented by the courts.

3. Under the constitution of the United States, the right to make choices is implied as a component of the Bill of Rights. For example, under the Bill of Rights, a citizen of the United States has an unalienable right to freedom of speech, religion, and assembly. The courts have deduced that the refusal of treatment is an extension of this right.

Although the patient was inebriated at the time (**choice A**), it is extremely difficult to prove in a court of law that the patient was at the time mentally incapable of making an appropriate decision. Thus, a person who is an adult and is mentally capable of making a decision has the right to refuse treatment, provided he understands the consequences of such refusal. The courts will take into consideration a competent patient's right to refuse treatment and override it only when the interest of the state is paramount.

Therefore, you will not be disciplined by the American Medical Association (**choice C**) or the state medical board (**choice D**) if you fail to treat him.

Repairing the laceration under the umbrella of beneficence (**choice E**)—in this case, implied consent—would not be tenable. This is because although the patient was brought to the emergency room, the nature of the injury was not life threatening; therefore, charges of battery could be successfully brought to bear against the physician.

32. **The correct answer is C.** The clinical history and physical examination are consistent with traumatic rupture of the urethra. In men, blood at the urethral meatus indicates urethral injury; catheterization per urethra (**choice E**) should *never* be attempted if blood is present at the urethral meatus. Attempting to pass a catheter in a patient with urethral injury may result in infection of a periprostatic and perivesical hematoma or possibly convert an incomplete laceration into a complete one. Retrograde urethrogram is the diagnostic modality of choice to evaluate a patient suspected of having urethral injury. This procedure is performed by placing a small Foley catheter into the meatus and inflating the balloon with approximately 2 cc of water in the fossa navicularis. Contrast is then injected slowly through the catheter to outline the entire length of the urethra.

Urethral injuries are uncommon and occur most often in men. They are rare in women. Various parts of the urethra may be lacerated, transected, or contused. Injuries are divided into two categories based on anatomic divisions. There are anterior urethral injuries, which involve the pendulous and bulbar urethra, and there are posterior urethral injuries involving the prostatic and membranous portions of the urethra. This patient has injured his anterior urethra, causing blood extravasation deep to Colles fascia. Colles fascia in the perineum is continuous with dartos fascia in the penis/scrotum and Scarpa fascia over the anterior abdominal wall. Colles fascia is not continuous with the fascia lata of the thigh. Therefore, blood from an anterior urethral injury may track into the perineum but not laterally; this creates the typical "butterfly" pattern. This blood can also extend up the scrotum and anterior abdominal wall, all the way up to the clavicles, where Scarpa fascia inserts. Posterior urethral injuries are usually associated with pelvic fractures. The urethra is sheared off just proximal to the urogenital diaphragm. This causes the prostate to be displaced superiorly by the developing hematoma in the periprostatic and perivesical spaces.

Evaluating the patient's hemoglobin and hematocrit (**choice A**) is important in those patients with hemodynamic instability or multiple injuries. This patient is stable and these values will not contribute to his immediate care. Even if his BUN/creatinine are elevated this should easily correct itself once his retention has been resolved. If this patient is in distress secondary to urinary retention, it would be appropriate to place a suprapubic cystostomy tube prior to obtaining any studies.

Scrotal ultrasound and CT scan (**choices B and F**) will not allow you to evaluate the urethra appropriately. While the scrotum may show ecchymosis, it is important to realize that blood at the meatus indicates that the problem is within the urethra, and the appropriate studies should be ordered.

Cystogram (**choice D**) allows for complete visualization of the bladder to check for extravasation. This test may ultimately be necessary in a patient with some types of urethral injury. However, it is not the most appropriate initial study in the evaluation of patients with blood at the meatus.

33. **The correct answer is D.** This patient is suffering from acute urinary retention with associated acute renal failure, most likely secondary to an enlarged, obstructing prostate. The mass appreciated on physical examination is the patient's bladder, which has

increased in size secondary to urinary retention. This distended bladder has made the patient uncomfortable. The most important and emergent intervention is to relieve his obstruction to prevent any further renal damage. The easiest method to achieve this goal is to place a Foley catheter in the emergency room.

It is not uncommon for the serum PSA to be elevated during an acute episode of urinary retention. This number is falsely elevated (**choice A**) and needs to be reevaluated once the acute episode is resolved. Investigations for prostate cancer will only delay appropriate intervention.

The patient's complaints of hesitancy, urgency, and weak stream are common in patients with BPH. This patient was being treated with pharmacologic agents with some success until this episode. Increasing his medication (**choice B**) will not provide him with the immediate relief he requires to prevent further renal failure and possible uremia.

While sedatives (**choice C**) may make the patient more comfortable, they can be completely avoided with placement of a catheter. Relieving this patient's obstructed bladder will relax him without any medication at all. Sedation will only mask the urgency of the situation.

Radiographic studies will only delay this patient from receiving the treatment he really needs. Images of the kidneys (**choice E**) will be important to evaluate for hydronephrosis, decreased renal parenchyma, etc. But to delay bladder drainage for this test is inappropriate.

TURP (**choice F**) is not the method of choice for relieving obstruction in the acute setting. Once the patient has received adequate bladder drainage and his renal function has normalized (hopefully) then he can be evaluated for possible surgical intervention. All initial intervention should be directed toward immediate bladder drainage.

Urinary tract infections (**choice G**) may precipitate episodes of acute urinary retention, and it will be important to obtain urine for analysis and culture. This can be done once the catheter is placed under sterile conditions. The patient has already proven that he will not be able to provide a urine sample on his own. Continuing to wait would simply make the patient even more uncomfortable and worsen his renal failure.

34. **The correct answer is B.** The clinical picture is most consistent with an acute parotitis, or inflammation of the parotid gland. Acute parotitis is characterized by a painful swelling of the affected gland with associated fever. In some cases, a purulent discharge can be expressed by the parotid (Stensen) duct. This condition is often seen in the setting of dehydration. An acute parotitis may result either from obstruction of the ductile system by a mucous plug or stone, or from stasis of salivary flow. This is then complicated by bacterial infection, most commonly due to *Staphylococcus aureus*. Other medical conditions predisposing to acute parotitis include hepatic or renal failure, diabetes mellitus, hypothyroidism, malnutrition, HIV, and AIDS. Medications such as anticholinergics can also be predisposing factors. Treatment generally involves hydration and antibiotics. Warm compresses and sialogogues (such as sour candies) are also used to improve salivary flow. Cases that progress to abscess formation, or coalesce, may require incision and drainage in addition to intravenous antibiotics. Chronic or recurrent disease may require a parotidectomy with careful sparing of the facial nerve, although this can prove difficult in the setting of previous inflammation and infection. Other causes of parotid gland enlargement include viral parotitis, autoimmune diseases (e.g., Sjögren syndrome), granulomatous diseases (e.g., tuberculosis, sarcoidosis), bulimia, and chronic fatty infiltration secondary to alcoholism.

The most common benign salivary gland neoplasms (**choice A**) affecting the parotid are pleomorphic adenoma and Warthin tumor (or papillary cystadenoma lymphomatosum). These are more commonly associated with a palpable nontender nodule or mass of the parotid gland.

While HIV (**choice C**) has not been excluded in this patient, the more classic parotid gland finding in patients with HIV infection is a benign lymphoepithelial cyst. This would present as a unilateral or bilateral, somewhat fluctuant, parotid enlargement. Lymphoepithelial cysts are generally nontender, unless complicated by superinfection. CT scan findings confirming a cystic structure can be diagnostic. Fine needle aspiration (FNA) can also be used to help exclude malignancy.

Mumps (**choice D**), a once-common childhood disease, leads to a viral parotitis with associated bilateral painful parotid swelling, trismus, and malaise. Mumps is caused by a paramyxovirus and is usually self-limited with conservative treatment.

Squamous cell carcinoma of the parotid gland (**choice E**) is rare and often due to metastatic spread from a primary scalp or facial skin cancer. It would likely present as a nontender parotid mass or enlargement. The most common primary malignancy of the parotid gland is mucoepidermoid carcinoma.

35. **The correct answer is A.** Malocclusion after facial trauma is one of the most common symptoms of a facial fracture, usually a mandible fracture. While splinting of muscles involved in mastication, such as the masseter muscle, can produce malocclusion, a thorough evaluation including mandible x-rays must be performed. Because many muscles attach to the mandible and pull this bone in multiple directions, mandible fractures commonly result in displacement of the bony fragments. Mandible fractures of all kinds are best treated early after the fracture before the bones have been allowed to heal in their new anatomic position.

Providing the name and phone number of dentists for the patient to make an appointment and followup on her dental concerns (**choice B**) is incorrect because although the mandible does contain teeth, this is not primarily a dental concern. Mandible fractures should be treated by an oral surgeon, otolaryngologist, or plastic surgeon familiar with facial trauma.

Reassuring her that her dental malocclusion is common after crashes and that it should resolve spontaneously within a month (**choice C**) is not correct because these injuries must be recognized and treated early to produce the best long-term outcome.

Reexamining her oral cavity to make sure there are no fractures of her mandible (**choice D**) is not correct because mandible fractures can occur in segments of the mandible that do not have teeth and can be present without obvious signs of fracture visible on the oral cavity exam.

36. **The correct answer is C.** This patient has muscle invasive adenocarcinoma of the colon. Adenocarcinoma of the colon that penetrates the muscularis mucosa is considered invasive, and colectomy is the treatment of choice. Tumors of the cecum and ascending colon are resected with right hemicolectomy. The ileocolic, right colic, and right branches of the middle colic artery are ligated. The remaining bowel is then anastomosed. If no complications are encountered during the procedure, then a colostomy is not required (**choice F**). It is not necessary to remove the entire colon for his cancer in the ascending colon (**choice B**).

Almost all cancers of the large intestine are adenocarcinomas. Some of the more rare histological types are squamous cell, adenosquamous, lymphomas, sarcomas, and carcinoid tumors (**choice A**).

As previously stated, colonic polyps that contain malignancy and penetrate the muscularis mucosa require colectomy (**choice D**). The likelihood is high that not all of this patient's cancer was removed with his biopsy because it is muscle invasive.

The natural progression of adenocarcinoma of the colon is spread via local invasion, lymphatics, and hematogenously. Local progression is usually transverse, causing circumferential involvement. Lymphatic spread correlates with the extent of local invasion. Hematogenous spread is most commonly to the liver, then lung. It is unusual for other sites to become involved without liver and lung metastases (**choice E**).

37. **The correct answer is E.** This patient has a collapsed left lung, most likely a hemopneumothorax (when the chest fills with air and blood). His history of being struck on the left side, and the multiple abrasions and bruises on the left side, in association with absent breath sounds, all point in this direction. The treatment for this hemopneumothorax is placement of a left-sided chest tube to allow drainage of the blood, reinflation of the left lung, and stabilization of his pulmonary status.

Asking the patient if he uses tobacco (**choice A**) has no direct benefit to his management at this point. His shortness of breath is related to an acute injury and not a chronic condition.

Increasing the oxygen (**choice B**) delivered to the patient will only help minimally with his oxygen saturation. It will not be what he definitively needs to treat his hemopneumothorax.

An arterial blood gas (**choice C**) will only confirm what you already know clinically, which is that the patient is not saturating as well as he should be. This patient is quickly becoming unstable, and delaying treatment of his collapsed lung will only place him in further danger.

CT scan of the chest (**choice D**) may ultimately be necessary to evaluate the complete extent of the patient's injuries. However, to delay definitive treatment of his underlying source of respiratory distress during his acute decompensation would be a critically wrong maneuver.

While a chest x-ray (**choice F**) is necessary at some point in this patient's evaluation, the type of x-ray chosen is important. To obtain a PA and lateral chest x-ray requires that the patient stand up. Having this patient stand before all of his injuries are completely evaluated and his spine is cleared, is wrong. In some trauma patients with a small pneumothorax, a chest x-ray may be necessary for diagnosis. These films are usually done with AP technique with the patient on a back board. That technique is necessary because most trauma patients must have their pulmonary status addressed prior to having the rest of their injuries completely evaluated. In this case, however, a chest tube should be placed, as it is clinically evident that he has a collapsed left lung.

38. **The correct answer is A.** This patient is suffering from varicose veins. These are dilated tortuous superficial veins that result from the defective structure and function of the valves of the saphenous veins. It is due to an intrinsic weakness of the vein wall and high intraluminal pressure. Primary varicose veins originate in the superficial system and are more frequent in women. Secondary varicose veins result from deep venous insufficiency and incompetent perforating veins or from deep venous occlusion causing enlargement of superficial veins that are serving as collaterals (**choice C**). Symptoms consist of dull ache or pressure sensation in the legs after prolonged standing. Compression stockings and leg elevation provides relief, not walking (**choice E**). Examination should be performed with the patient standing. If the varicosities become extensive then skin ulcerations may occur. Rarely, they may rupture and bleed (**choice D**). Conservative measures provide initial treatment. Symptoms often decrease when legs are elevated periodically, prolonged standing is avoided, and elastic support hose are worn. External compression stockings provide a counterbalance to the hydrostatic pressure within the veins and may be helpful (**choice A**). If symptoms progress, then small veins may be injected with a sclerosing agent a process called sclerotherapy (**choice B**). Other surgical options include ligation and stripping of the greater and lesser saphenous veins.

39. **The correct answer is C.** This patient is suffering from Budd-Chiari syndrome. This syndrome is defined as occlusion of the hepatic veins and/or suprahepatic inferior vena cava. This produces postsinusoidal portal hypertension that develops secondary to obstruction of hepatic venous drainage. It is characterized by the onset of ascites, abdominal pain, and tender hepatomegaly. If untreated, most patients die of progressive liver failure or complications of portal hypertension. The most commonly affected age group is women in their 30s. Liver function is relatively normal initially with normal transaminase and bilirubin levels. Elevated protein in the ascitic fluid suggests the syndrome.

Acute cholecystitis (**choice A**) is usually associated with persistent and unremitting right upper quadrant pain. There is frequently elevated temperature, anorexia, nausea, and vomiting. Most patients prefer to lay completely still secondary to peritoneal irritation. There may be an associated leukocytosis.

Alcoholic liver cirrhosis (**choice B**) patients have a history of chronic alcohol consumption. In the acute phase, there is failing health with muscle wasting, jaundice, and ascites. Laboratory data shows elevated bilirubin, alkaline phosphatase, anemia, and prolonged prothrombin time. In the chronic phase, patients complain of fatigue, anorexia, and weight loss.

Cancer of the gallbladder (**choice D**) occurs more commonly in women than men and usually in those over the age of 65. Signs and symptoms may mimic gallstones, i.e., right-upper-quadrant pain, discomfort, and dyspepsia. Frequently, these patients present late in the course of their disease with malaise, weight loss, anorexia, or obstructive jaundice.

Hepatitis C (**choice E**) is a virus that attacks the liver. The most common source in the U.S. is the transfusion of blood or blood products and the illicit use of intravenous drugs. Initial rise in serum alanine aminotransferase (ALT) may be associated with little or no clinical disturbance. Many patients progress to chronic hepatitis C and may show no ill effects other than mildly fluctuating elevations in liver enzymes. Those patients who progress to incapacitating liver failure may be treated with liver transplantation.

40. **The correct answer is E.** The most likely diagnosis is mesenteric ischemia. He presents a classic story of chronic mesenteric ischemia. His "fear of food" is because of intestinal angina. Oral intake increases blood flow to the intestine; however, in the setting of visceral arterial stenosis an appropriate amount of blood cannot be delivered to the organ, leading to "intestinal angina," especially after meals. As patients discover that they have pain after meals, they tend to avoid food and subsequently lose weight. The diagnosis is made by visceral angiography. Mesenteric ischemia may be acute or chronic, and occlusive or nonocclusive. Angiography allows for evaluation of the celiac, superior mesenteric, and inferior mesenteric arteries. Treatment is individualized to the patient and depends on the severity of symptoms, patient's co-morbidities, and the risk/benefit ratio of angiography or surgery.

Celiac sprue (**choice A**) is characterized by an intolerance to gluten. Severity of disease varies and some patients are completely asymptomatic. The majority of the patients are women and there is a familial tendency. Complaints include weight loss, abdominal distention, and bloating with diarrhea. Eighty percent of patients improve with the institution of a gluten-free diet.

Crohn disease (**choice B**) is an incurable chronic inflammatory disorder of the alimentary tract. The terminal ileum and proximal colon are the areas affected most often. The disease usually arises between 15 to 35 years of age. Patients complain of abdominal pain, diarrhea, and weight loss. Signs and symptoms may mimic acute appendicitis.

Gastroenteritis (**choice C**) is a viral infection associated with vomiting and diarrhea.

Irritable bowel syndrome (**choice D**) is characterized by chronic, intermittent symptoms, including recurrent abdominal pain, usually in the left lower quadrant, altered defecation, stool urgency, and a sense of incomplete evacuation. It is a disease of young or middle-aged adults with a female-to-male ratio of 4:1.

41. **The correct answer is E.** When one is confronted with a lesion that appears to be transitional cell carcinoma of the bladder, initial treatment is resection of the mass (transurethral resection of bladder tumor, TURBT). This procedure will allow for staging and possibly cure. Transitional cell carcinoma (TCC) is responsible for approximately 90% of all bladder cancer. Adenocarcinoma and squamous cell carcinoma compromise the other 10%. After the tumor has been resected, it should be evaluated microscopically for depth of invasion and grade. In general, those tumors that do not invade past the lamina propria and into the bladder muscle may not require further treatment. If the TCC invades into the muscle, then radical cystectomy with urinary diversion is necessary to cure the patient. Patients who have their bladder tumors resected require continued surveillance, as there is a high rate of recurrence (potentially >50%).

Chemotherapy (**choice A**) and radiation therapy (**choice F**) are not first-line treatments for early stage bladder cancer. These treatment modalities are utilized in patients with locally advanced and metastatic disease.

Biopsy of the lesion (**choice B**) will provide you with a diagnosis but leaves the patient without definitive therapy. Performing only a biopsy will require that the patient return to the operating room for resection.

BCG (**choice C**) and thiotepa (**choice D**) are agents that can be distilled directly into the bladder. In general, these agents are used for patients with either carcinoma in situ of the bladder (CIS) or in patients with multiple areas of TCC when all of the tumor cannot be resected or the patient refuses cystectomy for muscle invasive cancer.

42. **The correct answer is B.** This patient is suffering from a thrombosed external hemorrhoid. Hemorrhoids are classified as either internal or external based on their location. They occur when the veins of either the internal or external hemorrhoid plexus become enlarged and the supporting muscles deteriorate. Both types are very common and are associated with increased hydrostatic pressure in the portal venous system, such as during pregnancy, straining at stool, or cirrhosis. The most common manifestation of hemorrhoids is painless, bright red rectal bleeding that occurs with bowel movement. Some patients complain of a feeling of incomplete evacuation. Definitive diagnosis is made by physical examination. If possible, the patient is asked to strain as if defecating and the anus is examined for prolapsing veins. Anoscopy and proctoscopy may be performed to rule out coexisting pathology. This patient is suffering from one of the complications of hemorrhoids, which is thrombosis. The hemorrhoid has prolapsed and the normal blood within the vein has become acutely thrombosed. This leads to severe pain. The treatment for an acutely thrombosed hemorrhoid is incision and extraction of the clot followed by compression of the incised area.

Aspiration of the thrombus will most likely be difficult (**choice A**). The clotted blood will not move through a fine needle.

Any procedure that requires manipulation of the anus will be impossible in this patient. He cannot tolerate a digital examination, let alone a barium enema or colonoscopy (**choices C and D**). Neither of these tests will help in the diagnosis or treatment of this patient's acute condition.

Conservative measures such as sitz baths (**choice E**) are appropriate in patients with symptomatic hemorrhoids that are not thrombosed. This can be combined with other modalities such as moist heat, suppositories, stool softeners, and bedrest.

43. **The correct answer is C.** This patient has a sigmoid volvulus. This occurs when the sigmoid colon twists more than 180 degrees about its mesentery. The sigmoid colon is the most common site for this to occur. Volvulus is a form of closed-loop obstruction. As with all forms of colonic obstruction, volvulus is associated with pain, vomiting, and tenderness. The most obvious sign in large bowel obstruction is marked abdominal distention. The common radiographic feature in sigmoid volvulus is a "bent inner tube" appearance of the sigmoid. The treatment of sigmoid volvulus is with endoscopic decompression. This is performed by advancing a flexible sigmoidoscope into the rectum until a rush of air and feces indicates that the torsion has been relieved. After, a rectal tube can be placed into

the loop as a stent to prevent retorsion. After detorsion, the patient should undergo sigmoid resection if he is a surgical candidate, otherwise the volvulus is likely to recur. However, exploration with bowel resection is not the initial treatment modality. It is in the patient's best interest if endoscopic decompression can be performed and then he can be resuscitated and stabilized prior to open surgery (**choice E**).

The patient definitely needs admission to the hospital. However, he requires detorsion of the sigmoid volvulus as this will not occur spontaneously. Therefore, serial abdominal examinations (**choice A**) would be inappropriate for this patient.

An upper GI series with small bowel followthrough (**choice B**) is not indicated in this case. It is typically used for patients where there is suspicion or concern for Crohn disease and sometimes to evaluate a possible gastric or small bowel obstruction.

In patients with a competent ileocecal valve, the abdominal distention with gas is mainly confined to the large bowel. For this reason, a nasogastric tube will provide little relief in this patient. The patient has no dilated small bowel loops or distended stomach. Therefore, an NGT with repeat x-rays will not help in the diagnosis or treatment of this patient (**choice D**).

44. **The correct answer is B.** The patient is presenting with a lower gastrointestinal (GI) bleed, the differential for which is broad. Upper GI bleeds will usually present with melena; however, if they are extraordinarily brisk, red blood can be expelled per rectum. The lower the bleed, the more likely it is to present with red blood per rectum. A CT scan was performed to help narrow the differential diagnosis, and it shows hyperemic and thickened small bowel. This finding is very concerning for inflammation or ischemia, and in the setting of GI bleeding, crampy, abdominal pain, elevated lactate, and particularly untreated atrial fibrillation, ischemia becomes the leading culprit. In this setting, the ischemia is usually from an acute embolus to a mesenteric artery. Treatment is very tricky because the patient has both thrombosis and hemorrhage. Thus, treating simply with systemic anticoagulation is often dangerous. Visualization of the clot via arteriogram can allow the interventional radiologist to deliver direct thrombolysis.

Simply admitting to the medical service for rehydration (**choice A**) in the setting of ischemic bowel has a greater than 90% mortality.

Colonoscopy (**choice C**) and endoscopic gastroduodenoscopy (**choice D**) are important tests in the setting of acute GI bleeding; however, they do not address problems in the mid-small bowel where the problem is in this case.

A small bowel followthrough study (**choice E**) may show the thickening of bowel wall of the ischemic region; however, that would be redundant information at that point, and furthermore, time to treatment is of the essence.

45. **The correct answer is B.** The most immediate concern after the metacarpal fracture is an avulsion fracture of the extensor digiti minimi at the middle or distal phalanges of the little finger. This is evidenced by the inability to extend the little finger. This injury is also a common sporting injury and usually missed on physical examination. It does not always show up on x-ray and therefore cannot entirely be dismissed if the x-ray does not demonstrate an avulsion fracture.

A compartment syndrome (**choice A**) presents as pain with physical examination. It typically presents in the larger upper and lower limb areas surrounded by fascial sheaths. It can sometimes present after trauma, although it is less likely here in view of the localized tenderness and the ability to move the fingers.

A radial head fracture (**choice C**) would likely be seen on x-ray and manifest as pain on supination and pronation at the radial head with associated joint swelling.

A scaphoid fracture (**choice D**) is unlikely in view of the lack of scaphoid tenderness. It can present 2 weeks later. It is always important to have a high index of suspicion for it due to the risk of avascular necrosis. It can be alleviated with splints or operative repair with a Herbert screw.

Movement of digits and lack of paresthesia make nerve ligation (**choice E**) unlikely.

46. **The correct answer is B.** The recommendation that would have the greatest benefit in the perioperative stage of this patient's hip replacement would be to discontinue the aspirin. This would reduce the diathesis to bleeding. This allows less bleeding in the operative field, which is beneficial to the surgeon and results in reduced blood loss for the patient.

Strict diabetic control can be achieved before the operation with an insulin sliding scale, along with the metformin. Therefore, it is not necessary for metformin (**choice A**) to be discontinued at this stage.

The patient's blood pressure is appropriate at this time and there would be no need to increase the antihypertensive medication (**choices C and D**). This is particularly true if it took months to control his hypertension in the first place.

Weight reduction (**choice E**) would be ideal for any surgical candidate. In this case it is highly unrealistic to see a beneficial reduction in weight only 2 weeks before the operation.

47. **The correct answer is E.** The current objective is to maintain the patient's blood pressure at a normotensive status and to prevent him from becoming hypoglycemic before the operation.

Strictly speaking, a patient is supposed to be kept nil by mouth before the operation in the event of him requiring general anesthesia. Therefore, allowing a midnight snack (**choice A**) is incorrect.

However, the patient is supposed to take his medications and especially his antihypertensive medications. (If necessary, small sips of water are permissible in order to allow him to swallow the medications.) This eliminates the option of discontinuing all of his remaining his medications as part of the *nil per os* status (**choice B**) and discontinuing all of his medications as part of his *nil per os* status except the metformin (**choice C**).

In addition, the patient should not take the metformin since it is a hypoglycemic and may drop his serum glucose significantly on the morning of the operation.

48. **The correct answer is B.** The patient described is likely demonstrating rude and inflexible behavior in response to his recent debilitation and disfigurement from surgery. Empathically discussing the effects of these significant changes on his life may help the patient to develop insight and acceptance to his illness.

The patient is evidencing behaviors consistent with a defense of displacement, the diversion of emotional content from one situation to another designed to avoid emotional pain. A change of hospital team or location (**choice A**) does not address that which is truly distressful to this patient.

Directly telling the patient how fortunate he is to have had a surgery that has greatly disfigured and depressed him is likely only to upset the patient, make him even more defensive, and contribute to his perception that the hospital staff does not care about his needs (**choice C**).

Attributing the patient's demanding behavior to steroid therapy (**choice D**) would serve as a validation and rationalization of the patient's rudeness. Additionally, it would divert the patient from his actual problem, the insecurity he feels following major surgery and having a colostomy placement.

The patient does not manifest symptoms of a body dysmorphic disorder. His disfigurement is real, not imagined. Additionally, haloperidol (**choice E**) is not an accepted treatment for body dysmorphic disorder.

49. **The correct answer is B.** A Gleason grade 7 carcinoma represents an intermediate grade tumor. Intermediate cancers may behave like low-grade or high-grade cancers and thus have unpredictable growth. The cells' behavior may depend on the volume of the cancer and the prostate specific antigen (PSA) level. This is the most common grade of prostate cancer and there is a risk of metastasis. A bone scan is necessary to evaluate for bony metastasis from prostate cancer. Pending this result, if the patient desires treatment, surgery or hormonal therapy can be considered.

An antitestosterone agent (**choice A**) may be necessary to treat this patient's recently diagnosed prostate cancer, but it is not the most appropriate next step. Prior to starting any type of chemotherapy, complete staging of the tumor should be performed. Staging in prostate cancer involves obtaining a bone scan to evaluate for metastatic disease since prostate cancer frequently metastasizes to bone.

Prior to initiating any type of therapy for prostate cancer, whether it is surgery (**choices C and D**) or chemotherapy, complete staging of the tumor should be performed. A bone scan is necessary to evaluate for metastases since prostate cancer frequently metastasizes to bone. Pending this result, if the patient desires treatment, surgery or hormonal therapy should be considered.

50. **The correct answer is C.** Complications of cholecystectomy, whether performed laparoscopically or by open surgery, include retained gallstones, biliary leak, and biloma. This patient's symptoms of intermittent right upper quadrant pain in the absence of fever is suspicious for a retained gallstone, causing biliary obstruction. For further evaluation, it is important to obtain an ultrasound of the abdomen, which will provide information regarding intrahepatic biliary duct dilatation, and fluid in the gallbladder fossa, and may sometimes demonstrate a common bile duct stone. If the ultrasound confirms the presence of a common bile duct stone, the patient will need an endoscopic retrograde cholangiopancreatography (ERCP) for stone removal.

Liver function tests (**choice A**) are not the most important part of evaluating this patient. These laboratory values are useful for determining liver synthetic function as well as to evaluate for hepatitis. This patient most likely has a retained gallstone and needs an ultrasound of the abdomen to look for both a stone as well as secondary signs, such as biliary duct dilatation.

A CT scan of the abdomen and pelvis (**choice B**) is a good alternative to an ultrasound for evaluation of the hepatobiliary system. It is not the diagnostic imaging study of choice to evaluate for gallstones or biliary dilatation. A CT is useful if biliary leak or biloma is suspected.

Reassuring the patient that some abdominal pain following surgery is to be expected (**choice D**) is appropriate immediately following the procedure. However, at this time her symptoms of pain, are 3 weeks after surgery and are likely secondary to a retained gallstone.

Referring the patient back to surgery for possible bile leak (**choice E**) is premature at this time. A bile leak, as well as a biloma, are potential complications of cholecystectomy, whether it is performed laparoscopically or as an open procedure. Patients will a bile leak develop a bile peritonitis and usually present with diffuse abdominal pain, distention, and fever. This patient most likely has a retained gallstone and needs an ultrasound of the abdomen to evaluate for both a stone as well as secondary signs, such as biliary duct dilatation. If the ultrasound demonstrates a lot of fluid in the gallbladder fossa, a bile leak is still possible. At that time, referral to surgery is appropriate.

Surgery: Test Two

1. A 54-year-old man comes to the office because of a neck mass that he first noticed 2 weeks ago while shaving. He denies any pain in his neck, dysphagia, odynophagia, or fever. He has no significant medical problems and does not take any medications. On physical examination, you palpate an approximately 2-cm round firm nodule in the right lobe of the thyroid. He does not have significant cervical lymphadenopathy. The physical examination or imaging finding that is most suggestive of malignancy is

   (A) a CT scan of the neck showing multiple 1 cm cervical lymph nodes

   (B) a nodule that is fixed in place and no movement on swallowing

   (C) radioactive iodine scan that shows a "hot" lesion in the region of the nodule

   (D) ultrasonography of the thyroid that shows multiple solid nodules in both lobes of the thyroid

   (E) ultrasonography of the thyroid that shows that the palpable nodule is a cyst

2. You are working in the emergency department evaluating a 19-year-old woman with complaints of "back pain near her tailbone." Upon questioning, the patient reports pain on the right side of her "low back" for the past 3 days. She has taken acetaminophen and ibuprofen with only minimal relief of the pain. Today she noticed that there was swelling and she thought that she should come in to be evaluated. She feels otherwise well and denies trauma, fever, or change in her bowel or bladder function. She does report that occasionally she will have painful bowel movements and has had more pain with this illness, but was unsure if they were related. She also says that she thinks that one of her uncles had the same problem in the past but is unsure. Her temperature is 37.0 C (98.6 F), blood pressure is 115/65 mm Hg, pulse is 80/min, and respirations are 16/min. Examination reveals a tender, erythematous, fluctuant mass on the patient's right buttock. It measures 3 cm in size and is 2 cm from her rectum. Rectal examination is normal except for mild tenderness on the right. There is no mass, no fluctuance, and no pus seen during rectal examination. At this time you inform the patient that

   (A) she will need to have the area drained immediately

   (B) you suspect that she may have Crohn disease and will need an immediate colonoscopy

   (C) you suspect that she has Crohn disease and this area is likely rectal cancer that needs to be surgically removed

   (D) you suspect that she may have Crohn disease and will prescribe steroids to help control the inflammatory response

   (E) you will prescribe stronger pain medication and eventually this will resolve without further treatment

3. A 65-year-old man is admitted to the hospital because of moderate abdominal discomfort and guaiac-positive stool. He has had poor appetite and a 15-lb weight loss over the past 6 months and a pruritic skin rash. He has not seen a doctor for the longest time because in the past they just annoyed him immensely with their recommendations to stop drinking, start eating healthy and exercising. In his line of work, which is an Italian delicatessen food store, you had to taste all the goodies to know what you are selling to customers. After work, he always goes out with his buddies from the "old country" for a nightcap, and there is just no time for exercise. But now he has finally become concerned for his health because he believes that there is "really something wrong." Apart from the terribly itchy "barnacles" on his back that appeared suddenly about 6 months ago and had been keeping him up at night, he can no longer enjoy his tasty treats; they make him nauseous after just a few bites. On physical examination you notice hundreds of greasy looking dark brown to black plaques on the patient's back and many more on other parts of the body with excoriations on the skin surrounding them. They range in size from 0.2 mm to 1.1 cm. This patient is at greatest risk of having

(A) gastric adenocarcinoma
(B) hepatoma
(C) leukemia
(D) melanoma
(E) osteogenic sarcoma

4. A 50-year-old man is involved in a motor vehicle accident. He has been thrown out of the car and is lying on the road. You are amazed to note that he has no apparent major injuries. He is breathing adequately, has no evidence of hemorrhage, and is conscious. During your examination, however, you inadvertently move his neck, which results in quadriparesis. You would most likely

(A) be disciplined by the American Medical Association
(B) be disciplined by the state medical board
(C) be protected by the Good Samaritan statute, because you were under no obligation to render assistance
(D) be sued because you were negligent
(E) not be sued, as you had the best interests of the patient in mind

5. A 60-year-old man of Irish descent is admitted to the hospital for an acute exacerbation of chronic obstructive pulmonary disease. You have been taking care of him for the past few years and have managed to convince him to abandon a 40-year-long cigarette smoking habit only last summer after a prolonged hospital stay for his pulmonary disease. He has also been treated with liquid nitrogen application for multiple actinic keratoses on his face and arms, a souvenir of many years spent in the sun during his naval career. During morning rounds you note a small, ulcerated nodule on his lower lip covered with an adherent hemorrhagic crust. The patient says it has appeared only recently and he thought he had cut himself shaving. On palpation of this 3-mm lesion the base is firm and fixed to the underlying soft tissue. There are no palpable lymph nodes in the area of lymphatic drainage of the lower lip. The surrounding vermilion border shows signs of chronic actinic damage. A biopsy of the lesion will most likely show

(A) hyperkeratosis, wedge shaped hypergranulosis, acanthosis with "saw toothing" of the dermoepidermal junction, and a dense lichenoid infiltrate in the papillary dermis
(B) irregular nests of pleomorphic epidermal cells with horn pearl formation invading the dermis to varying degrees
(C) many aggregations of sebaceous lobules directly communicating with the overlying epidermis
(D) nests of darkly staining polyhedral cells in the dermis with columnar cells characteristically arranged in a palisade at the periphery
(E) pagetoid spread of atypical melanocytes in the epidermis

6. A 24-year-old man is admitted to the hospital with a comminuted left femur fracture after a motorcycle accident. He had some abdominal pain on presentation; however, a CT scan was totally unremarkable. You are called to see the patient the night of admission due to complaints of sudden onset of tachypnea. On physical examination, he has alteration in his level of consciousness. His temperature is 37.0 C (98.6 F), blood pressure is 100/68 mm Hg, pulse is 110/min, and respirations are 28/min. Pulse oximetry reading is 88%. His lungs are clear to auscultation and his heart is tachycardic with no murmurs, rubs, or gallops. Skin examination shows numerous petechial hemorrhages on the upper body. The fracture of the left femur also appears to be improperly immobilized. An electrocardiogram is normal. Laboratory studies show a hematocrit of 32%, platelet count of 100,000/mm^3, and PaO_2 is 60 mm Hg. You place him on supplemental oxygen and his pulse oximeter now reads 95%. A chest x-ray is normal. The most appropriate initial step in management is to

   (A) begin a heparin drip
   (B) immobilize the fracture appropriately
   (C) provide no specific therapy at this time
   (D) start systemic thrombolytics
   (E) start the patient on prednisone

7. A 60-year-old man comes to the office with a 6-month history of dysphagia with solids, regurgitation of undigested food, halitosis, and a fullness of the left neck during meals. He denies a decrease in appetite, abdominal pain, weight loss, or change in bowel habits. His only significant past medical history is a total hip replacement. Laboratory studies show

Hemoglobin	14 g/dL
Hematocrit	43%
Leukocyte count	6000/mm^3
Platelets	300,000/mm^3
Sodium	35 mmol/L
Potassium	4.0 mEq/L
Urea	6 mEq/L
Creatinine	0.6 mEq/L
Glucose	98 mg/dL
Chloride	100 mEq/L
Bicarbonate	25 mEq/L

   His liver panel is normal.

   The most appropriate initial step in evaluation is

   (A) a barium esophagogram
   (B) esophageal manometry
   (C) MRI of the head and neck
   (D) radionuclide scanning
   (E) upper endoscopy

Items 8-9

A 39-year-old woman comes to the office because of "achy" legs. She is a surgical scrub nurse and says that by the end of each day, she has the "heaviest feeling" in her legs. For the past few months she has had to ask other scrub nurses to "take over" for a few minutes while she goes to the locker room and sits on the bench with her legs elevated against the lockers. She frequently sees other nurses doing to the same thing and they laugh that "it must be the job." She has no other symptoms. She eats a low fat diet, has an "occasional" glass of wine, does not smoke cigarettes, and goes to an aerobic exercise class twice a week after work. Her grandmother and mother, who were also nurses, have the same symptoms. She is 185 cm (6 ft 1 in) tall and weighs 70 kg (154 lb). Her temperature is 37.0 C (98.6 F), blood pressure is 110/70 mm Hg, and pulse is 60/min. Physical examination shows a dilated, tortuous saphenous vessel. The remainder of the physical examination is unremarkable.

8. This patient should be advised to

   (A) discontinue her exercise regimen
   (B) lose weight
   (C) quit her job
   (D) take a daily aspirin to prevent thromboemboli
   (E) wear external compression stockings

9. The patient returns 3 months later because of a painful, red left thigh. Physical examination shows a warm, erythematous tender area along a tortuous vessel. The surrounding skin is erythematous and edematous. There is no pain when she dorsiflexes her left foot. Pulses are equal on both lower extremities. The most likely diagnosis is

   (A) acute arterial insufficiency
   (B) deep vein thrombosis
   (C) lymphangitis
   (D) postphlebitic syndrome
   (E) superficial vein thrombosis

10. A 21-year-old construction worker comes to the emergency department after falling from a ladder. He believes he fell about 5 feet off the ladder and landed on his outstretched right hand. He denies any loss of consciousness prior to or after the fall and can recall the entire accident. He denies any right shoulder or elbow pain. On physical examination, the patient's vital signs are unremarkable and he appears in no distress. He has some small abrasions on his elbow and forearm. The wrist is moderately swollen and a slight deformity of the forearm just proximal to the wrist is present. There is no evidence of skin compromise overlying the deformity. The patient is unable to flex and extend his wrist because of the pain. Sensation to light touch is intact throughout the right upper extremity and he has a 2+ radial pulse with adequate capillary refill in all of the fingers in the right hand. The most appropriate next step in management is to

    (A) contact the orthopedic surgeon on call for an emergency consult
    (B) forcibly correct the deformity of the right wrist
    (C) obtain lateral and PA radiographs of the right wrist and forearm
    (D) prescribe pain medication for the patient and tell him to return if his pain does not improve in 2 weeks
    (E) splint the affected extremity and give him a phone number for a local orthopedic surgeon

11. A 63-year-old man comes to the emergency department with generalized abdominal pain and diarrhea. He states that the diarrhea has been going on for several days and initially was accompanied by nausea and vomiting. On physical examination, he has a temperature of 37.2 C (99.0 F) and mild abdominal tenderness, which is slightly worse in the right lower quadrant. Laboratory studies are pending. A non-contrast CT scan of the abdomen to rule out appendicitis is ordered, which reveals a normal appendix with no evidence of periappendiceal fat stranding; however, an incidental 3 cm right adrenal mass is identified. It has a Hounsfield unit measurement of –13. If a noncontrast CT scan is 98% specific for an adrenal adenoma when the Hounsfield unit measurement is less than zero, then

(A) CT scanning is 98% likely to identify a mass of the adrenal gland
(B) if the Hounsfield unit measurement of an adrenal mass is greater than 10, then it is 98% likely not to be an adenoma
(C) it is 98% likely that a mass in the adrenal gland with Hounsfield units less than 0 is an adenoma
(D) 98% percent of adrenal masses seen on CT scans are adenomas
(E) 2% percent of adrenal masses are cancerous

12. A 52-year-old man is admitted to the hospital with diabetic ketoacidosis and altered mental status. On rounds in the morning, he is more alert and states that he has been having some sinus congestion over the past few days, and a dry cough. He denies any abdominal pain or urinary symptoms. His temperature is 38.5 C (101.3 F), blood pressure is 122/78 mm Hg, pulse is 99/min, and respirations are 22/min. Visual acuity is normal and extraocular movements are intact. He has pain to palpation over the left maxillary sinus. Some dark discoloration is seen on the mucosal of the left middle nasal turbinate on direct nasal examination. Oropharynx is normal. Lungs are clear and heart is normal. Abdomen is benign. Laboratory studies show a leukocyte count of 11,500/mm^3, creatinine of 0.9 mg/dL, and blood urea nitrogen of 16 mg/dL. A urinalysis is normal. A chest x-ray is also normal. The most appropriate next step in management is to

(A) obtain an emergent otolaryngology consult
(B) prescribe amoxicillin/clavulanate 875 mg orally twice per day
(C) prescribe ciprofloxacin 500 mg orally twice per day
(D) prescribe vancomycin 15 mg/kg intravenously every 12 hours
(E) reassure him that no additional treatment is necessary

13. A 70-year-old woman who is scheduled to have a hip replacement operation for long-standing degenerative arthritis is referred to you by her orthopedic surgeon for preoperative clearance. The woman is well, active, and motivated to have surgery so that she can resume her walking exercise program. Except for arthritis, her medical history is unremarkable. She has never smoked cigarettes and has no known cardiac, pulmonary, or renal conditions. On physical examination she appears ruddy in appearance. Her temperature is 37.0 C (98.6 F), blood pressure is 150/70 mm Hg, and pulse is 74/min and regular. There is no peripheral lymphadenopathy, the thyroid is normal in size and without nodules, and mild jugular venous distention is noted in the upright position. Chest examination is normal. There is no hepatomegaly; however, the spleen is distinctly palpable 4 cm below the left costal margin. The extremities are free of edema and without clubbing or cyanosis. Her latest laboratory studies show

Hemoglobin	17.1 g/dL
Hematocrit	53%
Platelet count	475,000/mm^3
Leukocyte count	13,400/mm^3
Uric acid	11.5 mg/dL

At this time the most appropriate recommendation to the orthopedic surgeon is to

(A) delay surgery and determine red blood cell mass
(B) delay surgery and perform a bone marrow biopsy
(C) proceed to surgery, keeping the patient well hydrated, and during the procedure obtain a biopsy specimen of the bone marrow
(D) proceed to surgery, keeping the patient well hydrated, and once surgery is completed start anticoagulation with intravenous heparin
(E) proceed to surgery, keeping the patient well hydrated, and once surgery is completed start aspirin 325 mg/day

14. An 18-year-old man comes to the urgent care clinic after a motor vehicle accident 24 hours earlier. He was brought to the hospital immediately following the accident and examination revealed an isolated tibial fracture in the lower part of the tibia. A cast was applied from below the knee to the metatarsophalangeal joints and his toes were exposed. He was sent home with analgesics after the pain was controlled in the hospital. He is now complaining of severe, persistent pain in his foot and toes that is not relieved by analgesics or by elevation. On examination, the patient seems to be in distress. His blood pressure is 100/80 mm Hg and pulse is 70/min. Examination of the right lower extremity shows decreased toe movement and severe tenderness on passive movements of the toes. The most likely cause of his pain is

(A) inadequate immobilization of the fractured fragments of tibia
(B) ischemia
(C) muscle spasm
(D) neural compression
(E) pressure point necrosis

15. A 71-year-old man is admitted to the hospital because of chest pain. On the day of admission, he had been having nausea intermittently and then vomited just prior to the onset of his chest pain, which he describes as substernal and sharp. There was no significant dyspnea or change in the pain with inspiration. A chest x-ray on admission shows some minimal basilar atelectasis. A myocardial infarction is ruled out with serial cardiac enzymes and electrocardiograms. On day 2 of hospitalization he develops a low-grade fever 37.8 C (100.0 F). His vitals signs are: blood pressure 138/92 mm Hg, pulse 98/min, and respirations 20/min. Cardiac examination is normal, the lungs have decreased breath sounds at left base with dullness to percussion, and the extremities have no edema. A chest x-ray shows a moderate sized left pleural effusion. A thoracentesis and laboratory studies show

Pleural fluid	Thick yellow
Pleural LDH	75 U/L
Serum LDH	100 U/L
Pleural total protein	4 g/dL
Serum total protein	6 g/dL
Pleural amylase	2000 U/L
Serum amylase	50 U/L
Pleural WBCs	20/HPF
Pleural RBCs	50/HPF
Sodium	140 mEq/L
Potassium	3.8 mEq/L
BUN	26 mg/dL
Creatinine	0.9 mg/dL

The most appropriate next step in management is to

(A) order a Gastrografin esophagram
(B) order a ventilation perfusion
(C) place a chest tube
(D) send him for cardiac catheterization to rule out three vessel coronary artery disease
(E) start course of intravenous ceftriaxone for complicated pneumonia

Items 16-20

A 67-year-old woman with severe peripheral vascular disease and non-insulin dependent diabetes mellitus is postoperative day 2 from an aortic-bifemoral bypass procedure. She presented 3 days ago to the emergency clinic with severe calf claudication bilaterally. On initial presentation her feet were cool to the touch and her dorsalis pedis pulses were nonpalpable. An angiogram showed severe distal aortic-iliac disease with poor filling of her superficial femoral and anterior tibial arteries bilaterally. Postoperatively she has had excellent pain control with an epidural catheter that is infusing morphine. Her vital signs have been stable. You are now called by the nurse because the patient is complaining of abdominal pain that has been worsening over the last few days. On physical examination, her blood pressure is 100/50 mm Hg and her pulse is 100/min and regular. Her abdomen is soft, but with diffuse tenderness on palpation. Her stools are positive for blood. Laboratory studies show

Sodium	145 mEq/L
Potassium	3.8 mEq/L
Chloride	102 mEq/L
Bicarbonate	16 mEq/L

Arterial blood gas obtained on 3 liters oxygen:

PO_2	144 mm Hg
PCO_2	34 mm Hg
pH	7.22

16. The most important diagnostic test at this time is

    (A) an abdominal CT scan
    (B) a digital rectal examination
    (C) an exploratory laparotomy
    (D) flexible sigmoidoscopy
    (E) rigid sigmoidoscopy

17. The laboratory abnormality most likely associated with this patient's acid-base disturbance is an elevated

    (A) blood acetone level
    (B) blood glucose level
    (C) blood lactate level
    (D) blood urea nitrogen level
    (E) urinary pH

18. On further evaluation of this patient, her creatinine is noticed to be 1.8 mg/dL while her preoperative value was noted to be 0.8 mg/dL. Her urine output is between 5 and 15 mL per hour. Her postoperative hematocrit is 34%. The most appropriate intervention is to

    (A) give furosemide, intravenously
    (B) give intravenous crystalloid
    (C) give intravenous packed red blood cells
    (D) order a pelvic ultrasound
    (E) send a urine sample for sediment analysis

19. After 4 liters of intravenous fluids and 1 unit of packed red blood cells are given over the next 8 hours, the patient's urine output continues to be poor. Laboratory studies show

BUN	34 mg/dL
Creatinine	1.9 mg/dL
CPK	3400 mg/dL
Potassium	5.1 mmol/L

On reviewing the patient's operative record, there was no evidence of hypotension and the total cross clamp time was 43 minutes per side. The most likely cause of her renal failure is

(A) abdominal compartment syndrome
(B) acute tubular necrosis secondary to angiographic dye
(C) acute tubular necrosis secondary to ongoing ischemia
(D) acute tubular necrosis secondary to rhabdomyolysis
(E) prerenal azotemia secondary to volume depletion

20. The patient is taken emergently to the operating room for continued abdominal pain. Her arterial blood gas continued to show a pH of less than 7.25 and her stools were grossly blood streaked. The most likely finding at surgery is

    (A) aorto-enteric fistula
    (B) infarcted small bowel
    (C) sigmoid infarction
    (D) sigmoid volvulus
    (E) small bowel obstruction secondary to adhesions

21. A 47-year-old Chinese born woman comes to the clinic with complaints of "some yellowness" in her eyes, abdominal swelling, and vague right upper quadrant pain that has been progressive over the past several months but is now worse over the last 10 days. Until now she has been healthy and is on no medications. Her temperature is 37.2 C (99.0 F), blood pressure is 108/72 mm Hg, and pulse is 86/min. Her sclera are slightly icteric, abdomen is moderately distended for her size with a fluid wave present and mild right upper quadrant tenderness. Bowel sounds are normal. The extremities have 2+ pitting edema. Laboratory studies show a leukocyte count of $5300/mm^3$, platelets $270,000/mm^3$, hematocrit 34%, BUN 20 mEq/L, creatinine 0.7 mEq/L, ALT 88 IU/L, AST 103 IU/L, alkaline phosphatase 120 U/L, bilirubin (total) 3.4 mg/dL, bilirubin (direct) 3.0 mg/dL. Alpha-fetoprotein is 610 μg/L and a hepatitis viral panel is pending. An abdominal shows a course nodular liver with a heterogenous 4.8-cm lesion in the right lobe of the liver, which is invading the right portal vein, and there is no Doppler color flow within the vessel. The hepatic veins are normal with good Doppler color flow. The spleen is 14 cm and there is a moderate amount of ascites seen. The most likely etiology of her liver mass is

(A) Budd-Chiari syndrome causing necrosis
(B) hepatic adenoma
(C) hepatocellular carcinoma (HCC)
(D) metastatic colon adenocarcinoma
(E) metastatic squamous cell carcinoma of the lung

22. A 53-year-old woman comes to the acute care clinic with left lower quadrant pain worsening over the last 36 hours. She has felt febrile with some chills and her appetite is markedly decreased. Her past medical history is significant for mild hypertension and hypercholesterolemia. Her only medication is metoprolol. Her temperature is 38.5 C (101.3 F), blood pressure is 142/90 mm Hg, pulse is 102/min, and respirations are 18/min. She is in moderate distress from abdominal discomfort, her heart is tachycardic, regular, and no murmurs are present, and her lungs are clear. Her abdomen is soft, with voluntary guarding and moderate tenderness over the left lower quadrant and hypoactive bowel sounds. Rectal examination shows brown guaiac-positive stool. Laboratory studies show a hematocrit of 40%, a platelet count of $300,000/mm^3$, and a leukocyte count of $15,300/mm^3$. The most likely cause of this patient's pain is

(A) appendicitis
(B) diverticulitis
(C) epiploic appendagitis
(D) ovarian carcinoma
(E) perforated duodenal ulcer

23. A 36-year-old man is admitted to the hospital for left inguinal hernia repair. On admission he is asymptomatic and has a normal chest x-ray, electrocardiogram, complete blood count, and electrolytes. Postoperatively, he is given subcutaneous heparin at 7500 units bid for prophylaxis of deep vein thrombosis, and 1 g of cefazolin to prevent infection with skin flora. On postoperative day 3, he is fully ambulatory and eating regular meals. Laboratory studies show a platelet count of $62,000/mm^3$, down from $178,000/mm^3$ on admission. His hematocrit is unchanged at 44%. He has no complaints and there is no evidence of bleeding on physical examination. He has no family history of any blood disorders. The most appropriate next step in management is to

(A) change therapy from subcutaneous heparin to lepirudin
(B) change therapy from subcutaneous heparin to low-molecular-weight heparin
(C) decrease the dose of subcutaneous heparin to 5000 units bid
(D) discontinue the subcutaneous heparin
(E) make no changes in his current therapy

24. A 32-year-old woman comes to the emergency department with a 2-day history of abdominal distention and discomfort. She had been to Mexico last weekend, at which time she had similar symptoms. She attributed the symptoms to food poisoning and treated herself with oral hydration. The symptoms improved temporarily but abdominal distention and diffuse discomfort reappeared over the past 2 days. She also complains of nausea and vomited once. She has had diarrhea with watery, loose stools, not mixed with blood. She underwent an appendectomy at the age of 6 years. Her temperature is 38.6 C (101.4 F), blood pressure is 110/70 mm Hg, and pulse is 82/min. On physical examination, she is noted to have abdominal distention and diffuse tenderness with no peritoneal signs. Chest and abdominal x-rays reveal distended small bowel loops with air fluid levels with some air in the colon. Laboratory studies show a leukocyte count of $14,700/mm^3$. She is diagnosed with a partial intestinal obstruction and a nasogastric tube is inserted and intravenous hydration is initiated. After nasogastric tube decompression, she feels better but continues to have diarrhea. A CT scan of the abdomen and pelvis shows distended small bowel loops with thickened small bowel wall, especially in the terminal ileum. The bowel loops are displaced from each other and a dense mass is noted in the center of the abdomen. There is no leakage of contrast that can be seen on the CT scan. She is admitted to the hospital and is started on therapy with intravenous antibiotics. The most appropriate study at this time is

(A) a barium enema
(B) colonoscopy
(C) a gastrointestinal series with small bowel followthrough
(D) stool for ova and parasites
(E) upper gastrointestinal endoscopy

Items 25-26

25. A just completed study sponsored by the National Institutes of Health examined differences in rates of survival for men ages 65 to 75 who were diagnosed with prostate cancer. For all cases, the cancer was first identified based on PSA readings and then confirmed by biopsy. The following chart shows 10-year survival rates for patients receiving standard radiation treatment, targeted radiation pellets, and surgical intervention.

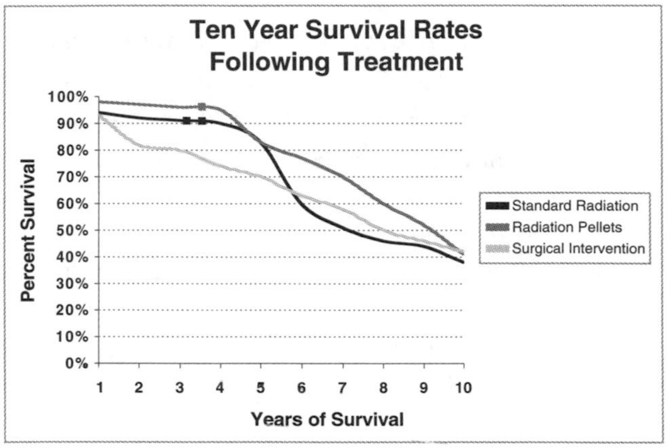

Based on the data derived from this study, life expectancy for patients diagnosed with prostate cancer who elect surgical intervention is best estimated as

(A) 3 years
(B) 4 years
(C) 5 years
(D) 6 years
(E) 7 years
(F) 8 years
(G) 9 years
(H) 10 years

26. A 65-year-old man is diagnosed with prostate cancer and elects therapy with radiation pellets. After his initial treatment he seems pleased at the process, but asks with some concern whether he "will be alive in 10 years to see my son graduate from college?" Based on the available data, the most appropriate response is:

(A) "Don't you feel that we have done the best we can for you?"

(B) "If that is your wish, I will hope for it with you."

(C) "If you had chosen a different treatment option, I would have given you a better chance."

(D) "I never give patients predictions about the future."

(E) "It is possible, but less than a 50-50 chance."

(F) "I want you to not think so much about the future, but concentrate on getting everything you can out of each passing day."

(G) "Tell your son you will be there so he does not worry."

(H) "That's a long way away. Let's not even worry about that now."

(I) "That's really in the hands of God."

(J) "Why do you ask?"

(K) "With careful, continued treatment, I think we can assure you that you will be able to be there."

27. A previously healthy 13-year-old boy is brought to the emergency department by his mother because of a 5-hour history of acute right testicular pain. The patient denies a history of trauma and he has never experienced this type of dull, achy visceral pain before. He has tried some nonsteroidal anti-inflammatory drugs that his mother gave him with marginal relief. A urinalysis is negative. His temperature is 37.0 C (98.6 F). His right testicle is tender to palpation and larger as compared to the other side. There is a probable blue dot sign with a normal lie to the testicle. The cremasteric reflex is not observed. The most appropriate next step is to

(A) admit him overnight for pain control and intravenous antibiotics

(B) get an immediate ultrasound of the testicles

(C) order an immediate nuclear testicular scan to assess for vascular compromise

(D) prepare the patient for immediate surgery for exploration

(E) send the patient home with scheduled ibuprofen, with orders to elevate the scrotum and followup in the clinic in 3 days

28. You see a 35-year-old woman who was involved in a motor vehicle accident. You institute resuscitative measures and maintain her vital signs. You do not, however, make a correct diagnosis before transferring the patient. The woman's husband decides to sue you because you did not make a correct initial diagnosis. The most likely outcome would be that the

(A) attorneys for the plaintiff and the defendant will try to settle it out of court

(B) courts will hold you liable for failing to make a correct initial diagnosis

(C) courts will not hold you liable for failing to make a correct initial diagnosis

(D) courts will order the state medical board to revoke your license

29. A 34-year-old previously healthy man comes to the office because of a 2-week history of rectal bleeding that he describes as blood mixed with stool. The bleeding has been intermittent and not associated with nausea, vomiting, abdominal pain, or any other symptomatology. He denies any previous history of rectal bleeding, diarrhea, or recent foreign travel. On eliciting the family history, he says that he is worried about this rectal bleeding because his father had similar complaints and underwent a total colectomy when he was 47 years old. Family history is also suggestive of breast carcinoma in his mother at the age of 52 years and his mother's sister at the age of 56 years. His father had prostate carcinoma, for which he underwent resection and received chemotherapy. He also vaguely remembers that there was a history of polyps in the colon in his family members, requiring surgery by the age of 40. Clinical examination is unremarkable and laboratory studies are within normal limits. Rectal examination does not reveal any mass. A flexible sigmoidoscopy performed in the office reveals numerous polyps that cannot be counted. Most of these polyps are less than 1 cm in size. Two of the lesions are biopsied and the pathology shows benign adenomas. One week after the office visit, the patient returns for the pathology report and subsequent advice. At this time the most correct statement about his condition is:

(A) A CT scan of the abdomen and pelvis is necessary to rule out any metastases.

(B) Genetic testing is unnecessary, as he does not have a genetic disease.

(C) He should be referred to a surgeon for a colectomy.

(D) He should be rescreened in 1 year.

(E) It is necessary to biopsy and remove all the polyps.

30. A 72-year-old man with hypertension, insulin-dependent diabetes mellitus, and congestive heart failure is admitted to the hospital because of nausea and persistent back pain. He has been treated with intravenous fluids since admission last evening. His vital signs have been stable; however, at 3 o'clock in the afternoon, the nurse calls you because the patient is complaining of persistent abdominal pain that has increased in severity. On approaching the patient, you notice that he is in distress. His blood pressure is 80/palpable and pulse is 92/min. His abdomen is distended and there is a nontender central fullness. Examination of the flanks shows bruises on both sides. The most appropriate immediate intervention is to

    (A) order abdominal ultrasonography
    (B) order a CT scan of the abdomen and pelvis
    (C) resuscitate with intravenous fluids and blood and request a routine surgical consult
    (D) request an immediate surgical consult
    (E) transfer him to the intensive care unit

31. A 46-year-old woman is diagnosed with hyperparathyroidism and is scheduled for surgery. While awaiting surgery she rapidly develops muscular weakness, nausea, vomiting, and confusion and is brought to the emergency department. Appropriate immediate management of her current condition is

    (A) intravenous calcitonin
    (B) intravenous hydration with normal saline
    (C) intravenous mithramycin
    (D) intravenous potassium
    (E) surgical consultation for immediate parathyroid exploration

32. A previously healthy 40-year-old man comes to the office complaining of a 1-week history of left scrotal swelling. He initially noticed it shortly after moving furniture for his new living room. He denies any nausea, vomiting, change in bowel habits, abdominal pain, or urinary tract symptoms. On examination, he has an enlarged left hemi-scrotum with a reducible mass that is clearly distinct from the testicle. With the mass reduced, you ask the patient to perform the Valsalva maneuver and you feel a protrusion at the external inguinal ring. Also, the testicles appear normal in size and consistency when the mass is reduced. The most correct statement regarding this patient's condition is:

    (A) Definitive treatment includes an abdominal binder.
    (B) Emergent surgery is necessary.
    (C) The mass is caused by compression of his left renal vein.
    (D) This mass may become strangulated.
    (E) Tumor markers should be drawn before surgery.

33. A 49-year-old man comes to the emergency department complaining of severe abdominal pain. He tells you that he has had intermittent epigastric pain for several months, but today the pain suddenly worsened. He has been taking an increased amount of ibuprofen over the last 6 months to help control the pain from a knee injury he suffered during a company softball game. He denies any other medical or surgical history. He takes no other medications. He does drink on a social basis. His temperature is 38.3 C (101.0 F), blood pressure is 118/76 mm Hg, and pulse is 110/min. He is clearly uncomfortable. On abdominal examination you find that he has decreased bowel sounds and a diffusely tender abdomen with rebound tenderness and guarding. His leukocyte count is 17,000/mm^3. Upright radiographs show free air under the diaphragm. The most appropriate next step in management is to

    (A) begin a morphine drip and admit for observation
    (B) order a CT scan of the abdomen and pelvis
    (C) perform colonoscopy
    (D) prepare him for emergent exploratory laparotomy
    (E) schedule a barium enema

34. A 26-year-old man comes to the office complaining of a "new mole" on his right shoulder. He is a pale man with blond hair and he enjoys staying outside in the sun. He vaguely recalls that an uncle "had some cancer removed from his face once." Physical examination shows a 2-cm, slightly raised lesion with irregular borders on his shoulder. There are no significantly palpable lymph nodes and no other similar lesions anywhere else on his body. You perform an excisional biopsy of the lesion, which the pathologist informs you is a melanoma. The most correct statement about this condition is:

(A) It is the most common form of skin cancer.
(B) A negative surgical margin of 2 mm is adequate.
(C) A shave biopsy would also have been appropriate for diagnosis.
(D) The Clark microstaging system will most accurately determine prognosis.
(E) Tumor thickness most accurately determines therapy and prognosis.

35. A 28-year-old man feels a sudden, sharp pain in the lower calf after jumping for a basketball during a neighborhood game. Examination reveals weak plantar and dorsiflexion of the ankle with diffused ecchymosis in the left lower extremity. The patient is able to stand on both feet but experiences discomfort. Examination with the patient in a prone position with his legs over the ends of the examining table shows no palpable defect. Squeezing of the calf muscle fails to produce ankle plantar flexion. The most likely explanation for this patient's condition is a

(A) subfascial hematoma
(B) torn Achilles tendon
(C) torn plantaris tendon
(D) torn gastrocnemius
(E) torn posterior tibial tendon

36. A 71-year-old man with hypertension, hypercholesterolemia, coronary artery disease, and BPH comes to the office for routine physical examination. He has no complaints today. His physical examination is essentially unchanged from previous visits, except for a palpable pulsatile abdominal mass. You perform an abdominal ultrasound in the office and diagnose a 6-cm abdominal aortic aneurysm (AAA). At this time, the most correct statement about his condition is:

(A) Atherosclerosis plays an insignificant role in this disease process.
(B) He does not have increased risk for aneurysms at other sites in his body.
(C) The AAA involves all three layers of the arterial wall.
(D) There is no danger with the size of this AAA.
(E) These aneurysms do not involve the renal arteries.

37. A 68-year-old man with hypertension and coronary artery disease comes to the office complaining of a sore on his left lower lip that he thinks has been present for about a month. His wife thinks it is probably more like 2 months. He has a 60-pack year history of smoking and drinks alcohol socially. You perform a biopsy that comes back as squamous cell carcinoma of the oral cavity. At this time the most correct statement about his condition is:

(A) Endoscopic evaluation of his larynx and hypo/nasopharynx is indicated.
(B) His history of tobacco use is not a significant risk factor.
(C) Lymph node spread is to the midjugular chain first.
(D) Surgery plays no role in the therapy of this cancer.
(E) This is a rare form of head and neck cancer.

38. You are asked to evaluate a 72-year-old woman who is 6 days status post-placement of a screw in the right hip. She has had no stool or flatus since surgery. She does not complain of any abdominal pain when questioned; however, her history is limited because of her lethargy. She is afebrile with normal vital signs. Her abdomen is distended with decreased bowel sounds. There are no old abdominal scars. She is nontender on palpation and tympanitic to percussion. Her potassium level is 2.9 mEq/L. Plain films of the abdomen show marked gaseous distention of the colon localized to the right colon. At this time the most correct statement about her condition is:

(A) Colonoscopy plays no role in management.
(B) Normally this process involves the descending colon.
(C) Perforation of the cecum is a feared complication.
(D) She requires emergent exploratory laparotomy.
(E) The etiology is a "kink" in the large bowel.

39. A 36-year-old woman is brought to the emergency department after jumping out of a fourth floor window and landing on her feet. Physical examination is normal except for point tenderness on her bony prominences. Initial laboratory studies are normal. A chest x-ray, pelvic x-ray, and cervical spine x-ray do not reveal any abnormalities. Further evaluation of this patient should include

(A) a CT scan of the abdomen and pelvis
(B) a CT scan of the head
(C) repeat chest x-ray in 6 hours
(D) x-rays of the lower extremities and spine
(E) x-rays of the knees and ankles

40. A 31-year-old healthy man with no significant past medical history comes to the emergency department complaining of upper abdominal pain and bloody diarrhea for the past 6 weeks. He denies any prior similar episodes, travel history, similar symptoms in close contacts, or risk factors for an immunocompromised state. His temperature is 38.1 C (100.6 F). He has diffuse abdominal tenderness without rebound or guarding and a peri-umbilical mass with exudative discharge. Other than local erythema and tenderness, there is no abdominal wall crepitus or fluctuance. Rectal examination is nontender but stool is guaiac-positive. His leukocyte count is 17,400/mm^3, hemoglobin is 11.4 g/dL, and hematocrit is 30%. Mean corpuscular volume is 76. A CT scan of the abdomen shows a thickened terminal ileum with inflammatory changes and a focal area of contrast and fluid that extends anteriorly through the subcutaneous tissue near the umbilicus. This clinical picture is most commonly associated with

(A) appendicitis
(B) an enterocutaneous fistula
(C) Fournier gangrene
(D) an incarcerated umbilical hernia
(E) a patent urachal cyst

41. A 28-year-old healthy man comes to the employee health clinic complaining of a 2-week history of a constant dull, achy feeling in his left testicle. He denies any trauma, dysuria, fevers or chills, unprotected sexual activity, or prior similar episodes. On physical examination you find that the right testicle is normal in location, size, and consistency. The left testicle is enlarged, hard, irregular, and nontender to palpation. There is no trans-illumination of light through this scrotal mass. Serum beta hCG (human chorionic gonadotropin) and AFP (alpha-fetal protein) levels are elevated. At this time the most correct statement about his condition is:

(A) Chemotherapy is required before surgery.
(B) He should undergo exploration through an incision in the scrotum.
(C) His condition has a poor prognosis.
(D) Orchiectomy will make him infertile.
(E) Radiation therapy is required before surgery.
(F) Radical orchiectomy is the first line of treatment.

42. A 61-year-old alcoholic man returns to the emergency department in obvious discomfort during your shift late one night. He was discharged from the hospital 3 weeks earlier, after recovering from a severe episode of pancreatitis. Vital signs are: temperature 38.2 C (100.8 F), blood pressure 82/40 mm Hg, pulse 108/min. His abdomen has decreased bowel sounds and is tender in the epigastric area with guarding. There is a palpable mass over the center of the abdomen with an audible bruit. Distal extremity pulses are intact. Complete blood count shows a decrease in hemoglobin by 4 g since discharge. There are no other signs of internal or external bleeding. The most appropriate next step in management is to

(A) aspirate the mass
(B) order an ultrasound to be performed when staff arrives in the morning
(C) perform endoscopic retrograde cholangiopancreatography (ERCP)
(D) prepare him for an exploratory laparotomy
(E) stabilize and discharge him with outpatient followup

43. A 58-year-old woman with hypertension, noninsulin-dependent diabetes, and a history of a perforated gastric ulcer requiring surgery 16 years earlier comes to the office complaining of pain over the middle of her "stomach above the belly button." It has been present for many months but recently got worse and has become constant, non-radiating, and not associated with food intake. She has no change in bowel habits, weight loss, nausea, vomiting, fevers, or chills. Her vital signs are normal and heart and lung examinations are unchanged from prior visits. There is a supra-umbilical midline incision that is well healed. Bowel sounds are present and normal. There is a tender mass approximately 5 cm at the superior aspect of her incision. There is no overlying erythema, crepitus, or drainage. It is difficult, but you are able to reduce the mass back into the abdominal cavity. With the mass reduced, you appreciate a defect approximately 3 cm in the abdominal wall. She expressed that she feels better after you reduce the mass. The most appropriate step in the management of this patient's abdominal pain is to

(A) check liver function tests
(B) order upper endoscopy
(C) prescribe an abdominal binder only
(D) recommend surgical repair of the defect
(E) schedule an outpatient liver/gallbladder ultrasound

44. A 58-year-old man comes to the office complaining of pain during bowel movements. This pain has been present for the past 6 weeks but has recently gotten extremely uncomfortable. He occasionally notices blood on the toilet paper after bowel movements. He also has constipation but denies weight loss, fever, or chills. He has no other significant surgical or medical history and a colonoscopy 2 years earlier was normal. On examination, his abdomen is soft and nontender without masses. Examination of the anus reveals a linear defect in the anal mucosa that began bleeding slowly during the exam. Digital rectal examination is difficult owing to patient discomfort but there were no masses or stool in the rectal vault. The most appropriate next step in the management is to

(A) incise and drain anal area
(B) perform stool guaiac testing
(C) prescribe sitz baths, anal cleaning, and stool bulk-forming agents
(D) refer him for hemorrhoidectomy
(E) schedule chemotherapy

45. During hospital rounds, you are asked to evaluate an 81-year-old woman who was recently admitted for pneumonia. The day nurse noted an abnormality of the anus while changing the patient's diaper. The patient is comfortable and her fevers have improved once antibiotics were started. She is a poor historian and did not realize there was anything wrong with her "backside." She does admit to constipation that she attributes to being old. She is unable to provide any other contributory history. On examination her abdomen is soft, nontender, and without organomegaly. On visual inspection there is a mass of red mucosa with folds that is seen protruding from the anus. There is no bleeding from this mass and it is soft and smooth. You are able to gently push the mass back into the rectal vault. The most appropriate treatment for this patient's condition is to

(A) insert a pessary
(B) perform anal manometry
(C) perform colonoscopy
(D) perform rectosigmoid resection and rectopexy
(E) send her for an immediate barium enema

46. A 60-year-old man comes to the office to discuss treatment options for his recently diagnosed prostate cancer. Further evaluation with an MRI and a radionuclide bone scan reveals that the cancer appears to be localized to the prostate and there is no evidence of metastatic disease. Given the patient's age and the aggressive nature of his cancer, you recommend surgical removal of the prostate. Just the mention of this option makes him clearly upset. At this point in the discussion, he pulls out an article that he found while searching at his local library. In the article, researchers went back through medical records of 120 patients who had been diagnosed with prostate cancer. Fifty of these patients underwent surgical interventions and the remaining 70 received radiation treatments. The 3-year survival rate for the patients who underwent surgery was 88%, and the 3-year survival rate for the patients who received radiation was 97%. This difference was significant at the level of $p<0.01$. The article was published within the previous year in a reputable medical journal. The patient asks if the article does not prove that radiation is a better treatment. Faced with the information presented in this research article the most appropriate response is:

(A) "I'll be happy to look at it more carefully and tell you what I think the next time we talk."
(B) "I see why you would ask that. Unfortunately, the study is flawed. I suspect that patients were given different treatments based on the severity of their disease."
(C) "Is there some reason that you are uncomfortable with my judgment?"
(D) "Look, I've treated many patients in my day, and for someone in your condition, surgery will give you the best chance of a long and happy life."
(E) "Maybe you would like some time to talk about your options with your family before we proceed?"
(F) "The difference in outcomes in the article is not really enough to matter when making treatment decisions."
(G) "There is no need to make any decision right now. Why don't you take a few days and think about your options."
(H) "This is just one study. I've read many in my time, and on balance, the research points to surgery for you."
(I) "Why don't you leave the research to me and concentrate on getting yourself better."
(J) "You know, you may have found something there. Let's try radiation if that is really what you want."
(K) "You seem a bit anxious. Before I answer, let's talk about that first."

Items 47-48

A 30-year-old man is brought to the emergency department after a motor vehicle accident in which he sustained serious trauma, including a massive hemothorax. It is obvious to you that he has blood within the thoracic cavity, and maybe it's helping to tamponade the source of bleeding. You draw blood for an urgent type and cross-match and contact the laboratory, informing them that you must have the blood available immediately. To your dismay the laboratory technician informs you that no blood is available at all. Despite your pleas, the laboratory is unable to comply and has suggested that you call back in an hour's time when they would have the requisite blood. They apologize for the error that occurred because of a corruption of the database in their computer, and, as a result, inadvertently showed adequate stocks. In fact, they inform you that they are frantically trying to locate donors. You are infuriated about this and concerned about its implications.

47. The most appropriate next step is to

(A) continue resuscitation with the fluids you are presently giving until blood is available
(B) drain the hemothorax
(C) inform the hospital attorney in case of a lawsuit
(D) notify the local TV station about this lapse
(E) notify your partner

48. The appropriate step has been taken. The most appropriate next step in management is to

(A) give blood
(B) go with the attorney to the laboratory and confront the technician
(C) go with your partner to the laboratory and confront the technician
(D) speed up the fluids you are giving to the maximum rate possible
(E) spruce yourself up to face the television cameras

49. A 36-year-old man who works at an automobile assembly plant is brought to the emergency department with stab wounds to the abdomen. It appears that he got into an altercation with a colleague who had borrowed $100.00 from him and now denied ever having done so. As a result, his friend got angry and stabbed him several times while he was leaving the factory gates. You learn that he has a wife, who is a homemaker, and two young children. He informs you that he does not want any treatment and would prefer to die. Your response would be based on the premise that the

(A) patient has a right to refuse treatment
(B) patient's older brother has a right to intervene
(C) patient's parents have a right to intervene
(D) patient's wife has a right to intervene
(E) state has a right to enforce treatment

50. A 72-year-old man with diabetes mellitus, chronic emphysema, and cor pulmonale is admitted to the hospital for sigmoid resection secondary to recurrent volvulus. His resting pulse is persistently more than 110/min and his pulse oxygen saturation varies between 85-90% on 2 L/min of oxygen by way of nasal cannula, making any kind of physical therapy difficult to accomplish. His hemoglobin A1c level is estimated at 6%. Three weeks after surgery he develops asymptomatic blisters on his lower extremities. On physical examination you notice that there is symmetric 3+ pitting edema of the lower extremities with *peau d'orange* appearance of the skin on the lower legs. In addition, there are multiple, grouped, translucent, thick-roofed bullae around the ankles and shins bilaterally. The most likely cause of the skin lesions is

(A) beta hemolytic group A *Streptococcus*
(B) chronic venous insufficiency
(C) lymphedema
(D) persistent hyperglycemia
(E) superficial vein thrombosis

Surgery Test Two: **Answers and Explanations**

ANSWER KEY

1. B
2. A
3. A
4. D
5. B
6. B
7. A
8. E
9. E
10. C
11. C
12. A
13. A
14. B
15. A
16. D
17. C
18. B
19. B
20. C
21. C
22. B
23. D
24. C
25. F
26. E
27. D
28. C
29. C
30. D
31. B
32. D
33. D
34. E
35. B
36. C
37. A
38. C
39. D
40. B
41. F
42. D
43. D
44. C
45. D
46. B
47. B
48. A
49. E
50. C

1. **The correct answer is B.** The finding that is most suggestive of a thyroid cancer is a nodule that is fixed in place and does not move with swallowing. Other physical examination features suggestive of malignancy include a firm or irregular nodule and a rapidly growing lesion. Malignant lesions in the thyroid or other organ systems tend to infiltrate the adjacent tissues and often seem fixed in place on physical exam.

    The finding of multiple 1-cm cervical lymph nodes on a CT of the neck (**choice A**) is not suggestive of malignancy. Lymph nodes are not considered pathologic unless they are greater than 1 cm in their short axis. Finding small lymph nodes anywhere in the lymphatic chain is normal or may represent a recent inflammatory or infectious process that is resolving. If the CT demonstrated cervical lymph nodes greater than 1 cm in size in this patient, this would be suggestive of a malignant process.

    A "hot" lesion on a radioactive iodine scan of the thyroid (**choice C**) is suggestive of a benign process. A "hot" lesion is indicative of increased radioactive tracer uptake in that particular region and may be secondary to a functioning thyroid adenoma. Most malignant tumors of the thyroid are seen as "cold" lesions on the scan since the malignant cells do not function like normal thyroid cells and thus do not uptake iodine. Although "cold" lesions are more suggestive of malignant tumors, only 10% of "cold" lesions are found to be malignant at pathology.

    The finding of multiple solid nodules in both lobes of the thyroid (**choice D**) is suggestive of a benign process. The finding of multiplicity is usually associated with a benign process. This sonographic finding is suggestive of a multinodular goiter. Most malignant tumors of the thyroid are single solid lesions on ultrasonography.

    If ultrasonography of the nodule demonstrates that it is a cyst (**choice E**), this is consistent with a benign lesion. The thyroid gland is normally homogeneous in echotexture on ultrasound. There are, however, many other sonographic appearances that are still considered benign. Some thyroid glands may appear diffusely heterogeneous and some may have multiple solid and cystic areas. The cystic areas may represent colloid cysts or degenerating thyroid tissue in a multinodular goiter.

2. **The correct answer is A.** This patient has a perirectal abscess that will need to be drained as soon as possible to prevent complications, which include fistula formation and systemic infection. The patient will likely need stronger pain relief after the procedure and should be instructed in local wound care. However, pain relief alone would not be adequate treatment (**choice E**). Recurrent perirectal abscesses with fistula formation can be seen in Crohn disease and the chronic history of bowel complaints and possible family history warrant further evaluation. However, the need for colonoscopy (**choice B**) is not urgent and should wait until the patient has symptomatic relief of her pain. Crohn flare-ups may necessitate treatment with steroids (**choice D**). However, that diagnosis has not been established. Crohn disease does increase the patient's risk of colon cancer and frequent colon cancer screening is recommended. However, this presentation is not consistent with rectal cancer (**choice C**), which would be very rare in this age group even in patients with Crohn disease.

3. **The correct answer is A.** This patient presented with the classic sign of Leser-Trélat associated with a gastric adenocarcinoma, i.e., the sudden appearance of numerous itchy seborrheic keratoses in an adult with internal malignancy. Sixty percent of the neoplasms have been adenocarcinoma, primarily of the stomach. The other most common malignancies found are lymphoma, breast cancer, and squamous cell carcinoma of the lung. Other less common associations are with melanoma, neurofibrosarcoma, leukemia, hepatoma, ovarian adenocarcinoma, other gastrointestinal malignancies, and osteogenic sarcoma. To be accepted as having the sign of Leser-Trélat the keratoses should begin approximately the same time as development of the cancer and run a parallel course in regard to growth and remission. Gastric cancers, when superficial and surgically curable, usually produce no symptoms. As the tumor becomes more extensive patients may complain of an insidious upper abdominal discomfort varying in intensity from a vague, postprandial fullness to a severe, steady pain. Anorexia, often with slight nausea, is very common but is not the usual presenting complaint. The risk of gastric cancer is greater among lower socioeconomic classes. Migrants from high- to low-incidence nations maintain their susceptibility to gastric cancer, while the risk for their offspring approximates that of the new homeland. These findings suggest that an environmental exposure, probably beginning early in life, is related to the development of gastric cancer, with dietary carcinogens considered the most likely factor(s). The long-term ingestion of high concentrations of nitrates in dried, smoked, and salted foods appears to be associated with a higher risk.

    Hepatoma (**choice B**) clinically presents with right upper quadrant pain and the presence of a palpable mass or features of intratumoral hemorrhage (pain and circulatory collapse). It is infrequently associated with the sign of Leser-Trélat.

Even though leukemia (**choice C**) has been reported with the sign of Leser-Trélat, the association is much less frequent and presenting signs are usually fatigue or weakness at the time of diagnosis. Anorexia and weight loss are common. Fever with or without an identifiable infection is the initial symptom in ~10% of patients. Signs of abnormal hemostasis (bleeding, easy bruising) are noted first in 5% of patients. On occasion, bone pain, lymphadenopathy, nonspecific cough, headache, or diaphoresis is the presenting symptom.

Melanoma (**choice D**) most commonly presents as a slowly enlarging brown or black asymmetrical patch with an irregular, scalloped border and color variegation. Again, it is infrequently associated with the sign of Leser-Trélat.

Osteosarcoma (**choice E**) has a predilection for metaphyses of long bones; the most common sites of involvement are the distal femur, proximal tibia, and proximal humerus. Patients typically present with pain and swelling of the affected area. It is infrequently associated with the sign of Leser-Trélat.

4. **The correct answer is D.** A lawsuit would result because the rescuer was negligent, and the plaintiff would win. There are four elements of negligence. The plaintiff has to prove that the physician was wrong in all four of them to sue successfully. The first is to establish the standard of care appropriate in the given situation. This is obtained by expert medical testimony. The second is to establish that the physician has breached the standard of care. This has two components, either of which will be upheld—errors of commission or errors of omission (i.e., either that the defending physician acted negligently or negligently failed to act). The third is that the plaintiff should have a demonstrable physical injury. Finally, the fourth is to establish that the breach of standard was the logical and legal cause of the injury claimed by the plaintiff. In this situation, the standard of care that would be established would be that of a physician reasonably competent in advanced trauma life support. The essence of standard of care as determined by the courts is "in the same class in which he belongs." This definition is operational on a national basis. The application of advanced trauma life support standard is not based on right or wrong, but on what a reasonably competent physician with appropriate skills based on advanced trauma life support should do in a given situation. The courts would accept the plaintiff's plea that the physician was grossly negligent in the discharge of his duties. The physician had breached the accepted standard of care because every physician should know that movement of the neck could be extremely hazardous as an underlying cervical spinal injury must be presumed until proved otherwise. The negligent act in breach of the accepted standard of care precluded to the patient developing a demonstrable physical injury in the form of a quadriplegia that was not present before this.

   Disciplinary action by the state medical board (**choice B**) or American Medical Association (**choice A**) does not apply.

   The Good Samaritan statute (**choice C**) does not condone acts of negligence. Good Samaritan statutes are operational in every state in the United States to encourage potential rescuers who would otherwise stay away for fear of being sued to render emergency aid to victims. The possibility of a successful outcome in a lawsuit against a physician or healthcare provider acting under the Good Samaritan statute is very minuscule indeed, unless of course there has been a gross act of negligence, as has been demonstrated in this case.

   No matter how good the rescuer's intent (**choice E**) may have been, it caused avoidable injury brought about by an act of negligence.

5. **The correct answer is B.** This patient has developed a squamous cell carcinoma on the lower lip. Primary cutaneous squamous cell carcinoma is a malignant neoplasm of keratinizing epidermal cells. Unlike basal cell carcinoma, which has a very low metastatic potential, squamous cell carcinoma can metastasize and grow rapidly. The clinical features of squamous cell carcinoma vary widely. Commonly, squamous cell carcinoma appears as an ulcerated nodule or a superficial erosion on the skin or lower lip, but it may present as a verrucous papule or plaque. Unlike basal cell carcinoma, overlying telangiectasias are uncommon. The margins of this tumor may be ill defined and fixation to underlying structures may occur. Cutaneous squamous cell carcinoma may develop anywhere on the body, but it usually arises on sun-damaged skin. Squamous cell carcinoma has several premalignant forms (actinic keratosis, actinic cheilitis, and some cutaneous horns that are confined to the epidermis). Actinic keratoses and cheilitis are hyperkeratotic papules and plaques that occur on sun-exposed areas. While the potential for malignant degeneration is low in any individual lesion, the risk of squamous cell carcinoma increases with larger numbers of lesions. Treatment of premalignant lesions reduces the subsequent risk of invasive disease. On histopathologic examination, squamous cell carcinoma is characterized by irregular nests of

pleomorphic epidermal cells with horn pearl formation invading the dermis to varying degrees. The degree of cell differentiation has been used to grade squamous cell carcinoma and horn pearl formation is considered a sign of advanced differentiation toward keratinizing epidermal cells from which this tumor stems. Although interpretations vary, it is considered the better the differentiation, the less the invasive tendency, thereby the better the prognosis.

Hyperkeratosis, wedge-shaped hypergranulosis, acanthosis with "saw toothing" of the dermoepidermal junction, and a dense lichenoid infiltrate in the papillary dermis (**choice A**) is seen in lichen planus. Lichen planus is a papulosquamous disorder in which the primary lesions are pruritic, polygonal, flat-topped, violaceous papules. Close examination of the surface of these papules often reveals a network of gray lines (Wickham striae). The skin lesions may occur anywhere but have a predilection for the wrists, shins, lower back, and genitalia. Involvement of the scalp may lead to hair loss. Lichen planus commonly involves mucous membranes, particularly the buccal mucosa, where it can present as a white netlike eruption.

Many aggregations of sebaceous lobules directly communicating with the overlying epidermis are the histopathologic finding of Fordyce spots (**choice C**), which are ectopic sebaceous glands typically located on non-glabrous skin of the lips and glans penis. They present as 1 to 2-mm, asymptomatic, translucent, yellowish papules that require no treatment.

Nests of darkly staining polyhedral cells in the dermis with columnar cells characteristically arranged in a palisade at the periphery (**choice D**) are characteristic of nodular basal cell carcinoma, the most common type. The natural history is that of a slowly enlarging, locally invasive neoplasm. It begins as a small, pearly nodule, often with small telangiectatic vessels on its surface. Location on the central face (e.g., the nose, the nasolabial fold, or the periorbital or perioral area) is typical.

Pagetoid spread of atypical melanocytes in the epidermis (**choice E**) is seen in melanoma in situ (lentigo maligna). Lentigo maligna presents as a slowly enlarging hyperpigmented patch with irregular and sometimes notched borders, variation in pigment pattern, and variation in color. It is most commonly located on the head. An increase in size or change in color is noted by the patient in 70% of early lesions. Bleeding, ulceration, and pain are late signs (of progression to invasive melanoma) and are of little help in early recognition.

6. **The correct answer is B.** This patient is presenting with classic fat embolism. The treatment for this entity is primarily supportive; however, the most important first step is to appropriately immobilize all fractures to prevent further embolism. Diagnosis is difficult and largely based on clinical grounds. One thing that this patient did not exhibit which can often be seen is fat globules actually within the blood specimen.

Systemic anticoagulation (**choice A**), as would be used in traditional venous thromboembolism, is not used, nor would systemic thrombolytics (**choice D**) be beneficial as this is most likely a fat embolism.

Clearly no treatment (**choice C**) is incorrect as the case states that the fracture appears to be improperly immobilized and he is symptomatic.

Some studies have shown benefit with corticosteroid therapy (**choice E**), and this patient will likely benefit from this. However, as mentioned previously, the most important thing is to first immobilize the fracture.

7. **The correct answer is A.** The patient may have a Zenker diverticulum, which may predispose the patient to aspiration pneumonia. The diagnosis is likely to be Zenker diverticulum since the patient has halitosis during feeding along with the fullness *after* the meal. The best method to establish the diagnosis is a barium esophagogram initially. Then, as part of the workup before surgery to reduce the size of the diverticulum, an upper endoscopy (**choice E**) should be ordered to rule out esophageal cancer.

Esophageal manometry (**choice B**) would not be useful in this instance. It is normally used in evaluating patients with noncardiac chest pain, motor disorders of the esophagus, achalasia, or gastroesophageal reflux disease.

An MRI of the head and neck (**choice C**) would expose the patient to a lot of radiation compared to a barium swallow and would not be feasible as the first diagnostic test for evaluating a diverticulum. In any case, the total hip replacement would be a contraindication of an MRI, as would any metal arthroplasty, surgical clips, or pacemaker to name a few.

Radionuclide scanning (**choice D**) would be used in evaluating the patient for thyroid tumors, which is low on the differential list for this patient based on his symptoms (e.g., fullness of neck after a meal, lack of weight loss, or appetite loss).

8. **The correct answer is E.** This patient has varicose veins, which are most likely the result of valvular dysfunction, a weakness in the walls, or elevated intraluminal pressure. They are very common in women and are often familial. Individuals with varicose veins complain of heavy, achy, crampy feelings in their legs after prolonged standing that is relieved by elevating the legs. Treatment involves leg elevation, external compression stockings, and the avoidance of long periods of standing. Surgery may be indicated in cases with severe pain and discomfort, and for cosmetic reasons.

It is inappropriate to advise her to discontinue her exercise regimen (**choice A**) because the exercise regimen twice a week most likely does not negatively affect her varicose veins. Also the overall benefits of exercise are well documented, and she can probably get relief by wearing external compression stockings.

This patient is certainly not overweight, therefore she should not be advised to lose weight (**choice B**).

She should not be told to quit her job (**choice C**). External compression stockings and periodic small breaks for leg elevation should provide her with some symptomatic relief.

Since superficial vein thrombi do not lead to pulmonary emboli (deep vein thrombi do), the routine use of aspirin (**choice D**) for the prevention of thromboembolism in patients with varicose veins is not usually indicated.

9. **The correct answer is E.** This patient most likely has a superficial vein thrombosis, which is a thrombosis of the lesser or greater saphenous vein, and in this case, is associated with her history of varicose veins. The history and physical examination are classic for a superficial vein thrombosis, a warm, tender, erythematous cord along a superficial varicose vein. The treatment includes leg elevation, warm compresses, and painkillers. Anticoagulants may be considered; however, the risk of a pulmonary embolism is very small.

Acute arterial insufficiency (**choice A**) typically presents with the six P's—pain, pallor, pulselessness, paralysis, paresthesia, and poikilothermia. This patient's clinical presentation is not consistent with this diagnosis.

A deep vein thrombosis (**choice B**), which is caused by stasis, endothelial injury, or a hypercoagulable state, may be asymptomatic, or may be associated with calf tenderness, calf pain with dorsiflexion of the foot, tenderness, and swelling. A duplex venous ultrasonography, impedance plethysmography, and venography are all diagnostic tests used to evaluate a deep vein thrombosis (DVT). DVTs are not usually associated with varicose veins.

Lymphangitis (**choice C**) is an infection of the lymphatic system, and is typically caused by streptococci or filariasis. It may lead to lymphedema, which is characterized by the enlargement of the affected extremity with localized inflammation. Soft pitting edema becomes "woody", indurated, and fibrotic over time. It presents with a dull, heavy sensation in the extremity. Treatment includes antibiotics, leg elevation, and bed rest. It is not usually associated with varicose veins.

Post-phlebitic syndrome (**choice D**) is caused by venous valvular incompetence and often follows a deep venous thrombosis. It is characterized by chronic swelling, hyperpigmentation, and ulcerations, most commonly near the ankle. Patients complain of a "heavy" feeling. The treatment includes leg elevation, support stockings, compressive medicated boots, and possibly ligation of incompetent veins. It is not usually associated with varicose veins.

10. **The correct answer is C.** This patient likely has a distal radius fracture. Distal radius fractures are very common following a fall on an outstretched hand. They are very common in both children (playground accidents) and the elderly. Other possibilities in this case scenario would include a wrist dislocation (much less common), a severe wrist sprain, or a fracture within the carpus itself. To make a definitive diagnosis radiographs are required and should be obtained in at least two planes; this holds true for nearly all orthopedic radiographs.

The patient likely will require an orthopedic surgery consultant (**choice A**) but not until the appropriate diagnostic studies (radiographs) have been obtained.

A reduction of this patient's deformity may eventually be required **(choice B)**, but it should be performed only after further defining the pathology with radiographs and by a physician familiar with appropriate reduction techniques.

Simply prescribing pain medicine is inadequate for this patient as a displaced fracture may not heal or heal incorrectly if not treated **(choice D)**.

Splinting the extremity may be appropriate but not until the injury has been defined by radiographs and an orthopedic surgeon has been directly contacted. Untreated displaced forearm and wrist fractures can have disastrous functional outcomes (**choice E**).

11. **The correct answer is C.** The easiest way to think about specificity is that it is used to rule in the presence of a certain entity (in this case, the presence of an adenoma rather than a malignancy). Sensitivity on the other hand is used to rule out a certain entity. A Hounsfield unit measurement less than zero, which implies fat is present in the lesion, is highly suggestive of an adenoma. In this particular question, the CT scan has a specificity of 98%, which is very high, thus "ruling in" the presence of an adenoma.

CT scanning is 98% likely to identify a mass of the adrenal gland (**choice A**) is more a question of sensitivity. It is implying (although not stated in the question) that a CT scan should identify 98% of adrenal masses. Thus, if you want to rule out the presence of an adenoma, then a CT scan of the abdomen would not be likely to miss it.

If the Hounsfield unit measurement of an adrenal mass is greater than 10, then it is 98% likely not to be an adenoma (**choice B**), although it may seem to hold true, is not necessarily the case. Just because an adrenal mass with Hounsfield unit measurements less than 10 is highly suggestive of an adenoma, it may also be the case that a mass with higher Hounsfield unit measurements could be an adenoma as well. The level of confidence about this is unclear from the given information.

Ninety-eight percent of adrenal masses seen on CT scans are adenomas (**choice D**) is much too broad of an assumption to be made from the given information. It also does not take into account the measurement of Hounsfield units.

Two percent of adrenal masses are cancerous (**choice E**) also is too broad of an assumption (and an incorrect one at that) to be made from the information given.

12. **The correct answer is A.** In any patient with diabetes presenting with ketoacidosis, the underlying precipitant of the acidosis must be sought out. Often times the precipitating factor is infection. One infection that is extremely concerning and must be identified and treated emergently is mucormycosis of the sinuses. Diabetics are relatively immunocompromised and at a high risk for this type of infection. The finding of sinusitis in a diabetic should already heighten your clinical suspicion, but to see dark discoloration of the mucous membranes or skin of the face is particularly concerning. The mainstay of therapy is biopsy/culture followed by surgical debridement emergently. Amphotericin B is integral but purely adjunctive in therapy.

Amoxicillin/clavulanate (**choice B**) is a good therapy for standard community-acquired sinusitis, and vancomycin (**choice D**) and to a lesser extent ciprofloxacin (**choice C**) are employed in nosocomially acquired sinusitis; however, in this case neither of these is the most important issue at hand.

Clearly, no treatment (**choice E**) is inappropriate management as this is possibly a surgical emergency.

13. **The correct answer is A.** The patient has a ruddy appearance and splenomegaly noted on exam. The patient has increased levels of hemoglobin, hematocrit, platelets, and leukocytes. The patient is likely to have polycythemia rubra vera. This is a neoplastic (clonal) stem cell disorder, which leads to excessive production of all myeloid cell lines, but predominantly red cells. The increase in whole blood viscosity causes vascular occlusion and ischemia compounded by the increase in platelets. Patients with polycythemia rubra vera are at risk of thrombosis, headaches, pruritus, vascular occlusion, TIA, and stroke. It is diagnosed by determining the red cell mass using a radioactive tracer. From there, one would rule out any secondary causes of polycythemia. Treatment choices of polycythemia rubra vera can be with phlebotomy to a target hematocrit of less than 0.45, low-dose aspirin (controversial) 325 mg/day or less, and hydroxyurea if necessary.

Diagnosis with a bone marrow biopsy (**choice B**) is unnecessary and invasive and is the incorrect choice.

There is a high risk of thrombosis in polycythemia rubra vera and when a patient has a total hip replacement it places the patient at greater risk of developing a deep venous thrombosis or pulmonary embolism. Therefore, proceeding to surgery without adequate diagnosis *and treatment* of the condition is incorrect (**choices C, D, and E**).

14. **The correct answer is B.** Several factors can be responsible for limb pain after casting, but severe, persistent, and unrelenting pain after adequate immobilization is suggestive of ischemia. This ischemia should be promptly diagnosed and the plaster cast be relieved with splitting of the cast by parallel cuts through the padding on both sides of the extremity. Failure to do so might result in persistent ischemia, causing complications. The complications could include muscle necrosis resulting in serious disability. After plaster casting, the extremity should be elevated and the digits exposed so that further examination to rule out ischemia is possible.

Adequate immobilization is essential to treat a fracture (**choice A**) and also relieve pain from the fracture, but inadequate immobilization should not result in severe, persistent pain.

Muscle spasms (**choice C**) are possible when fractures are immobilized in a plaster cast. These muscle spasms can present as discomfort or mild-to-moderate pain, but this pain can be relieved usually with analgesics and muscle relaxants.

Neural injury associated with the fracture can cause tingling and numbness and burning sensation but not severe, persistent, unrelenting pain (**choice D**).

Pressure point necrosis can present as localized burning pain (**choice E**). This pressure point necrosis usually occurs over a bony prominence and is treated by cutting a cast window.

15. **The correct answer is A.** A swallow study would show a contained esophageal rupture. The key to this question is to first realize that the patient's chest pain occurred after he vomited. This is often hard to sort out clinically and esophageal rupture (Boerhaave syndrome) should always be in your mind as a possible differential diagnosis of acute chest pain. He also has a very high amylase in the pleural fluid, which usually is seen in pancreatitis, but the patient has no symptoms of this and his serum amylase is normal. It is important to note that more often than not these patients are very ill; however, if the rupture gets walled off and contained, they will present in a more subacute manner.

    A ventilation perfusion scan (**choice B**) could be used to rule out pulmonary emboli (PE), which can cause chest pain and pleural effusions. However, the patient has never had any significant shortness of breath and the lab values of the effusion are not consistent with PE.

    Chest tube placement (**choice C**) will likely be required in this patient's care; however, the most pressing manner is to diagnose what is actually going on with the patient.

    Although the patient could have coronary artery disease, this is not likely the cause of his acute presentation and cardiac catheterization (**choice D**) is not the next appropriate step.

    Intravenous antibiotics (**choice E**) will also likely be required in this patient's care, but his problem is not consistent with a complicated pneumonia.

16. **The correct answer is D.** One of the most important things to understand when evaluating a patient post-operatively is that depending on the procedure, specific issues and concerns must be addressed at the visit. Simply looking in on the patient without thinking clearly about the issues facing that patient can result in serious morbidity and even death. In the case of this patient, her surgical procedure likely involved ligation of the inferior mesenteric artery. Depending upon the patient's blood supply via the superior mesenteric artery, she may become ischemic. Her electrolytes and arterial blood gas reveal an anion gap metabolic acidosis. Her abdominal pain is persistent despite analgesia and her stools are trace positive for blood. This is mesenteric ischemia. The appropriate diagnostic test is to visualize the sigmoid colon with a flexible sigmoidoscope.

    An abdominal CT scan (**choice A**) is a poor imaging modality for early ischemia and the bowel would need to be infarcted before any changes could be detected.

    A digital rectal examination (**choice B**) may confirm the blood in the stool but adds little diagnostic benefit in terms of diagnosing mesenteric ischemia.

    An exploratory laparotomy (**choice C**) is reserved for patients in whom the suspicion of an intra-abdominal process continues to be high despite negative evaluations with other modalities such as flexible sigmoidoscopy.

    A rigid sigmoidoscopy (**choice E**) is not correct since the distance reached by the scope is not adequate to visualize the area of the sigmoid colon likely affected by the surgery.

17. **The correct answer is C.** Looking at this patient's labs, it can be seen that she has an anion gap metabolic acidosis. Although the causes for such an acidosis are numerous, given this patient's recent surgical procedure and likely complication, she is most likely to have elevated lactate levels.

    An elevated blood glucose level (**choice B**) is almost certain in this patient given her history of diabetes. However, she is non-insulin requiring so her sugar is not likely to be significantly elevated and is not likely to be causing ketoacidosis and an elevated acetone level (**choice A**).

    An elevated blood urea nitrogen level (**choice D**) can be seen in renal failure and during reabsorption of a gastrointestinal bleed. Because this patient is acidotic, her renal response should be to secrete an acid load. Her urinary pH (**choice E**) should therefore be low.

18. **The correct answer is B.** Although this patient is post-surgical, the approach to renal failure should always be the same. The incidence of peri-operative renal insufficiency and failure is high and meticulous attention to renal and fluid status is critical to successful post-operative care. There are many reasons why this patient is likely to have pre-renal azotemia: NPO status, surgery

of the abdomen, and inability to take oral fluid. In general, a fluid challenge is always appropriate in the initial evaluation of declining renal function. Some contend that if urine output fails to increase after 3 liters of intravenous crystalloid, the patient does not have pre-renal azotemia.

To give furosemide intravenously (**choice A**) could cause significant harm in this patient. The kidneys are extremely "smart" and their failure to produce urine in a patient that has pre-renal azotemia should be viewed as "acute renal success." Furosemide will certainly allow urine to be seen in the Foley catheter bag, but this urine is a false indicator of the patient's renal function. Patients with healthy kidneys should not need a diuretic to produce urine.

If this patient were also anemic, giving intravenous packed red blood cells (**choice C**) would be an excellent way in which to administer volume.

Since the differential diagnosis of acute renal failure includes post-renal obstruction, a pelvic ultrasound (**choice D**) would be indicated after pre-renal causes have been excluded.

If a patient continues to be anuric or oliguric after an appropriate fluid challenge has been offered, it is then appropriate to send a urine sample for sediment analysis (**choice E**) since the patient almost certainly has acute tubular necrosis.

19. **The correct answer is B.** This patient most likely has acute tubular necrosis secondary to angiographic dye. Although this patient is post-surgical, the approach to renal failure should always be the same. The incidence of peri-operative renal insufficiency and failure is high and meticulous attention to renal and fluid status is critical to successful post-operative care. There are many reasons why this patient is likely to have pre-renal azotemia: NPO status, surgery of the abdomen, and inability to take oral fluid. In general, a fluid challenge is always appropriate in the initial evaluation of declining renal function. Some contend that after 3 liters of intravenous crystalloid, if urine output fails to increase, the patient does not have pre-renal azotemia. In this patient, this has been done and therefore another cause of her renal failure must be sought. The incidence of contrast-induced renal failure is about 1% in all patients, but given this patient's diabetes, her risk is substantially greater. It is not uncommon to have transient renal failure due to ATN in these patients after vascular procedures that necessitate a dye load preoperatively.

There is no evidence that this patient has abdominal compartment syndrome (**choice A**). The surgical procedure should not have caused massive swelling of abdominal contents. ACS is most often seen after trauma in patients who require laparotomy for massive bowel resections and manipulation.

Since we have no evidence of any significant hypotension and the patient is not currently hypo-perfusing her kidneys, acute tubular necrosis secondary to ischemia (**choice C**) is unlikely.

This patient has a CPK of less than 10,000 mg/dL. Therefore acute tubular necrosis secondary to rhabdomyolysis (**choice D**) is unlikely. A CPK of 10,000 mg/dL is generally the level at which ATN from myoglobin becomes a concern.

Since this patient had an appropriate crystalloid and colloid fluid challenge and her urine output failed to improve, pre-renal azotemia secondary to volume depletion (**choice E**) is not the cause of her renal failure.

20. **The correct answer is C.** This patient most likely has a sigmoid infarction. As detailed above in the case of this patient, her surgical procedure likely involved ligation of the inferior mesenteric artery. Depending upon the patient's blood supply via the superior mesenteric artery, she may become ischemic. Her electrolytes and arterial blood gas reveal an anion gap metabolic acidosis. Her abdominal pain is persistent despite analgesia and her stools are trace positive for blood. This is mesenteric ischemia.

An aorto-enteric fistula (**choice A**) would present with massive exsanguination and although a complication of this procedure, it often takes weeks to develop near the internal suture sites.

Given the blood supply to the small bowel is celiac and superior mesenteric, infarcted small bowel (**choice B**) is unlikely.

A sigmoid volvulus (**choice D**) certainly would culminate in bowel infarction. However, given this patient's surgical procedure a superimposed volvulus is very unlikely.

Small bowel obstruction secondary (SBO) to adhesions (**choice E**) would not present in this manner. SBO generally presents with vomiting and obstructive symptoms, not acidemia and bloody stool.

21. **The correct answer is C.** The first key to this question is to realize that the patient is Chinese and is presenting with findings of cirrhosis that is acutely worsening. Hepatitis B and C are very common in China and are

often transmitted vertically at the time of birth as opposed to in the United States where HCV and HBV are more often transmitted sexually or by IV drug use. In these patients, the most common liver tumor is primary hepatocellular carcinoma. Alpha-fetoprotein is also commonly elevated above 500 μg/L with these tumors and can be used in screening. HCC also classically invades the portal venous system, and this may be the reason her jaundice is acutely worsening.

Budd-Chiari syndrome (**choice A**) is thrombosis of the hepatic veins, which were normal by Doppler color flow on the ultrasound.

Hepatic adenomas (**choice B**) can cause large hepatic lesions; however, they are benign entities and would not be seen invading the portal vein. In general, they are more common in females and often are associated with use of oral contraceptives. They are usually asymptomatic unless they internally hemorrhage.

Metastatic colon cancer (**choice D**) and metastatic squamous cell carcinoma of the lung (**choice E**), as most metastatic tumors to the liver are, are often multiple, but do not have to be. It would be very rare for them to invade the portal venous system, and in the clinical setting of a Chinese immigrant with findings of cirrhosis, hepatocellular carcinoma is a much more likely etiology.

22. **The correct answer is B.** In a patient of this age presenting with left lower quadrant pain, fever, and elevated WBC count, the first consideration should always be diverticulitis. This is the classic clinical presentation of this disease. Diverticulitis can occur on the right side but this is much less common, as most diverticula are located in the descending and sigmoid colon. Diverticulitis can often be confirmed with CT scanning; however, empiric treatment with antibiotics is certainly reasonable. If the patient does not improve, a CT scan can be used to rule out complicating factors such as abscess formation. Once the patient has recovered, a colonoscopy or barium enema should be performed to rule out an underlying adenocarcinoma of the colon.

If this clinical history had been exactly the same but with right lower quadrant pain, appendicitis (**choice A**) would be the correct answer. The only thing that might not fit very well would be the heme positive stool.

Epiploic appendagitis (**choice C**) is a torsion of one of the fatty appendages of the colon. It is a self-limited disorder and does not require antibiotics. It is typically diagnosed by a CT scan. Epiploic appendagitis certainly could present exactly like this; however, it is far less common than diverticulitis and should not be considered the most likely diagnosis.

The clinical history in this case suggests an acute infectious/inflammatory process occurring in the abdomen. Ovarian carcinoma (**choice D**) can present with pain, but typically in a much more subacute fashion.

Perforated ulcers (**choice E**) can also present with acute abdominal pain; however, the pain will usually begin in the epigastric region and then if perforation occurs will likely have symptoms of a diffuse peritonitis.

23. **The correct answer is D.** This patient has most likely developed heparin-induced thrombocytopenia. Because he is fully ambulatory and appears ready for discharge, and because his platelet count of 62,000/mm^3 is not dangerously low, he can safely be followed as an outpatient after heparin is discontinued.

Although this would be correct if he must be anticoagulated, he doesn't need further anticoagulation (**choice A**). Lepirudin and danaparoid are "heparinoids" believed not to be associated with heparin-induced thrombocytopenia. If this patient was still not ambulatory or had another reason for needing anticoagulation (e.g., known DVT), this would be the right thing to do.

Low-molecular-weight heparin (**choice B**) still is associated with heparin-induced thrombocytopenia, albeit at a much lower incidence. Anyway, this patient no longer requires anticoagulation.

Again, he no longer requires anticoagulation (**choice C**). If he did, simply decreasing the dose would be inappropriate and would put him at risk for worsening thrombocytopenia and clotting (*not* bleeding—HIT causes a paradoxical procoagulant state).

Making no changes in his therapy (**choice E**) is wrong on several levels. The point of this question is what to do about heparin-induced thrombocytopenia, and again this patient should simply be taken off the heparin because he doesn't need it anymore.

24. **The correct answer is C.** The patient most likely has Crohn disease. Although 10% of patients with Crohn disease present acutely with symptoms similar to appendicitis, in most instances the onset is insidious. The patients present with intermittent pain and discomfort most commonly. Diarrhea is the next most frequent symptom and it is not associated with mucus, pus, or blood. One third of patients present with weight loss, weakness, and easy fatigability. Complete obstruction is uncommon in Crohn disease. Partial obstruction is com-

mon, and when high grade requires an elective operation. The partial obstruction in Crohn disease is initially treated with nasogastric decompression and intravenous hydration. Gastrointestinal series with small bowel followthrough should be obtained in evaluating patients suspected of having Crohn disease. Luminal narrowing of the terminal ileum as a result of acute edema or chronic fibrosis produces the string sign of canter seen on barium examination. Thickening of the bowel wall and the mesentry increases the space between the adjacent loops of bowel. Fistulas may be seen either in connection to the skin or with the adjacent bowel loops. Skip areas of diffused bowel with intervening normal bowel segments also may be detected and can help differentiate Crohn disease from ulcerative colitis.

A barium enema (**choice A**) is useful to evaluate the colon for any polyps, carcinoma, ulcerative colitis, or Crohn colitis. In this patient, however, with the absence of colon involvement on the CT scan of the abdomen and pelvis, barium enema is not the investigation of choice.

Colonoscopy (**choice B**) is indicated in patients suspected of ulcerative colitis or Crohn colitis. In patients suspected of having Crohn disease of the small bowel with no significant signs of colon involvement on the CT scan of the abdomen and pelvis, a colonoscopy is not indicated.

In a young patient with a history of foreign travel and having abdominal pain, distention, and loose stools, examination of the stool for ova and parasites (**choice D**) is indicated. In this patient, however, with evidence of small bowel involvement with extensive edema, Crohn disease should be suspected and should be ruled out by further investigation.

Crohn disease involving the duodenum and stomach is rare compared with that found in the small intestine. Upper gastrointestinal endoscopy (**choice E**) is mainly performed for the diagnostic purpose of visualizing the esophagus, stomach, and duodenum, and may not be helpful in this patient.

25. **The correct answer is F.** Life expectancy is a synonym for median survival time. At 8 years after surgery, 50% of the patients have died and 50% have yet to die.

Since the life expectancy is 8 years, all of the other choices (**choices A, B, C, D, E, G, and H**) are incorrect.

26. **The correct answer is E.** Based on median survival time, the patient is more likely to be dead before 10 years than to still be alive. The physician must not dance around the issue, but answer the patient's question directly. Other options that lie (**choices C, I, and K**), create false hope (**choice G**), or evade the question (**choices A, B, D, F, H, and J**) are wrong because they do not treat the patient as a full partner who has the right to know. Remember, tell the patient what you know and as soon as you know it. The physician's task is to prepare the patient to cope with reality, not shield the patient from that reality.

27. **The correct answer is D.** The most common lawsuit brought against a urologist is the failure to diagnose acute torsion of the testicle. Torsion occurs most frequently in the age group between 12 to 20. There is some conflicting information in this clinical vignette between a differential diagnosis of acute testicular torsion versus torsed appendix testis or epididymis versus epididymitis. The bottom line is, unless the clinician is 100% certain that it is not testicular torsion, this should be considered an emergency and the patient should be taken to the operating room for surgical exploration and possible orchiopexy. There is a window of 6 hours time after which irreversible damage to the testicle occurs.

Admission for pain control (**choice A**) is done after the surgical exploration. Admitting him for pain control and antibiotics is inappropriate without first performing surgical exploration.

An ultrasound (**choice B**) is incorrect because although important information could be obtained, precious time is lost if indeed there is real torsion.

Nuclear study (**choice C**) can help in assessing vascular compromise but is rarely used in the acute setting.

Send him home with ibuprofen (**choice E**) is incorrect because the diagnosis of torsed appendix testis is not certain. This would be a serious mistake.

28. **The correct answer is C.** The physician is not liable for failing to make a correct initial diagnosis. A malpractice suit can only be brought if the physician had been negligent. In this instance, you had carried out the appropriate procedures and maintained the vital signs. There had been no deterioration in the patient's condition. If failure to make the initial diagnosis had jeopardized the patient's vital signs or led to further complications, then a case of negligence could be brought to bear on the defendant physician. Often, it is not possible to make a correct initial diagnosis, and one has to have a differential diagnosis in mind. Thus, the plaintiff will be unable to establish that there has been a breach of the standard of care. Therefore **choices A, B, and E** are incorrect.

29. **The correct answer is C.** Familial polyposis syndrome is well known with presence of colonic polyps within the family members. These patients and the family members should be screened early in their life with a complete colonoscopy for the diagnosis of familial polyposis syndrome. With increase in duration, the risk for carcinoma in these colonic polyps is increased. It is not possible to annually screen these patients and take diagnostic biopsy from the representative polyps. Hence, a total colectomy should be recommended for all patients over the age of 30 years. The patients with familial polyposis may also have associated cancers like cancer of the prostate, stomach, ovary, or breast. Screening should include evaluation of these patients to exclude the above cancers.

The presence of polyps is not an indication for further workup to rule out metastatic lesions (**choice A**). Only when the pathology after biopsy of the polyp or the final pathology shows a colonic carcinoma is a further workup required in this age group.

Genetic testing (**choice B**) is recommended not only to the patient but also for the rest of the family members.

With a suspicion of familial polyposis syndrome, rescreening in 1 year is not recommended (**choice D**). There is an increased chance of developing a carcinoma or missing a carcinoma in one of these polyps; hence, total colectomy should be recommended on the first visit.

Biopsy and removal of all the polyps (**choice E**) is practically impossible when the colon is packed with polyps. Even carrying out subsequent sessions of colonoscopy for polypectomy is not practical in this patient.

30. **The correct answer is D.** Elderly patients with abdominal or back pain associated with hypotension suggest a ruptured abdominal aortic aneurysm. In this patient, with an increase in the abdominal distension, hypotension, and persistent back pain, an emergency surgical consult should be obtained so that the patient can be taken to the operating room to be explored to rule out ruptured abdominal aortic aneurysm.

Ultrasonography (**choice A**) is useful in the screening and initial evaluation of the patient to rule out abdominal aortic aneurysm. In an emergency situation, ultrasonography is not required. Clinical suspicion alone should provoke an emergency surgical consult as delay in diagnosis therapy might result in mortality.

A CT scan of the abdomen and pelvis (**choice B**) is indicated in elective investigation of aneurysm. In an emergency workup of ruptured abdominal aortic aneurysm, further investigations will only delay the operative intervention.

In a suspected ruptured abdominal aortic aneurysm, intravenous access (**choice C**) should be obtained in both antecubital fossas. The patient should be transferred immediately to the operating room without much fluid resuscitation or intubation. Any measures to increase the pressure by means of endotracheal intubation, nasotracheal intubation, or insertion of the Foley catheter might cause more pain and increase the blood pressure, which might have a devastating effect on the ruptured abdominal aortic aneurysm and should be avoided.

Transfer to the intensive care unit (**choice E**) and resuscitation with intravenous fluid and blood may be necessary if it is determined that this patient does not have a ruptured abdominal aortic aneurysm.

31. **The correct answer is B.** Hypercalcemic crisis occurs when the serum calcium level rises to 14.5 mg/dL or greater. Symptoms of hypercalcemic crisis include weakness, nausea, vomiting, and confusion, which, if untreated, may lead to coma. Hypercalcemic crisis is a medical emergency. Initial management should be designed to lower the serum calcium level acutely. Lowering of the serum calcium level is best accomplished by vigorous intravenous saline infusion to expand the intravascular volume, followed by administration of loop diuretic, such as furosemide, to increase the urinary calcium excretion. Hypercalcemia can cause cardiac arrhythmias and hence, cardiac monitoring is required, especially when the calcium level is higher than 16 mg/dL.

When the calcium level remains elevated, hypocalcemic agents should be used, such as calcitonin (**choice A**). Calcitonin given intravenously or subcutaneously has a rapid effect in reversing hypercalcemia.

Intravenous mithramycin (**choice C**) inhibits bone resorption and can effectively lower the serum calcium concentration within 24 hours of administration. It has potential hematologic, renal, and hepatic toxicity and hence, it is used only in palliation of malignancy or in cases in which conventional therapy for hypercalcemia is ineffective or contraindicated.

Intravenous potassium (**choice D**) is not indicated except in hypokalemia that presents with muscle weakness.

Parathyroid exploration (**choice E**) with resection of the offending gland represents the definitive treatment of hypercalcemia, but it should be delayed until the serum calcium level is reduced to a safer level.

32. **The correct answer is D.** This patient has an inguinal hernia. A hernia is a protrusion of a structure, usually intestine, through tissue that normally contains it. Inguinal hernias are either direct or indirect. Indirect inguinal hernias occur through the internal inguinal ring in a protrusion of peritoneum along the spermatic cord in the internal spermatic fascia. Direct inguinal hernias occur through the floor of the inguinal canal, separate from the spermatic cord, as a result of breakdown of the transversus abdominis aponeurosis and transversalis fascia. If the mass (i.e., hernia) is easily returned to its normal position, it is called reducible. If the mass is not reducible, it is called incarcerated. If the mass becomes incarcerated and develops a compromised blood supply, it is termed strangulated. Strangulated hernias require emergent repair as the intestinal contents will necrose and cause the patient to become sick. As long as the mass is reducible, surgical repair can be performed on an outpatient basis (**choice B**).

    Surgery is the treatment of choice. Abdominal binders (**choice A**) may control symptoms but will not fix the defect.

    A varicocele, dilatation of the pampiniform venous plexus of the spermatic cord, may be caused by compression of the left renal vein caused by renal cell cancer with thrombus extending in to the left renal vein. A varicocele typically appears as a mass of dilated, tortuous veins lying posterior to and above the testis. It is more prominent in the standing position and may abate in the recumbent position. Any elderly man who presents with a left-sided varicocele should be evaluated for renal cell carcinoma causing obstruction of the gonadal vein that drains into the left renal vein (**choice C**).

    If a scrotal mass is suspicious for testicular cancer, then tumor markers should be drawn before surgery. This patient clearly has an inguinal hernia and therefore it is unnecessary to draw serum tumor markers (**choice E**).

33. **The correct answer is D.** The diagnosis of "free air under the diaphragm" indicates that this patient has perforated a hollow viscous in the abdominal cavity. Based on his history of increased ibuprofen use, the source is most likely a perforated gastric ulcer. This patient is clearly sick and suffering from an acute abdomen and therefore an emergent exploratory laparotomy is indicated.

    Providing the patient with analgesia will only mask his pain (**choice A**). There is no need for observation or further studies with this clinical scenario.

    A CT scan will only delay treatment (**choice B**). Once free air is seen on radiographic films, a CT scan will not provide any information that cannot be picked up at the time of laparotomy.

    Colonoscopy (**choice C**) and barium enema (**choice E**) will also delay therapy. Again, the point is emphasized that his history, physical examination, and plain radiographic findings provide a clear picture that this patient requires exploration.

34. **The correct answer is E.** For melanoma, the Clark microstaging system involves histologic examination to determine the level of invasion into the dermal layers or subcutaneous fat. The Breslow staging system involves measurement of the primary melanoma thickness with an ocular micrometer. Tumor thickness as determined with the Breslow system is the most accurate index of metastatic potential and provides the best system to determine therapy and prognosis (**choices D and E**).

    The most common form of skin cancer is basal cell carcinoma. These tumors rarely metastasize but instead undergo local growth with invasion (**choice A**).

    Surgical margins vary according to the thickness of the melanoma. In general, for melanoma in situ, a margin of 5 mm should be obtained. As the thickness of tumor increases, so does the size of the margin (**choice B**).

    A shave biopsy should not be performed because it prevents adequate assessment of depth. A full thickness excisional biopsy is the preferred form of biopsy. A border of non-involved skin should be included (**choice C**).

35. **The correct answer is B.** Sudden contraction of the calf muscles in men, typically those in their 30s and 40s, can result in lower leg muscle and tendon injuries. Occasional participation in recreational sports can increase the risk of these injuries. The Thompson test, performed by squeezing the calf muscles and producing no ankle plantar flexion with the patient in a prone position, is pathognomonic for the Achilles tendon. Hence, these patients, in addition to evaluation of the lower extremity and neurologic examinations, should be specifically examined in a prone position.

    A subfascial hematoma (**choice A**) usually produces a tense swelling at the calf muscle region associated with severe tenderness and palpation. This hematoma can also be associated with bruising of the skin and soft tissues.

    A torn plantaris tendon (**choice C**) is possible, but does not produce weak plantar and dorsiflexion of the ankle and loss of ankle plantar flexion on squeezing the calf muscles.

A torn gastrocnemius muscle (**choice D**) produces more proximal swelling and a Thompson test would produce ankle plantar flexion.

A torn posterior tibial tendon (**choice E**) does not produce the above-mentioned signs and symptoms.

36. **The correct answer is C.** True aneurysms of the aorta are expansions or dilatations of the aorta that involve all three layers of the wall, intima, media, and adventitia. They can be fusiform or saccular in configuration. False aneurysms can cause aortic enlargement and exhibit intimal and medial disruption; luminal blood is contained only by adventitial layers and surrounding reactive fibrosis.

Aneurysms are caused by atherosclerosis, connective tissue degeneration (i.e., Marfan syndrome or Ehlers-Danlos syndrome), or aortic dissection (**choice A**).

It is not uncommon for AAAs to be associated with aneurysms at other sites (i.e., iliac, femoral, or popliteal arteries) (**choice B**).

There is a definite danger in a patient with an aneurysm of this size. The most worrisome complication is potential rupture, which is associated with a high morbidity and mortality rate (**choice D**).

AAAs may involve the renal arteries and are classified according to their location relative to the renal arteries. Infrarenal AAA begins below the level of the renal arteries. A juxtarenal AAA involves the entire segment of infrarenal aorta but the renal arteries are not involved. A pararenal AAA has extension cephalad to the renal arteries and includes the renal arteries (**choice E**).

37. **The correct answer is A.** These cancers require an exhaustive work-up. Panendoscopy with visualization of the larynx, hypopharynx, nasopharynx, and esophagus is necessary to avoid missing small lesions. A CT scan may help with staging, and liver enzymes help to determine metastatic disease.

Risk factors associated with squamous cell cancers include heavy tobacco use, heavy alcohol use, poor oral hygiene, ultraviolet radiation, and a variety of viruses (**choice B**).

Lymph node spread of squamous cancer of the oral cavity is to the nodes of the submental and submandibular areas and then to the midjugular chain (**choice C**).

In general, cancers of the oral cavity are treated with wide resection. Those tumors that are more locally advanced or have clinically positive nodes require radical neck dissection (**choice D**). Radiation therapy may be used to shrink tumors that have microscopically positive margins or margins close to the tumor, and to prevent metastatic disease to the contralateral side.

Squamous cell accounts for approximately 90% of head and neck malignancies (**choice E**).

38. **The correct answer is C.** This patient presents with acute pseudo-obstruction (Ogilvie syndrome). The condition is dangerous because of increasing distention of the cecum that can perforate when its diameter expands beyond 10 to 12 cm. Painless distention is a common finding. Risk factors include severe blunt trauma, orthopedic trauma or procedures, cardiac disease, acute neurologic disease, and acute metabolic derangements.

Observation while correcting metabolic derangements and minimizing narcotics is acceptable initially, but when the cecum becomes overly distended, immediate decompression is necessary. Decompression can be performed with colonoscopy or neostigmine (**choice A**).

The disease usually involves the proximal colon, but may extend through the transverse colon and rarely the descending colon (**choice B**).

Surgical intervention is necessary when either colonoscopy does not work or if perforation occurs (**choice D**).

This condition is the result of a failure of propulsive forces to overcome normal resistance to flow (i.e., a paralytic ileus, not a kink in the large bowel) (**choice E**).

39. **The correct answer is D.** Jumping from a height and landing on one's feet predisposes the patient to ankle fractures, knee fractures, knee dislocation, posterior dislocation of the hip, and spinal compression fractures. These patients should be examined and radiographically evaluated to rule out these fractures. This patient has several non-specific points of tenderness, but did not have any specific abnormality from systemic examination. Hence, the previously-mentioned fractures should be ruled out by specific x-rays.

In the absence of abdominal signs and stable vitals with normal laboratory values, a CT scan of the abdomen and pelvis (**choice A**) is not indicated.

In a stable patient with no neurologic deficit and a Glasgow coma scale of 15, a CT scan of the head (**choice B**) is not indicated.

This patient had a normal clinical examination of the chest with bilateral breath sounds and stable vitals, so a repeat chest x-ray (**choice C**) is not indicated.

A skeletal survey should include x-rays to rule out all possible injuries rather than just knee and ankle x-rays (**choice E**).

40. **The correct answer is B.** This patient has an enterocutaneous fistula, most likely an extraintestinal manifestation of Crohn disease. These fistulas follow tissue planes of least resistance from the ileum to the colon. They may emerge through the thin fascial layer around the umbilicus or along the psoas muscle. Fistula tracks can also develop between the small and large intestines to the colon, vagina, bladder, and other areas of the small intestine. The most common site of fistula track formation is the terminal ileum. Because they rarely close spontaneously they are often difficult to treat medically and require surgical intervention with colostomy and subsequent reanastomosis.

Appendicitis (**choice A**) occurs secondary to luminal obstruction of the appendiceal lumen. This leads to appendiceal inflammation and acute appendicitis. Patients complain of abdominal pain and anorexia. There is no associated bloody diarrhea or umbilical drainage as was noted in this patient.

Fournier gangrene (**choice C**) is an infection of the fascia by gas-forming organisms. Infection frequently occurs in the perineum or scrotum. The infection may spread quickly and track up the abdominal wall. Clinically, patients develop warmth, erythema, and crepitus over the infected sites. Treatment is wide surgical debridement of all infected tissue.

Umbilical hernias (**choice D**) commonly occur at birth and are diagnosed in the pediatric population. Incarcerated hernias are associated with bowel obstruction, nausea, and vomiting, none of which were observed in this patient. There is localized tenderness with an umbilical mass that cannot be reduced.

A patent urachal cyst (**choice E**) is diagnosed by finding urinary flow through the umbilicus. Embryologically, the allantois connects the urogenital sinus with the umbilicus. Normally, the allantois is obliterated and represented by a fibrous cord (urachus) extending from the dome of the bladder to the navel. If incomplete obliteration occurs, then a draining umbilical sinus may be noted.

41. **The correct answer is F.** This patient has a testicular tumor. The classic history of a dull, aching, and heavy testicle along with elevated serum tumor markers make the diagnosis clear. Malignant tumors of the testis are rare, with approximately two to three new cases per 100,000 men in the United States each year. Ninety to ninety-five percent of these tumors are germ cell (seminoma and nonseminoma). Radical orchiectomy is the first line of treatment.

Chemotherapy (**choice A**) and radiation therapy (**choice E**) play a role in the treatment of testicular tumors. They should not, however, be used before removal of the cancerous testicle. Which modality is used after orchiectomy varies based on pathology (seminoma versus nonseminoma) and serum tumor levels.

Inguinal exploration with cross clamping of the spermatic cord vasculature is the mainstay of exploration for possible testis tumor. If cancer cannot be excluded by examination of the testis, radical orchiectomy is warranted. Incisions through the scrotum or open testicular biopsy should be avoided (**choice B**), as these approaches carry the theoretic possibility of disrupting the normal lymphatic drainage of the testis.

Overall 5-year survival rates have increased in recent years and are now greater than 90% (**choice C**).

Removing one testicle does not make a man infertile. There is no reason to believe that this man with a normal appearing right testicle will be unable to make adequate sperm for reproduction (**choice D**).

42. **The correct answer is D.** This patient most likely has a ruptured pancreatic pseudocyst. Pseudocysts of the pancreas are collections of tissue, fluid, debris, pancreatic enzymes, and blood that develop over a period of 1 to 4 weeks after the onset of acute pancreatitis. In contrast to true cysts, pseudocysts do not have an epithelial lining and the walls consist of necrotic, granulation, and fibrous tissues. Most are located in the body/tail of the pancreas. Abdominal pain with or without radiation to the back is the usual presenting complaint. Pseudocysts resolve in 25 to 40% of patients; however, those greater than 5 cm or those that persist longer than 6 weeks rarely disappear on their own. Rupture of a pancreatic pseudocyst is a particularly serious complication. Shock usually supervenes and the mortality rate is 15 to 60%. Findings with rupture include an increase in the size of the mass, a localized bruit over the mass, and a sudden decrease in blood count without obvious signs of external blood loss. These patients require operative exploration to control hemorrhage.

Aspiration of pseudocysts (**choice A**) is reserved for persistent, sterile, chronic masses. In this scenario, the patient would be ill served with percutaneous drainage.

Delaying evaluation and treatment until the morning (**choice B**) will increase this patient's already high risk for mortality. Ultrasound may be used to monitor the status of known pseudocysts and can also be used to assist in cyst drainage, neither of which is beneficial to this patient.

ERCP (**choice C**) has a variety of uses in the diagnosis and treatment of pancreatic disease processes. The internal hemorrhage that this patient has, however, cannot be stopped with ERCP.

Although it may be possible to stabilize this patient (e.g., volume resuscitation, central line placement) before surgical exploration, allowing him to leave the hospital without definitive treatment is wrong (**choice E**). His source of shock must be identified and treated appropriately.

43. **The correct answer is D.** This patient has an incisional hernia. Sometimes called a ventral hernia, it is caused by a defect in the abdominal wall. As with all hernias, the risk is that any abdominal contents may protrude through the defect and not be able to be reduced. If this occurs, the term used is incarcerated hernia. If the incarcerated abdominal contents lose their blood supply then the hernia has become strangulated. A strangulated hernia is a surgical emergency as patients may become septic. If a hollow viscus becomes incarcerated or strangulated, then signs of bowel obstruction may occur. The only definitive treatment for this condition is surgical repair of the defect. Small defects can be repaired by reapproximating the abdominal wall. Larger defects may require the placement of a piece of mesh to cover the defect. This patient's diagnosis is based on history and physical. That her pain improves with reduction of the hernia confirms the diagnosis.

Liver function tests (**choice A**) will not contribute to the diagnosis. These values should be normal in this patient.

Upper endoscopy (**choice B**) is beneficial in patients with a variety of abdominal complaints similar to our patient's. There is no role for this test in the diagnosis of a ventral/incisional hernia, however.

An abdominal binder (**choice C**) will provide some support and may help the patient's symptoms. Her history provides the information that she is at risk for incarceration and strangulation of her hernia. These conditions will not be prevented by the abdominal binder. Because of her diabetes, the risk for strangulation is even more worrisome, as she may get sicker than an otherwise "healthy" patient.

As with the other diagnostic tests in this patient, liver/gallbladder ultrasound (**choice E**) will not provide any new helpful information. This answer emphasizes the importance of a good history and physical. Without examining this patient, it would appear that any of the diagnostic tests offered would seem reasonable. Her physical examination, however, makes the diagnosis clear.

44. **The correct answer is C.** This patient has an anal fissure. Anal fissure is an ulcer in the lower part of the anal canal. Primary fissures occur without other local systemic disease. Secondary fissure develops in association with diseases such as Crohn disease, leukemia, aplastic anemia, and agranulocytosis. Most tears of the anal canal are traced to passage of a large, hard stool or explosive diarrhea, trauma to the anus, or tearing during vaginal delivery. Clinical manifestations include burning, throbbing, or dull aching anal pain, particularly during and after bowel movement. Pain is severe and incapacitating. Bleeding is common and constipation may occur. Diagnosis is confirmed at examination. Digital rectal examination reveals a small, fibrotic defect and tightness of the anal canal. Anoscope is useful for visualization. Initial treatment of acute anal fissure includes pain relief, anal cleaning, warm sitz baths to relax the anal canal, and use of bulk-forming agents to relieve constipation. Application of a topical anesthetic jelly directly to the fissure before a bowel movement is helpful. Chronic fissures usually require intervention with a lateral internal sphincterotomy.

Incision and drainage (**choice A**) are reserved for those patients who have an abscess. An abscess usually presents acutely with a tender, fluctuant, erythematous mass. This patient does not have the signs or symptoms of an abscess.

Performing a guaiac (**choice B**) on this patient's stool may be misleading. The blood from the fissure will give you a positive result. If one is concerned about carcinoma in this patient, then a colonoscopy should be scheduled.

Hemorrhoidectomy (**choice D**) is used in those patients suffering from hemorrhoids. Hemorrhoids are dilated venules within the anal canal caused by downward displacement of the anal cushion.

Chemotherapy (**choice E**) is used in patients with carcinoma. One must always be concerned about carcinoma in a patient with a change in bowel habits and blood per rectum. Prescribing chemotherapy without a diagnosis, however, is incorrect.

45. **The correct answer is D.** This patient has a diagnosis of rectal prolapse. This occurs when the full thickness of the rectal wall turns inside out and passes into or through the anal canal. The extruded rectum is seen as concentric rings of mucosa. Rectal prolapse is an intussusception that usually starts in the anterior part of the lower rectum approximately 6 to 7 cm from the anal verge or at the rectosigmoid junction. Many patients give a history of straining with intractable constipation. This condition occurs more frequently in women than men and is associated with anorectal discomfort during defecation, difficulty in initiating bowel movements, and a feeling of incomplete evacuation. Diagnosis is easy if the prolapse has come through the anus but can be difficult if the prolapse remains in the rectum or anal canal. Treatment of rectal prolapse is by way of rectosigmoid resection and rectopexy.

A pessary (**choice A**) is a removable, manually inserted device that can be placed in the vagina to provide support for those patients suffering from pelvic floor prolapse with protrusion of the uterus or the bladder.

Anal manometry is helpful in the evaluation of incontinence and for followup testing of anal sphincteric function after repair (**choice B**).

Colonoscopy (**choice C**) and barium enema (**choice E**) are indicated to rule out an associated lesion, especially in patients with a recent episode of constipation. These tests are helpful in diagnosis but are unable to provide definitive treatment.

46. **The correct answer is B.** The correct answer requires understanding the research described and selecting the best response to the patient. Although a number of options do one or the other, only one answer does both. "I see why you would ask that. Unfortunately, the study is flawed. I suspect that patients were given different treatments based on the severity of their disease" begins by recognizing the perspective of the patient, but then communicates the essential problem, namely, that the study is likely biased. Bias is common in the type of studies described here. The problem is that patients who are treated by surgery are likely to be different (and likely sicker) than patients treated by radiation. Because of this, there is no clear way to tell if the difference in survival rates is attributable to disease severity between groups or to the different efficacy of the two treatments. This type of bias, called confounding, is impossible to eliminate completely, but a better research design, one that makes sure the groups are of equal severity of illness, would make the study results more valid.

Although "I'll be happy to look at it more carefully and tell you what I think the next time we talk" (**choice A**) is a sensitive, professional response, it misses the chance to discuss the article with the patient when it is presented. The patient will leave without a sense of resolution, perhaps feeling that the article will convince the physician, and so the patient may not consider any other treatment options.

"Is there some reason that you are uncomfortable with my judgment?" (**choice C**) is confrontative and makes the patient's treatment decision a matter of the physician's ego rather than an objective discussion of the available options. This also avoids discussing the research article with the patient.

"Look, I've treated many patients in my day, and for someone in your condition, surgery will give you the best chance of a long and happy life" (**choice D**) is the paternalistic, "doctor knows best" response. It rejects input from the patient and acts as if the treatment decision is the physician's rather than the patient's to make.

"Maybe you would like some time to talk about your options with your family before we proceed?" (**choice E**) is a nice suggestion, but out of context here. There is no recognition of the article presented and no direct answer to the patient's question.

"The difference in outcomes in the article is not really enough to matter when making treatment decisions" (**choice F**) is incorrect because a 9% increase in survival rate is not trivial. This means that out of every 100 patients, an additional nine would be alive at the end of 3 years. There is enough clinical significance to warrant a further look.

"There is no need to make any decision right now. Why don't you take a few days and think about your options" (**choice G**) is nonresponsive to the patient's direct question. It avoids the issue the patient presents and sidesteps a discussion of the issues the patient is raising.

"This is just one study. I've read many in my time, and on balance, the research points to surgery for you" (**choice H**) and "Why don't you leave the research to me and concentrate on getting yourself better" (**choice I**) are paternalistic responses. They reject input from the patient and act as if the treatment decision is the physician's rather than the patient's to make.

Accepting the research at face value by saying, "You know, you may have found something there. Let's try radiation if that is really what you want" (**choice J**) does a disservice to the patient and the practice of medicine in general. The study is likely biased and the conclusions are, therefore, suspect.

"You seem a bit anxious. Before I answer, let's talk about that first" (**choice K**) is not the best response. Being sensitive to the patient's emotional state is a good positive quality in a physician. In the present case, however, this response avoids answering the direct question asked by the patient. Any anxiety felt by the patient can and should be addressed after a discussion of the research article.

47. **The correct answer is B.** The hemothorax should be drained. Massive hemothorax involves rapid collection of more than 1500 mL of blood within the thoracic cavity. The most common condition leading to this is penetrating injury that tears the hilar vessels. Less often it could result from blunt trauma. Apart from severe hypotension that results, a large hemothorax can compromise respiration.

Continuing resuscitation until blood is available (**choice A**) would jeopardize the patient's life.

Notifying the attorney (**choice C**), your partner (**choice E**), or even the media (**choice D**) of an inadvertent lapse in the blood bank is inappropriate at this time when the patient needs immediate management.

48. **The correct answer is A.** Blood should be given. Initial management is comprised of restoration of lost blood and simultaneous decompression of the chest. Blood obtained from the thoracic cavity is retransfused with the help of an autotransfusion device. It cannot be used if the blood has clotted within the thoracic cavity. If more than 1500 mL of blood is expressed rapidly, a thoracotomy is most probably indicated at the earliest, to stem hemorrhage. Other indications for a thoracotomy include:

Continued loss of blood at the rate of at least 200 mL per hour.

Paraspinal penetrating wounds and penetrating wounds medial to the nipple. These wounds usually involve great vessels and may result in cardiac tamponade.

If bleeding had occurred within the peritoneal cavity, it could also be retransfused provided it had not been tainted with material from a perforated viscus.

Confronting the technician with the attorney (**choice B**) or your partner (**choice C**) by your side is inappropriate, as is inviting the media (**choice E**).

Speeding up the rate of infusion (**choice D**) will not address the problem of blood replacement.

49. **The correct answer is E.** Although a patient has a right to self-determination, and therefore the right to refuse treatment, the state can override this request if its interests are paramount. In this situation there is a compelling reason for the state to enforce treatment, and that is because it has a duty to protect an innocent third party. This patient is the sole breadwinner for his wife and two minor children. Refusal of treatment that would end in death would leave the family bereft of a person who is valuable to the family.

The patient cannot refuse treatment (**choice A**), as the state has a compelling reason for forcing him to accede to it.

The family (**choice C**) has a right to consent to treatment as a surrogate decision maker only if there is a durable power of attorney or if the patient is a minor. Thus, intervention by the wife or other members of the family such as the brother (**choice B**) will not be upheld in a court of law.

In general, one spouse cannot consent for another spouse to undergo treatment (**choice D**), and this includes consenting to a wife having an abortion during the first trimester.

50. **The correct answer is C.** This patient is predisposed to developing lymphedema through his long-term immobilization caused by abdominal surgery, enhanced by his inability to undergo physical therapy because of chronic emphysema and cor pulmonale. Lymphedema typically presents with pitting edema that causes the classic *peau d'orange* appearance of involved skin. When lymphedema develops acutely, distension of the skin and extreme edema of the dermal connective tissue eventuates in the formation of subepidermal blisters (that is why they have a thick roof) filled with clear fluid (that is why they are translucent). They will first develop in the areas of greatest distension, usually located around the ankles because of gravity, or on the anterior shins where there is little subcutaneous tissue and the skin is tightly adherent to underlying bony structures. Treatment involves diuresis and compression of the lower extremities with ace wraps or compression hoses. Mobilization of the patient and physical therapy is paramount for the pump function of the leg

muscles and drainage of excess fluid. If the lymphedema is persistent, chronic changes will supervene with thickening of the overlying skin and development of elephantiasis. At this stage, it is difficult to treat and complete resolution is improbable. It is important to know that trauma to lymphedematous tissue or surgical procedures will be very slow to heal and prone to infection. Biopsy of such tissue should be avoided unless necessary.

Beta hemolytic group A *Streptococcus* (**choice A**) infection causes erysipelas that clinically presents with well-demarcated erythema, edema, and tenderness accompanied by fever, chills, and malaise. It is almost always unilateral. The most common location for erysipelas is the face or the ear, but it can occur on the lower extremity also.

Chronic venous insufficiency (**choice B**) can be the cause of stasis dermatitis accompanied by edema, but it is of insidious onset and clinically characterized with varicosities or telangiectasias, petechiae that eventuate in hemosiderin pigmentation and a brown discoloration. It would be very unusual for it to manifest when a patient is immobilized and the lower extremities are not exposed to dependent edema caused by prolonged standing or sitting.

Persistent hyperglycemia (**choice D**) as seen in untreated or poorly controlled diabetes makes patients vulnerable to long-term complications, one of which is bullosis diabeticorum. Tense, fluid-filled blisters appear on skin that has been marred by microvascular change over the years. This patient's hemoglobin A1c level indicates excellent control of his blood sugar level during prolonged periods of time, however, and there are no indications that his skin has any chronic damage that would predispose him to bullosis diabeticorum.

Superficial vein thrombosis (**choice E**) commonly develops in preexisting varicose veins on the lower extremities and presents as a painful, tender, cord-shaped induration with elevation of local temperature over the thrombosed vein and, often, dusky erythema of the overlying skin.

STANDARD REFERENCE LABORATORY VALUES

	REFERENCE RANGE	SI REFERENCE INTERVALS
BLOOD, PLASMA, SERUM		
* Alanine aminotransferase (ALT, GPT at 30°C)	8-20 U/L	8-20 U/L
Amylase, serum	25-125 U/L	25-125 U/L
* Aspartate aminotransferase (AST, GOT at 30°C)	8-20 U/L	8-20 U/L
Bilirubin, serum (adult) Total // Direct	0.1-1.0 mg/dL // 0.0-0.3 mg/dL	2-17 µmol/L // 0-5 µmol/L
* Calcium, serum (Total)	8.4-10.2 mg/dL	2.1-2.8 mmol/L
* Cholesterol, serum	140-250 mg/dL	3.6-6.5 mmol/L
Cortisol, serum	0800 h: 5-23 µg/dL // 1600 h: 3-15 µg/dL	138-635 nmol/L // 82-413 nmol/L
	2000 h: 50% of 0800 h	Fraction of 0800 h: ≤ 0.50
Creatine kinase, serum (at 30°C) ambulatory	Male: 25-90 U/L	25-90 U/L
	Female: 10-70 U/L	10-70 U/L
* Creatinine, serum	0.6-1.2 mg/dL	53-106 µmol/L
Electrolytes, serum		
Sodium	135-147 mEq/L	135-147 mmol/L
Chloride	95-105 mEq/L	95-105 mmol/L
* Potassium	3.5-5.0 mEq/L	3.5-5.0 mmol/L
Bicarbonate	22-28 mEq/L	22-28 mmol/L
Estriol (E_3) total, serum (in pregnancy)		
24-28 weeks // 32-36 weeks	30-170 ng/mL // 60-280 ng/mL	104-590 // 208-970 nmol/L
28-32 weeks // 36-40 weeks	40-220 ng/mL // 80-350 ng/mL	140-760 // 280-1210 nmol/L
Ferritin, serum	Male: 15-200 ng/mL	15-200 µg/L
	Female: 12-150 ng/mL	12-150 µg/L
Follicle-stimulating hormone, serum/plasma	Male: 4-25 mIU/mL	4-25 U/L
	Female: premenopause 4-30 mIU/mL	4-30 U/L
	midcycle peak 10-90 mIU/mL	10-90 U/L
	ostmenopause 40-250 mIU/mL	40-250 U/L
Gases, arterial blood (room air)		
pO_2	75-105 mm Hg	10.0-14.0 kPa
pCO_2	33-44 mm Hg	4.4-5.9 kPa
pH	7.35-7.45	$[H^+]$ 36-44 nmol/L
Glucose, serum	Fasting: 70-110 mg/dL	3.8-6.1 mmol/L
	2-h postprandial: < 120 mg/dL	< 6.6 mmol/L
Growth hormone – arginine stimulation	Fasting: < 5 ng/mL	< 5 µg/L
	provocative stimuli: > 7 ng/mL	> 7 µg/L
Immunoglobulins, serum		
IgA	76-390 mg/dL	0.76-3.90 g/L
IgE	0-380 IU/mL	0-380 kIU/mL
IgG	650-1500 mg/dL	6.5-15 g/L
IgM	40-345 mg/dL	0.4-3.45 g/L
Iron	50-170 µg/dL	9-30 µmol/L
Lactate dehydrogenase (L → P, 30°C)	45-90 U/L	45-90 U/L
Luteinizing hormone, serum/plasma	Male: 6-23 mIU/mL	6-23 U/L
	Female: follicular phase 5-30 mIU/mL	5-30 U/L
	midcycle 75-150 mIU/mL	75-150 U/L
	postmenopause 30-200 mIU/mL	30-200 U/L
Osmolality, serum	275-295 mOsmol/kg	275-295 mOsmol/kg
Parathyroid hormone, serum, N-terminal	230-630 pg/mL	230-630 ng/L
* Phosphatase (alkaline), serum (p-NPP at 30°C)	20-70 U/L	20-70 U/L
* Phosphorus (inorganic), serum	3.0-4.5 mg/dL	1.0-1.5 mmol/L
Prolactin, serum (hPRL)	< 20 ng/mL	< 20 µg/L
* Proteins, serum		
Total (recumbent)	6.0-7.8 g/dL	60-78 g/L
Albumin	3.5-5.5 g/dL	35-55 g/L
Globulins	2.3-3.5 g/dL	23-35 g/L
Thyroid-stimulating hormone, serum or plasma	0.5-5.0 µU/mL	0.5-5.0 mU/L
Thyroidal iodine (^{123}I) uptake	8-30% of administered dose/24 h	0.08-0.30/24 h
Thyroxine (T_4), serum	5-12 µg/dL	64-155 nmol/L
Triglycerides, serum	35-160 mg/dL	0.4-1.81 mmol/L
Triiodothyronine (T_3), serum (RIA)	115-190 ng/dL	1.8-2.9 nmol/L
Triiodothyronine (T_3), resin uptake	25-35%	0.25-0.35
* Urea nitrogen, serum (BUN)	7-18 mg/dL	1.2-3.0 mmol urea/L
* Uric acid, serum	3.0-8.2 mg/dL	0.18-0.48 mmol/L

(*) Included in the Biochemical Profile (SMA-12)

	REFERENCE RANGE	SI REFERENCE INTERVALS
CEREBROSPINAL FLUID		
Cell count	0-5 cells/mm^3	0-5 x 10^6/L
Chloride	118-132 mmol/L	118-132 mmol/L
Gamma globulin	3-12% total proteins	0.03-0.12
Glucose	40-70 mg/dL	2.2-3.9 mmol/L
Pressure	70-180 mm H_2O	70-180 mm H_2O
Proteins, total	< 40 mg/dL	< 0.40 g/L
HEMATOLOGIC		
Bleeding time (template)	2-7 minutes	2-7 minutes
Erythrocyte count	Male: 4.3-5.9 million/mm^3	4.3-5.9 x 10^{12}/L
	Female: 3.5-5.5 million/mm^3	3.5-5.5 x 10^{12}/L
Hematocrit	Male: 41-53%	0.41-0.53
	Female: 36-46%	0.36-0.46
Hemoglobin, blood	Male: 13.5-17.5 g/dL	2.09-2.71 mmol/L
	Female: 12.0-16.0 g/dL	1.86-2.48 mmol/L
Hemoglobin, plasma	1-4 mg/dL	0.16-0.62 μmol/L
Leukocyte count and differential		
Leukocyte count	4500-11,000/mm^3	4.5-11.0 x 10^9/L
Segmented neutrophils	54-62%	0.54-0.62
Band forms	3-5%	0.03-0.05
Eosinophils	1-3%	0.01-0.03
Basophils	0-0.75%	0-0.0075
Lymphocytes	25-33%	0.25-0.33
Monocytes	3-7%	0.03-0.07
Mean corpuscular hemoglobin	25.4-34.6 pg/cell	0.39-0.54 fmol/cell
Mean corpuscular hemoglobin concentration	31-36% Hb/cell	4.81-5.58 mmol Hb/L
Mean corpuscular volume	80-100 μm^3	80-100 fl
Partial thromboplastin time (nonactivated)	60-85 seconds	60-85 seconds
Platelet count	150,000-400,000/mm^3	150-400 x 10^9/L
Prothrombin time	11-15 seconds	11-15 seconds
Reticulocyte count	0.5-1.5% of red cells	0.005-0.015
Sedimentation rate, erythrocyte (Westergren)	Male: 0-15 mm/h	0-15 mm/h
	Female: 0-20 mm/h	0-20 mm/h
Thrombin time	< 2 seconds deviation from control	< 2 seconds deviation from control
Volume		
Plasma	Male: 25-43 mL/kg	0.025-0.043 L/kg
	Female: 28-45 mL/kg	0.028-0.045 L/kg
Red cell	Male: 20-36 mL/kg	0.020-0.036 L/kg
	Female: 19-31 mL/kg	0.019-0.031 L/kg
SWEAT		
Chloride	0-35 mmol/L	0-35 mmol/L
URINE		
Calcium	100-300 mg/24 h	2.5-7.5 mmol/24 h
Chloride	Varies with intake	Varies with intake
Creatinine clearance	Male: 97-137 mL/min	
	Female: 88-128 mL/min	
Estriol, total (in pregnancy)		
30 weeks	6-18 mg/24 h	21-62 μmol/24 h
35 weeks	9-28 mg/24 h	31-97 μmol/24 h
40 weeks	13-42 mg/24 h	45-146 μmol/24 h
17-Hydroxycorticosteroids	Male: 3.0-10.0 mg/24 h	8.2-27.6 μmol/24 h
	Female: 2.0-8.0 mg/24 h	5.5-22.0 μmol/24 h
17-Ketosteroids, total	Male: 8-20 mg/24 h	28-70 μmol/24 h
	Female: 6-15 mg/24 h	21-52 μmol/24 h
Osmolality	50-1400 mOsmol/kg	
Oxalate	8-40 μg/mL	90-445 μmol/L
Potassium	Varies with diet	Varies with diet
Proteins, total	< 150 mg/24 h	< 0.15 g/24 h
Sodium	Varies with diet	Varies with diet
Uric acid	Varies with diet	Varies with diet

NOTES

NOTES

NOTES

NOTES

NOTES

NOTES

NOTES

NOTES

NOTES

How Did We Do? Grade Us.

Thank you for choosing a Kaplan Medical book. Your comments and suggestions are very useful to us. Please answer the following questions to assist us in our continued development of high-quality resources to meet your needs. Or go online and complete our interactive survey form at **kaplansurveys.com/books**.

The title of the Kaplan Medical book I read was: ______________________________

My name is: ______________________________

My address is: ______________________________

____

My e-mail address is: ______________________________

What overall grade would you give this book? (A) (B) (C) (D) (F)

How relevant was the information to your goals? (A) (B) (C) (D) (F)

How comprehensive was the information in this book? (A) (B) (C) (D) (F)

How accurate was the information in this book? (A) (B) (C) (D) (F)

How easy was the book to use? (A) (B) (C) (D) (F)

How appealing was the book's design? (A) (B) (C) (D) (F)

What were the book's strong points? ______________________________

How could this book be improved? ______________________________

Is there anything that we left out that you wanted to know more about?

Would you recommend this book to others? ☐ YES ☐ NO

Other comments: ______________________________

____

____

Do we have permission to quote you? ☐ YES ☐ NO

Thank you for your help.
Please tear out this page and mail it to:

Kaplan Medical
Kaplan, Inc.
1440 Broadway, 8th floor
New York, NY 10018

KAPLAN MEDICAL

Thanks!